Clinical Practice of Dialysis
(Interventional Nephrology)

Clinical Practice of Dialysis (Interventional Nephrology)

Edited by Sean Eastwood

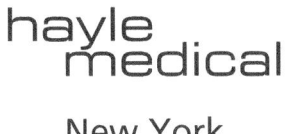

New York

Hayle Medical,
750 Third Avenue, 9th Floor,
New York, NY 10017, USA

Visit us on the World Wide Web at:
www.haylemedical.com

ISBN: 978-1-63241-929-3

Cataloging-in-Publication Data

Clinical practice of dialysis (interventional nephrology) / edited by Sean Eastwood.
   p. cm.
Includes bibliographical references and index.
ISBN 978-1-63241-929-3
1. Dialysis. 2. Nephrology. I. Eastwood, Sean.
RC903 .C55 2020
616.61--dc23

Table of Contents

Preface

Over the recent decade, advancements and applications have progressed exponentially. This has led to the increased interest in this field and projects are being conducted to enhance knowledge. The main objective of this book is to present some of the critical challenges and provide insights into possible solutions. This book will answer the varied questions that arise in the field and also provide an increased scope for furthering studies.

Dialysis is a medical procedure which is performed in people with acute kidney failure or Stage 5 chronic kidney disease. In this procedure the excess solutes, toxins and water from the blood are removed externally. This is also known as renal replacement therapy. It can be permanent or temporary. It is generally temporary in cases where kidney transplantation is due. The procedure can be classified into three primary and two secondary types. Peritoneal dialysis, hemodialysis and hemofiltration are the primary types, while intestinal dialysis and hemodiafiltration are the secondary types. Dialysis is initiated based on a number of acute and chronic indications. The presence of acidemia, fluid overload, uremia and electrolyte abnormality indicates the need for dialysis. There have been major advances both in terms of technology and clinical management of dialysis. This book traces the progress of interventional nephrology and highlights some of its key practices. The various sub-types of dialysis along with technological progress that have future implications are glanced at herein. This book is meant for students who are looking for an elaborate reference text on dialysis.

I hope that this book, with its visionary approach, will be a valuable addition and will promote interest among readers. Each of the authors has provided their extraordinary competence in their specific fields by providing different perspectives as they come from diverse nations and regions. I thank them for their contributions.

Editor

The Association of Mid-Regional Pro-Adrenomedullin and Mid-Regional Pro-Atrial Natriuretic Peptide with Mortality in an Incident Dialysis Cohort

Ghazaleh Gouya[1]**⁹, Gisela Sturm**[2]**⁹, Claudia Lamina**[2]**, Emanuel Zitt**[3]**, Otto Freistätter**[4]**, Joachim Struck**[5]**, Michael Wolzt**[1]**, Florian Knoll**[3]**, Friederike Lins**[4]**, Karl Lhotta**[3,4]**, Ulrich Neyer**[3,4]**, Florian Kronenberg**[2]*****

1 Department of Clinical Pharmacology, Medical University Vienna, Vienna, Austria, 2 Division of Genetic Epidemiology, Department of Medical Genetics, Molecular and Clinical Pharmacology, Innsbruck Medical University, Innsbruck, Austria, 3 Department of Nephrology and Dialysis, Academic Teaching Hospital Feldkirch, Feldkirch, Austria, 4 Vorarlberg Institute for Vascular Investigation and Treatment (VIVIT), Feldkirch, Austria, 5 Research Department, B.R.A.H.M.S GmbH (Part of ThermoFisher Scientific), Hennigsdorf/Berlin, Germany

Abstract

High levels of the plasma peptides mid-regional pro-adrenomedullin (MR-proADM) and mid-regional pro-atrial natriuretic peptide (MR-proANP) are associated with clinical outcomes in the general population. Data in patients with chronic kidney disease are sparse. We therefore investigated the association of MR-proANP and MR-proADM levels with all-cause and cardiovascular (CV) mortality, CV events and peripheral arterial disease in 201 incident dialysis patients of the INVOR-Study prospectively followed for a period of up to more than 7 years. The overall mortality rate was 43%, thereof 43% due to CV events. Both baseline MR-proANP and MR-proADM were associated with higher risk of all-cause (HR = 1.44, p = 0.001 and HR = 1.32, p = 0.002, respectively) and CV mortality (HR = 1.75, p<0.001 and HR = 1.41, p = 0.007, respectively) after adjustment for age, sex, previous CV events, diabetes mellitus and time-dependent type of renal replacement therapy. We then stratified patients in high risk (both peptides in the upper tertile), intermediate risk (only one of the two peptides in the upper tertile) and low risk (none in the upper tertile). Although demographic, clinical and laboratory variables were similar among the intermediate and high risk group, to be with both parameters in the upper tertile was associated with a 3-fold higher risk for all-cause (HR = 2.87, p<0.001) and CV mortality (HR = 3.58, p = 0.001). In summary, among incident dialysis patients MR-proANP and MR-proADM were shown to be associated with all-cause and CV mortality, with the highest risk when both parameters were in the upper tertiles.

Editor: Stefan Kiechl, Innsbruck Medical University, Austria

Funding: Joachim Struck is an employee of the Research Department of B.R.A.H.M.S GmbH (who provided reagents free of charge for this project) and was scientifically involved in the project. There were no other funders of the project and human resources were provided from the academic institutions.

Competing Interests: The authors have read the journal's policy and declare the following concerning conflicts of interest: Joachim Struck is an employee of the Research Department of B.R.A.H.M.S GmbH and was scientifically involved in that project; he is coauthor of the paper and did not influence the authors in terms of interpretation of the results or its writing. B.R.A.H.M.S GmbH holds patent rights on MR-pro ANP and MR-pro ADM. These are EP 03785634 "Sandwich immunoassay for identifying partial proANP peptides" (priority date: 20.11.2002) and EP 04700013 "Identifying a midregional proadrenomedullin partial peptide in biological liquids for diagnostic purposes, and immunoassays for conducting an identification of this type" (priority date: 10.04.2003). The authors confirm that this does not alter their adherence to all the PLoS ONE policies on sharing data and materials, as detailed online in the guide for authors http://www.plosone.org/static/policies.action#sharing. The remaining authors are all from academic institutions and were absolutely independent from that company to perform the analysis of the data.

* E-mail: Florian.Kronenberg@i-med.ac.at

⁹ These authors contributed equally to this work.

Introduction

Patients with chronic kidney disease (CKD) are at increased risk for death. Cardiovascular and non-cardiovascular mortality are 8 to 9 times higher in incident dialysis patients when compared to the general population [1]. Biomarkers which predict these fatal outcomes and provide insight into the pathogenesis are poorly established but highly required for an early risk stratification of this high risk cohort of patients [2,3].

There is evidence that peptides involved in maintaining the cardiovascular and renal homeostasis such as atrial natriuretic peptide (ANP) and adrenomedullin (ADM) may play a key role in the compensatory mechanisms of CKD. Both hormones are elevated in the early stages of CKD [4,5] and were shown to be highly predictive for progression of CKD in nondiabetic patients [6,7]. Elevated levels of ANP [8–12] and ADM [13] have been reported to be associated with cardiac events, overall and cardiovascular mortality in patients already on dialysis. Increased levels of ANP and ADM have been associated with higher mortality rates in cohorts of cardiac patients as well as in patients with type 2 diabetes mellitus [14–17]. The two peptides might provide additional help to estimate volume status and are probably also an early alarm signal of deteriorating hemodynamic changes in CKD patients. Since both peptides increase with deteriorating kidney function [6], it is unclear whether recently established thresholds [18] can be applied for prediction of all-cause and cardiovascular mortality in patients with renal disease.

Table 1. Clinical characteristics of patients.

	All patients (n = 201)	Survivors (n = 115)	Non-Survivors (n = 86)
Sex (male/female), n (%)	124/77 (62/38%)	69/46 (60/40%)	55/31 (64/36%)
Age (years)	61±14	56±15	69±10[d]
Diabetes mellitus, n (%)	75 (37%)	29 (25%)	46 (54%)[d]
Current smokers, n (%)	44 (22%)	29 (25%)	15 (17%)
Body Mass Index (kg/m^2)	26.1±4.4	25.9±4.4	26.2±4.5
Start of dialysis with			
Hemodialysis, n (%)	169 (84%)	93 (81%)	76 (88%)
Central venous catheter, n (%)	25 (15%)	8 (9%)	17 (22%)[a]
Native fistula, n (%)	114 (67%)	73 (79%)	41 (54%)[c]
Graft, n (%)	30 (18%)	12 (13%)	18 (24%)
Peritoneal dialysis, n (%)	32 (16%)	22 (19%)	10 (12%)
Year of start of dialysis			
2000–2003, n (%)	98 (49%)	51 (44%)	47 (55%)
2004–2006, n (%)	103 (51%)	64 (56%)	39 (45%)
Echocardiography			
Missing, n (%)	15 (7%)	5 (4%)	10 (12%)
Ejection fraction ≤60%, n (%)	86 (43%)	42 (37%)	44 (51%)[b]
Ejection fraction >60%, n (%)	100 (50%)	68 (59%)	32 (37%)[b]
Systolic blood pressure (mmHg)	153±23	154±22	153±24
Diastolic blood pressure (mmHg)	83±12	86±11	79±13[d]
Laboratory parameters			
MR-proANP (pmol/L)	798±524 [461; 669; 946]	662±439 [326; 571; 787]	981±573[d] [544; 786; 1405]
MR-proADM (nmol/L)	2.97±1.29 [2.20; 2.69; 3.52]	2.72±1.33 [2.05; 2.49; 3.13]	3.29±1.17[d] [2.49; 3.02; 3.88]
Albumin (g/dL)	3.7±0.8	3.9±0.8	3.5±0.6[d]
C-reactive protein (mg/dL)	3.0±5.4 [0.3; 0.8; 2.5]	2.6±4.3 [0.3; 0.7; 2.7]	3.8±6.5[a] [0.5; 1.0; 2.5]
Calcium (mmol/L)	2.12±0.28	2.16±0.27	2.08±0.28[a]
Phosphorus (mmol/L)	2.00±0.61 [1.57; 1.94; 2.33]	1.96±0.61 [1.51; 1.90; 2.25]	2.04±0.61 [1.60; 2.00; 2.39]
Hemoglobin (g/dL)	11.2±1.7	11.5±1.7	10.8±1.6[b]
Creatinine (mg/dL)	7.3±2.7 [5.5; 6.8; 8.7]	7.3±2.5 [5.5; 6.8; 8.7]	7.3±2.9 [5.3; 6.8; 8.4]
HbA1c (%)	6.43±1.55	6.15±1.32	6.70±1.71
Total cholesterol (mg/dL)	189±52	190±49	187±55
LDL cholesterol (mg/dL)	118±44	121±44	114±42
HDL cholesterol (mg/dL)	46.4±13.4	47.8±13.4	44.5±13.1
Triglycerides (mg/dL)	166±102 [106; 139; 192]	164±86 [106; 139; 193]	169±120 [105; 137; 189]
Comorbidities before dialysis			
CAD*, n (%)	36 (17.9%)	13 (11.3%)	23 (26.7%)[b]
CVD**, n (%)	61 (30.3%)	23 (20.0%)	38 (44.2%)[d]
PAD***, n (%)	35 (17.4%)	8 (7.0%)	27 (31.4%)[d]
Follow-up			
Follow-up time (months)‡	55.7±28.7	71.3±19.2	34.8±26.0[d]
Transplantation, n (%)	59 (29.4%)	53 (46.1%)	6 (7.0%)[d]

Mean±SD [25., 50. und 75. percentile in case of non-normal distribution] or number (%).
[a]p<0.05;
[b]p<0.01;
[c]p<0.005;
[d]p<0.001 – comparison between survivors and non-survivors.

Table 1. Cont.

***Coronary artery disease (CAD)**: myocardial infarction, percutaneous transluminal coronary angioplasty, aortocoronary bypass.
****Cardiovascular disease (CVD)**: myocardial infarction, percutaneous transluminal coronary angioplasty, aortocoronary bypass, angiographically-proven coronary stenosis ≥50%, ischemic cerebral infarction, transient ischemic attack.
*****Peripheral arterial disease (PAD)**: significant ultrasound- or angiographically-proven vascular stenosis, percutaneous transluminal angioplasty, peripheral bypass, amputation.
‡Follow-up time was calculated as the time from the start of dialysis until the patient died or the end of the observation period was reached.

The aim of this study was therefore to investigate whether MR-proANP and MR-proADM plasma concentrations at the start of dialysis treatment are associated with risk of cardiovascular or all-cause mortality in a prospective cohort study of incident dialysis patients.

Methods

INVOR-Study

The INVOR-Study [19] (Study of Incident Dialysis Patients in Vorarlberg) is a single-center, prospective, observational cohort study of incident Caucasian hemodialysis and peritoneal dialysis patients in Vorarlberg, the westernmost province of Austria counting approximately 400,000 inhabitants.

Ethic statement: The study was approved by the ethics committee of the Innsbruck Medical University and all patients enrolled in the study provided written informed consent.

All incident dialysis patients from this province starting chronic dialysis treatment between May 1st, 2000 and April 30th, 2006 were consecutively enrolled with the advantage that all patients of this region are treated by the same care provider. During this period of 6 years a total number of 235 incident dialysis patients were included and followed until the study endpoint was reached or follow-up was censored at December 31st, 2009. Ten patients having a malignant tumor at initiation of dialysis were not recruited defined by the exclusion criteria. Due to inappropriate or

missing blood samples MR-proANP and MR-proADM was measured in 201 out of 235 patients. All data and analyses described in this manuscript are based on these 201 patients.

Data description

Clinical, laboratory and medication data were collected prospectively starting at the time of initiation of dialysis. These data included age, sex, height, weight, body mass index, diabetes status and current smoking status. Type of and change in renal replacement therapy (hemodialysis, peritoneal dialysis and kidney transplantation) were recorded and considered as time-dependent treatment status for data analysis. Vascular access procedures and the type of vascular access (native fistula, graft or central venous catheter) for hemodialysis were also evaluated.

Information on the following clinical events were collected before initiation of dialysis and during the entire observation period thereafter: coronary artery disease (including myocardial infarction, percutaneous transluminal coronary angioplasty, aortocoronary bypass), cardiovascular disease (including myocardial infarction, percutaneous transluminal coronary angioplasty, aortocoronary bypass, angiographically-proven coronary stenosis ≥50%, sudden cardiac death, ischemic or hemorrhagic cerebral infarction, transient ischemic attack, carotid stenosis and carotid endarterectomy), peripheral arterial disease (significant ultrasound- or angiographically-proven vascular stenosis, percutaneous transluminal angioplasty, peripheral bypass, amputation).

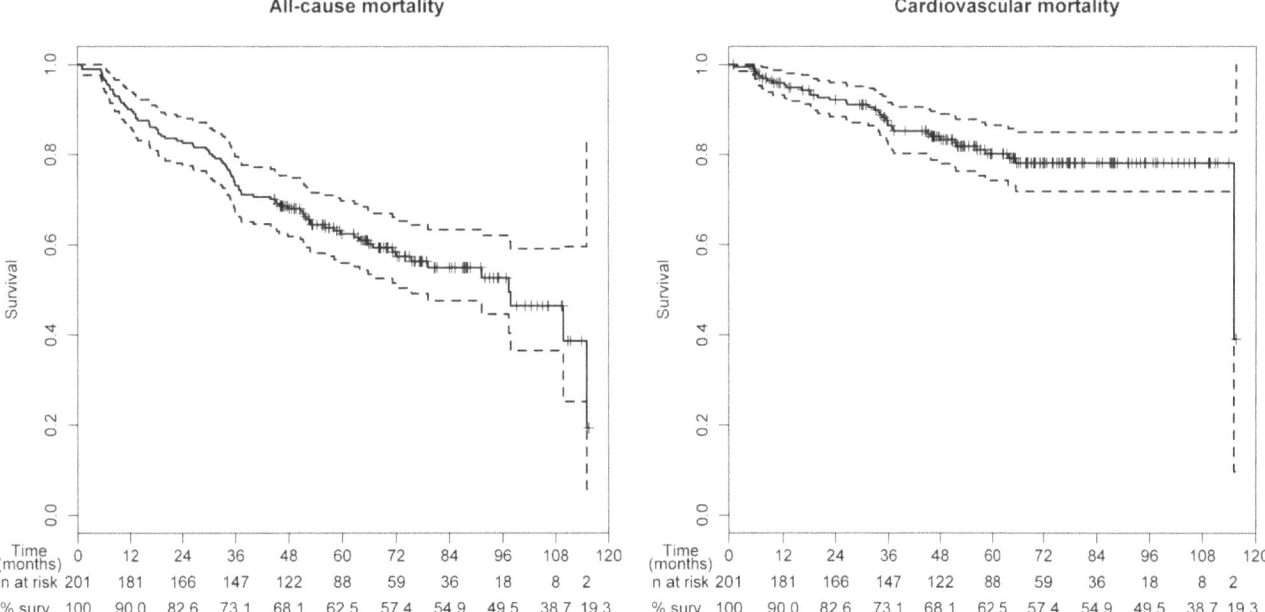

Figure 1. Kaplan-Meier survival curves with 95% confidence bands for all-cause and cardiovascular mortality. "% surv" stands for the percentage of survivors at each 12-month interval.

Biochemical analysis

We used two novel commercially available fully automated sandwich immunoassays for the measurement of MR-proANP (B.R.A.H.M.S MR-proANP KRYPTOR) and MR-proADM (B.R.A.H.M.S MR-proADM KRYPTOR) according to the manufacturer's instruction manuals (B.R.A.H.M.S GmbH, Hennigsdorf Germany). The design of these assays is based on immunoluminometric assays described previously [20,21]. Both parameters were measured in plasma collected at the time immediately before the initiation of the first dialysis therapy and kept frozen at $-80°C$ until measurement in a single batch. Other laboratory parameters reported here were measured from the same blood collection immediately before the first dialysis therapy.

As described earlier, the limit of quantitation was 4.5 pmol/L for the MR-proANP assay with a within-run imprecision coefficient of variation (CV) of <4.5% between 10 and 20 pmol/L and <2.5% between 20 and 1000 pmol/L, and between-run imprecision CV of <6.5% between 10 and 1000 pmol/L [21]. The limit of quantification was 0.23 nmol/L for the MR-proADM assay with a within-run imprecision CV of <4% between 0.5 and 2 nmol/L and <2% between 2 and 6 nmol/L, and a between-run imprecision CV of <11% between 0.5 and 2 nmol/L and <10% between 2 and 6 nmol/L [20]. All blood samples were processed by personnel blinded from any patient data.

Study Outcomes

The first outcome of interest was all-cause mortality and cardiovascular mortality. We also investigated other endpoints such as cardiovascular disease and peripheral arterial disease. Cardiovascular mortality was defined as death of myocardial infarction, heart failure, sudden death, ischemic or hemorrhagic stroke. Cardiovascular disease (CVD) events were defined as fatal and non-fatal myocardial infarction, percutaneous transluminal coronary angioplasty (PTCA), aortocoronary bypass (ACBP), angiographically-proven coronary stenosis ≥50%, ischemic cerebral infarction or transient ischemic attack. For peripheral arterial disease (PAD) at least one of the following events was existent: significant ultrasound- or angiographically-proven vascular stenosis, percutaneous transluminal angioplasty (PTA), peripheral bypass or amputation. An incident PAD event was only considered as a first time manifestation or a deterioration of PAD in terms of e.g. a change in PAD stage according to Fontaine. Two patients were lost to follow-up, one regained renal function and the other one moved away.

Statistical Methods

At baseline, categorical data were compared using χ^2-test and continuous variables were analyzed using an unpaired t-test or the non-parametric Wilcoxon rank-sum test. Data are presented as mean$\pm$SD and as median and 25th and 75th percentiles for skewed variables where appropriate.

To investigate the influence of MR-proANP and MR-proADM on all-cause mortality, cardiovascular mortality, cardiovascular disease and peripheral arterial disease, multivariable adjusted Cox-proportional hazards regression models were performed. In all analyses a p-value of 0.05 was considered significant. Variables were chosen for the multiple Cox regression analysis since they were either well-known risk factors for all-cause or CV mortality or they showed correlations with MR-proADM or MR-proANP. The first model was adjusted for age, sex, previous cardiovascular events, diabetes mellitus and type of renal replacement therapy, which was modeled time-dependently (Model 1). The second model (Model 2) was additionally adjusted for albumin, C-

reactive protein, current smoking status, native fistula and echocardiographic data (ejection fraction ≤60% versus >60%). Due to sparseness of the data and risk of overfitting, this fully-adjusted model should only be considered as a sensitivity analysis to Model 1, which is taken as the main model in this investigation. Linear relationship assumption of MR-proANP and MR-proADM in the Cox models was tested, as well as the proportional hazards assumption. One standard deviation (SD) was taken as the unit of measure for each of the continuous outcome variables to ensure comparability of Hazard Ratios. For ease of interpretation, additional fully adjusted Cox-proportional hazards regression models were calculated by dividing MR-proANP and MR-proADM into tertiles and also by stratifying patients in groups of high risk (both MR-proANP and MR-proADM in the upper tertile), intermediate risk (only one of the two parameters in the upper tertile) and low risk (none of the two parameters in the upper tertile). Adjusted survival curves are given for each of these risk groups and for each of the tertiles, holding all covariates fixed at their mean level. We also performed a sensitivity analysis with censoring at the time of transplantation. All analyses were conducted in SPSS version 16.0 software (SPSS Inc., Chicago, IL, USA) and R using the package "survival".

Results

Table 1 provides an overview on the demographic and laboratory parameters of our study cohort including MR-proANP, and MR-proADM plasma concentrations. Causes of CKD were

Table 2. Correlations between mid-regional pro-atrial natriuretic peptide (MR-proANP) and mid-regional pro-adrenomedullin (MR-proADM) and different parameters.

	Correlation coefficient (r)	
	MR-proANP	MR-proADM
Sex (male/female)	−0.032	−0.042
Age (years)	0.368[c]	0.298[c]
Diabetes mellitus (no/yes)	0.227[b]	0.091
Current smokers (no/yes)	−0.084	0.016
Body Mass Index (kg/m²)	−0.090	0.157[a]
Left ventricular ejection fraction (≤60%/>60%)	−0.262[c]	−0.257[c]
Systolic blood pressure (mmHg)	0.133	0.056
Diastolic blood pressure (mmHg)	−0.078	−0.082
Laboratory parameters		
Albumin (g/dL)	−0.198[b]	−0.223[b]
C-reactive protein (mg/dL)	0.003	0.084
Hemoglobin (g/dL)	−0.164[a]	−0.223[b]
Creatinine (mg/dL)	−0.070	0.032
Comorbidities before dialysis		
CAD*	0.168[a]	0.082
CVD**	0.150[a]	0.075
PAD***	0.168[a]	0.101

For footnotes see Table 1.
[a]p<0.05;
[b]p<0.01;
[c]p<0.001.

diabetic nephropathy (32%), vascular nephropathy (25%), glomerulonephritis (15%), interstitial and reflux nephropathy (9%), polycystic kidney disease (9%) and other causes (10%). During the entire observation period of up to more than 7 years 86 of the 201 patients (43%) passed away, 43% of them due to cardiovascular events (Figure 1). Patients who did not survive were older and had more severe illness compared to their event-free counterparts as indicated by lower serum albumin levels and impaired left ventricular systolic function, a higher frequency of diabetes as well as higher prevalence of comorbidities such as coronary and peripheral artery disease at baseline when compared to survivors. Almost all patients (99%) had MR-proANP levels ≥120 pmol/L, a recently investigated cut point for diagnosis of acute heart failure in patients with acute dyspnea [18]. 82% of all patients had at baseline MR-proADM levels above 1.985 nmol/L which was recently shown as optimal cut point to predict all-cause mortality in patients with acute dyspnea [18]. MR-proANP and MR-proADM levels were significantly higher among the non-survivors compared to the survivors (981±573 pmol/L vs. 662±439 pmol/L, p<0.001 and 3.29±1.17 nmol/L vs. 2.72±1.33 nmol/L, p<0.001, respectively). Table 2 lists the correlations between MR-proANP, MR-proADM and relevant parameters. Both parameters were moderately correlated with each other ($r^2 = 0.62$).

Cox-proportional hazards models for continuous variables of MR-proANP and MR-proADM

Table 3 presents the results from Cox-proportional hazards models for MR-proANP and MR-proADM, and all-cause and cardiovascular mortality as well as CVD and PAD events. Hazards ratios are adjusted for age, sex, previous CVD events, diabetes mellitus and time-dependent type of renal replacement therapy (Model 1) and an extended adjustment additionally for albumin, CRP, current smoking, native fistula and ejection fraction (Model 2 as sensitivity analysis). On a continuous scale, both MR-proANP and MR-proADM were significantly associated with all-cause and with cardiovascular mortality but not with the entire group of fatal and non-fatal cardiovascular disease events. When PAD was used as outcome variable only plasma MR-proANP but not MR-proADM levels showed a significant association. These results were only marginally influenced if further adjusted for albumin, CRP, current smoking, native fistula and ejection fraction determined by echocardiography (Model 2).

Table 3. The association of MR-proANP and MR-proADM as well as MR-proANP tertiles and MR-proADM tertiles and furthermore for patients with high risk (both MR-proANP and MR-proADM in the highest tertile) with different endpoints using multiple Cox-proportional hazards models.

	All-cause mortality (n events = 86)			Cardiovascular mortality* (n events = 37)			Cardiovascular disease** (n events = 85)			Peripheral arterial disease*** (n events = 54)		
	HR	95%CI	p-value	HR	95%CI	p-value	HR	95%CI	p-value	HR	95%CI	p-value
MR-proANP (per 1 SD increase)[a]												
Model 1	1.44	(1.17, 1.78)	0.001	1.75	(1.28, 2.39)	<0.001	1.15	(0.92, 1.45)	0.221	1.34	(1.02, 1.77)	0.037
Model 2	1.32	(1.04, 1.68)	0.021	1.73	(1.23, 2.44)	0.002	1.06	(0.83, 1.36)	0.642	1.35	(0.99, 1.84)	0.058
MR-proADM (per 1 SD increase)[a]												
Model 1	1.32	(1.11, 1.58)	0.002	1.41	(1.10, 1.82)	0.007	1.17	(0.98, 1.39)	0.092	1.08	(0.83, 1.41)	0.556
Model 2	1.23	(1.00, 1.50)	0.051	1.43	(1.07, 1.91)	0.015	1.11	(0.90, 1.36)	0.331	1.08	(0.80, 1.46)	0.603
MR-proANP (tertiles)[b]												
≤522 pmol/L	1			1			1			1		
523–794 pmol/L	1.07	(0.55, 2.05)	0.847	1.55	(0.50, 4.77)	0.446	0.97	(0.53, 1.78)	0.931	0.90	(0.40, 2.02)	0.802
≥795 pmol/L	1.76	(0.93, 3.33)	0.082	2.96	(0.99, 8.89)	0.053	1.07	(0.57, 1.98)	0.839	1.10	(0.49, 2.46)	0.815
MR-proADM (tertiles)[b]												
≤2.40 nmol/L	1			1			1			1		
2.41–3.10 nmol/L	1.04	(0.56, 1.92)	0.909	1.09	(0.41, 2.90)	0.862	1.03	(0.59, 1.80)	0.910	1.16	(0.59, 2.27)	0.674
≥3.11 nmol/L	2.39	(1.33, 4.28)	0.003	3.16	(1.27, 7.83)	0.013	1.53	(0.88, 2.67)	0.130	1.40	(0.68, 2.85)	0.360
MR-proANP- MR-proADM- Score[b]												
Low & intermediate risk	1			1			1			1		
High risk	2.87	(1.77, 4.65)	<0.001	3.58	(1.73, 7.43)	0.001	1.45	(0.87, 2.44)	0.156	1.59	(0.85, 2.97)	0.147

MR-proANP, mid-regional pro-atrial natriuretic peptide; MR-proADM, mid-regional pro-adrenomedullin.
Model 1: adjusted for age, sex, previous CVD**, diabetes mellitus, time-dependent type of renal replacement therapy.
Model 2: adjusted as in model 1 and additionally for albumin, CRP, current smoking, native fistula, echocardiography (ejection fraction ≤60% and >60%).
[a]For MR-proANP and MR-proADM 1 standard deviation (SD) increment was 524 pmol/L and 1.29 nmol/L, respectively. One SD was taken as the unit of increment for each of the continuous outcome variables to ensure comparability of Hazard Ratios.
[b]Adjusted for age, sex, previous CVD**, diabetes mellitus, time-dependent type of renal replacement therapy.
*CV mortality: myocardial infarction, heart failure, sudden cardiac death, ischemic stroke, hemorrhagic stroke.
**CVD: myocardial infarction, percutaneous transluminal coronary angioplasty, aortocoronary bypass, angiographically-proven coronary stenosis ≥50%, ischemic or hemorrhagic cerebral infarction, transient ischemic attack, carotid stenosis and carotid endarterectomy.
***PAD: significant ultrasound- or angiographically-proven vascular stenosis, percutaneous transluminal angioplasty, peripheral bypass, amputation.

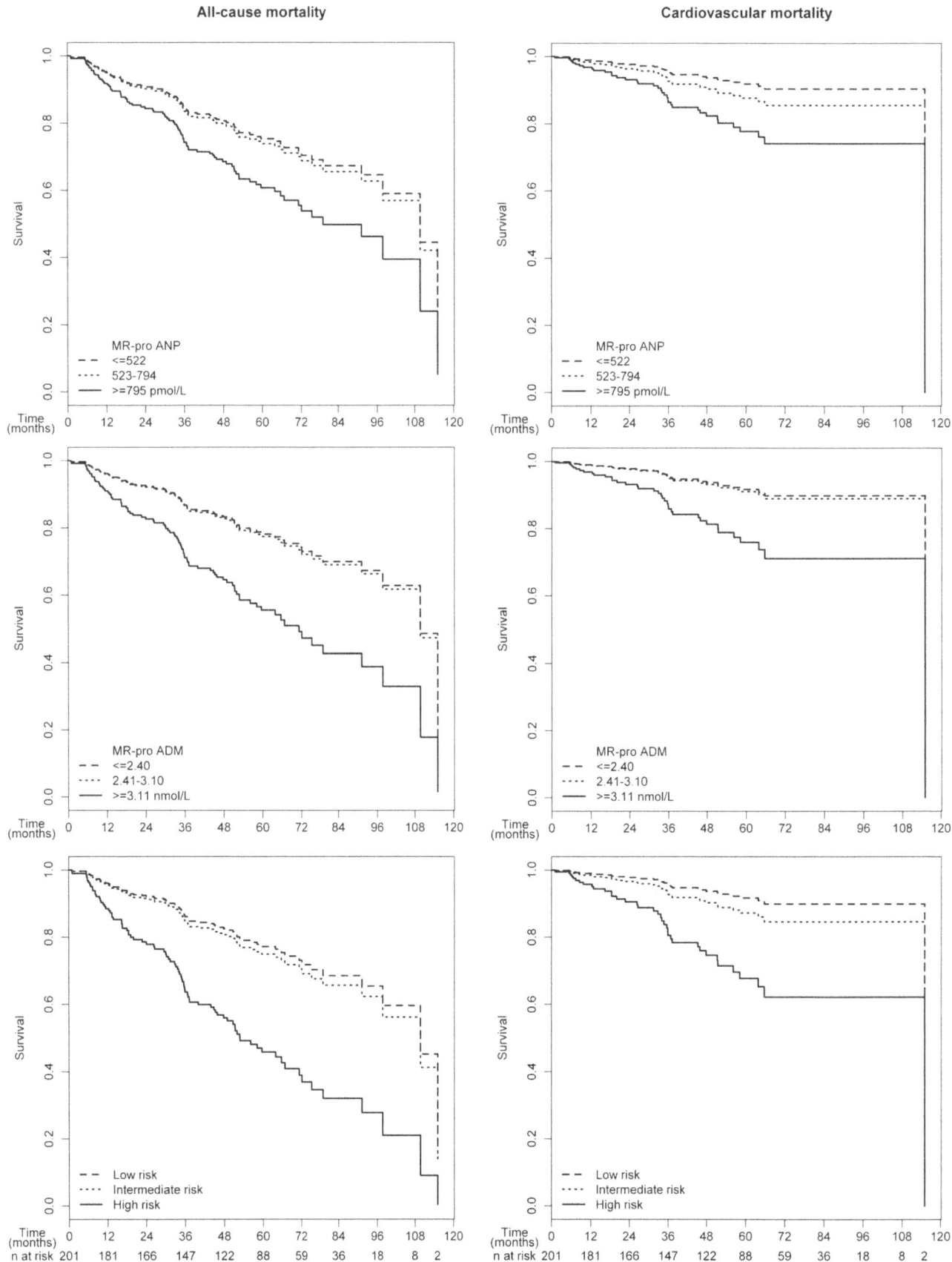

Figure 2. Survival curves for all-cause and cardiovascular mortality adjusted for age, sex, previous cardiovascular events, diabetes mellitus and time-dependent type of renal replacement therapy for mid-regional pro-atrial natriuretic peptide (MR-proANP)

tertiles (top), mid-regional pro-adrenomedullin (MR-proADM) tertiles (middle) and patients stratified for high risk (both MR-proANP and MR-proADM in the upper tertile), intermediate risk (only one of the two parameters in the upper tertile) and low risk (none of the two parameters in the upper tertile) (bottom). Tertiles for MR-proANP were ≤522, 523–794, and ≥795 pmol/L, respectively. Tertiles for MR-proADM were ≤2.40, 2.41–3.10, and ≥3.11 nmol/L, respectively.

Cox-proportional hazards models for categorical analysis of MR-proANP and MR-proADM

When we analyzed the data according to tertiles of MR-proANP and MR-proADM (Table 3), a non-significant trend for the upper tertile of MR-proANP for all-cause (HR = 1.76, p = 0.082) and cardiovascular mortality (HR = 2.96, p = 0.053) was observed. However, patients in the upper tertile of MR-proADM had a significantly increased risk for all-cause (HR = 2.39, p = 0.003) as well as cardiovascular mortality (HR = 3.16, p = 0.013). Survival curves for all-cause and cardiovascular mortality demonstrated that the first and second tertile of MR-proANP and MR-proADM were similar and only the third tertile discriminated between survivors and non-survivors (Figure 2).

This increased risk was clearly identified using a stratification based on the tertiles of the two peptides by combining the highest tertiles of MR-proANP (≥794 pmol/L) and MR-proADM (≥3.11 nmol/L). Table 4 provides the demographic and clinical characteristics of patients stratified in high risk (both MR-proANP and MR-proADM in the upper tertile), intermediate risk (only one of the two parameters in the upper tertile) and low risk (none of the two parameters in the upper tertile). The increase in risk with respect to all-cause mortality was almost identical when we compared the high risk group versus intermediate risk group (HR = 2.70, p = 0.001) and the high risk group versus low risk group (HR = 3.02, p<0.001). The risk was only increased when a patient had both parameters in the upper tertile, although demographic, clinical and laboratory variables were similar among the intermediate and high risk group. The high risk group was associated with an about 3-fold higher risk for all-cause mortality (HR = 2.87, p<0.001) and cardiovascular mortality (HR = 3.58, p = 0.001) when compared to the remaining patients (Table 3 and Figure 2).

Sensitivity analysis

It might introduce some considerable bias to the data analysis when a patient is selected for transplantation and follow-up time is censored at the time of transplantation. For this reason the above main analysis was performed by a time-dependent modeling of the renal replacement therapy status as discussed earlier [22,23]. To exclude that this procedure has influenced our main findings, we performed a sensitivity analysis with classical censoring at the time of transplantation which did, however, not reveal any substantial differences in HRs compared to the primary analysis (see Table S1). Due to sparseness of the data and risk of overfitting we also calculated a simple model only adjusting for age and sex that did not show major differences in estimates compared to Model 1. A further sensitivity analysis was calculated where Model 1 was additionally adjusted for hemoglobin. No substantial differences in estimates could be observed.

Discussion

The study at hand investigated the two peptides MR-proANP and MR-proADM in a prospective long-term cohort study of incident dialysis patients. We observed that increased concentrations of both peptides are associated with an increased risk of all-cause as well as cardiovascular mortality and this risk was about threefold elevated when both parameters were in the upper tertile of the entire patient group. This elevation of both parameters discriminated especially patients with intermediate and high risk which were otherwise similar in terms of clinical and laboratory parameters. Therefore, the incremental benefit to identify high risk patients is achieved by the combined evaluation of these two biomarkers. If a patient had an isolated increase in one of the two parameters, the risk was similar compared to patients which did show an increase at all (see Figure 2). Obviously, both peptides accumulate as a result of a series of pathophysiological parameters detrimental to survival. Our results indicate that cut points for the diagnosis of acute heart failure or for the prediction of mortality established in cohorts of patients not recruited because of end-stage renal disease (ESRD) do not necessarily apply for ESRD patients. In the present study MR-proANP and MR-proADM values above these cut-off points were demonstrated in a very high proportion of patients which might not only reflect the hemodynamic disturbances and risk prediction. Both peptides are produced in the kidney with important biological functions for the kidney. A compensatory increase in concentrations as well as a reduced clearance of both peptides requires searching for suitable cut points in patients with ESRD. Interestingly, we observed in the present study not only higher cut points of the two peptides but also a combination of both parameters to be predictive for outcomes.

Presumably, ANP reflects the central volume overload and intrinsic heart disease, whereas ADM reflects the decompensated reaction to the multifactorial stress state in preserving the integrity of the cardiovascular system in ESRD (22). It is of interest that we observed a strong association with all-cause and cardiovascular mortality but not with cardiovascular events combining fatal and non-fatal events. The slight increase in risk for CVD events (HR = 1.45, 95%CI 0.87–2.44) if both peptides were in the upper tertile was driven by the fatal CVD events. If these fatal events were excluded, the estimates for non-fatal CVD events did not show in any direction (HR = 1.04, 95%CI 0.45–2.39). This underscores that the pronounced increases of both peptides might reflect more the hemodynamic disturbances related to cardiac dysfunction rather than atherosclerotic processes resulting in non-fatal CVD events without hemodynamic decompensation. The combined measurement of these two peptides might provide surrogate variables for volume status but also act as an early indicator of deteriorating hemodynamic changes.

The diagnostic and prognostic utility of MR-proADM has been shown in various non-CKD cohorts and for different endpoints such as heart failure, cardiovascular events, and all-cause mortality [15–18]. In hemodialysis patients plasma ADM levels were associated with clinical conditions such as cardiac dysfunction, excessive blood volume and systemic inflammation but also with cardiovascular outcomes and mortality [13,24]. There is strong evidence that MR-proADM is produced in the kidney to exert hemodynamic actions on renal function [4]. That might be an explanation why MR-proADM was one of the strongest predictors for the progression of early stages of kidney impairment, which was even independent from baseline GFR measured by iohexol clearance [6,7].

It is currently unclear whether the systemic and renal haemodynamic effects are caused by MR-proADM itself or predomi-

Table 4. Clinical characteristics of patients stratified in high risk (both MR-proANP and MR-proADM in the upper tertile), intermediate risk (only one of the two parameters in the upper tertile) and low risk (none of the two parameters in the upper tertile).

	Low risk (n = 107)	Intermediate risk (n = 51)	High risk (n = 43)
Sex (male/female), n (%)	69/38 (64/36%)	32/19 (63/37%)	23/20 (53/47%)
Age (years)	57±15	67±11	66±11
Diabetes mellitus, n (%)	34 (32%)	22 (43%)	19 (44%)
Current smokers, n (%)	26 (24%)	9 (18%)	9 (21%)
Body Mass Index (kg/m^2)	26.0±4.1	26.6±4.4	25.5±5.4
Start of dialysis with			
Hemodialysis, n (%)	81 (76%)	49 (96%)	39 (91%)
Central venous catheter, n (%)	9 (11%)	9 (18%)	7 (18%)
Native fistula, n (%)	58 (72%)	32 (65%)	24 (62%)
Graft, n (%)	14 (17%)	8 (16%)	8 (21%)
Peritoneal dialysis, n (%)	26 (24%)	2 (4%)	4 (9%)
Year of start of dialysis			
2000–2003, n (%)	55 (51%)	26 (51%)	17 (40%)
2004–2006, n (%)	52 (49%)	25 (49%)	26 (60%)
Echocardiography			
Missing, n (%)	5 (5%)	4 (8%)	6 (14%)
Ejection fraction ≤60%, n (%)	36 (34%)	27 (53%)	23 (53%)
Ejection fraction >60%, n (%)	66 (62%)	20 (39%)	14 (33%)
Systolic blood pressure (mmHg)	151±22	154±21	157±25
Diastolic blood pressure (mmHg)	84±12	81±11	82±15
Laboratory parameters			
MR-proANP (pmol/L)	488±188 [322; 512; 625]	905±521 [546; 788; 1055]	1443±455 [975; 1422; 1811]
MR-proADM (nmol/L)	2.19±0.55 [1.84; 2.31; 2.57]	3.28±0.78 [2.71; 3.15; 3.69]	4.51±1.54 [3.46; 4.15; 4.93]
Albumin (g/dL)	3.8±0.6	3.7±0.6	3.5±0.7
C-reactive protein (mg/dL)	2.6±4.5 [0.3; 0.8; 2.1]	4.3±7.4 [0.3; 0.9; 4.4]	2.9±4.3 [0.4; 1.6; 3.1]
Calcium (mmol/L)	2.18±0.28	2.08±0.28	2.05±0.24
Phosphorus (mmol/L)	2.02±0.62 [1.59; 1.95; 2.40]	1.90±0.54 [1.54; 1.90; 2.14]	2.04±0.66 [1.57; 1.97; 2.39]
Hemoglobin (g/dL)	11.5±1.7	11.1±1.6	10.5±1.8
Creatinine (mg/dL)	7.3±2.7 [5.5; 6.8; 8.7]	7.4±2.5 [5.8; 7.1; 8.1]	7.2±2.9 [5.3; 6.4; 8.5]
HbA1c (% Hb)	6.51±1.44	6.57±2.02	6.16±1.21
Total cholesterol (mg/dL)	192±54	192±52	173±44
LDL cholesterol (mg/dL)	122±46	120±43	107±38
HDL cholesterol (mg/dL)	46.2±14.2	44.8±13.0	49.2±11.1
Triglycerides (mg/dL)	170±90 [111; 143; 212]	178±136 [109; 139; 194]	142±76 [100; 121; 161]
Comorbidities before dialysis			
CAD*, n (%)	15 (14%)	12 (23.5%)	9 (20.9%)
CVD**, n (%)	28 (26%)	19 (37.3%)	14 (32.6%)
PAD***, n (%)	18 (17%)	5 (9.8%)	12 (27.9%)
Follow-up			
Follow-up time (months)‡	63.2±26.6	56.3±28.5	36.1±25.3
All-cause mortality, n (%)	32 (30%)	26 (51%)	28 (65%)
Transplantation, n (%)	44 (41%)	8 (15.7%)	7 (16.3%)

For footnotes see Table 1.
doi:10.1371/journal.pone.0017803.t004

Table 5. Prospective studies in dialysis patients investigating the association between atrial natriuretic peptide (ANP) and adrenomedullin (ADM) on clinical outcomes.

Study	Design	Follow-up	Endpoint and number of patients with endpoint	HR (95% CI)
Atrial natriuretic peptide (ANP)				
Zoccali et al. 2001 [11]	Cohort study: 246 patients with end-stage renal disease without heart failure	26 mos.	All-cause mortality: 63 CV mortality: 35	All-cause mortality: 2.39 (1.59–3.59) for ln ANP adjusted for Kt/V, age, ln albumin, ln cholesterol, diabetes. 4.22 (1.79–9.92) for patients in the 3rd vs. the 1st tertile of ANP. CV mortality: 2.13 (1.29–3.52) for ln ANP adjusted for calcium, Kt/V, age. 3.80 (1.44–10.03) for patients in the 3rd vs. the 1st tertile of ANP.
Goto et al. 2002 [12]	Cohort study: 53 hemodialysis patients	11.3 mos.	Cardiac events: 13	118±21 vs. 56±5 pg/mL in patients in compared to without cardiac events.
Nakatani et al. 2003 [8]	Cohort study: 105 hemodialysis patients	24 mos.	Cardiac death: 11	32 (4–252) for ANP>50 pg/mL vs. <50 pg/mL. 3.5 (1.6–7.4) for ln ANP (adjusted for LVMI and CRP).
Odar-Cederlöf et al. 2003 [9]	Cohort study: 33 hemodialysis patients	47 mos.	All-cause mortality: 18 Early deaths (<1 year): 6	All-cause mortality: ANP (predialysis) 1.004 (1.000–1.007); ANP (postdialysis): 1.006 (1.000–1.012). Early deaths: ANP (predialysis) 1.007 (1.001–1.013); ANP (postdialysis) 1.006 (0.995–1.016).
Yoshihara et al. 2005 [13]	Cohort study: 67 hemodialysis patients	1 yr.	7 patients died and 8 CV events	Mortality and CV events combined: 1.41 (0.36–5.56) for ANP≥230 (median) compared to ANP<230.
Rutten et al. 2006 [10]	Cohort study: 68 peritoneal dialysis patients	1.5–4.5 yrs.	All-cause mortality: 10	11.3 (1.4–91.9) for ANP>median compared to ANP<median. 7.9 (0.9–72.1) adjusted for age, comorbidity, residual GFR.
This study	Incident cohort study: 201 dialysis patients	56 mos.	All-cause mortality: 86 CV mortality: 37	All-cause mortality: 1.44 (1.17–1.78) per SD increase of ANP. CV mortality: 1.75 (1.28–2.39) per SD increase of ANP.
Adrenomedullin (ADM)				
Yoshihara et al. 2005 [13]	Cohort study: 67 hemodialysis patients	1 yr.	7 patients died and 8 CV events	Mortality and CV events combined: 4.55 (1.23–16.80) for ADM≥4.55 (median) compared to ADM<4.55.
This study	Incident cohort study: 201 dialysis patients	56 mos.	All-cause mortality: 86 CV mortality: 37	All-cause mortality: 1.32 (1.11–1.58) per SD increase of ADM. CV mortality:1.41 (1.10–1.82) per SD increase of ADM.
Combination of the upper tertiles of ANP and ADM compared to other tertiles				
This study	Incident cohort study: 201 dialysis patients	56 mos.	All-cause mortality: 86 CV mortality: 37	All-cause mortality: 2.82 (1.76–4.53) per SD increase of ANP. CV mortality: 3.30 (1.62–6.70) per SD increase of ANP.

CV, cardiovascular; SD, standard deviation.

nantly through its active peptide ADM since an active role of MR-proADM is currently unclear. However, the eligible measurement of the active hormone ADM was doubted largely mainly due to the short half-life of 22 minutes and the partial binding to complement factor H [25–27]. Since MR-proADM and ADM are stoichiometrically generated and MR-proADM is more stable [28], MR-proADM seems to be at least a reliable surrogate marker for the active hormone ADM. The same holds true for MR-proANP and ANP. A perfect correlation between the midregional parts of the prohormones and the respective active hormones can not be expected since differences in the metabolic rates are assumed. Nevertheless, the midregional parts of the prohormones seem to mirror the hard to measure active hormones, otherwise the manifold associations with clinical endpoints would not be observed.

Our findings complement and extend previously reported cohort studies of end-stage renal disease for the biomarkers ANP [8–12] and ADM [13] (Table 5). Most of these studies were done in small cohorts and/or short observation periods and only one study considered ADM. Our cohort differs from these earlier studies since we investigated baseline levels in patients before first dialysis treatment. It therefore avoids a potential survival bias caused by the higher mortality rates during the first year of dialysis treatment which are not considered in cross-sectional cohorts or mixed cohorts of prevalent and incident dialysis patients.

MR-proANP concentrations were substantially increased in our cohort of dialysis patients when compared to patients with mild to moderate impairment of kidney function [6] as well as to a high risk cohort of heart failure patients [14]. While the role of ANP as regulator of the cardiovascular system is established, its physiological regulatory role on transport processes in the nephron is under debate [5]. ANP has been known to be primarily produced in the cardiac atrium, however, up-regulation of ANP mRNA expression has been demonstrated in extra-atrial tissues such as the kidneys [29]. The exact pathophysiological significance of kidney-synthesized ANP has not been defined yet.

To date prognostic biomarkers which predict outcome in this high risk cohort of CKD patients are sparse but highly demanded. However, as we discussed recently [6] the measurement of the active hormones has little clinical utility due to the short half life of most of the bioactive peptides, their immediate binding to receptors [27], their interaction with binding proteins [30] and several technical difficulties [30]. This is even more important when long-term stored samples are analysed because the active hormones undergo degradation even in frozen samples which is not the case for their propeptides. Therefore, replacing the problematic measurement of bioactive rapidly cleared peptides by measuring the non-functional, stable peptides MR-proANP and MR-proADM derived from their precursors represents a valuable advance for clinical practice. Interestingly, proteolytic degradation of pro-ANP seems to be mainly directed to the N- and C-terminal parts, whereas the midregion is significantly more stable [28] promoting this region to a suitable target of measurement. In addition, circulating mid-regional fragments are not influenced by a binding protein, making it suitable for immunometric analysis.

Strengths and limitations of the study

The prospective recruitment of all patients starting dialysis treatment over a period of six years in a clearly described area allowed a complete recruitment of patients requiring renal replacement therapy with almost no loss to follow-up during a long observation period. We can therefore exclude the most important bias of cross-sectional studies with a mix of prevalent and incident cases and the resulting survival bias. We furthermore considered even the observation period following kidney transplantation by modeling the treatment status in a time-dependent model, but on the other hand excluded by sensitivity analysis, that this procedure has obscured our results.

There are also some limitations of this study. A first limitation is the relatively small number of patients and events. We therefore could only adjust our analyses for a small number of variables (6 variables in Model 1). An extended adjustment with more variables (Model 2 and additional sensitivity analyses) was provided but should only be considered as sensitivity analysis. Interestingly, the estimates for MR-proADM and MR-proANP remained widely stable in Models 1 and 2, the additional sensitivity analyses and a very simple model only adjusted for age and sex. This argues for a pronounced independence of the two investigated variables for the prediction of endpoints. Second, we examined patients at the time immediately before renal replacement therapy was started. Therefore, some patients might not have been in a steady metabolic or extracellular volume state of the parameters evaluated. Concentrations of these hormones might therefore not necessarily be applicable to other cohorts of

patients with CKD. On the other hand, values measured after the start of dialysis treatment as done in other mostly smaller studies might represent dialysis dose or dialysis efficacy and thus answer a different question. Third, our study includes only Caucasian patients of a clearly described geographical region with almost complete ascertainment of incident dialysis patients over a defined period of time. It therefore lacks generalizability to other ethnic populations as well as other recruitment procedures. Finally, since the measurements of the two peptides are not rigorously standardized, concentrations measured by various assays are not necessarily comparable.

Conclusion

Among incident dialysis patients MR-proANP and MR-proADM were shown to be associated with all-cause mortality and cardiovascular mortality, with the highest risk when both parameters were in the upper tertiles.

Acknowledgments

We thank B.R.A.H.M.S GmbH (Hennigsdorf/Berlin, Germany) for providing reagents free of charge.

Author Contributions

Conceived and designed the experiments: GG GS CL UN F. Kronenberg. Performed the experiments: GS CL F. Kronenberg. Analyzed the data: GS CL F. Kronenberg. Contributed reagents/materials/analysis tools: GS CL EZ JS MW F. Knoll FL KL UN F. Kronenberg. Wrote the paper: GG GS CL EZ F. Knoll KL UN F. Kronenberg. Recruitment and follow-up of patients: EZ OF F. Knoll FL KL UN.

References

1. de Jager DJ, Grootendorst DC, Jager KJ, van Dijk PC, Tomas LM, et al. (2009) Cardiovascular and noncardiovascular mortality among patients starting dialysis. JAMA 302: 1782–1789.

2. Kronenberg F, Neyer U, Lhotta K, Trenkwalder E, Auinger M, et al. (1999) The low molecular weight apo(a) phenotype is an independent predictor for coronary artery disease in hemodialysis patients: a prospective follow-up. J Am Soc Nephrol 10: 1027–1036.

3. Kwan BCH, Kronenberg F, Beddhu S, Cheung AK (2007) Lipoprotein metabolism and lipid management in chronic kidney disease. J Am Soc Nephrol 18: 1246–1261.

4. Nishikimi T (2007) Adrenomedullin in the kidney-renal physiological and pathophysiological roles. Curr Med Chem 14: 1689–1699.

5. Franz M, Woloszczuk W, Horl WH (2001) Plasma concentration and urinary excretion of N-terminal proatrial natriuretic peptides in patients with kidney diseases. Kidney Int 59: 1928–1934.

6. Dieplinger B, Mueller T, Kollerits B, Struck J, Ritz E, et al. (2009) Pro-A-type natriuretic peptide and pro-adrenomedullin predict progression of chronic kidney disease: the MMKD Study. Kidney Int 75: 408–414.

7. Kronenberg F (2009) Emerging risk factors and markers of chronic kidney disease progression. Nat Rev Nephrol 5: 677–689.

8. Nakatani T, Naganuma T, Masuda C, Sugimura T, Uchida J, et al. (2003) The prognostic role of atrial natriuretic peptides in hemodialysis patients. Blood Purif 21: 395–400.

9. Odar-Cederlof I, Ericsson F, Theodorsson E, Kjellstrand CM (2003) Neuropeptide-Y and atrial natriuretic peptide as prognostic markers in patients on hemodialysis. ASAIO J 49: 74–80.

10. Rutten JH, Korevaar JC, Boeschoten EW, Dekker FW, Krediet RT, et al. (2006) B-type natriuretic peptide and amino-terminal atrial natriuretic peptide predict survival in peritoneal dialysis. Perit Dial Int 26: 598–602.

11. Zoccali C, Mallamaci F, Benedetto FA, Tripepi G, Parlongo S, et al. (2001) Cardiac natriuretic peptides are related to left ventricular mass and function and predict mortality in dialysis patients. J Am Soc Nephrol 12: 1508–1515.

12. Goto T, Takase H, Toriyama T, Sugiura T, Kurita Y, et al. (2002) Increased circulating levels of natriuretic peptides predict future cardiac event in patients with chronic hemodialysis. Nephron 92: 610–615.

13. Yoshihara F, Horio T, Nakamura S, Yoshii M, Ogata C, et al. (2005) Adrenomedullin reflects cardiac dysfunction, excessive blood volume, and inflammation in hemodialysis patients. Kidney Int 68: 1355–1363.

14. Moertl D, Berger R, Struck J, Gleiss A, Hammer A, et al. (2009) Comparison of midregional pro-atrial and B-type natriuretic peptides in chronic heart failure: influencing factors, detection of left ventricular systolic dysfunction, and prediction of death. J Am Coll Cardiol 53: 1783–1790.

15. Khan SQ, O'Brien RJ, Struck J, Quinn P, Morgenthaler N, et al. (2007) Prognostic value of midregional pro-adrenomedullin in patients with acute myocardial infarction: the LAMP (Leicester Acute Myocardial Infarction Peptide) study. J Am Coll Cardiol 49: 1525–1532.

16. Maier C, Clodi M, Neuhold S, Resl M, Elhenicky M, et al. (2009) Endothelial markers may link kidney function to cardiovascular events in type 2 diabetes. Diabetes Care 32: 1890–1895.

17. Melander O, Newton-Cheh C, Almgren P, Hedblad B, Berglund G, et al. (2009) Novel and conventional biomarkers for prediction of incident cardiovascular events in the community. JAMA 302: 49–57.

18. Maisel A, Mueller C, Nowak R, Peacock WF, Landsberg JW, et al. (2010) Mid-region pro-hormone markers for diagnosis and prognosis in acute dyspnea: results from the BACH (Biomarkers in Acute Heart Failure) trial. J Am Coll Cardiol 55: 2062–2076.

19. Sturm G, Lamina C, Zitt E, Lhotta K, Lins F, et al. (2010) Sex-specific association of time-varying hemoglobin values with mortality in incident dialysis patients. Nephrol Dial Transplant 25: 2715–2722.

20. Morgenthaler NG, Struck J, Alonso C, Bergmann A (2005) Measurement of midregional proadrenomedullin in plasma with an immunoluminometric assay. Clin Chem 51: 1823–1829.

21. Morgenthaler NG, Struck J, Thomas B, Bergmann A (2004) Immunoluminometric assay for the midregion of pro-atrial natriuretic peptide in human plasma. Clin Chem 50: 234–236.

22. Schwaiger JP, Lamina C, Neyer U, König P, Kathrein H, et al. (2006) Carotid plaques and their predictive value for cardiovascular disease and all-cause mortality in hemodialysis patients considering renal transplantation - A decade follow-up. Am J Kidney Dis 47: 888–897.

23. Schwaiger JP, Neyer U, Sprenger-Mähr H, Kollerits B, Mündle M, et al. (2006) A simple score predicts future cardiovascular events in an inception cohort of dialysis patients. Kidney Int 70: 543–548.

24. Yoshihara F, Ernst A, Morgenthaler NG, Horio T, Nakamura S, et al. (2007) Midregional proadrenomedullin reflects cardiac dysfunction in haemodialysis patients with cardiovascular disease. Nephrol Dial Transplant 22: 2263–2268.

25. Meeran K, O'Shea D, Upton PD, Small CJ, Ghatei MA, et al. (1997) Circulating adrenomedullin does not regulate systemic blood pressure but increases plasma prolactin after intravenous infusion in humans: a pharmacokinetic study. J Clin Endocrinol Metab 82: 95–100.

26. Hinson JP, Kapas S, Smith DM (2000) Adrenomedullin, a multifunctional regulatory peptide. Endocr Rev 21: 138–167.

27. Pio R, Martinez A, Unsworth EJ, Kowalak JA, Bengoechea JA, et al. (2001) Complement factor H is a serum-binding protein for adrenomedullin, and the resulting complex modulates the bioactivities of both partners. J Biol Chem 276: 12292–12300.

28. Ala-Kopsala M, Magga J, Peuhkurinen K, Leipala J, Ruskoaho H, et al. (2004) Molecular heterogeneity has a major impact on the measurement of circulating N-terminal fragments. Clin Chem 50: 1576–1588.

29. Lo CS, Chen CH, Hsieh TJ, Lin KD, Hsiao PJ, et al. (2009) Local action of endogenous renal tubular atrial natriuretic peptide. J Cell Physiol 219: 776–786.

30. Lewis LK, Smith MW, Yandle TG, Richards AM, Nicholls MG (1998) Adrenomedullin(1–52) measured in human plasma by radioimmunoassay: plasma concentration, adsorption, and storage. Clin Chem 44: 571–577.

2

Sequence-Based Polymorphisms in the Mitochondrial D-Loop and Potential SNP Predictors for Chronic Dialysis

Jin-Bor Chen[1], Yi-Hsin Yang[2], Wen-Chin Lee[1], Chia-Wei Liou[3], Tsu-Kung Lin[3], Yueh-Hua Chung[4], Li-Yeh Chuang[5], Cheng-Hong Yang[6]*, Hsueh-Wei Chang[7,8]*

1 Division of Nephrology, Department of Internal Medicine, Mitochondrial Research Unit, Kaohsiung Chang Gung Memorial Hospital, Chang Gung University College of Medicine, Kaohsiung, Taiwan, **2** School of Pharmacy, Kaohsiung Medical University, Kaohsiung, Taiwan, **3** Department of Neurology and Mitochondrial Research Unit, Kaohsiung Chang Gung Memorial Hospital and Chang Gung University College of Medicine, Kaohsiung, Taiwan, **4** Institute of Biomedical Sciences, National Sun Yat-Sen University, Kaohsiung, Taiwan, **5** Department of Chemical Engineering & Institute of Biotechnology and Chemical Engineering, I-Shou University, Kaohsiung, Taiwan, **6** Department of Electronic Engineering, National Kaohsiung University of Applied Sciences, Kaohsiung, Taiwan, **7** Department of Biomedical Science and Environmental Biology, Kaohsiung Medical University, Taiwan, **8** Center of Excellence for Environmental Medicine, Cancer Center, Kaohsiung Medical University Hospital, Kaohsiung Medical University, Kaohsiung, Taiwan

Abstract

Background: The mitochondrial (mt) displacement loop (D-loop) is known to accumulate structural alterations and mutations. The aim of this study was to investigate the prevalence of single nucleotide polymorphisms (SNPs) within the D-loop among chronic dialysis patients and healthy controls.

Methodology and Principal Findings: We enrolled 193 chronic dialysis patients and 704 healthy controls. SNPs were identified by large scale D-loop sequencing and bioinformatic analysis. Chronic dialysis patients had lower body mass index, blood thiols, and cholesterol levels than controls. A total of 77 SNPs matched with the positions in reference of the Revised Cambridge Reference Sequence (CRS) were found in the study population. Chronic dialysis patients had a significantly higher incidence of 9 SNPs compared to controls. These include SNP5 (16108Y), SNP17 (16172Y), SNP21 (16223Y), SNP34 (16274R), SNP35 (16278Y), SNP55 (16463R), SNP56 (16519Y), SNP64 (185R), and SNP65 (189R) in D-loop of CRS. Among these SNPs with genotypes, SNP55-G, SNP56-C, and SNP64-A were 4.78, 1.47, and 5.15 times more frequent in dialysis patients compared to controls ($P<0.05$), respectively. When adjusting the covariates of demographics and comorbidities, SNP64-A was 5.13 times more frequent in dialysis patients compared to controls ($P<0.01$). Furthermore, SNP64-A was found to be 35.80, 3.48, 4.69, 5,55, and 4.67 times higher in female patients and in patients without diabetes, coronary artery disease, smoking, and hypertension in an independent significance manner ($P<0.05$), respectively. In patients older than 50 years or with hypertension, SNP34-A and SNP17-C were found to be 7.97 and 3.71 times more frequent ($P<0.05$) compared to patients younger than 50 years or those without hypertension, respectively.

Conclusions and Significance: The results of large-scale sequencing suggest that specific SNPs in the mtDNA D-loop are significantly associated with chronic dialysis. These SNPs can be considered as potential predictors for chronic dialysis.

Editor: Yury E. Khudyakov, Centers for Disease Control and Prevention, United States of America

Funding: This study was partly supported by grants from Kaohsiung Chang Gung Memorial Hospital under contract nos. CMRPG850271, CMRPG850272, CMRPG850242, and CMRPG850252, the Department of Health, Executive Yuan, Republic of China (DOH101-TD-C-111-002), and the Kaohsiung Medical University Research Foundation (KMUER014 and KMU-M110001) and the National Sun Yat-sen University-KMU Joint Research Project (#NSYSUKMU 101-006). The funders had no role in study design, data collection and analysis, decision to publish, or preparation of the manuscript.

Competing Interests: The authors have declared that no competing interests exist.

* E-mail: changhw@kmu.edu.tw (HWC); chyang@cc.kuas.edu.tw (CHY)

Introduction

Mitochondria (mt) are organelles that are susceptible to oxidative stress. The presence of excessive amounts of reactive oxidative species (ROS) results in mitochondrial oxidative damage and inefficient repair of mtDNA [1–3]. This can contribute to pathophysiological processes, including aging, degenerative disease [4–6] and cancer [7]. In these circumstances, somatic mutations are also generated [8].

The displacement loop (D-loop) regions of mtDNA does not encode any functional proteins [9,10] and is known to accumulate mutations at a higher frequency than other regions of mtDNA in

the setting of increased oxidative stress [11]. The D-loop contains the initial site of heavy chain replication and the promoters for heavy chain replication and light chain transcription. Therefore, it is responsible for the regulation of mtDNA replication and transcription [10,11]. The D-loop is highly polymorphic, and some polymorphisms are associated with aging [12–15], coronary artery disease [16], and a variety of tumors, including lung [17], colorectal [18], liver [19], gastric [20], breast [21], cervical [22], melanoma [23], head and neck [24], oral [25], and kidney [26] cancers. However, D-loop polymorphisms are not associated with prostate cancer [27,28]. Most of these D-loop studies focus on some cancer-associated single nucleotide polymorphisms (SNPs) for mtDNA, which were accompanied by poly-C tract alterations [21,24,25,29,30]. However, D-loop polymorphisms have not been systematically characterized in chronic dialysis patients.

Complications of chronic kidney disease (CKD) promote morbidity and mortality [31]. CKD patients can be classified according to kidney function along a continuum from mild renal dysfunction to irreversible kidney failure. CKD increases oxidative stress [32] which has been demonstrated to influence mtDNA content in CKD patients [33,34].

Because the D-loop region susceptible to oxidative stress, we hypothesized that specific SNP patterns in the D-loop of chronic dialysis patients may serve as potential genetic markers for chronic dialysis. To examine this hypothesis, we performed D-loop sequencing and used bioinformatic tools to identify SNPs that were associated with chronic dialysis when compared to healthy controls.

Materials and Methods

Subjects

We enrolled 704 unrelated Taiwanese of ethnic Chinese background in this study through the hospital health examination center after giving consent. Participants included 312 men and 392 women with a mean age of 51.9 years. We enrolled 193 dialysis patients from the outpatient dialysis unit of the same hospital. They were composed of 78 men and 115 women with a mean age of 49 years. Venous blood samples were collected after overnight fasting. The serum was separated using a centrifuge and stored at −80°C. DNA was isolated from leucocytes using PUREGENE®

Table 1. Basic demographic characteristics of patients and controls.

			patients		controls		Chi-square
		total	n	%	n	%	P value
Total		897	193	21.5	704	78.5	
Sex	female	427	115	59.6	312	44.3	0.0002
	male	470	78	40.4	392	55.7	
Age	≤50	422	97	50.3	325	46.2	0.3127
	>50	475	96	49.7	379	53.8	
	Mean (SD)		49.0	(13.9)	51.9	(12.9)	0.0055
DM	N	836	161	83.4	675	98.3	<0.0001
	Y	44	32	16.6	12	1.7	
CHD	N	854	170	88.1	684	98.4	<0.0001
	Y	34	23	11.9	11	1.6	
HT	N	593	109	56.5	484	69.6	0.0006
	Y	295	84	43.5	211	30.4	
Smoke	N	698	170	88.1	528	75.0	0.0001
	Y	199	23	11.9	176	25.0	
BMI	Mean (SD)		22.3	(3.8)	24.5	(3.5)	<0.0001
TBARS	Mean (SD)		1.1	(0.6)	1.2	(0.8)	0.0801
Thiols	Mean (SD)		1.5	(0.5)	2.0	(0.4)	<0.0001
TG	Mean (SD)		169.5	(128.1)	130.4	(85.7)	<0.0001
Chol	Mean (SD)		189.4	(35.7)	202.1	(37.9)	<0.0001

Abbreviations and/or units: CHD: coronary heart disease, HT: hypertension, BMI: body mass index, TBARS: thiobarbituric acid reactive substance (μM), Thiols (μM); TG: triglyceride (mg/dL), Chol: cholesterol (mg/dL).

DNA Purification kit (Gentra, Minneapolis, MN, USA) and stored at −20°C. The protocol for the present study was approved by the Committee on Human Research at Kaohsiung Chang Gung Memorial Hospital (CMRPG850271, CMRPG850272, CMRPG850242, CMRPG850252, IRB 95-0395B) and conducted in accordance with the Declaration of Helsinki. All participants signed a written informed consent form to obtain the approval for participation in this study.

Assessment of Oxidative and Anti-oxidative Stress Capacities

Serum free thiols were determined by direct reaction of the thiols with 5,5-dithiobis(2-nitrobenzoic acid) (DTNB) to form 5-thio-2-nitrobenzoic acid (TNB). The amount of thiols was calculated from the absorbance determined using the extinction coefficient of TNB (A412 = 13,600 M^{-1} cm^{-1}). The serum thiobarbituric acid reactive substance (TBARS) concentration was assessed according to the method of Ohkawa *et al.* [35]. Results are expressed as micromoles of TBARS per liter. A standard curve of TBARS was obtained by hydrolysis of 1,1,3,3-tetraethoxypropane (TEPP).

D-loop Sequencing

The mtDNA control region segment (relative to nucleotide (nt) regions 15911–16569 and 1–602 in the Revised Cambridge Reference Sequence ("rCRS") [36]; NC_012920) was amplified using the forward primer L15911 (5′-ACCAGTCTTG-TAAACCGGAG-3′) and the reverse primer H602 (5′-GCTTTGAGGAGGTAAGCTAC-3′). The products were purified with gel extraction kits (Watson BioMedicals Inc.) and sequenced using primer L15911 and primer L29 (5′-CTCACGG-GAGCTCTCCATGC-3′) on an ABI 377XL DNA Sequencer (Applied Biosystems, Foster, CA, USA). However, due to the conversion of thymine to cytosine and the presence of homopolymeric cytosine tracts at nt16184–16193 and nt303–315 within the D-loop region of some subjects, the sequencing procedure was prematurely terminated. Therefore, we also performed reverse sequencing using 2 additional sets of primers, H81 (5′-CAGCGTCTCGCAATGCTATC-3′) and H528 (5′-TTCGGGGTATGGGGTTAGCA-3′). The polymerase chain reaction (PCR) conditions used were as follows: an initial denaturation step at 95°C for 5 min, followed by 35 cycles of denaturation at 95°C for 1 min, annealing at 60°C for 1 min, and extension at 68°C for 2 min, with a final extension of 10 min at 72°C. The PCR fragments were analyzed by electrophoresis on a 2% agarose gel and visualized by staining with ethidium bromide.

SNP Identification

DNA sequences were analyzed by using the DNASTAR software and Bio Edit Sequence Alignment Editor freeware (http://www.mbio.ncsu.edu/bioedit/bioedit.html). After multiple sequence alignments were performed, both 5′ and 3′ ends of the sequences were trimmed into blunt ends. The SNPs were identified by calculating each nucleotide (A, T, C, or G) for each position in the trimmed and aligned sequences by "count if = " in Excel software. SNP frequencies greater than 1% were selected for further investigation. The SNPs were compared to the D-loop polymorphisms in rCRS as shown in MITOMAP [37] (http://www.mitomap.org/MITOMAP/PolymorphismsControl).

Statistical Analysis

Chi-square tests were used to compare basic characteristics between patients and controls. A sequence of analyses was adopted

Table 2. SNP identification from aligned sequences of cases and controls and their positional information.

SNP No.	Align-position*1	D-loop position*2	IUPAC code	SNP No.	Align-position*1	D-loop position*2	IUPAC code
1	51	16051	R	40	298	16298	Y
2	86	16086	Y	41	304	16304	Y
3	92	16092	H	42	309	16309	R
4	93	16093	Y	43	311	16311	Y
5	108	16108	Y	44	316	16316	R
6	111	16111	Y	45	319	16319	R
7	126	16126	Y	46	324	16324	Y
8	129	16129	R	47	327	16327	Y
9	136	16136	Y	48	335	16335	R
10	140	16140	Y	49	355	16355	Y
11	145	16145	R	50	356	16356	Y
12	148	16148	Y	51	357	16357	Y
13	157	16157	Y	52	362	16362	Y
14	162	16162	R	53	390	16390	R
15	164	16164	R	54	399	16399	R
16	167	16167	Y	55	463	16463	R
17	172	16172	Y	56	519	16519	Y
18	209	16209	Y	57	662	93	R
19	217	16217	Y	58	672	103	R
20	218	16218	Y	59	715	146	H
21	223	16223	Y	60	719	150	Y
22	227	16227	R	61	720	151	Y
23	234	16234	Y	62	721	152	Y
24	235	16235	R	63	722	153	R
25	243	16243	H	64	754	185	R
26	248	16248	Y	65	758	189	R
27	249	16249	Y	66	763	194	Y
28	256	16256	Y	67	764	195	Y
29	257	16257	H	68	768	199	Y
30	260	16260	Y	69	769	200	R
31	261	16261	Y	70	773	204	Y
32	266	16266	N	71	776	207	R
33	272	16272	R	72	779	210	R
34	274	16274	R	73	786	217	Y
35	278	16278	Y	74	803	234	R
36	290	16290	Y	75	804	235	R
37	291	16291	Y	76	885	317	Y
38	295	16295	Y	77	1019	461	Y
39	297	16297	Y				

*1.The positions are defined by the aligned sequences from cases and controls. Due to the poor quality at both 5′ and 3′ ends for PCR amplified by primers L15911/H602 as described in materials and methods, the sequences of nt15911–16000 and nt486–602 of the NC_012920 were excluded. nt249/353/354 of the NC_012920 were not included because they were not found in our sequencing data.

*2.The position for the D-loop in the Revised Cambridge Reference Sequence ("rCRS"; NC_012920).

for SNP selection. The Chi-square tests were first used to compare distributions of SNPs between patients and controls. Nine SNPs with significant differences and with sufficient cell sizes were chosen for further analysis. These 9 SNPs were included in a logistic regression model with backward selection. Only statistically significant SNPs were selected by logistic regression. The same logistic regression selection process was also conducted for several subgroups. Lastly, the adjusted odds ratios (AOR) from selected SNPs were computed on the basis of logistic regression with additional covariates of basic demographic characteristics (Table 1). The statistical data were expressed as mean ± SD. A P value of less than 0.05 was considered as statistically significant.

Table 3. The 9 SNPs with significantly different genotype distributions between patients and controls.

Variable[*1]	Variable[*2]		total	patients		controls		Chi-square
				n	%	n	%	P value
total			897	193		704		
SNP 5	16108Y	C	877	185	95.9	692	98.3	0.0419
		T	20	8	4.1	12	1.7	
SNP 17	16172Y	C	126	36	18.7	90	12.8	0.0376
		T	771	157	81.3	614	87.2	
SNP 21	16223Y	C	394	97	50.3	297	42.2	0.0453
		T	503	96	49.7	407	57.8	
SNP 34	16274R	A	13	6	3.1	7	1.0	0.0294
		G	884	187	96.9	697	99.0	
SNP 35	16278Y	C	843	188	97.4	655	93.0	0.0238
		T	54	5	2.6	49	7.0	
SNP 55	16463R	A	888	188	97.4	700	99.4	0.0125
		G	9	5	2.6	4	0.6	
SNP 56	16519Y	C	488	119	61.7	369	52.4	0.0224
		T	409	74	38.3	335	47.6	
SNP 64	185R	A	25	14	7.3	11	1.6	0.0000
		G	872	179	92.7	693	98.4	
SNP 65	189R	A	874	184	95.3	690	98.0	0.0373
		G	23	9	4.7	14	2.0	

*1The annotation of these SNPs is listed in Table 2.
*2SNPs in rCRS position with IUPAC code.

Results

Basic Demographic Characteristics

The study participants included 193 dialysis patients and 704 healthy controls, and their basic characteristics are shown in Table 1. Most of these characteristics were found to be significantly different, except for age groups and blood TBARS levels. The patients were 3 years younger (49.0±13.9 vs. 51.9±12.9) than the controls and had lower values of body mass index (BMI), blood thiols, and cholesterol levels. The mean triglyceride (TG) level was higher in patients than in controls. There was a significantly higher incidence of comorbidities of

Table 4. The OR and AOR for the 3 SNPs selected by backward logistic regression.

Variable[*1]	OR[*2]	95% CI	P value	AOR[*3]	95% CI	P value
SNP 55 G vs. A	4.78	1.26–18.09	0.0212	1.35	0.15–12.41	0.7886
SNP 56 C vs. T	1.47	1.06–2.04	0.0225	1.41	0.89–2.24	0.1441
SNP 64 A vs. G	5.15	2.29–11.60	0.0001	5.13	1.61–16.35	0.0057

*1.The annotation of these SNPs is listed in Table 2.
*2.Odds ratios (ORs) were computed by having only SNP variables in the logistic regression.
*3.Adjusted odds ratios (AORs) were computed by having SNP variables in the analysis model with covariates of sex, diabetes mellitus, coronary heart disease, smoker, hypertension, age, body mass index, thiobarbituric acid reactive substance, thiols, triglyceride, and cholesterol.

diabetes, hypertension (HT), and coronary heart disease (CHD) in dialysis patients compared to controls.

D-loop Sequencing, Alignment, and SNP Identification

There are 2 poly-C regions in the mitochondrial D-loop that stretch between nt16180–16195 [38] and nt303–315 [9]. Because the length of these mononucleotide repeats varies, they may interfere the sequence alignment processing or lead to error alignment in part. Accordingly, the sequences for these 2 repeat regions were replaced with the corresponding sequences for the reference CRS to improve the performance of sequence alignment. The sequencing data from the 5′ and 3′ ends of nt15911–16000 and nt486–602 were of poor quality and, therefore, were trimmed after confirmation of sequence alignment. Finally, aligned sequences were trimmed to the same length ranging from nt16000–16569 and nt1–485 for further SNP identification (Table S1 and Table S2; all D-loop trimmed sequences for cases and controls and their alignment visualization, respectively). After examining each nt for each position of the trimmed sequence, 77 SNPs with frequencies greater than 1% were identified (Table S3). The relationships between positions of the aligned sequences and D-loop in the reference CRS as well as the SNP types in the IUPAC code are listed in Table 2.

Significance Analysis for 77 Individual SNPs

The P values for 77 individual SNPs with A, G, C, and T distribution data were analyzed (Table S4). Nine SNPs were selected from 77 SNPs by Chi-square tests with significant differences and sufficient cell sizes; their genotype distributions are compared in Table 3. For each SNP, the genotype that appeared at a higher frequency in patients was selected as the

Table 5. The OR and AOR for the 9 SNPs selected by backward logistic regression for subgroups related to several basic demographic characteristics.

(no adjust) *1	female			male			age<=50			age>50		
effect *2	OR	95% CI	P	OR	95% CI	P	OR	95% CI	P	OR	95% CI	P
SNP 5 T vs. C				5.88	1.78–19.44	**0.004**						
SNP 17 C vs. T							1.81	1.01–3.28	**0.048**			
SNP 21 C vs. T				2.06	1.22–3.47	**0.007**						
SNP 34 A vs. G										5.26	1.15–24.00	**0.032**
SNP 35 C vs. T												
SNP 55 G vs. A	6.10	1.10–33.79	**0.039**				11.43	1.17–111.50	**0.036**			
SNP 56 C vs. T												
SNP 64 A vs. G	15.24	3.29–70.73	**0.001**							5.59	1.89–16.57	**0.002**
SNP 65 G vs. A				8.14	1.57–42.28	**0.013**						

(no adjust) *1	no DM			no CHD			non smoker			no HT			having HT		
effect *2	OR	95% CI	P	OR	95% CI	P	OR	95% CI	P	OR	95% CI	P	OR	95% CI	P
SNP 5 T vs. C							2.81	1.09–7.25	**0.033**						
SNP 17 C vs. T													3.10	1.48–6.51	**0.003**
SNP 21 C vs. T															
SNP 34 A vs. G	3.20	1.02–10.00	0.046												
SNP 35 C vs. T				3.97	1.22–12.91	**0.022**				4.62	1.10–19.41	**0.037**			
SNP 55 G vs. A	4.59	1.14–18.58	**0.033**	5.14	1.36–19.37	**0.016**	5.85	1.38–24.77	**0.016**	6.06	1.33–27.54	**0.020**			
SNP 56 C vs. T															
SNP 64 A vs. G	4.13	1.66–10.23	**0.002**	4.52	1.89–10.85	**0.001**	7.02	2.59–19.02	**0.000**	5.20	1.84–14.68	**0.002**			
SNP 65 G vs. A													4.46	1.05–18.98	**0.043**

(Adjust) *3	female			male			age<=50			age>50		
effect *4	AOR	95% CI	P	AOR	95% CI	P	AOR	95% CI	P	AOR	95% CI	P
SNP 5 T vs. C				4.53	0.80–25.65	0.088						
SNP 17 C vs. T							1.48	0.55–3.96	0.435			
SNP 21 C vs. T				2.05	0.95–4.40	0.067						
SNP 34 A vs. G										7.97	1.25–50.94	**0.028**
SNP 35 C vs. T												
SNP 55 G vs. A	0.97	0.02–41.98	0.986				14.39	0.30–685.42	0.176			
SNP 56 C vs. T												
SNP 64 A vs. G	35.80	3.23–396.84	**0.004**							3.67	0.78–17.25	0.100
SNP 65 G vs. A				4.84	0.35–67.24	0.240						

(Adjust) *3	no DM			no CHD			non smoker			no HT			having HT		
effect *4	AOR	95% CI	P	AOR	95% CI	P	AOR	95% CI	P	AOR	95% CI	P	AOR	95% CI	P
SNP 5 T vs. C							3.02	0.80–11.42	0.102						
SNP 17 C vs. T													3.71	1.10–12.55	**0.035**
SNP 21 C vs. T															
SNP 34 A vs. G	4.53	1.02–20.21	0.048												
SNP 35 C vs. T				3.76	0.84–16.81	0.083				5.95	0.73–48.65	0.096			
SNP 55 G vs. A	1.55	0.15–15.83	0.713	1.45	0.16–13.54	0.742	2.06	0.16–27.11	0.582	1.97	0.16–24.08	0.595			
SNP 56 C vs. T															
SNP 64 A vs. G	3.48	0.97–12.55	0.056	4.69	1.44–15.27	**0.010**	5.55	1.38–22.28	**0.016**	4.67	1.02–21.24	**0.046**			

Table 5. Cont.

(Adjust) *3	no DM			no CHD			non smoker			no HT			having HT		
effect *4	AOR	95% CI	P	AOR	95% CI	P	AOR	95% CI	P	AOR	95% CI	P	AOR	95% CI	P
SNP 65 G vs. A													4.19	0.41–42.36	0.225

*1.Odds ratios (ORs) were computed by having only SNP variables in the logistic regression.
*2.Significant SNPs were selected by backward logistic regression for subgroups.
*3.Adjusted odds ratios (AORs) were computed by having SNP variables in the analysis model with covariates of sex, diabetes mellitus, coronary heart disease, smoker, hypertension, age, body mass index, thiobarbituric acid reactive substance, thiols, triglyceride, and cholesterol.
*4.Adjusted covariates were added in models with significant SNPs.
P = P value.

indicator. Hence, the indicators for the SNPs 5, 17, 21, 34, 35, 55, 56, 64, and 65 (16108Y, 16172Y, 16223Y, 16274R, 16278Y, 16463R, 16519Y, 185R, and 189R) were T, C, C, A, C, G, C, A, and G, respectively. These 9 indicators were further added into a logistic regression by employing the backward selection method.

Backward Logistic Regression Analysis for 9 SNPs

As shown in Table 4, we identified 3 statistically significant indicators (SNP55 G, SNP56 C, and SNP64 A). Individuals with the SNP55 G increase risk of chronic dialysis by 4.78 times (OR, 95% CI = 1.26~18.09, P = 0.0212). SNP56 C or SNP64 A subjects increase risk of chronic dialysis by 1.47 (95% CI = 1.06~2.04, P = 0.0225) or 5.15 (95% CI = 2.29~11.60, P = 0.0001) times. The AORs of the 3 SNPs were further computed by adding the covariates shown in Table 1 into the logistic regression analysis. Following this, only SNP64 A remained significant (OR = 5.13, 95% CI = 1.61~16.35, P = 0.0057). Hence, SNP64 is only an independent SNP for disease as well as for the patients' basic characteristics. On the other hand, while SNP55 and SNP56 found in the backward logistic regression could only be considered as independent SNPs among the 77 SNPs, they were affected by covariates.

Stepwise Regression for Subgroups Related to Several Basic Demographic Characteristics

Similar procedures were also conducted in several subgroups (Table 5). While the frequencies of SNP55 and SNP64 were found to be significantly higher in women, only those with SNP64 A genotype had a statistically significant higher risk of chronic dialysis (AOR = 35.80, 95% CI = 3.23~396.84, P = 0.004). In subjects older than 50 years, SNP34 A genotype was significantly associated with chronic dialysis (AOR = 7.97, 95% CI = 1.25~50.94, P = 0.028). For subjects without diabetes, without CHD, no smoking habit, or without HT, SNP64 A was the independent SNP in association with chronic dialysis (AOR = 3.48, 4.69, 5.55, and 4.67, P = 0.010, 0.016, and 0.046, respectively). For subjects with history of hypertension, SNP17 C was significantly associated with chronic dialysis (AOR = 3.71, 95% CI = 1.10~12.55, P = 0.035).

Discussion

To date, most association studies of chronic dialysis focus on the nuclear genome [39–43] rather on mtDNA. In our previous report [9], we addressed the association between polymorphisms in the poly-C tract (D310) of the mtDNA D-loop and probability of dialysis treatment. However, we found that the poly-C tract was not significantly different in dialysis patients compared with healthy controls. In

addition to the poly-C tract, SNPs are also found in the D-loop. Therefore, we decided to determine whether there was any association between chronic dialysis and SNPs in the D-loop in this study.

Using sequence alignment, we found 9 SNPs present at significantly higher frequency in dialysis patients (SNP5, 17, 21, 34, 35, 55, 56, 64, and 65). Among them, 3 significant indicators (SNP55 G, SNP56 C, and SNP64 A) were independently associated with a high risk of chronic dialysis. Furthermore, only women with the SNP64 A genotype were statistically significant to be associated with chronic dialysis. SNP34 A was significantly associated with chronic dialysis in subjects older than 50 years. For subjects without diabetes, CHD, or hypertension, or in non-smokers, SNP64 A was statistically associated with chronic dialysis. Individuals with history of hypertension were significantly associated with chronic dialysis if they carried SNP17 C.

In this study, we focused solely on the question of whether individual SNPs within the D-loop were associated with chronic dialysis. However, the consideration of interdependence among SNPs was found to improve the association of genetic variations with several diseases [44,45] and cancers [46–54]. Therefore, we cannot exclude the possibility that some rare SNPs may still contribute to the synergistic association with chronic dialysis.

According to the diseases-associated mtSNPs in the D-loop locus in MITOMAP [37] (http://www.mitomap.org/bin/view.pl/MITOMAP/MutationsCodingControl), only 7 mtSNPs were reported. With reference to the rCRS, these are C114T, C150T, T195C, C309CC, T16189C, A16300G, and C16519T. We only identified C150T (SNP60), T195C (SNP67), and C16519T (SNP56) in our study (Table 2), and of these, only C16519T (SNP56) was significantly associated with chronic dialysis (Table 3 and Table 4). Similarly, C16519T was reported to be associated with "cyclic vomiting syndrome with migraine" [55,56]. When stratification of genotypes by demographic characteristics was considered, C16519T did not appear to be a marker associated with chronic dialysis (Table 5). On the contrary, we identified several novel mtSNPs associated with chronic dialysis, suggesting that these mtSNPs are potential genetic markers for this disease.

The acquisition of ROS-induced mutations in CKD may be a consequence of increased oxidative burden in patients with chronic renal failure [9,32,33,57]. For example, elevated oxidative stress in chronic peritoneal dialysis patients may lead to alterations in the mtDNA copy number in peripheral leukocytes [33]. In our current study, the mtSNPs listed in Table 3 were homoplasmic, as revealed by sequencing chromatograms (data not shown) [58–60]. However, we cannot exclude the possibility that a minor fraction of heteroplasmic mutations, below the level of sensitivity of the sequencing method that we used, may be present. We suggest that additional PCR/restriction fragment length polymorphism (RFLP) analysis may assist in the identification of mitochondrial hetero-plasmy [61,62]. In light of this, we are unable to identify mtSNPs that are suitable as progression markers for CKD with our current data, since our sequencing method lacked sufficient sensitivity to detect ROS-induced mutations. Therefore, the biological and clinical significance of the homoplasmic mtSNPs are more suitable as potential genetic markers for chronic dialysis, rather than progression markers of CKD.

To the best of our knowledge, this is the first report of SNPs in the mtDNA D-loop showing that they are significantly associated with chronic dialysis. The study also demonstrated the relationship of SNPs with comorbidities in dialysis patients. One may postulate that the presence of these SNPs is a risk factor for the development of end-stage renal disease, and that they may be used as markers to predict the likelihood of dialysis. In the future, further studies are needed to establish the role of these SNPs in the pathophysiology of CKD and to validate their clinical application.

Supporting Information

Table S1   Case (n = 193)-D-loop trimmed sequences in FSATA format.

Table S2   Control (n = 704)-D-loop trimmed sequences in FSATA format.

Table S3   77 SNP genotype raw data for cases and controls.

Table S4   *P* values of 77 individual SNPs for cases and controls.

Acknowledgments

We appreciate the valuable technical assistance of Miss Yi-Ju Tsai, Miss Jia-Ying Yang, and Mr. Yu-Da Lin.

Author Contributions

Conceived and designed the experiments: JBC CHY HWC. Performed the experiments: JBC YHC WCL CWL TKL. Analyzed the data: YHY LYC CHY HWC. Contributed reagents/materials/analysis tools: JBC YHC WCL CWL TKL. Wrote the paper: JBC HWC.

References

1. do Rosario Marinho AN, de Moraes MR, Santos S, Ribeiro-Dos-Santos A (2011) Human aging and somatic point mutations in mtDNA: A comparative study of generational differences (grandparents and grandchildren). Genet Mol Biol 34: 31–34.

2. Khaidakov M, Heflich RH, Manjanatha MG, Myers MB, Aidoo A (2003) Accumulation of point mutations in mitochondrial DNA of aging mice. Mutat Res 526: 1–7.

3. Rose G, Passarino G, Franceschi C, De Benedictis G (2002) The variability of the mitochondrial genome in human aging: a key for life and death? Int J Biochem Cell Biol 34: 1449–1460.

4. Mao P, Reddy PH (2011) Aging and amyloid beta-induced oxidative DNA damage and mitochondrial dysfunction in Alzheimer's disease: implications for early intervention and therapeutics. Biochim Biophys Acta 1812: 1359–1370.

5. Kashihara N, Haruna Y, Kondeti VK, Kanwar YS (2010) Oxidative stress in diabetic nephropathy. Curr Med Chem 17: 4256–4269.

6. Karbowski M, Neutzner A (2012) Neurodegeneration as a consequence of failed mitochondrial maintenance. Acta Neuropathol 123: 157–171.

7. Sotgia F, Martinez-Outschoorn UE, Lisanti MP (2011) Mitochondrial oxidative stress drives tumor progression and metastasis: should we use antioxidants as a key component of cancer treatment and prevention? BMC Med 9: 62.

8. He Y, Wu J, Dressman DC, Iacobuzio-Donahue C, Markowitz SD, et al. (2010) Heteroplasmic mitochondrial DNA mutations in normal and tumour cells. Nature 464: 610–614.

9. Chen JB, Lin TK, Liao SC, Lee WC, Lee LC, et al. (2009) Lack of association between mutations of gene-encoding mitochondrial D310 (displacement loop) mononucleotide repeat and oxidative stress in chronic dialysis patients in Taiwan. J Negat Results Biomed 8: 10.

10. Penta JS, Johnson FM, Wachsman JT, Copeland WC (2001) Mitochondrial DNA in human malignancy. Mutat Res 488: 119–133.

11. Clayton DA (2000) Transcription and replication of mitochondrial DNA. Hum Reprod 15 Suppl 2: 11–17.

12. Michikawa Y, Mazzucchelli F, Bresolin N, Scarlato G, Attardi G (1999) Aging-dependent large accumulation of point mutations in the human mtDNA control region for replication. Science 286: 774–779.

13. Coskun PE, Ruiz-Pesini E, Wallace DC (2003) Control region mtDNA variants: longevity, climatic adaptation, and a forensic conundrum. Proc Natl Acad Sci U S A 100: 2174–2176.

14. Wang Y, Michikawa Y, Mallidis C, Bai Y, Woodhouse L, et al. (2001) Muscle-specific mutations accumulate with aging in critical human mtDNA control sites for replication. Proc Natl Acad Sci U S A 98: 4022–4027.

15. Zhang J, Asin-Cayuela J, Fish J, Michikawa Y, Bonafe M, et al. (2003) Strikingly higher frequency in centenarians and twins of mtDNA mutation causing remodeling of replication origin in leukocytes. Proc Natl Acad Sci U S A 100: 1116–1121.

16. Mueller EE, Eder W, Ebner S, Schwaiger E, Santic D, et al. (2011) The mitochondrial T16189C polymorphism is associated with coronary artery disease in Middle European populations. PLoS One 6: e16455.

17. Suzuki M, Toyooka S, Miyajima K, Iizasa T, Fujisawa T, et al. (2003) Alterations in the mitochondrial displacement loop in lung cancers. Clin Cancer Res 9: 5636–5641.

18. Lievre A, Chapusot C, Bouvier AM, Zinzindohoue F, Piard F, et al. (2005) Clinical value of mitochondrial mutations in colorectal cancer. J Clin Oncol 23: 3517–3525.

19. Wang C, Zhang F, Fan H, Peng L, Zhang R, et al. (2011) Sequence polymorphisms of mitochondrial D-loop and hepatocellular carcinoma outcome. Biochem Biophys Res Commun 406: 493–496.

20. Wu CW, Yin PH, Hung WY, Li AF, Li SH, et al. (2005) Mitochondrial DNA mutations and mitochondrial DNA depletion in gastric cancer. Genes Chromosomes Cancer 44: 19–28.

21. Parrella P, Xiao Y, Fliss M, Sanchez-Cespedes M, Mazzarelli P, et al. (2001) Detection of mitochondrial DNA mutations in primary breast cancer and fine-needle aspirates. Cancer Res 61: 7623–7626.

22. Goia-Rusanu CD, Iancu IV, Botezatu A, Socolov D, Huica I, et al. (2011) Mitochondrial DNA mutations in patients with HRHPV-related cervical lesions. Roum Arch Microbiol Immunol 70: 5–10.

23. Ebner S, Lang R, Mueller E, Eder W, Oeller M, et al. (2011) Mitochondrial haplogroups, control region polymorphisms and malignant melanoma: A study in Middle European Caucasians. PLoS One 6: e27192.

24. Ha PK, Tong BC, Westra WH, Sanchez-Cespedes M, Parrella P, et al. (2002) Mitochondrial C-tract alteration in premalignant lesions of the head and neck: a marker for progression and clonal proliferation. Clin Cancer Res 8: 2260–2265.

25. Liu SA, Jiang RS, Chen FJ, Wang WY, Lin JC (2011) Somatic mutations in the D-loop of mitochondrial DNA in oral squamous cell carcinoma. Eur Arch Otorhinolaryngol: in press.

26. Nagy A, Wilhelm M, Kovacs G (2003) Mutations of mtDNA in renal cell tumours arising in end-stage renal disease. J Pathol 199: 237–242.

27. Mueller EE, Eder W, Mayr JA, Paulweber B, Sperl W, et al. (2009) Mitochondrial haplogroups and control region polymorphisms are not associated with prostate cancer in Middle European Caucasians. PLoS One 4: e6370.

28. Kim W, Yoo TK, Shin DJ, Rho HW, Jin HJ, et al. (2008) Mitochondrial DNA haplogroup analysis reveals no association between the common genetic lineages and prostate cancer in the Korean population. PLoS One 3: e2211.

29. Nomoto S, Yamashita K, Koshikawa K, Nakao A, Sidransky D (2002) Mitochondrial D-loop mutations as clonal markers in multicentric hepatocellular carcinoma and plasma. Clin Cancer Res 8: 481–487.

30. Wada T, Tanji N, Ozawa A, Wang J, Shimamoto K, et al. (2006) Mitochondrial DNA mutations and 8-hydroxy-2'-deoxyguanosine content in Japanese patients with urinary bladder and renal cancers. Anticancer Res 26: 3403–3408.

31. Lenz O, Fornoni A (2006) Chronic kidney disease care delivered by US family medicine and internal medicine trainees: results from an online survey. BMC Med 4: 30.

32. Himmelfarb J, Stenvinkel P, Ikizler TA, Hakim RM (2002) The elephant in uremia: oxidant stress as a unifying concept of cardiovascular disease in uremia. Kidney Int 62: 1524–1538.

33. Chen JB, Lin TK, Liou CW, Liao SC, Lee LC, et al. (2008) Correlation of oxidative stress biomarkers and peritoneal urea clearance with mitochondrial DNA copy number in continuous ambulatory peritoneal dialysis patients. Am J Nephrol 28: 853–859.

34. Wang YC, Lee WC, Liao SC, Lee LC, Su YJ, et al. (2011) Mitochondrial DNA copy number correlates with oxidative stress and predicts mortality in nondiabetic hemodialysis patients. J Nephrol 24: 351–358.

35. Ohkawa H, Ohishi N, Yagi K (1979) Assay for lipid peroxides in animal tissues by thiobarbituric acid reaction. Anal Biochem 95: 351–358.

36. Andrews RM, Kubacka I, Chinnery PF, Lightowlers RN, Turnbull DM, et al. (1999) Reanalysis and revision of the Cambridge reference sequence for human mitochondrial DNA. Nat Genet 23: 147.

37. Ruiz-Pesini E, Lott MT, Procaccio V, Poole JC, Brandon MC, et al. (2007) An enhanced MITOMAP with a global mtDNA mutational phylogeny. Nucleic Acids Res 35: D823–828.

38. Liou CW, Lin TK, Chen JB, Tiao MM, Weng SW, et al. (2010) Association between a common mitochondrial DNA D-loop polycytosine variant and alteration of mitochondrial copy number in human peripheral blood cells. J Med Genet 47: 723–728.

39. Zheng ZL, Hwang YH, Kim SK, Kim S, Son MJ, et al. (2009) Genetic polymorphisms of hypoxia-inducible factor-1 alpha and cardiovascular disease in hemodialysis patients. Nephron Clin Pract 113: c104–111.

40. Sperati CJ, Parekh RS, Berthier-Schaad Y, Jaar BG, Plantinga L, et al. (2009) Association of single-nucleotide polymorphisms in JAK3, STAT4, and STAT6 with new cardiovascular events in incident dialysis patients. Am J Kidney Dis 53: 845–855.

41. Sigrist MK, McIntyre CW (2008) Vascular calcification is associated with impaired microcirculatory function in chronic haemodialysis patients. Nephron Clin Pract 108: c121–126.

42. Kalousova M, Germanova A, Jachymova M, Mestek O, Tesar V, et al. (2008) A419C (E111A) polymorphism of the glyoxalase I gene and vascular complications in chronic hemodialysis patients. Ann N Y Acad Sci 1126: 268–271.

43. Wetmore JB, Johansen KL, Sen S, Hung AM, Lovett DH (2006) An angiotensin converting enzyme haplotype predicts survival in patients with end stage renal disease. Hum Genet 120: 201–210.

44. Yao L, Zhong W, Zhang Z, Maenner MJ, Engelman CD (2009) Classification tree for detection of single-nucleotide polymorphism (SNP)-by-SNP interactions related to heart disease: Framingham Heart Study. BMC Proc 3 Suppl 7: S83.

45. Lin GT, Tseng HF, Chang CK, Chuang LY, Liu CS, et al. (2008) SNP combinations in chromosome-wide genes are associated with bone mineral density in Taiwanese women. Chin J Physiol 51: 32–41.

46. Briollais L, Wang Y, Rajendram I, Onay V, Shi E, et al. (2007) Methodological issues in detecting gene-gene interactions in breast cancer susceptibility: a population-based study in Ontario. BMC Med 5: 22.

47. Bostrom MA, Kao WH, Li M, Abboud HE, Adler SG, et al. (2011) Genetic association and gene-gene interaction analyses in African American dialysis patients with nondiabetic nephropathy. Am J Kidney Dis: in press.

48. Yen CY, Liu SY, Chen CH, Tseng HF, Chuang LY, et al. (2008) Combinational polymorphisms of four DNA repair genes XRCC1, XRCC2, XRCC3, and XRCC4 and their association with oral cancer in Taiwan. J Oral Pathol Med 37: 271–277.

49. Zheng SL, Sun J, Wiklund F, Smith S, Stattin P, et al. (2008) Cumulative association of five genetic variants with prostate cancer. N Engl J Med 358: 910–919.

50. Lin GT, Tseng HF, Yang CH, Hou MF, Chuang LY, et al. (2009) Combinational polymorphisms of seven CXCL12-related genes are protective against breast cancer in Taiwan. OMICS 13: 165–172.

51. Yang CH, Chuang LY, Chen YJ, Tseng HF, Chang HW (2011) Computational analysis of simulated SNP interactions between 26 growth factor-related genes in a breast cancer association study. OMICS 15: 399–407.

52. Chuang LY, Chang HW, Lin MC, Yang CH (2012) Chaotic particle swarm optimization for detecting SNP-SNP interactions for CXCL12-related genes in breast cancer prevention. Eur J Cancer Prev 21: 336–342.

53. Chuang LY, Lin YD, Chang HW, Yang CH (2012) An improved PSO algorithm for generating protective SNP barcodes in breast cancer. PLoS One 7: e37018.

54. Yang CH, Chuang LY, Cheng YH, Lin YD, Wang CL, et al. (2012) Single nucleotide polymorphism barcoding to evaluate oral cancer risk using odds ratios-based genetic algorithms. Kaohsiung Journal of Medical Sciences 28: 362–368.

55. Boles RG, Zaki EA, Lavenbarg T, Hejazi R, Foran P, et al. (2009) Are pediatric and adult-onset cyclic vomiting syndrome (CVS) biologically different conditions? Relationship of adult-onset CVS with the migraine and pediatric CVS-associated common mtDNA polymorphisms 16519T and 3010A. Neurogastroenterol Motil 21: 936 e972.

56. Zaki EA, Freilinger T, Klopstock T, Baldwin EE, Heisner KR, et al. (2009) Two common mitochondrial DNA polymorphisms are highly associated with migraine headache and cyclic vomiting syndrome. Cephalalgia 29: 719–728.

57. Rao M, Li L, Demello C, Guo D, Jaber BL, et al. (2009) Mitochondrial DNA injury and mortality in hemodialysis patients. J Am Soc Nephrol 20: 189–196.

58. Reiner JE, Kishore RB, Levin BC, Albanetti T, Boire N, et al. (2010) Detection of heteroplasmic mitochondrial DNA in single mitochondria. PLoS One 5: e14359.

59. Tan DJ, Chang J, Chen WL, Agress LJ, Yeh KT, et al. (2003) Novel heteroplasmic frameshift and missense somatic mitochondrial DNA mutations in oral cancer of betel quid chewers. Genes Chromosomes Cancer 37: 186–194.

60. Andrew T, Calloway CD, Stuart S, Lee SH, Gill R, et al. (2011) A twin study of mitochondrial DNA polymorphisms shows that heteroplasmy at multiple sites is associated with mtDNA variant 16093 but not with zygosity. PLoS One 6: e22332.

61. McFarland R, Chinnery PF, Blakely EL, Schaefer AM, Morris AA, et al. (2007) Homoplasmy, heteroplasmy, and mitochondrial dystonia. Neurology 69: 911–916.

62. Wang Q, Boles RG (2006) Individual human hair mitochondrial DNA control region heteroplasmy proportions in mothers and children. Mitochondrion 6: 37–42.

3

Effect of Diuretic use on 30-Day Postdialysis Mortality in Critically Ill Patients Receiving Acute Dialysis

Vin-Cent Wu[1,9]⁹, Chun-Fu Lai[1]⁹, Chih-Chung Shiao[2], Yu-Feng Lin[3], Pei-Chen Wu[1], Chia-Ter Chao[1], Fu-Chang Hu[5], Tao-Min Huang[6], Yu-Chang Yeh[7], I-Jung Tsai[8], Tze-Wah Kao[1], Yin-Yi Han[3], Wen-Chung Wu[10], Chun-Cheng Hou[11], Guang-Huar Young[3], Wen-Je Ko[3,4]*, Tun-Jun Tsai[1], Kwan-Dun Wu[1]

1 Division of Nephrology, Department of Internal Medicine, National Taiwan University Hospital, Taipei, Taiwan, **2** Division of Nephrology, Department of Internal Medicine, Saint Mary's Hospital, and Saint Mary's Medicine, Nursing and Management College, Yilan, Taiwan, **3** Department of Traumatology, National Taiwan University Hospital, Taipei, Taiwan, **4** Department of Surgery, National Taiwan University Hospital, Taipei, Taiwan, **5** International Harvard Statistical Consulting Company, Taipei, Taiwan, **6** Division of Nephrology, Department of Internal Medicine, Yun-Lin Branch, Douliou City, Yun-Lin County, Taiwan, **7** Department of Anesthesiology, National Taiwan University Hospital, Taipei, Taiwan, **8** Department of Pediatrics, National Taiwan University Hospital, Taipei, Taiwan, **9** NSARF: National Taiwan University Hospital Study Group on Acute Renal Failure, Taipei, Taiwan, **10** Section of Internal Medicine, Miao-Li Hospital, Department of Health, Miao-Li, Taiwan, **11** Department of Internal medicine , Min-Sheng Hospital, Tao-Yuan, Taiwan

Abstract

Background: The impact of diuretic usage and dosage on the mortality of critically ill patients with acute kidney injury is still unclear.

Methods and Results: In this prospective, multicenter, observational study, 572 patients with postsurgical acute kidney injury receiving hemodialysis were recruited and followed daily. Thirty-day postdialysis mortality was analyzed using Cox's proportional hazards model with time-dependent covariates. The mean age of the 572 patients was 60.8 ± 16.6 years. Patients with lower serum creatinine ($p = 0.031$) and blood lactate ($p = 0.033$) at ICU admission, lower predialysis urine output ($p = 0.001$) and PaO_2/FiO_2 ($p = 0.039$), as well as diabetes ($p = 0.037$) and heart failure ($p = 0.049$) were more likely to receive diuretics. A total of 280 (49.0%) patients died within 30 days after acute dialysis initiation. The analysis of 30-day postdialysis mortality by fitting propensity score-adjusted Cox's proportional hazards models with time-dependent covariates showed that higher 3-day accumulated diuretic doses after dialysis initiation (HR = 1.449, $p = 0.021$) could increase the hazard rate of death. Moreover, higher time-varying 3-day accumulative diuretic doses were associated with hypotension ($p < 0.001$) and less intense hemodialysis ($p < 0.001$) during the acute dialysis period.

Background and Significance: Higher time-varying 3-day accumulative diuretic dose predicts mortality in postsurgical critically ill patients requiring acute dialysis. Higher diuretic doses are associated with hypotension and a lower intensity of dialysis. Caution should be employed before loop diuretics are administered to postsurgical patients during the acute dialysis period.

Editor: Pan-Chyr Yang, National Taiwan University Hospital, Taiwan

Funding: This study was supported by The Ta-Tung Kidney Foundation and Taiwan National Science Council (grant NSC 96-2314-B-002-164, NSC 96-2314-B-002-033-MY3, NSC 97-2314-B-002-155-MY2, NSC 98-2314-B-002-155-MY4) and NTUH.098-001177, NTUH 100-001667. The funders had no role in study design, data collection and analysis, decision to publish, or preparation of the manuscript.

Competing Interests: The authors have declared that no competing interests exist.

* E-mail: kowj@ntu.edu.tw

❥ These authors contributed equally to this work.

Introduction

Postoperative acute kidney injury (AKI) is a serious complication resulting in prolonged hospital stays and high mortality rates [1]. AKI develops in 5% to 30% of postsurgical patients and is associated with a mortality rate of 60% to 90% [2,3,4]. Prerenal azotemia and ischemic acute tubular necrosis (ATN) are the predominant causes of AKI [5]. During the perioperative period, fluid balance is one of the most important issues [6]. It is reasonable to consider that diuretic use could help preserve urine output and thereby shorten the dialysis period for better fluid management. Loop diuretics may convert oliguric into nonoliguric form of AKI, allowing easier fluid and/or nutritional support for

the patient. Furosemide is a loop diuretic and a vasodilator, which may decrease the metabolic work of the thick ascending limb [7]. Diuretic use in critically ill patients with acute kidney injury is reported not related to mortality [6]. High-dose furosemide (35 mg/kg/d orally) was used in patients with AKI requiring dialysis but did not have an impact on the survival and renal recovery rates [8]. It was reported diuretic might confer a survival advantage in patients on hemodialysis [9]. Loop diuretic use after dialysis in DOPPS study ranged from 9.2% in the United States to 21.3% in Europe, whereas use within 90 days of starting dialysis therapy ranged from 25.0% in the United States to 47.6% in Japan [9]. Preoperative diuretic use could be associated with postoperative AKI [10]; however, the association between patients' mortality and diuretic use in postoperative critical patients receiving acute dialysis has not been elucidated.

The concern about acute dialysis-related mortality usually focuses on the severity of the predialytic disease. However, predialysis risk factors may have different effects on short- and long-term survival, and the risk factors assessed at initial dialysis may change over time [11,12]. Thus, in view of the complex relationship between diuretic use and mortality in critically ill patients, we used a comprehensive approach with both time-independent and time-dependent predictor variables to test the hypothesis that diuretic use during acute dialysis affects mortality in postsurgical patients.

Results

Patients' basic demographic characteristics

A total of 572 critically ill patients (191 women; mean age, 60.8±16.6 years) who had received acute RRT after major surgical operations were recruited and followed daily (Figure 1). The mean APACHE II score was 11.3±6.0, and SOFA score was 8.3±3.5 at ICU admission. Among the patients, 424 (74.1%) used diuretics during the first three days of initial hemodialysis. The histogram of initially accumulated 3-day diuretic dose after RRT is shown in Figure 2. At dialysis initiation, the mean APACHE II and SOFA scores were 12.9±6.3 and 11.4±3.7, respectively. The mean time to dialysis from ICU admission was 6.6±18.0 days. Postoperatively,

283 (49.5%) patients died within 30 days after dialysis, which accounted for 77.3% of hospital mortality. After dialysis, only 193 (33.7%) patients were successfully withdrawn from acute dialysis.

Predialysis assessments

Before dialysis, 417 (72.9%) postsurgical patients received inotropics treatment, and 94 (16.4%) developed anuria. Most patients underwent cardiovascular surgery (203, 35.5%). Although there were multiple indications for starting hemodialysis, oliguria (51.6%) and fluid overload (15.7%) were the leading causes for acute hemodialysis. Most (73.6%) of the patients had a status that was more severe than the injury criteria of the RIFLE classification upon initial dialysis.

The indications of acute hemodialysis were the same between 3-day predialysis diuretic and nondiuretic use groups. The SOFA score was higher at ICU admission in the nondiuretic than the diuretic group ($p = 0.006$). However, there were no differences in duration from hospital admission to dialysis, duration from ICU admission to dialysis, comorbidities, operation types, indication of acute dialysis or disease severity at the beginning of dialysis between the two groups (Table 1, 2). Patients with diuretic use had lower PaO_2/FiO_2 ($p = 0.011$) before the first hemodialysis session.

At the initiation of dialysis, the survival patients had lower disease severity scores (APACHE II, SOFA, and SAPA, all $p<0.001$), but the ratio of diuretic use was the same between two groups, ($p = 0.775$) (Table 3,4).

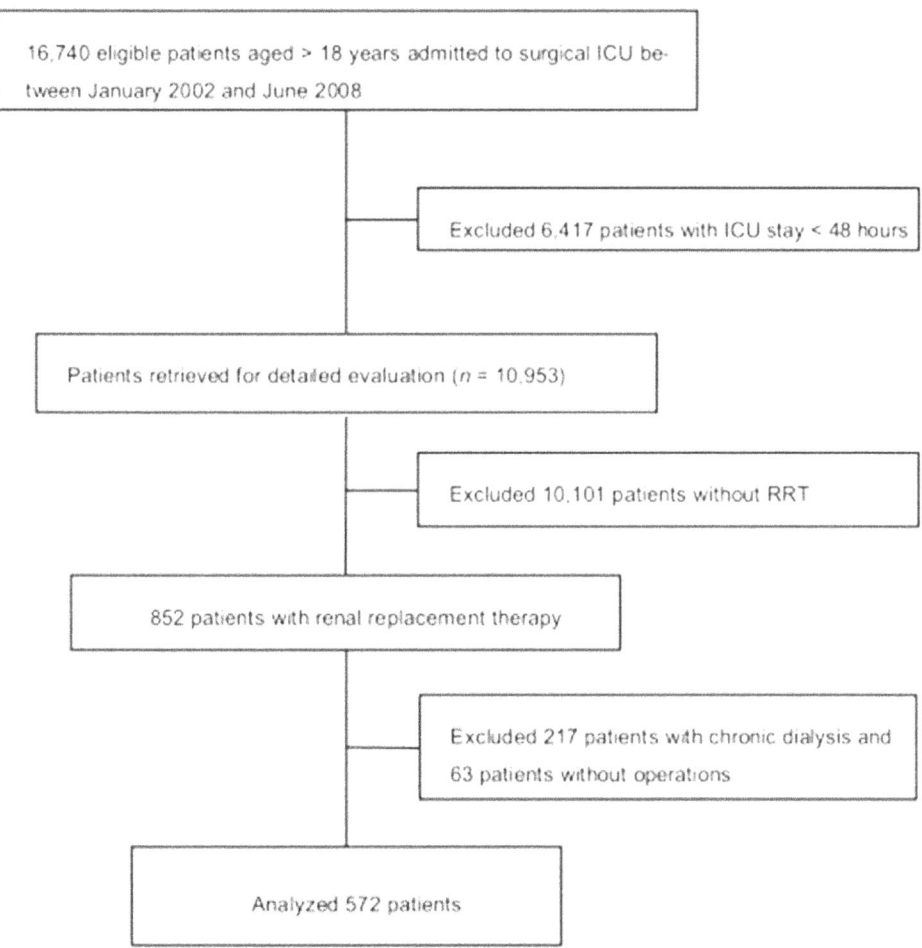

Figure 1. Flow diagram of the study population.

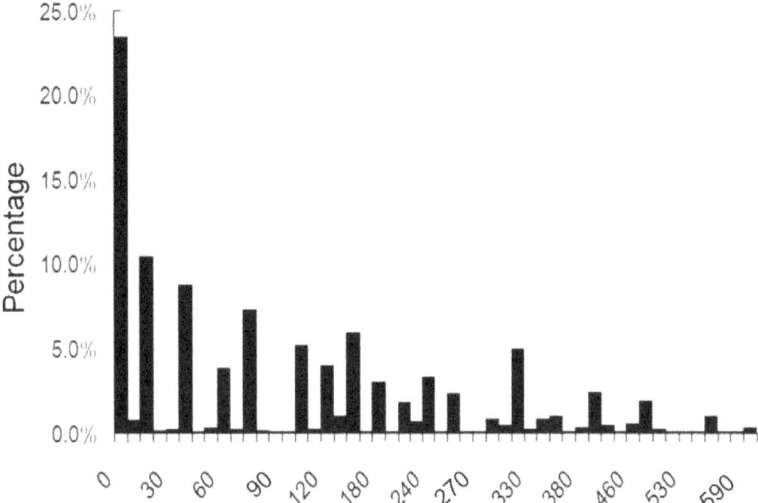

Accumulated 3 days diuretics dose before dialysis initiation, mg

Figure 2. Histogram of accumulated 3-day diuretic use before dialysis initiation (equivalent of furosemide, mg).

Propensity score model for diuretic use

To explore what types of patients would require diuretics upon dialysis initiation, we conducted a logistic regression analysis and established a propensity score model. Variables (Table 1,2) were included for inclusion in the new propensity score model.

Finally, based on the fitted logistic regression model (see Table 5), the propensity score for treatment with diuretic upon initializing acute dialysis was estimated (see File S1).

Factors associated with 30-day postdialysis mortality

The serial measurement of accumulated diuretics through the spectrum and duration of RRT was significant to predict 30-day postdialysis mortality ($p = 0.021$) during the dialysis period, using Cox's model adjusted with time-varying significant covariates (Table 6 and Figure 3). Regardless of diuretic use, patients who died were significantly more likely to have liver failure ($p<0.001$), and have a higher ratio of azotemia ($p = 0.038$) when dialysis began. Older age ($p<0.001$), higher APACHE II score ($p<0.001$), lower daily PaO_2/FiO_2 ($p<0.001$), higher daily lactate ($p<0.001$), and less daily IHD versus no dialysis ($p = 0.030$) were associated with 30-day postdialysis mortality (Table 4). The final Cox's model fit the observed data well; the adjusted generalized $R^2 = 0.495$.

In the sensitivity test, a higher accumulated diuretic dose predicted mortality in the postsurgical critically ill noncardiac surgery patients requiring acute dialysis ($p<0.01$).

Diuretic dose associated with daily variables

To examine the effect of diuretic use and decrease the residual confounding factors (e.g., fluid overload, oliguria, and tissue hypoxia), daily variable factors (body weight, urine output, mean blood pressure, PaO_2/FiO_2, lactate, BUN, and creatinine) were correlated to the time-varying three-day accumulative diuretic dose, as shown in the GEE model, and plotted by smoothed GAM plot after adjusting for all the covariates listed in Table 1. Diuretic use was significantly associated with the intensity of dialysis ($p<0.001$) (Table S1) and daily mean blood pressure ($p<0.001$) (Table S2 and Figure 4), but not with daily PaO_2/FiO_2 ($p = 0.293$),

lactate ($p = 0.948$), BUN ($p = 0.905$), body weight ($p = 0.449$), creatinine ($p = 0.653$), and urine output ($p = 0.075$).

Discussion

Given the high incidence of AKI in the ICU and its high morbidity, better evidence is needed to guide AKI treatment strategies. Few studies have demonstrated any material benefit of diuretic use in AKI apart from augmenting urine output, and some studies have suggested potential deleterious effects [13,14]. Although two of the previous controlled studies found a trend toward improvement in renal function recovery rates with diuretic use [15], one cohort analysis suggested that diuretics may delay renal recovery [13]. Diuretic use has not been found to shorten the duration of AKI, reduce the need for dialysis, or improve overall outcomes [16].

Our study evaluated the relationships between diuretic use and dose with subsequent mortality after dialysis, unlike the previous report by Uchino [6], which used distinct multivariate models. The current study adds to this previous work [13] in that it identifies a group of patients, who have increased mortality and not just delayed or diminished return of renal function. Firstly, to ensure that our results were reliable, we only included postsurgical AKI patients receiving acute dialysis in surgical ICUs. In our patient cohort, all patients received dialysis; however, only 70% patients in Uchino's study received dialysis. Secondly, to show the interactions between diuretics and dialysis settings, we recorded the daily dialysis modality and settings; Uchino recorded only diuretic use at the time of acute kidney injury or dialysis initiation [6].

Furosemide is nondialysable, and retained up to 6 to 8 hours in patients with chronic renal failure; however no specific dosage adjustment of furosemide is necessary for dialysis patients [17]. It is effective for the treatment of edema associated with renal failure [18]. Therefore, diuretic use and dosage is likely to have effects on patients' outcomes. In our study, similar to a previous study on high furosemide doses for established acute renal failure [8], renal recovery rates did not differ between the diuretic and nondiuretic

Table 1. Comparison of demographic of the nondiuretic and diuretic groups.

	Nondiuretic (n = 148)	Diuretic (n = 424)	p
Male gender	103 (69.6%)	278 (65.6%)	0.418
Age, mean (SD), years	59.8 (18.2)	61.2 (16.1)	0.386
BMI, mean (SD), Kg/M^2	23.6 (4.1)	23.5 (3.8)	0.780
Elective operation	48 (32.4%)	170 (40.1%)	0.115
IABP	28 (18.9%)	79 (18.3%)	0.999
ECMO	40 (27.0%)	87 (20.5%)	0.108
CPR	30 (20.3%)	64 (15.1%)	0.156
Comorbid diseases			
Diabetes mellitus	37 (25.0%)	141 (33.3%)	0.064
Hypertension	62 (41.9%)	188 (44.3%)	0.631
CHF	5 (3.4%)	17 (4.0%)	0.999
Cirrhosis	17 (11.5%)	47 (11.1%)	0.880
CKD	87 (58.8%)	234 (55.2%)	0.501
Sepsis	35 (23.6%)	87 (20.6%)	0.485
Systemic organ failure			
Central nervous system	28 (18.9%)	87 (20.5%)	0.722
Respiratory	27 (18.2%)	114 (26.9%)	0.036
Cardiac	42 (28.4%)	147 (34.7%)	0.187
Liver	29 (19.6%)	61 (14.4%)	0.149
Operation			
Abdominal	50 (33.8%)	129 (30.5%)	0.696
Cardiovascular	76 (51.4%)	207 (48.9%)	
Chest	14 (9.5%)	54 (12.8%)	
Neurology	4 (2.7%)	22 (5.2%)	
Urology	3 (2.0%)	8 (1.9%)	
Orthopedic	1 (0.7%)	3 (0.7%)	

NOTE. Data are no. (%) of patients, unless otherwise indicated.
Abbreviations: BMI, body mass index; CHF, congestive heart failure; CPR, cardiopulmonary resuscitation; CKD, chronic kidney disease; ECMO, extracorporeal membrane oxygenation; IABP, intraaortic balloon pump; SD, standard deviation.
§Data correspond to the worst value in the 24 hours preceding the time point.

Table 2. Comparison of predialysis clinical characteristics of the nondiuretic and diuretic groups.

	Nondiuretic (n = 148)	Diuretic (n = 424)	p
Indication for acute dialysis			
Azotemia	48 (32.4%)	117 (27.6%)	0.292
Fluid overload	23 (15.5%)	67 (15.9%)	0.999
Hyperkalemia	11 (7.4%)	32 (7.5%)	0.999
Oliguria	72 (48.6%)	223 (52.6%)	0.445
Acidosis	4 (2.7%)	17 (4.0%)	0.615
At dialysis initiation§			
Hospital admission to dialysis, mean (SD), days	18.1 (36.7)	17.7 (35.5)	0.913
ICU admission to dialysis, mean (SD), days	4.7 (8.3)	7.3 (20.9)	0.134
Ventilator	122 (82.4%)	361 (85.1%)	0.432
NPO	89 (60.1%)	248 (58.5%)	0.771
BUN, mean (SD), mg/dL	65.5 (36.2)	64.4 (37.8)	0.750
sCr, mean (SD), mg/dL	3.4 (2.0)	3.3 (1.8)	0.831
MAP, mean (SD), mmHg	80.1 (17.4)	81.2 (16.8)	0.498
CVP, mean (SD), cm	13.8 (6.0)	14.2 (5.6)	0.560
PaO2/FiO2, mean (SD), mmHg	320.6 (209.2)	279.6 (149.4)	0.011
Urine output, mean (SD), mL/24 hours	812.5 (840.5)	700.9 (755.1)	0.134
Anuria	29 (19.6%)	65 (15.5%)	0.250
Inotropic agents	99 (66.9%)	318 (75.2%)	0.053
Lactate, mean (SD), mmol/L	5.2 (4.5)	4.5 (2.2)	0.147
Sodium, mean (SD), mmol/L	139.8 (8.1)	139.6 (7.7)	0.721
Potassium, mean (SD), mmol/L	4.25 (0.86)	4.2 (0.8)	0.906
Disease severity score			
APACHE II at ICU admission	11.4 (5.9)	11.2 (6.0)	0.688
APACHE II at initial dialysis	12.9 (5.5)	12.4 (6.2)	0.380
SOFA at ICU admission	9.0 (3.7)	8.1 (3.4)	0.006
SOFA at initial dialysis	10.9 (3.9)	11.2 (3.6)	0.369
SAPS at ICU admission	111.3 (14.3)	107.9 (13.4)	0.010
SAPS at initial dialysis	116.7 (13.4)	114.4 (13.6)	0.081
RIFLE at initial dialysis:			
Risk	38 (25.7%)	113 (26.7%)	0.540
Injury	28 (18.9%)	74 (17.5%)	
Failure	82 (55.4%)	237 (55.9%)	
Dialysis modality at initial dialysis			
IHD	34 (23.0%)	82 (19.3%)	0.540
SLED	11 (7.4%)	27 (6.4%)	
CVVH	103 (69.6%)	315 (74.3%)	

NOTE. Data are no. (%) of patients, unless otherwise indicated.
§Data correspond to the worst value in the 24 hours preceding the time point.
Abbreviations: APACHE II, acute physiology and chronic health evaluation; BUN, blood urea nitrogen; CVP, central venous pressure; CVVH, continuous venovenous hemofiltration; ICU, intensive care unit; IHD, intermittent hemodialysis; MAP, mean arterial pressure; NPO, nil per os; RIFLE, risk of renal failure, injury to kidney, failure of kidney function, loss of kidney function and end-stage renal failure; SAPS, simplified acute physiological score; SD, standard deviation; SOFA, Sequential Organ Failure Assessment; sCr, serum creatinine; SLED, sustained low-efficiency dialysis.
‖Defined as 3-day predialysis diuretic use.

groups. Mehta et al. proposed that diuretic use could delay the recognition of AKI and might delay the timing of dialysis [13], which might be related to patient mortality. In our study, the duration between hospital admission to dialysis or ICU admission to dialysis did not differ among patients who were taking or not taking diuretics at initial dialysis, and no lead-time bias was found between the two groups. Our propensity score, lower predialysis PaO$_2$/FiO$_2$ saturation, reduced urine output, lower creatinine level, and lower lactate level at admission were predictors of diuretic use, which reflected the general features of the use of diuretics in critical care.

Using a time-dependent Cox's regression model that considers risk factors changing over time, rather than a traditional Cox's model with only fixed baseline risk factors, was an important analysis strategy, especially in critical patients with changing daily variables and inconsistent diuretic use [11]. Diuretic use when

Table 3. Comparison of demographic of the postdialysis 30-day survival and mortality patients.

	Survival (n = 289)	Mortality (n = 283)	p
Male gender	192 (66.4%)	189 (66.8%)	0.930
Age, mean (SD), years	59.7 (17.1)	62.0 (16.1)	0.100
BMI, mean (SD), Kg/M2	23.7 (3.7)	23.4 (4.1)	0.403
Elective operation	118 (40.8%)	100 (35.3%)	0.169
CPR	39 (13.5%)	55 (19.6%)	0.056
Diuretic use	213 (74%)	205 (72.4%)	0.376
Comorbid diseases			
Hypertension	131 (45.3%)	119 (42.0%)	0.449
DM	96 (32.9%)	82 (29.3%)	0.367
Cirrhosis	29 (10.0%)	35 (12.4%)	0.427
CKD	175 (60.6%)	146 (51.6%)	0.035
CHF	11 (3.8%)	11 (3.9%)	0.999
Sepsis	41 (14.2%)	81 (28.6)	<0.001
Systemic organ failure			
Central nervous system	36 (12.5%)	79 (27.9%)	<0.001
Respiratory	50 (17.3%)	91 (32.2%)	<0.001
Cardiac	82 (28.4%)	107 (37.8%)	0.021
Liver	30 (10.4%)	60 (21.2%)	0.001
Operation			
Abdominal	86 (29.6%)	93 (33.2%)	0.045
Cardiovascular	153 (52.6%)	130 (46.4%)	
Chest	25 (8.6%)	43 (15.4%)	
Neurology	16 (5.5%)	10 (3.6%)	
Urology	8 (2.7%)	3 (1.1%)	
Orthopedic	3 (1.0%)	1 (0.4%)	

NOTE. Data are number (%) of patients, unless otherwise indicated.
Abbreviation: BMI, body mass index; CPR, cardiopulmonary resuscitation; CKD, chronic kidney disease; CHF, congestive heart failure; DM, diabetics mellitus; SD, standard deviation.

Table 4. Comparison of predialysis characteristics of the postdialysis 30-day survival and mortality patients.

	Survival (n = 289)	Mortality (n = 283)	p
Indication for acute dialysis			
Azotemia	79 (27.3%)	86 (30.4%)	0.460
Fluid overload	31 (10.7%)	60 (21.2%)	<0.001
Hyperkalemia	21 (7.3%)	22 (7.8%)	0.875
Oliguria	143 (49.5%)	152 (53.7%)	0.317
Severe acidosis	7 (2.4%)	14 (4.9%)	0.123
At dialysis initiation§			
IABP	37 (12.8%)	70 (24.8%)	<0.001
ECMO	47 (16.3%)	80 (28.3%)	0.001
Diuretic use‖	216 (74.7%)	208 (73.5%)	0.775
Ventilator	230 (79.6%)	253 (89.4%)	0.001
NPO	156 (54.0%)	181 (64.0%)	0.017
Serum creatinine, mean (SD), mg/dL	3.6 (1.9)	3.1 (1.9)	0.002
Blood urea nitrogen, mean (SD), mg/dL	64.4 (33.4)	65.0 (41.1)	0.841
Potassium, mean (SD), mmol/L	4.3 (0.8)	4.2 (0.8)	0.483
MAP, mean (SD), mmHg	84.5 (17.1)	77.3 (15.9)	<0.001
APACHE II, mean (SD)	10.7 (5.3)	14.4 (6.1)	<0.001
SOFA, mean (SD)	9.9 (3.2)	12.5 (3.6)	<0.001
SAPS, mean (SD)	110.5 (11.9)	119.7 (13.4)	<0.001
PaO2/FiO2, mean (SD), mmHg	306.2 (161.6)	274.1 (172.7)	0.023
RIFLE			
Risk	79 (27.3%)	72 (25.4%)	0.848
Injury	52 (18.0%)	5 (17.7%)	
Failure	158 (54.7%)	161 (56.9%)	
Lactate, mean (SD), mmol/L	3.9 (4.1)	5.5 (5.1)	0.001
CVP, mean (SD), mmHg	13.6 (5.5)	14.5 (5.8)	0.053
Urine output, mean (SD), mL/24 hours	768 (792)	692 (766)	0.246
Dialysis modality at dialysis initiation			
IHD	78 (27.0%)	38 (13.4%)	<0.001
SLED	22 (7.6%)	16 (5.7%)	
CVVH	189 (65.4%)	229 (80.9%)	

NOTE. Data are number (%) of patients, unless otherwise indicated.
Abbreviation: APACHE II, acute physiology and chronic health evaluation; CVP, central venous pressure; CVVH, continuous venovenous hemofiltration; ECMO, extracorporeal membrane oxygenation; IABP, intraaortic balloon pump; MAP, mean arterail pressure; NPO, nil per os; RIFLE, risk of renal failure, injury to kidney, failure of kidney function, loss of kidney function, and end-stage renal failure (RIFLE) classification; SD, standard deviation; SOFA, Sequential Organ Failure Assessment; SAPS, simplified acute physiological score; IHD, intermittent hemodialysis; sCr, serum creatinine, SLED, sustained low-efficiency dialysis.
§Data correspond to the worst value in the 24 hours preceding the time point.
‖Defined as 3-day predialysis diuretic use.

dialysis was initiated was not associated with patient mortality; however, higher varying accumulated doses during the dialysis period were associated with higher mortality. The total dose of diuretics required to achieve the treatment goal might reflect the severity of renal impairment and patients' underlying clinical status. Accumulated diuretic dose was significantly associated with hypotension and mortality in a dose dependent manner. Compared with patients who were not taking diuretics, those taking diuretics had significant hypotension. (Table S2). This study produced a novel finding that patients taking diuretics had lower blood pressure in a dose-response manner, leading to a poor prognosis throughout the duration of RRT [19]. Nevertheless, the intensive high dose diuretic therapy should be tailored on the basis of a close assessment of baseline hemodynamic data and hemodynamic response to the medications, in addition to the careful diuretic dose titration and cautious evaluation of risk/benefit ratio [20].

Moreover, patients using diuretics during dialysis periods showed borderline increasing daily urine output (p = 0.075). ICU care providers may underestimate the severity of renal injury when urine output is sustained [13]. Our study has shown that loop diuretics have negative effects on the natural history of AKI, apart from a mild increase in urine output in the postsurgical critically ill group. Fluid overload was independently associated with mortality in patients with AKI [21]. However, the daily urine output and body weight in our study were not associated with diuretic dose or mortality in our cohort of dialysis patients. Fluid overload, in terms of oliguria and increased body weight, led to more intense dialysis, according to clinical adjustments made during the dialysis period (Table S1). Large doses of furosemide activate the renin-

Table 5. Multiple logistic regression model for estimating the propensity score of diuretic exposure at acute dialysis initiation.

Covariate	Estimate	Odds ratio	95% confidence	limits	p
Diabetes (yes)	0.522	1.685	1.032	2.751	0.037
CPR (yes)	−0.522	0.593	0.335	1.051	0.074
Predialysis urine output (mL/day)	−0.001	0.999	0.999	1.000	0.001
Congestive heart failure (yes)	0.531	1.700	1.000	2.888	0.050
Creatinine at ICU admission (mg/dL)	−0.134	0.874	0.774	0.988	0.031
Lactate (mmol/L)	−0.049	0.952	0.910	0.996	0.033
Predialysis PaO$_2$/FiO$_2$ (mmHg)	−0.001	0.999	0.998	1.000	0.039

Abbreviations: CPR, cardiopulmonary resuscitation; OR, odds ratio; ICU, intensive care unit.
Adjusted for gender, age, body mass index, elective operation, cardiopulmonary resuscitation, extracorporeal membrane oxygenation, cardiopulmonary resuscitation, ventilator use, days from hospital admission to dialysis, NPO status, total parenteral nutrition, blood pressure, BUN, creatinine, lactate, urine output, body weight, anuria, inotropic equivalent, lactate, sodium, potassium, APACHE II at initializing dialysis, diabetes mellitus, hypertension, congestive heart failure, cirrhosis, chronic kidney disease, systemic organ failure (central nervous system, respiratory, cardiac, liver), operation categories (abdominal, cardiovascular, chest, neurology, urology, orthopedic), and indication for dialysis (azotemia, fluid overload, hyperkalemia, oliguria, acidosis).

angiotensin system and sympathetic nervous system and aggravate left ventricular pump deterioration [22]. Actually, there is a risk that a tubular or glomerular injury can be generated and that a preexisting renal dysfunction can be aggravated, especially when excessive doses of loop diuretics are being erroneously administered [20]. Hence, caution should be taken when furosemide is administered to postsurgical patients undergoing dialysis.

In our report, daily dialysis with IHD demonstrated a survival benefit as compared with no dialysis; however, daily dialysis with CVVH was marginally associated with poor prognosis (Table 6). Although the results showed that CVVH had a survival disadvantage, this could reflect residual confounding by illness severity because we used CVVH in more severely, acutely ill patients. Moreover, lower dialysis intensity was related to higher accumulated diuretic use, a common observation in clinical practice. Initial clinical trial data on the use of UF have demonstrated promising cardiac outcomes with regard to fluid removal and symptom relief, without worsening renal function [23]. The addition of a solute clearance component by dialysis may provide additional benefits for these patients with varying degrees of renal impairment [24].

Moreover, our study analysis has several notable strengths. Firstly, the relationship between lower daily blood pressure and higher diuretic dose throughout the duration of RRT was a robust finding resistant to the influence of most variables. Therefore, future randomized trial studies that stratify patients according to diuretic use should stress the relationship between blood pressure and diuretic dose. Secondly, we focused on diuretic use in heterogeneous, multicenter postsurgical patients using a comprehensive statistical approach and a large prospective database of patients with acute dialysis; therefore, our results could be extrapolated to other critical care situations because the current use of diuretics depends on clinical judgment without consensus. Thirdly, the propensity score for diuretic use and the need for dialysis were adjusted for time variable models, allowing us to incorporate changes in disease progression after dialysis for AKI and potentially providing useful prognostic information regarding important complications in intensive care units. However, patient heterogencity could lead to confounding, and most of our patients were cardiovascular in nature. Future observational studies and clinical trials with regard to AKI should attempt to understand the long-term effects of diuretic-associated episodes.

Our study has shown that higher loop diuretic doses are associated with significant grave effects on critical patients who require acute RRT after major surgery. Higher diuretic doses were associated with hypotensive episodes after initializing dialysis, lower daily oxygen saturation and lactate level or poor kidney function parameters and was associated with higher patient mortality. Forced diuresis as an indicator of adequate renal function has less scientific rationale under such circumstances. Caution should be taken when loop diuretics is administered to postsurgical patients during acute dialysis. Future larger randomized clinical trials are required to confirm and validate the adverse effect of diuretic use in acute dialysis patients.

Methods

Study cohort

This study was based on a clinical cohort study of the renal failure patients in the database of the National Taiwan University Hospital Study Group for Acute Renal Failure (NSARF). The Institutional Review Board of the National Taiwan University Hospital approved the study (No. 31MD03) and waived the need of informed consent because there was neither breach of privacy nor interference with clinical decisions related to patient care.

This non-concurrent prospective cohort for quality assurance has been maintained since January 2002 in one medical center (National Taiwan University Hospital, Taipei, Taiwan) and its three branch hospitals in different cities [12,25,26,27,28]. A total of 16,740 adult patients (age>18 years) were admitted to the SICU, and 852 patients received renal replacement therapy (RRT) during their hospitalization before January 2008. Patients with chronic dialysis (n = 217) and without operations (n = 63) were excluded (Fig. 1). A total of 572 patients were included in this study. Surgical procedures were considered major if the length of the ICU stay for patients in a given diagnosis-related group exceeded two days [29].

Clinical evaluation

Demographics, clinical characteristics at ICU admission and predialysis were assessed. Clinical evaluations included medical history, physical examination, and identification of comorbid diseases. Medical history included the presence of diabetes mellitus (DM, defined as having been treated with oral hypoglycemic agents or insulin), peripheral vascular disease (defined as having had a previous vascular procedure, a history of claudication, or the presence of femoral bruits), hypertension (defined as having taken antihypertensive drugs or having systolic and diastolic blood pressures >145/95 mmHg at the time of hospitalization), and chronic kidney disease (CKD, defined as estimated glomerular filtration rate (eGFR)<60 mL/min/1.73 m^2 noted at ICU admission) [30]. Oliguria was defined as a urine volume<100 mL in 8 hours [31]. Sepsis was defined as the presence of both infection and systemic inflammatory response syndrome (SIRS) as in previous reports [32,33]. A diet of 1.0–1.2 g protein/kg/day was prescribed for these patients.

Critical scoring systems, hemodynamic data, biochemistry data, and urine output were assessed after SICU admission and followed prospectively from the day that hemodialysis began. Physiological calculations were performed using the worst physiologic values

Table 6. Cox's model with time-dependent covariates showing the estimated hazard ratios (HRs) for 30-day mortality in the postsurgical acute dialysis patients[§].

Covariate	Parameter estimate	Adjusted HR	95% confidence interval	p
Age (years)	0.015	1.015	1.018–1.023	<0.001
At dialysis initiation				
IABP	0.316	1.372	1.018–1.873	0.044
APACHE II	0.046	1.047	1.037–1.078	<0.001
Systemic organ failure				
Sepsis	0.432	1.541	1.183–2.015	0.001
Liver	0.699	2.011	1.476–2.763	<0.001
Indication for acute dialysis				
Azotemia	0.273	1.314	1.025–1.705	0.038
Time-varying hazard (daily)				
PaO2/FiO2 (mmHg)	−0.002	0.998	1.007–1.009	<0.001
Lactate (mmol/L)	0.171	1.186	1.144–1.236	<0.001
Time-varying three day accumulative diuretic dose (g/3day)	0.371	1.449	1.060–1.981	0.021
Varying daily dialysis modality				
Daily IHD vs. No dialysis	−0.420	0.657	0.453–0.960	0.030
Daily CVVH vs. No dialysis	0.222	1.248	0.934–1.684	0.141
Daily SLED vs. No dialysis	−0.430	0.651	0.397–1.106	0.107
Inotropic equivalents at ICU admission‖	−0.002	0.998	0.990–1.001	0.107
Inotropic equivalent at Dialysis‖	0.003	1.003	1.000–1.010	0.357
Propensity score adjusted diuretic use	−0.866	0.421	0.153–1.159	0.092

NOTE. Data are number (%) of patients, unless otherwise indicated.
Abbreviations: APACHE, acute physiology and chronic health evaluation; BUN, blood urea nitrogen; CVVH, continuous venovenous hemofiltration; IABP, intraaortic balloon pump; MBP, mean blood pressure; IHD, intermittent hemodialysis; TPN, total parenteral nutrition; SLED, sustained low-efficiency dialysis.
§Adjusted for gender, age, body mass index, elective operation, cardiopulmonary resuscitation, extracorporeal membrane oxygenation, cardiopulmonary resuscitation, ventilator use, days from hospital admission to dialysis, NPO status, total parenteral nutrition, time-varying variables (blood pressure, BUN, creatinine, lactate, urine output, body weight, time-varying three day accumulative diuretic dose, daily dialysis modality and dialysis intensity), anuria, inotropic equivalent, lactate, sodium, potassium, APACHE II at initial dialysis, diabetes mellitus, hypertension, congestive heart failure, cirrhosis, chronic kidney disease, sepsis, shock, systemic organ failure (central nervous system, respiratory, cardiac, liver), operation categories (abdominal, cardiovascular, chest, neurology, urology, orthopedic), and indication for dialysis (azotemia, fluid overload, hyperkalemia, oliguria, acidosis).
‖Inotropic equivalent = [(dopamine+dobutamine)+(milrinone×15)+[(epinephrine+norepinephrine+isoproterenol)×100] in mcg/kg/min [35,40].

assessed daily. Because of severe fluctuations in hemodynamic and biochemical data [34], we recorded patients' clinical parameters such as blood pressure, BUN, lactate, creatinine, urine output, body weight and dialysis intensity daily at 8:00 a.m.

The 30-day mortality, defined as death within 30 days after acute dialysis initiation, was the primary outcome variable. Vital signs, hemodynamic data, and laboratory data between groups were examined at the time of dialysis initiation. Anuria was defined as urine output of less than 100 mL/day. Diuretics were prescribed according to the clinical judgment in terms of patients' urine output and fluid status. Therefore the dose of diuretic was collected retrospectively. Diuretics were held if daily urine output is still less than 100cc after a single dose challenge of furosemide. The daily diuretic dose of each patient was recorded and calculated after hemodialysis was initiated. Only two types of loop diuretic, bumetanide and furosemide, were used in our unit. For the calculation, 1 mg of bumetanide was considered to be equivalent to 40 mg of furosemide [13,26]. Because the frequency and dose of diuretic varied during dialysis, the time-varying 3-day accumulative diuretic dose was integrated to analyze the effect of diuretic use and dosage on patient mortality [11]. The time-varying 3-day accumulative diuretic dose was recorded as the total dose of diuretic received within the 3-day prior to dialysis and every 3-days after dialysis initiation.

Renal replacement therapy (RRT)

The indication for RRT has been previously reported [25,26,27], namely, (1) azotemia (BUN>80 mg/dL) with uremic symptoms (165 patients); (2) fluid overload with a central venous pressure >12 mm Hg or pulmonary edema with a PaO$_2$/FiO$_2$<300 (90 patients); (3) hyperkalemia (serum K$^+$>5.5 mmol/L) despite medical treatment (43 patients); (4) oliguria (urine amount<100 mL/8 h) with or without diuretic use (295 patients); and (5) acidosis (pH<7.2 in arterial blood gas) (21 patients).

The RRT modality was chosen according to patient hemodynamics, as previously reported [12,25]. Continuous venovenous hemofiltration (CVVH) was used if an inotropic equivalent (IE) dose [35] of more than 15 points was required to keep systolic blood pressure (SBP) above 120 mmHg when RRT was initiated; or if SBP<120 mmHg despite inotropic agents. CVVH was performed with high-flux filters (Hemofilter, PAN-10, Asahi Kasei

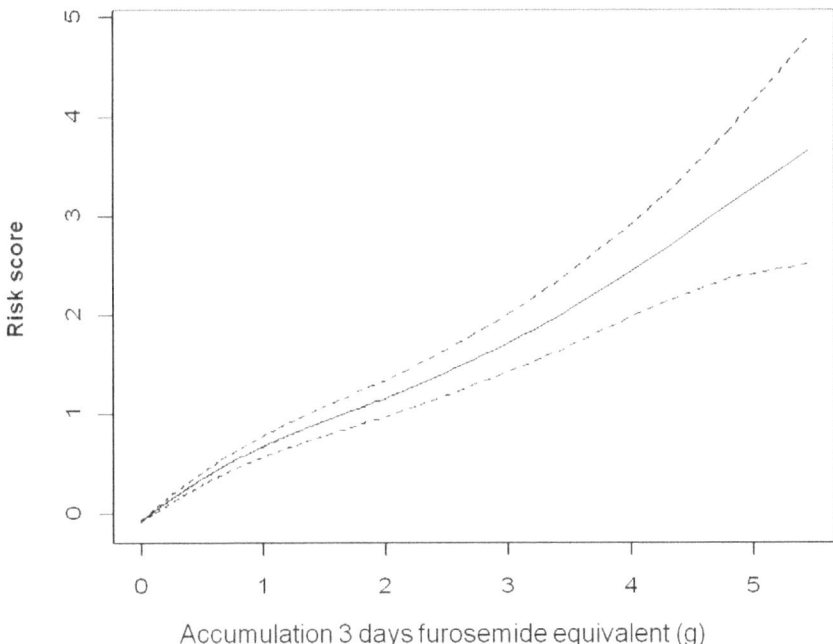

Figure 3. Accumulated diuretics dose predicts post dialysis mortality. Time-varying three-day accumulative diuretic dose (equivalent to furosemide dose) predicts 30 days mortality after undergoing acute dialysis. The smoothed plot of a generalized additive model included all demographic variables in the time-varying analyses, plus comorbid states (p<0.001).

Medical Company, Japan) using HF 400 (Infomed, Geneva, Switzerland) and a hemofiltration flow of 35 mL/kg/hour with a blood flow of 200 mL/min. Replacement fluid was bicarbonate-buffered and was administered predilutionally at a dynamically adjusted volume to achieve the desired fluid therapy goals.

Sustained low efficiency dialysis (SLED) was operated by the same group of technicians, nephrologists, and intensive care physicians as CVVH using a previously reported standard protocol [12]. SLED was delivered for 8 hours daily, from 9:00 a.m. to 5:00 p.m., using conventional HD machines (Fresenius 4008B, Fresenius Medical Care AG, Bad Homburg, Germany) and a Fresenius F8 dialyzer (Polysulfone, Fresenius Medical Care, Taipei, Taiwan). Blood flow was 200 mL/min, and the dialysate flow was 300 mL/min. Patients were eligible for SLED if they met one of the following two criteria [12]: (1) severe fluid overload (defined as an estimated ultrafiltration >2.5 L during a single dialysis session) and a central venous pressure level >15 mmHg or pulmonary edema with $PaO_2/FiO_2<200$ mmHg despite diuretic treatment, modified from a SOFA respiratory score of 3 or 4 [36], or (2) moderately unstable hemodynamics (defined as SBP 120–140 mmHg with inotropic equivalent (IE) score 5–15 [35]). Otherwise, intermittent hemodialysis was used. Typically, most patients were treated with more than one RRT modalities during an AKI episode. Because of the use of different RRT modalities (continuous and intermittent), the dialysis intensity was defined as the number of dialysis days divided by the dialysis period and determined by consensus among the attending intensivists and nephrologists.

Disease severity

Organ failure was classified according to the following findings [25,26]: respiratory failure, with ventilator support; coagulopathy, platelet count $\leq 50 \times 10^3/mm^3$; central nervous system failure, Glasgow coma score ≤9; cardiac failure, signs of low cardiac output with a central venous pressure >12 mm Hg and the administration of an IE>5 points; and liver dysfunction, total bilirubin ≥2.0 mg/dL

with INR>1.4. Sepsis was defined as the persistence or progression of signs and symptoms of the systemic inflammatory response syndrome with a documented or presumed persistence of infection [32].

Statistical analysis

Statistical analyses were performed using SAS software, Version 9.1.3 (SAS Institute Inc., Cary, NC, U.S.A.) and R software, Version 2.8.1 (Free Software Foundation, Inc., Boston, MA, U.S.A.). A two-sided p value≤0.05 was considered statistically significant. The continuous variables were summarized as mean ± standard deviation (SD) unless otherwise indicated, whereas the categorical variables were presented as proportions. A two-sample student's t-test was used to test the difference in the means of continuous variables between groups, and the chi-square test or Fisher's exact test was used to analyze the associations between two categorical variables.

Moreover, because diuretic use was randomly assigned, the potential selection bias was controlled by applying propensity score analysis (PSA) [37]. To estimate each patient's propensity score for diuretic use, we fitted a separate multivariable logistic regression model with the factors predicting diuretic use [6] (further seen at File S1).

In the multivariate analysis, Cox's regression model with time-dependent covariates [11] was used to test the associations between the prognostic factors and the hazard rate of mortality within 30 days. Patients were censored at the time of withdrawal from RRT or at the end of the 30-day observation period. The baseline values for mean arterial pressure, O_2 index, IE, lactate level, BUN, creatinine, and urine output when dialysis began and the time-varying values of their repeated measurements during the 30 days after RRT were also analyzed. Besides, the frequency and modality of RRT were also added as independent covariates to evaluate the effect of RRT intensity.

Additionally, to visualize the potential nonlinear effects of continuous covariates, such as the 3-day cumulative diuretic dose, a generalized additive models (GAM)-type approach was applied

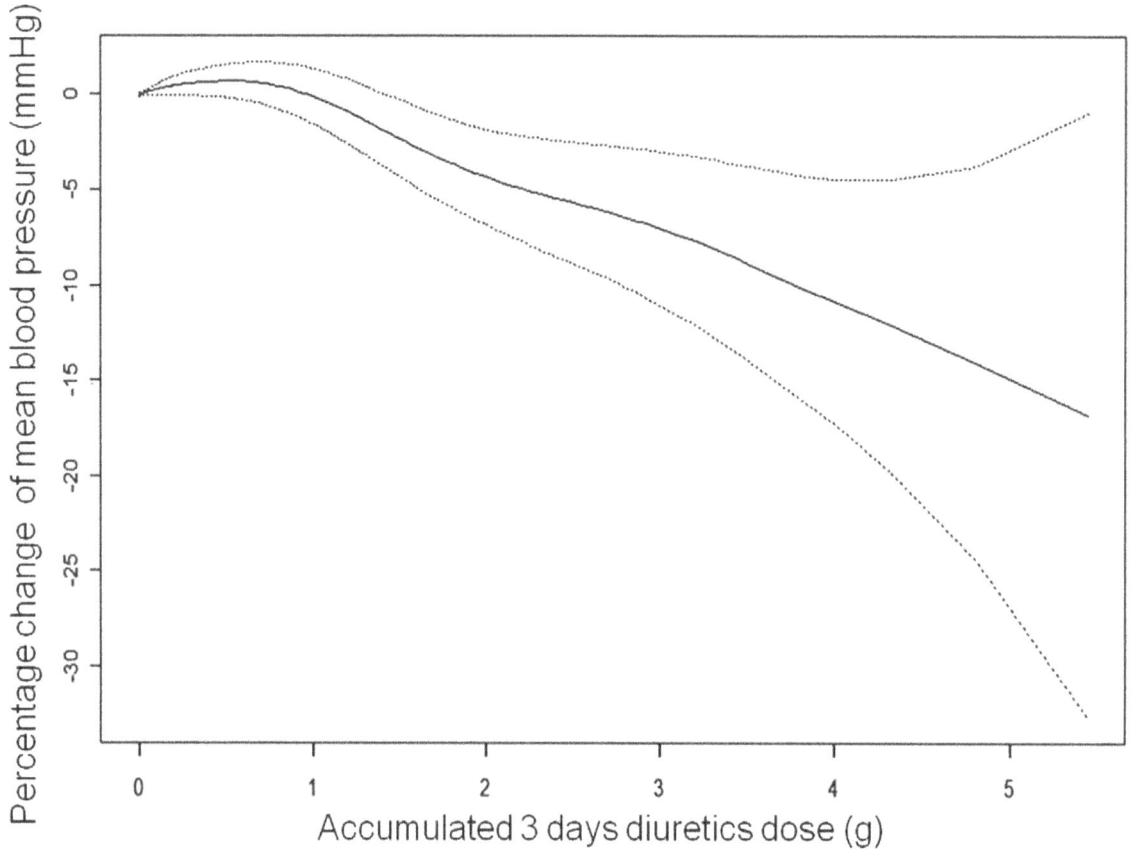

Figure 4. Accumulated diuretics related to blood pressure. The smoothed plot of a generalized additive model for the relationship between time-varying three-day accumulative diuretic dose and blood pressure difference in post-surgical dialysis patients with adjustments for possible linear and nonlinear effects* ($p < 0.001$).

to the Cox's proportional hazards model, with the aid of the loess regression and spline smoothing techniques [38].

Finally, to examine the effect of diuretic use on various time-dependent variables, marginal linear regression models were fitted to these repeatedly measured responses using the generalized estimating equations (GEE) method [39] (further seen at File S1). The estimated propensity score of diuretic exposure and the need for dialysis was also added into the GEE marginal linear regression models as a covariate to adjust for the selection bias from diuretic use [6].

Supporting Information

File S1 Statistics about Propensity score, Regression model and Generalized estimating equation (GEE) model.

Table S1 Diuretic dose and dialysis intensity. Generalized estimating equation (GEE) model after adjusting propensity score including diuretic dose and significant time-dependent covariates was used to evaluate intensity of daily dialysis through the spectrum and duration of dialysis.

Table S2 Diuretic dose and daily blood pressure. Generalized estimating equations (GEE) model after adjusting propensity score including diuretic dose and significant time-dependent covariates was used to evaluate daily blood pressure through the spectrum and duration of dialysis.

Acknowledgments

The authors would like to thank the staff of the Second Core Lab of Department of Medical Research in National Taiwan University Hospital for technical assistance.

National Taiwan University Hospital Study Group for Acute Renal Failure (NSARF) includes Wen-Je Ko, MD, PhD, Vin-Cent Wu, MD, Yu-Feng Lin, MD, Chun-Fu Lai, MD, Tao-Min Huang, MD, Yih-Sharng Chen, MD, PhD, Tzong-Shinn Chu, MD, PhD, Yung-Ming Chen, MD, Chih-Chung Shiao, MD, Wei-Jie Wang, MD, Cheng-Yi Wang, MD, Pei-Chen Wu, MD, Chia-Ter Chao, MD, Pi-Ru Tsai, RN, Hui-Chun Wang, RN, Hung-Bin Tsai, MD, Wen-Yi Li, MD, Yu-Chang Yeh, MD, Tao-Min Huang, MD, Fu-Chang Hu, MS, ScD, and Kwan-Dun Wu, MD, PhD.

Author Contributions

Conceived and designed the experiments: VCW. Performed the experiments: WJK CFL CCS GHY. Analyzed the data: YFL PCW FCH YYH WCW CCH. Contributed reagents/materials/analysis tools: CTC TMH YCY IJT TWK. Wrote the paper: VCW WJK TJT KDW.

References

1. Reddy VG (2002) Prevention of postoperative acute renal failure. J Postgrad Med 48: 64–70.
2. Levy EM, Viscoli CM, Horwitz RI (1996) The effect of acute renal failure on mortality. A cohort analysis. Jama 275: 1489–1494.
3. Mangano CM, Diamondstone LS, Ramsay JG, Aggarwal A, Herskowitz A, et al. (1998) Renal dysfunction after myocardial revascularization: risk factors, adverse outcomes, and hospital resource utilization. The Multicenter Study of Perioperative Ischemia Research Group. Ann Intern Med 128: 194–203.
4. Lassnigg A, Schmidlin D, Mouhieddine M, Bachmann LM, Druml W, et al. (2004) Minimal changes of serum creatinine predict prognosis in patients after cardiothoracic surgery: a prospective cohort study. J Am Soc Nephrol 15: 1597–1605.
5. Tang IY, Murray PT (2004) Prevention of perioperative acute renal failure: what works? Best Pract Res Clin Anaesthesiol 18: 91–111.
6. Uchino S, Doig GS, Bellomo R, Morimatsu H, Morgera S, et al. (2004) Diuretics and mortality in acute renal failure. Crit Care Med 32: 1669–1677.
7. Shilliday IR, Quinn KJ, Allison ME (1997) Loop diuretics in the management of acute renal failure: a prospective, double-blind, placebo-controlled, randomized study. Nephrol Dial Transplant 12: 2592–2596.
8. Cantarovich F, Rangoonwala B, Lorenz H, Verho M, Esnault VL (2004) High-dose furosemide for established ARF: a prospective, randomized, double-blind, placebo-controlled, multicenter trial. Am J Kidney Dis 44: 402–409.
9. Bragg-Gresham JL, Fissell RB, Mason NA, Bailie GR, Gillespie BW, et al. (2007) Diuretic use, residual renal function, and mortality among hemodialysis patients in the Dialysis Outcomes and Practice Pattern Study (DOPPS). Am J Kidney Dis 49: 426–431.
10. Metz LI, LeBeau ME, Zlabek JA, Mathiason MA (2009) Acute renal failure in patients undergoing cardiothoracic surgery in a community hospital. WMJ 108: 109–114.
11. Dekker FW, de Mutsert R, van Dijk PC, Zoccali C, Jager KJ (2008) Survival analysis: time-dependent effects and time-varying risk factors. Kidney Int 74: 994–997.
12. Wu VC, Wang CH, Wang WJ, Lin YF, Hu FC, et al. (2009) Sustained low-efficiency dialysis versus continuous veno-venous hemofiltration for postsurgical acute renal failure. Am J Surg 199: 466–476.
13. Mehta RL, Pascual MT, Soroko S, Chertow GM (2002) Diuretics, mortality, and nonrecovery of renal function in acute renal failure. Jama 288: 2547–2553.
14. Lassnigg A, Donner E, Grubhofer G, Presterl E, Druml W, et al. (2000) Lack of renoprotective effects of dopamine and furosemide during cardiac surgery. J Am Soc Nephrol 11: 97–104.
15. Cantarovich F, Galli C, Benedetti L, Chena C, Castro L, et al. (1973) High dose frusemide in established acute renal failure. Br Med J 4: 449–450.
16. van der Voort PH, Boerma EC, Koopmans M, Zandberg M, de Ruiter J, et al. (2009) Furosemide does not improve renal recovery after hemofiltration for acute renal failure in critically ill patients: a double blind randomized controlled trial. Crit Care Med 37: 533–538.
17. Cutler RE, Forrey AW, Christopher TG, Kimpel BM (1974) Pharmacokinetics of furosemide in normal subjects and functionally anephric patients. Clin Pharmacol Ther 15: 588–596.
18. Docci D (1984) Dopamine-furosemide in oliguric acute renal failure. Nephron 36: 74.
19. Bakker J, Coffernils M, Leon M, Gris P, Vincent JL (1991) Blood lactate levels are superior to oxygen-derived variables in predicting outcome in human septic shock. Chest 99: 956–962.
20. De Vecchis R, Ciccarelli A, Pucciarelli A (2010) Unloading therapy by intravenous diuretic in chronic heart failure: a double-edged weapon? J Cardiovasc Med (Hagerstown) 11: 571–574.
21. Bouchard J, Soroko SB, Chertow GM, Himmelfarb J, Ikizler TA, et al. (2009) Fluid accumulation, survival and recovery of kidney function in critically ill patients with acute kidney injury. Kidney Int 76: 422–427.
22. Francis GS, Siegel RM, Goldsmith SR, Olivari MT, Levine TB, et al. (1985) Acute vasoconstrictor response to intravenous furosemide in patients with chronic congestive heart failure. Activation of the neurohumoral axis. Ann Intern Med 103: 1–6.
23. Costanzo MR, Guglin ME, Saltzberg MT, Jessup ML, Bart BA, et al. (2007) Ultrafiltration versus intravenous diuretics for patients hospitalized for acute decompensated heart failure. J Am Coll Cardiol 49: 675–683.
24. Udani SM, Murray PT (2009) The use of renal replacement therapy in acute decompensated heart failure. Semin Dial 22: 173–179.
25. Wu VC, Ko WJ, Chang HW, Chen YS, Chen YW, et al. (2007) Early renal replacement therapy in patients with postoperative acute liver failure associated with acute renal failure: effect on postoperative outcomes. J Am Coll Surg 205: 266–276.
26. Wu VC, Ko WJ, Chang HW, Chen YW, Lin YF, et al. (2008) Risk factors of early redialysis after weaning from postoperative acute renal replacement therapy. Intensive Care Med 34: 101–108.
27. Huang TM, Wu VC, Young GH, Lin YF, Shiao CC, et al. (2010) Preoperative Proteinuria Predicts Adverse Renal Outcomes after Coronary Artery Bypass Grafting. J Am Soc Nephrol.
28. Wu VC, Huang DM, Ko WJ, Wu KD (2011) Acute-on-chronic kidney injury predicted long-term dialysis and mortality in critical patients after discharge. Kidney Intin press.
29. Lindenauer PK, Pekow P, Wang K, Mamidi DK, Gutierrez B, et al. (2005) Perioperative beta-blocker therapy and mortality after major noncardiac surgery. N Engl J Med 353: 349–361.
30. Wijeysundera DN, Karkouti K, Beattie WS, Rao V, Ivanov J (2006) Improving the identification of patients at risk of postoperative renal failure after cardiac surgery. Anesthesiology 104: 65–72.
31. Elahi MM, Lim MY, Joseph RN, Dhannapuneni RR, Spyt TJ (2004) Early hemofiltration improves survival in post-cardiotomy patients with acute renal failure. Eur J Cardiothorac Surg 26: 1027–1031.
32. Wu VC, Wang YT, Wang CY, Tsai IJ, Wu KD, et al. (2006) High frequency of linezolid-associated thrombocytopenia and anemia among patients with end-stage renal disease. Clin Infect Dis 42: 66–72.
33. Chou YH, Huang TM, Wu VC, Wang CY, Shiao CC, et al. (2011) Impact of timing of renal replacement therapy initiation on outcome of septic acute kidney injury. Crit Care 15: R134.
34. Berbece AN, Richardson RM (2006) Sustained low-efficiency dialysis in the ICU: Cost, anticoagulation, and solute removal. Kidney Int.
35. Chen YS, Ko WJ, Lin FY, Huang SC, Chou TF, et al. (2001) Preliminary result of an algorithm to select proper ventricular assist devices for high-risk patients with extracorporeal membrane oxygenation support. J Heart Lung Transplant 20: 850–857.
36. Palevsky PM, Zhang JH, O'Connor TZ, Chertow GM, Crowley ST, et al. (2008) Intensity of renal support in critically ill patients with acute kidney injury. N Engl J Med 359: 7–20.
37. Stenestrand U, Tabrizi F, Lindback J, Englund A, Rosenqvist M, et al. (2004) Comorbidity and myocardial dysfunction are the main explanations for the higher 1-year mortality in acute myocardial infarction with left bundle-branch block. Circulation 110: 1896–1902.
38. Woo MJ, Reiter JP, Karr AF (2008) Estimation of propensity scores using generalized additive models. Stat Med 27: 3805–3816.
39. Zeger SL, Liang KY (1986) Longitudinal data analysis for discrete and continuous outcomes. Biometrics 42: 121–130.
40. Ko WJ, Lin CY, Chen RJ, Wang SS, Lin FY, et al. (2002) Extracorporeal membrane oxygenation support for adult postcardiotomy cardiogenic shock. Ann Thorac Surg 73: 538–545.

4

Back to Basics: Pitting Edema and the Optimization of Hypertension Treatment in Incident Peritoneal Dialysis Patients (BRAZPD)

Sebastião R. Ferreira-Filho[1,2]*, **Gilberto R. Machado**[1,2], **Valéria C. Ferreira**[1], **Carlos F. M. A. Rodrigues**[1], **Thyago Proença de Moraes**[3], **José C. Divino-Filho**[4], **Marcia Olandoski**[3], **Christopher McIntyre**[5], **Roberto Pecoits-Filho**[3], on behalf of the BRAZPD study investigators

1 Nefroclínica de Uberlândia, Minas Gerais, Brazil, 2 Federal University of Uberlândia, Minas Gerais, Brazil, 3 Center for Health and Biological Sciences, Pontifícia Universidade Católica do Paraná, Curitiba, Brazil, 4 Baxter Healthcare, Division of Baxter Novum and Renal Medicine, CLINTEC, Karolinska Institute, Stockholm, Sweden, 5 Faculty of Medicine & Health Sciences, University of Nottingham, Nottingham, United Kingdom,

Abstract

Systemic arterial hypertension is an important risk factor for cardiovascular disease that is frequently observed in populations with declining renal function. Initiation of renal replacement therapy at least partially decreases signs of fluid overload; however, high blood pressure levels persist in the majority of patients after dialysis initiation. Hypervolemia due to water retention predisposes peritoneal dialysis (PD) patients to hypertension and can clinically manifest in several forms, including peripheral edema. The approaches to detect edema, which include methods such as bioimpedance, inferior vena cava diameter and biomarkers, are not always available to physicians worldwide. For clinical examinations, the presence of pitting located in the lower extremities and/or over the sacrum to diagnose the presence of peripheral edema in their patients are frequently utilized. We evaluated the impact of edema on the control of blood pressure of incident PD patients during the first year of dialysis treatment. Patients were recruited from 114 Brazilian dialysis centers that were participating in the BRAZPD study for a total of 1089 incident patients. Peripheral edema was diagnosed by the presence of pitting after finger pressure was applied to the edematous area. Patients were divided into 2 groups: those with and without edema according to the monthly medical evaluation. Blood arterial pressure, body mass index, the number of antihypertensive drugs and comorbidities were analyzed. We observed an initial BP reduction in the first five months and a stabilization of blood pressure levels from five to twelve months. The edematous group exhibited higher blood pressure levels than the group without edema during the follow-up. The results strongly indicate that the presence of a simple and easily detectable clinical sign of peripheral edema is a very relevant tool that could be used to re-evaluate not only the patient's clinical hypertensive status but also the PD prescription and patient compliance.

Editor: Emmanuel A. Burdmann, University of Sao Paulo Medical School, Brazil

Funding: The authors have no funding or support to report.

Competing Interests: Baxter Healthcare sponsored this study. During the data collection and analysis, JCDF was employed by Baxter. RPF received a consulting fee and speaker honorarium from Baxter Healthcare. There are no patents, products in development or marketed products to declare. This does not alter the authors' adherence to all the PLoS ONE policies on sharing data and materials, as detailed online in the guide for authors.

* E-mail: sebahferreira@gmail.com

Introduction

Cardiovascular disease is the most common cause of morbidity and mortality in patients with chronic kidney disease (CKD) [1–3]. Systemic arterial hypertension (SAH) is an important risk factor for cardiovascular disease and is frequently observed in this population along with a decline of renal function [4]. Although overload and renal replacement therapy (RRT) with dialysis usually improve fluid balance and partially remove uremic toxins, high blood pressure levels may persist after the initiation of dialysis, and hypertension is present in the majority of both peritoneal and hemodialysis patients [5,6].

The reduction in blood pressure levels observed in peritoneal dialysis (PD) patients can be attributed to the continuous effective control of fluid balance and, consequently, extracellular volume [7]; however, this reduction is not always sustained. In fact, higher than normal blood pressure levels are observed in many patients during dialysis therapy, mainly due to the limitations in achieving normal fluid status [8–10]. Hypervolemia due to water retention predisposes PD patients to hypertension [11,12] and can manifest clinically in several forms, including peripheral edema [9]. Detecting occult edema often involves the measurement of metrics such as bioimpedance, inferior vena cava diameter and biomarkers, but these methods are not available to all physicians. To detect edema in their patients, many doctors have at their disposal only the presence of pitting located in the lower extremities and/or over the sacrum.

Despite the fact that some patients present SAH independently of volemic status, it is recognized that hypervolemia, with or without the presence of edema, is one of the principal factors responsible for the resistance of PD patients to SAH treatment [13,14]. Blood pressure normalization often requires modifications to the ultrafiltration target, an increase in sodium removal, a decrease in fluid and sodium intake, blood sugar control and/or an increase in the number of prescribed hypertension drugs [6,7,15,21]. Considering that the expansion of extracellular volume can occur during dialysis and that peripheral edema detectable on a physical exam can be the result of a hypervolemic state [13], little is known about the correlations between pitting edema and blood pressure control in hypertensive patients receiving PD treatment.

We hypothesized that the presence of pitting edema is associated with the worsening of SAH, which leads to the cardiovascular impact observed in fluid-overloaded patients. Thus, in the present study, we evaluated the impact of peripheral edema on hypertensive control in incident PD patients with SAH during the first year of dialysis treatment.

Methods

Each consecutive incident patient recruited from 114 Brazilian dialysis centers participating in the BRAZPD study from December 2004 through October 2007 was included, totaling 3439 patients. Incident patients were defined as patients who originated from pre-dialysis conservative treatment or HD, who started treatment with PD during the study period and who remained on the therapy for at least 90 days. In Brazil, 60% of the patients start treatment in APD and 40% in CAPD. Details of the BRAZPD study design and characteristics of the cohort are described elsewhere [16]. Briefly, after being selected to participate in the study, each clinic submitted the project to its local ethics committee (the protocol was approved by the ethics committees of Federal University of Uberlandia), and all patients signed an informed consent. Physician and nurses at each dialysis center were trained by the study monitors to use the clinical research software *PDnet*, which was designed specifically to collect data for this study. From a total of 3439 incident patients, 239 were excluded because they were less than 18 years old, 1650 were excluded for not completing 12 full months of follow up (i.e., patients who missed at least one medical evaluation monthly for 12 consecutive months, or who dropped out due to hemodialysis, transplant or death), 430 were excluded because they were normotensive with or without previously using any antihypertensive drugs and because they did not have peripheral edema at the beginning of the PD treatment, and 31 were excluded due to missing data. After exclusion criteria were applied, 1089 hypertensive patients were included in the analysis.

The variables analyzed included anthropomorphic data, comorbidities, systolic arterial pressure (SAP), diastolic arterial pressure (DAP), mean arterial pressure (MAP), erythropoietin use, PD modality (CAPD or APD), and physical examination. During the physical examination, peripheral edema was characterized by the presence of pitting after finger pressure was applied to the edematous area for at least five seconds. The nephrologists graded pitting edema on a scale from 1+ to 4+. The urea and plasma creatinine, serum potassium, and hemoglobin values of the patients were measured to be used as annual means.

For all patients, the dialysis nurse or the nephrologist measured blood pressure during their monthly visits to the dialysis clinic. For the diagnosis of systemic hypertension, the following WHO/ISH criteria were applied: SAP≥140 mmHg and/or DAP≥90 mmHg, with or without the use of hypertensive medication. SAP levels were verified using an oscillating method. Mean arterial pressure was calculated using the formula MAP=(2DAP+SAP)/3. The number of anti-hypertensive drug classes used monthly by the patients (NAC) was also reported. The classes considered were

diuretics, beta-blockers, ACE inhibitors, angiotensin II receptor blockers, centrally and peripherally acting alpha-blockers, and calcium channel blockers. Each class listed was counted as one unit, and the NAC represented the mathematical mean of the number of anti-hypertensive drug classes used per patient for each subgroup.

After the exclusion criteria were applied, the final sample consisted of 1089 hypertensive patients. These patients were subdivided into those with (E+) and without (E−) clinically detectable pitting edema, according to the monthly medical evaluation at both the beginning of the observation period and during the twelve months of follow up. The number of patients in each subgroup varied monthly depending on the presentation of edema at that particular evaluation (Figure 1). In order to analyze the trend for edema and high blood pressure levels, we also monitored for 12 months the patients classified E+ and E− based on the first month classification.

Statistical Analysis

Categorical variables are presented as frequencies and percentages. Continuous variables are presented as the mean ± standard deviation (mean ± SD). In the figures, continuous variables are presented as the mean ± standard error. The chi-squared test and analysis of variance (ANOVA), with repeat measures and measures of position and distribution, were utilized for the comparison between the E+ and E− subgroups. The parallelism analysis of both groups was performed to verify the trends and similarities between the groups, for the initial defined groups at month 1. For all analyses, a p-value of <0.05 was considered statistically significant. All statistical analyses were performed using SPSS version 8.0 (Chicago, IL, USA).

Results

Descriptive data at baseline PD treatment level (after the first month on PD) for all patients included in this study are shown in Table 1. The mean patient age was 58.2±15.3 years, and more than half (56.9%) of the patients were female. The mean SBP was 156.7±18.7 mmHg, the mean DBP was 90.0±12.7 mmHg, and the mean MAP was 112.2±12.8 mmHg. The mean body mass index (BMI) was 25.4±5.0 kg/m^2. The correlation between BMI and the number of patients with edema was negative and significant (r = −0.83). The increase of blood pressure (SBP, DBP and MAP) correlated with the number of patients with

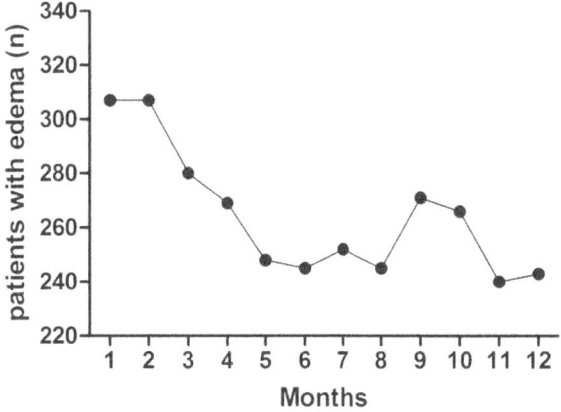

Figure 1. Number of patients/month with clinically detectible edema.

edema: 0.76; 0.69 and 0.52 respectively (p<0.001).Overall, 42.6% of study participants were diabetic, and the mean number of anti-hypertensive class drugs (NAC) used was 2.1±1.0 drugs/patient. Forty-three percent of patients were on APD using Home-choice[TM] (Baxter Healthcare) as the cycler, and all patients were prescribed only glucose-based PD solutions (Dianeal, Baxter Healthcare).

Analysis of groups divided by the presence of clinically detectible edema

Subgroup analysis of patients with clinically detectible edema (E+)

During the study, subgroup E+ (n = 307) presented a decrease in SAP between the 1st and 5th month (from 159.5±19.6 to 150.0±25.3 mmHg, $p<0.05$), and SAP remained constant from the 5th month until the end of the study (151.2±30.3 mmHg, $p>0.05$). DAP did not change significantly between the 1st and 12th month (from 90.7±13.3 to 89.0±17.7 mmHg, $p>0.05$). SAP decreased significantly between the 1st and 5th month (from 113.7±13.4 to 108.0±17.2 mmHg, $p<0.05$), and MAP remained constant from the 5th month through the 12th month (109.7±19.8 mmHg, $p>0.05$). NAC did not change between the 1st and 12th months (from 2.3±1.0 to 2.2±1.0 drugs/patient,

$p>0.05$). The number of patients with edema decreased between the 2nd and 6th months from 307 to 245 individuals; this number varied through the end of the evaluation period, at which point 243 patients were clinically diagnosed with edema (Figure 1). BMI

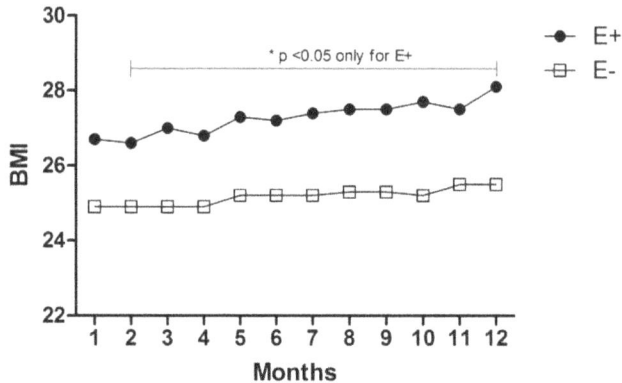

Figure 2. Twelve-month evolution of the body mass index (BMI) in the patient cohort.

Table 1. Demographic, clinical and laboratory characteristics of patients at the baseline evaluation.

Variable	Total population	Patients with edema (E+)	without edema (E−)	P value
Number of patients (n)	1089	307	782	<0.001
Age (year)	58.2±15.3	59. 6±14.3	57.7±15.6*	0.03
Female (%)	56.9	55.7	57.4	0.61
Diabetes (%)	42.6	56.0	37.3*	<0.0001
Race (%)				
Asian	2.7	3.2	2.8	0.92
White	61.7	61.6	61.1	0.96
Black	35.6	35.2	36.1	0.93
Height (cm)	161.6±10.0	161.6±10.5	161.7±9.8	0.44
Weight (Kg)	66.7±15.0	69.8±14.5	65.5±15.1*	<0.0001
Body mass index (Kg/m2)	25.4±5.0	26.7±5.1	24.9±4.9*	<0.0001
SAP (mmHg)	156.7±18.7	159.5±19.6	155.6±18.2*	0.001
DAP (mmHg)	90.0±12.7	90.7±13.3	89.7±12.5	0.11
MAP (mmHg)	112.2±12.8	113.7±13.4	111.7±12.6*	0.01
NCA	2.1±1.0	2.3±1.0	2.0±0.7*	<0.0001
Erythropoietin (%)	44.0	51.0	41.2*	0.003
CAPD/APD (%)	57.0/43.0	63.5/36.5	55.5*/44.5*	0.01/0.02
Conservative treatment (%)	56.2	60.4	54.7	0.093
Serum Albumin (g/dL)(n)	3.6±0.69	3.54±0.78	3.64±0.64	0.295
Hemodialysis previously (%)	44.5	44.4	44.6	0.933
Serum urea (mg/dl)	101.2±24.8	124.5±26.2	101.8±24.9	0.34
Serum creatinine (mg/dl)	8.0±3.1	7.8±3.1	8.1±3.1	0.12
Serum potassium (mEq/L)	4.3±0.6	4.3±0.6	4.4±0.6	0.08
Haemoglobin (g/dl)	11.5±4.0	11.4±3.7	11.5±4.1	0.44

NCA, number of classes of anti-hypertensives in use;
*(E−) vs (E+);
SAP: systolic arterial pressure; DAP: diastolic arterial pressure;
MAP: mean arterial pressure.

increased from the 2nd to the 12th month of evaluation (from 26.7 ± 5.1 to 28.1 ± 5.6 kg/m2, $p<0.05$) (Figure 2).

Subgroup analysis of patients without clinically detectible edema (E−)

Subgroup E− (n = 782) presented a significant decrease in SAP between the 1st and 5th month (from 155.6 ± 18.2 to 142.7 ± 24.2 mmHg, $p<0.05$). After this initial period, SAP remained constant until the end of the study period (141.2 ± 26.6 mmHg, $p>0.05$). DAP did not change between the 1st and 12th months (89.7 ± 12.5 to 84.7 ± 15.8 mmHg, $p>0.05$). MAP decreased significantly between the 1st and 5th months (from 111.7 ± 12.6 to 104.1 ± 15.8 mmHg, $p<0.05$) and then remained constant from the 5th month through the 12th month (103.6 ± 17.9 mmHg, $P>0.05$). NAC did not vary throughout the study period; the mean at the 1st month was 2.0 ± 0.7, and the mean at the 12th month was 2.1 ± 1.1 ($p>0.05$). For subgroup E−, there was no difference in BMI during the 12 months of follow-up (Figures 3 and 4)).

Comparison between the two subgroups of patients

The descriptive characteristics of the two subgroups defined by the presence of edema at the start of dialysis are shown in Table 1. At baseline, subgroup E+ consisted of 307 patients and E− consisted of 782 patients; however, these numbers varied according to monthly clinical evaluations (Figure 1). When only the patients classified E+ and E− in the first month were monitored, the results confirmed the monthly patient classification. E+ and E− move in the same way for the SBP (p = 0.654) although with different mean profiles (p = 0.001). In other words, E+ group showed higher SAP values than E-group during the 12 months period. For the DAP and MAP the trend and mean profile did not show statistical diferences (Figure 4). A comparison of subgroups E+ and E− at the start of treatment (Table 1) revealed significant differences with respect to age (59.6 ± 14.3 vs. 57.7 ± 15.6 years, respectively; $p<0.03$), BMI (26.7 ± 5.1 vs. 24.9 ± 4.9 kg/m2, respectively; $p<0.0001$), SAP (159.5 ± 19.6 vs. 155.6 ± 18.2 mmHg, respectively; $P<0.001$), MAP (113.7 ± 13.4 vs. 111.7 ± 12.6 mmHg, respectively; $P<0.01$), NAC (2.3 ± 1.0 vs. 2.0 ± 0.7 drugs/patient, respectively; $P<0.05$) and erythropoietin use (51.0 vs. 41.2%, respectively; P = 0.003). In both subgroups, there were a greater percentage of patients on APD than on CAPD (63.5/36.5 vs. 55.5/44.5%, respectively; $p<0.01/0.02$). The percentage of patients with diabetes mellitus was greater in subgroup E+ than in subgroup E− (56.0 vs. 37.3%, respectively;

$P<0.0001$), and the number of patients with a history of cardiovascular disease at the start of PD was not significantly different between the two groups (Table 1). SAP, MAP, NAC, and BMI were significantly different between the two subgroups (E+ and E−) in the analysis of the entire follow up period ($p<0.05$).

Discussion

It is well known that the expansion of extracellular volume with or without detectible edema is one of the principal factors responsible for the increase in SAP in patients with CKD [3,9]. In the present study, we observed that SAP and MAP of both subgroups presented a significant decrease in values in the first five months after starting PD therapy and stabilization of these values through the end of the observation period. This behavior was also conferred by Menon et al. [17], who reported a reduction in systemic pressures at the start of PD and, contrary to our data, detected an increase in blood pressure levels after 6–12 months on PD. On the other hand, Saldanha et al. [7] reported a decrease in blood pressure levels during PD treatment over 5 years, which was associated with the concomitant increase in the number of anti-hypertensive drugs used. In the present study, the initial decline observed in the E+ and E − groups could be attributed to a reduction in extracellular volume as a result of PD [8,18] because NAC did not change during this period. However, it should be noted that NAC represents a number of anti-hypertensive classes of drugs, which allows for the possibility of variations in the measurement of anti-hypertensive drugs within the same class. On the other hand, NAC maintenance can reflect a non-worsening of SAH in these patients and/or the medical preference to use these drugs for other therapeutic goals such as cardio-protection and/or preservation of residual renal function. Despite the initial decline in arterial blood pressure levels observed in our study, they did not decrease to values within the normal limits; SAP levels were above 140 mmHg during the entire study period. There are other reasons that could explain in the relative control of blood pressure levels in both groups, which are increase activity of the sympathetic nervous system, increase endothelium-derived vaso-constrictors, vascular calcification and activation of the renin-angiotensin system.

Upon separate analysis of the E+ and E − groups, we observed a monthly variation throughout the study period in the number of patients. This variation was a consequence of bi-directional flow between these groups. Despite this, the number of patients in the E+ subgroup decreased significantly after 12 months, from 307 to 243 patients (Figure 1). Among the E+ subgroup, SAP and MAP levels decreased from baseline until the 5th month, at which time they stabilized until the 12th month (Figure 3 and 4), while DAP did not change significantly during the entire period. In our study, patients with edema exhibited greater blood pressure levels (SAP and MAP) than those observed in the E − subgroup (Figure 3 and 4). Gunal et al. [12] and Katzarski et al. [19] demonstrated that volume overload is an important factor in resistance to SAH treatment for dialysis patients, while Ates et al. [20] showed that SBP and DBP were negatively correlated with total fluid and sodium removal, as well as with sodium restriction. The increase of blood pressure values was correlated with the number of patients with edema. This association shows that the patients who belonged to the E+ had higher blood pressure levels than those of group E− (Figure 5).

Our data demonstrated that the NAC in the E+ subgroup, despite not varying throughout the study, was significantly greater than in the E − subgroup during the months evaluated. This observation may suggest a greater difficulty in SAH control in the

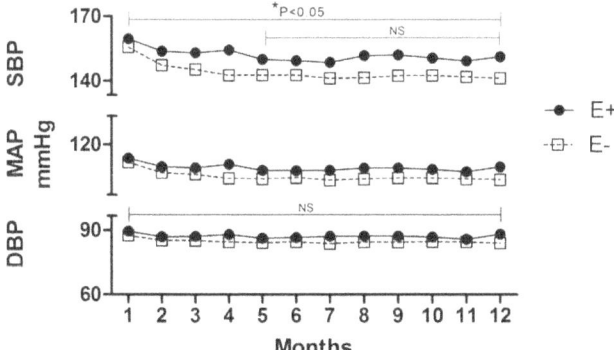

Figure 3. Systolic (SBP), Diastolic (DBP) and Mean Arterial Pressures (MAP) in incident PD patients during 12 months of follow up.

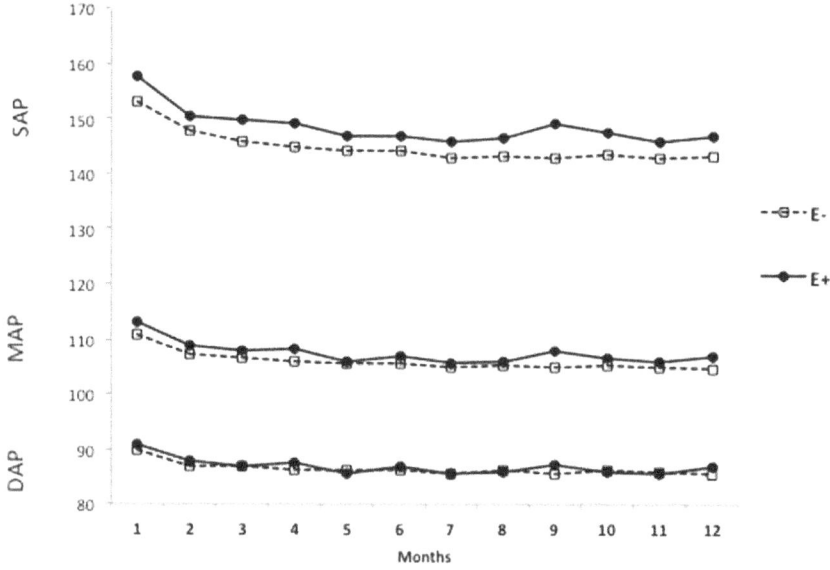

Figure 4. The initial groups (first month) were followed for 12 months.

E+ group. Furthermore, BMI in the E+ group increased progressively over the 12 month period. A strong and negative correlation between BMI and the number of patients with edema was observed. This association could be explained in two ways: a worsening of the edema status during PD therapy or a real gain of body mass. We believe that future studies with adequate designs will help to answer this question.

The progressive increase in body weight, likely caused to a large extent by the presence of edema, can be attributed to a water and salt imbalance, the patient's failure to follow medical recommendations, and/or an inadequate PD prescription. The progressive increase in body weight among PD patients might also be attributed to a gain of fat mass due to glucose absorption from the peritoneal cavity, as the patients may have been prescribed more hypertonic PD solutions to improve UF.

In the E− subgroup, blood pressure patterns followed the trend observed in the E+ group and decreased in the first months of PD before subsequently stabilizing (Figure 3). In the E− group, blood

pressure levels were lower than those observed in the E+ group during the entire observation period, whereas the NAC in the E− group did not vary significantly during the study period. However, blood pressure values did not reach the normal recommended levels. In general, there are several associated factors that make normalization of blood pressure levels difficult to attain in PD patients, including the presence of diabetes mellitus, aging, and the use of erythropoietin [11,14,18]. This was observed in the present study in the E+ group, in which the patients were significantly older and the percentage of patients with diabetes mellitus was significantly greater than in the E− group (Table 1). The significantly larger number of E+ patients who were treated with CAPD as opposed to APD may reflect an inadequate PD prescription, as many of these CAPD patients may be high transporters and/or have UF problems in the long run. Therefore, these patients should have been switched to APD. However, during the observation period, Extraneal was not available in Brazil. Moreover, blood pressures above the normal values could be caused by therapeutic inertia, where soft reasoning often leads to avoidance of intensified therapy by the medical staff [21].

The present study presents several limitations. Edema evaluation cannot be easily standardized, and the influence of expansion or retraction of volume on the systemic pressure levels could be better analyzed if it was evaluated by other methods, such as bioimpedance, inferior vena cava diameter [22], and biomarkers such as ANP [22,23]. This approach, however, is uncommon in daily medical practice due to the need for tools that are not always available. In addition, the analysis of fluid retention in PD patients is limited by the absence of data regarding residual renal function, the peritoneal membrane solute transport type and UF measurements [9]. Hypoalbuminemia, and consequent water and sodium retention, can explain the presence of edema and the difficulty in normalizing pressure levels; however, an evaluation of the causes of resistance to anti-hypertension therapy was not a focus of this study. It is important to note that the results of this observational study reflect PD practices in Brazil, which may be similar to treatment practices in a large number of countries around the world.

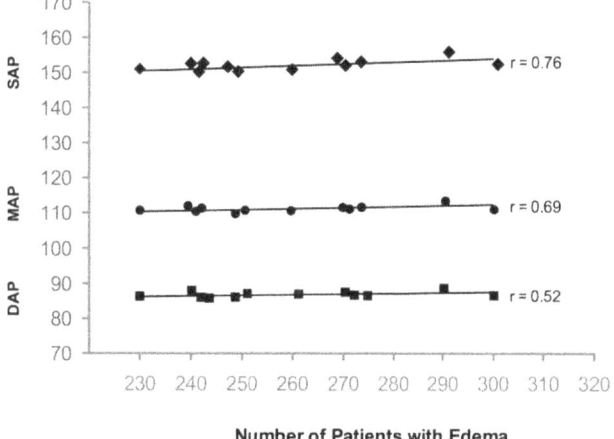

Figure 5. The increase in blood pressure levels correlates positively to the number of patients with edema.

Hypertensive CKD patients experienced a significant reduction in blood pressure levels after the initiation of PD, which was more pronounced in the first few months of therapy. However, most patients do not achieve normalization during the first year of treatment. This difficulty in reducing arterial blood pressure to normal levels is aggravated by the presence of edema, which points to a pivotal role of fluid overload in the hypertension of CKD patients on dialysis. The presence of clinically detectible pitting edema can be a useful clinical sign that could be used to guide the optimization of SAH treatment in patients undergoing continuous peritoneal dialysis.

In summary, volume status is of major importance to outcomes in patients undergoing PD. The lack of a robust edema evaluation and the limited availability of BIA and other objective measures of quantifying volume status make clinicians highly dependent on clinical evaluation. Clinically detectable pitting edema remains the most readily used clinical assessment tool. This study is the first to give a large-scale systematic description of pitting edema in the context of arterial hypertension in PD patients and to assess the effects of edema resolution in blood pressure values with PD initiation.

The results presented here strongly indicate that the presence of such a simple and easily detected clinical sign as pitting edema should be considered to be a relevant observational tool to assess a patient's clinical status, PD prescription and compliance with treatment. The term "back to basics" could mean, "examine your patients, look for edema and observe the blood pressure" and to do this sophisticated technologies are not needed.

Author Contributions

Conceived and designed the experiments: SRFF GRM RPF. Performed the experiments: GRM SRFF. Analyzed the data: SRFF GRM VCF CFMAR CM TPM MO JCDF. Wrote the paper: SRFF GRM. These authors contributed with important points in the discussion: JCDF.

References

1. Lynn KL, McGregor DO, Moesbergen T, Buttimore AL, Inkster JA, et al. (2002) Hypertension as a determinant of survival for patients treated with home dialysis. Kidney Int 62: 2281–2287.
2. Levey AS, Beto JA, Coronado BE, Eknoyan G, Foley RN, et al. (1998) Controlling the epidemic of cardiovascular disease in chronic renal disease: what do we know? What do we need to learn? Where do we go from here? National Kidney Foundation Task Force on Cardiovascular Disease. Am J Kidney Dis 32: 853–906.
3. van Dijk PC, Jager KJ, de Charro F, Collart F, Cornet R, et al. (2001) Renal replacement therapy in Europe: the results of a collaborative effort by the ERA-EDTA registry and six national or regional registries. Nephrol Dial Transplant 16: 1120–1129.
4. Barri YM (2008) Hypertension and kidney disease: a deadly connection. Current hypertension reports 10: 39–45.
5. Foley RN, Parfrey PS, Sarnak MJ (1998) Clinical epidemiology of cardiovascular disease in chronic renal disease. Am J Kidney Dis 32: S112–119.
6. Cocchi R, Degli Esposti E, Fabbri A, Lucatello A, Sturani A, et al. (1999) Prevalence of hypertension in patients on peritoneal dialysis: results of an Italian multicentre study. Nephrol Dial Transplant 14: 1536–1540.
7. Saldanha LF, Weiler EW, Gonick HC (1993) Effect of continuous ambulatory peritoneal dialysis on blood pressure control. Am J Kidney Dis 21: 184–188.
8. Lameire N (1993) Cardiovascular risk factors and blood pressure control in continuous ambulatory peritoneal dialysis. Perit Dial Int 13 Suppl 2: S394–395.
9. Tzamaloukas AH, Saddler MC, Murata GH, Malhotra D, Sena P, et al. (1995) Symptomatic fluid retention in patients on continuous peritoneal dialysis. J Am Soc Nephrol 6: 198–206.
10. Tang W, Cheng LT, Lu XH, Wang T (2009) Effect of nutrition on arterial stiffness in peritoneal dialysis patients. American journal of nephrology 30: 120–125.
11. Rahman M, Dixit A, Donley V, Gupta S, Hanslik T, et al. (1999) Factors associated with inadequate blood pressure control in hypertensive hemodialysis patients. American journal of kidney diseases : the official journal of the National Kidney Foundation 33: 498–506.
12. Gunal AI, Duman S, Ozkahya M, Toz H, Asci G, et al. (2001) Strict volume control normalizes hypertension in peritoneal dialysis patients. American journal

of kidney diseases : the official journal of the National Kidney Foundation 37: 588–593.
13. Van Biesen W, Verbeke F, Devolder I, Vanholder R (2008) The relation between salt, volume, and hypertension: clinical evidence for forgotten but still valid basic physiology. Perit Dial Int 28: 596–600.
14. Fishbane S, Natke E, Maesaka JK (1996) Role of volume overload in dialysis-refractory hypertension. Am J Kidney Dis 28: 257–261.
15. Slingeneyer A, Canaud B, Mion C (1983) Permanent loss of ultrafiltration capacity of the peritoneum in long-term peritoneal dialysis: an epidemiological study. Nephron 33: 133–138.
16. Fernandes N, Bastos MG, Cassi HV, Machado NL, Ribeiro JA, et al. (2008) The Brazilian Peritoneal Dialysis Multicenter Study (BRAZPD) : characterization of the cohort. Kidney Int Suppl: S145–151.
17. Menon MK, Naimark DM, Bargman JM, Vas SI, Oreopoulos DG (2001) Long-term blood pressure control in a cohort of peritoneal dialysis patients and its association with residual renal function. Nephrol Dial Transplant 16: 2207–2213.
18. Mailloux LU, Haley WE (1998) Hypertension in the ESRD patient: pathophysiology, therapy, outcomes, and future directions. Am J Kidney Dis 32: 705–719.
19. Katzarski KS, Charra B, Luik AJ, Nisell J, Divino Filho JC, et al. (1999) Fluid state and blood pressure control in patients treated with long and short haemodialysis. Nephrology, dialysis, transplantation : official publication of the European Dialysis and Transplant Association - European Renal Association 14: 369–375.
20. Ates K, Nergizoglu G, Keven K, Sen A, Kutlay S, et al. (2001) Effect of fluid and sodium removal on mortality in peritoneal dialysis patients. Kidney international 60: 767–776.
21. Basile J (2009) Clinical Inertia and Blood Pressure Goal Attainment. The Journal of Clinical Hypertension 11.
22. Leunissen KM, Kouw P, Kooman JP, Cheriex EC, deVries PM, et al. (1993) New techniques to determine fluid status in hemodialyzed patients. Kidney Int Suppl 41: S50–56.
23. Lang SM, Wolfram G, Gerzer R, Schiffl H (1999) Characterization of subtypes of hypertension in CAPD patients by cyclic guanosine monophosphate. Perit Dial Int 19: 143–147.

5

Endotoxaemia in Haemodialysis: A Novel Factor in Erythropoetin Resistance?

Laura E. A. Harrison[1], James O. Burton[1], Cheuk-Chun Szeto[2], Philip K. T. Li[2], Christopher W. McIntyre[1,3]*

1 Department of Renal Medicine, Royal Derby Hospital, Derby, United Kingdom, **2** Department of Medicine and Therapeutics, Chinese University of Hong Kong, Hong Kong, China, **3** School of Graduate Entry Medicine and Health, University of Nottingham, Derby, United Kingdom

Abstract

Background/Objectives: Translocated endotoxin derived from intestinal bacteria is a driver of systemic inflammation and oxidative stress. Severe endotoxaemia is an underappreciated, but characteristic finding in haemodialysis (HD) patients, and appears to be driven by acute repetitive dialysis induced circulatory stress. Resistance to erythropoietin (EPO) has been identified as a predictor of mortality risk, and associated with inflammation and malnutrition. This study aims to explore the potential link between previously unrecognised endotoxaemia and EPO Resistance Index (ERI) in HD patients.

Methodology/Principal Findings: 50 established HD patients were studied at a routine dialysis session. Data collection included weight, BMI, ultrafiltration volume, weekly EPO dose, and blood sampling pre and post HD. ERI was calculated as ratio of total weekly EPO dose to body weight (U/kg) to haemoglobin level (g/dL). Mean haemoglobin (Hb) was 11.3±1.3 g/dL with a median EPO dose of 10,000 [IQR 7,500–20,000] u/wk and ERI of 13.7 [IQR 6.9–23.3] ((U/Kg)/(g/dL)). Mean pre-HD serum ET levels were significantly elevated at 0.69±0.30 EU/ml. Natural logarithm (Ln) of ERI correlated to predialysis ET levels ($r = 0.324$, $p = 0.03$) with a trend towards association with hsCRP ($r = 0.280$, $p = 0.07$). Ln ERI correlated with ultrafiltration volume, a driver of circulatory stress ($r = 0.295$, $p = 0.046$), previously identified to be associated with increased intradialytic endotoxin translocation. Both serum ET and ultrafiltration volume corrected for body weight were independently associated with Ln ERI in multivariable analysis.

Conclusions: This study suggests that endotoxaemia is a significant factor in setting levels of EPO requirement. It raises the possibility that elevated EPO doses may in part merely be identifying patients subjected to significant circulatory stress and suffering the myriad of negative biological consequences arising from sustained systemic exposure to endotoxin.

Editor: Martin Gerbert Frasch, Université de Montréal, Canada

Funding: No external funding was received for this study.

Competing Interests: The authors have declared that no competing interests exist.

* E-mail: chris.mcintyre@nottingham.ac.uk

Introduction

Anaemia commonly occurs in patients with chronic kidney disease (CKD), as a result of insufficient production of erythropoietin (EPO) by the kidneys. Effective treatment of anaemia has been possible since the introduction of recombinant Human Erythropoietin therapy in 1986 [1].

Initial observational studies of EPO in CKD suggested a reduced risk of mortality with increasing haemoglobin levels, associated with improved quality of life [2,3,4]. However, several clinical trials in recent years have raised significant concerns regarding the optimum haemoglobin targets and erythropoietin stimulating agent (ESA) doses [5,6,7]. The randomised trials of Normal Haematocrit Cardiac Trial [8] and TREAT, comparing lower to higher haemoglobin (Hb) targets on composite endpoints, have demonstrated an increased risk of cardiovascular (CV) events. These include stroke and vascular access thrombosis and a potential increased risk of death and provide no clear signal concerning improved patient quality of life.

There remains controversy over whether the poorer outcomes are due to higher absolute levels of haemoglobin or elevated EPO dose, particularly in those patients who fail to achieve target haemoglobin [9]. Patients who do not achieve Hb targets despite elevated doses of EPO, or who require higher doses to maintain their Hb are considered to be Erythropoietin Resistant or Hyporesponsive [10,11].

Resistance to EPO, previously identified as a predictor of mortality risk [12], is widespread. Iron deficiency is recognised as a significant factor affecting ESA response, and is usually treated alongside erythropoietin replacement as part of co-ordinated anaemia management in the CKD population. Other important factors modulating the individual's response and potentially increasing ESA resistance include infection, hyperparathyroidism, inadequate dialysis, malnutrition and chronic inflammation [13,14].

Despite attempts to identify and treat known risk factors, ESA resistance cannot always be explained, suggesting that there may be alternative causes driving the condition. The drivers of systemic inflammation are often obscure. In order to more fully understand the complex relationship between EPO dose, Hb, clinical condition and the dialysis process itself, we identified circulating endotoxin as a potential factor influencing EPO response.

Endotoxin (without sepsis) was initially proposed as a stimulus for immune activation in the pro-inflammatory state of congestive heart failure (CHF) [15]. Endotoxin is released by bacterial cell wall breakdown, within and beyond the gut lumen, from effective host defence mechanisms and by autolysis. Endotoxin enters the circulation via bacterial translocation, passage of intact bacteria and macro-molecules such as endotoxin across the intestinal barrier [16].

Exposure to endotoxin, a profoundly pro-inflammatory stimulus, results in release of a wide variety of pro-inflammatory cytokines, and has been implicated in a broad range of other pathophysiological responses, including oxidative stress, endothelial dysfunction and impaired circulatory autoregulation [17,18]. We have recently reported significant incremental endotoxaemia with worsening renal function across the range of CKD, with levels roughly tripling after initiation of dialysis [19]. In HD patients the severity of endotoxaemia was associated with both the drivers (ultrafiltration volume and rate) and the consequences (dialysis induced myocardial injury) of dialysis induced circulatory stress.

We hypothesised that there was a potential link between endotoxaemia and EPO resistance in HD patients, and aimed to describe the relative contribution of circulating endotoxin levels to EPO resistance in HD patients.

Methods

Objectives

This study aims to explore the potential link between previously unrecognised endotoxaemia and EPO resistance in HD patients.

Ethics Statement

Ethical approval for the study was granted by Derbyshire Local Research Ethics Committee. Written informed consent was received from all participants.

Participants

Fifty prevalent HD patients were recruited from a single hospital-based haemodialysis unit. All patients were haemodialysed thrice weekly via native arterio-venous fistulae. Exclusion criteria comprised; change in target weight in the preceding six weeks, clinical evidence of blood loss, active infection or malignancy, bone marrow disease or haemoglobinopathy, or pre-existing severe LV systolic dysfunction (NYHA IV).

Methodology: Description of Procedures or Investigations Undertaken

Haemodialysis details. Dialysis was performed using Hospal Integra monitors (Hospal, Mirandola, Italy). Dialysate fluid contained sodium, 138 mmol/L; potassium, 1 mmol/L; calcium 1.25 mmol/L; magnesium, 0.5 mmol/L; bicarbonate, 32 mmol/L; glucose, 5.6 mmol/L; and acetate, 3 mmol/L. Dual pass water treatment was used with undetectable levels of endotoxin throughout study duration.

All studies were conducted after a 2 day interdialytic period. Anticoagulation was with unfractionated heparin. Dialysate flow was 500 mL/min, and dialysate temperature was set at 37°C. Net fluid removal was set on an individual basis according to ideal dry weight. Patients were permitted to eat during HD if this was their usual preference.

Ultrafiltration rate. The rate of volume removal at dialysis, expressed in ml/h/kg BW, measured by the weight change per duration of HD treatment using the post HD weight as denominator.

Data collection. The following basic demographic information was obtained: age (years), sex, dialytic vintage (months),

cardiovascular comorbidities, diabetes mellitus, body weight (BW; kg), body mass index (BMI; kg/m^2). The following factors were collected during the dialysis session: interdialytic weight gain (IDWG, kg), ultrafiltration volume (l), ultrafiltration rate (UFR: ml/h/kg body weight), pre-HD systolic and diastolic blood pressure, mean arterial blood pressure (MAP; mmHg), dialysis dose (Kt/V).

Erythropoietin dose. In order to normalize the amount of EPO required depending on the severity of anaemia, we calculated an EPO resistance (responsiveness) index (ERI), as described in previous studies [20], defined as the weekly EPO dose divided by Hb level (g/dl). Both the EPO dose and ERI were divided by target body weight to indicate the required EPO dose per kilogram of dry body weight.

Blood samples. All blood samples were taken before and after a dialysis session with rapid separation of serum and storage at −85°C before endotoxin measurement. Patients were not fasted prior to blood sampling. Haemoglobin (Hb), ferritin, reticulocytes, serum sodium, potassium, urea, creatinine, albumin, corrected calcium, albumin, and intact parathyroid hormone (PTH) were analyzed using standard autoanalyzer techniques (Roche diagnostics modular IIP®). Commercially available enzyme-linked immunosorbent assay (ELISA) kits (DRG instruments, Germany) were used to assess high-sensitivity C-reactive protein (hsCRP) and Interleukin-6 (IL-6), according to the manufacturer's protocol.

Circulating endotoxin level measurement. The method of lipopolysaccharide (LPS) quantification has been described previously [21]. Briefly, serum samples were diluted to 20% with endotoxin-free water and then heated to 70°C for 10 minutes to inactivate plasma proteins. Serum LPS was then quantified with a commercially available Limulus Amebocyte assay (Cambrex, Verviers, Belgium), according to the manufacturer's protocol. The detection limit of this assay was 0.01 EU/ml. Samples with LPS level below the detection limit were taken as 0.01 EU/ml. All samples were run in duplicate and background subtracted.

Statistical analysis. Results are presented as mean ± standard deviation (SD) or the median and interquartile range (IQR) unless otherwise stated. All data were tested for normality. Categorical data were compared using Chi-square test, continuous data using paired or unpaired Students t-test or one-way ANOVA with Tukey's correction as appropriate. Correlation between continuous variables was examined by Pearson's or Spearman's rank correlation coefficient. Factors associated with ERI/circulating endotoxin levels were further explored by a multivariable linear regression model. Analysis was performed using SPSS v16.0 (SPSS Inc, Chicago, IL). P value of less than 0.05 was considered significant. All probabilities were two-tailed.

Results

The patient characteristics and blood results are summarized in **Table 1**. Mean Hb was 11.3±1.3 g/dL with a median weekly EPO dose 169 IU/wk/kg [IQR 85–257]. EPO Resistance Index for the whole population was 13.7 IU/kg/wk/gm per dl [IQR 6.9–23.9]. Mean pre-HD serum endotoxin levels were appreciably elevated at 0.69±0.30 EU/ml, significantly higher than those of non-CKD patients (0.04±0.01 EU/ml, p<0.001) [22].

Predialysis endotoxin levels correlated to both EPO dose and natural logarithm (Ln) of ERI (r = 0.318, p = 0.03 and r = 0.324, p = 0.03 respectively). EPO dose and Ln ERI demonstrated a stronger relationship with ET than with traditional markers of inflammation, including high sensitivity C-Reactive Protein (hsCRP), Interleukin-6 (IL-6) and albumin. Endotoxin demonstrated a trend towards correlation with haemodynamic instability,

Table 1. Patient demographics, clinical characteristics and laboratory parameter results.

Parameter	Results
Age (yrs)	62.2±14.7
Gender (Male : Female)	36:14
Dialysis vintage (months; median [IQR])	38 [18,70]
Ethnicity (%)	
Caucasian	94
Asian	6
Cause of end-stage renal disease (%)	
Diabetic nephropathy	28
Glomerular disease	22
Adult polycystic kidney disease	12
Urological	10
Multiple myeloma	4
Tubulointerstitial nephritis	4
Unknown	10
Other	10
Diabetes Mellitus (%)	38
Cardiovascular Comorbidities (%)	42
EPO dose (IU/week)	10,000 [7,500–20,000]
ERI (IU/kg/wk/g/dl)	13.7 [6.9–23.9]
Weight (kg)	78.9±17
Body Mass Index (kg/m^2)	27±5.5
Kt/V $_{urea}$	1.3±0.2
Ultrafiltration volume (Litres)	1.97±0.76
Predialysis systolic BP (mmHg)	144±22
Predialysis diastolic BP (mmHg)	76±14
Haemoglobin (g/dl)	11.3±1.3 g
Haematocrit (%)	36±4
Ferritin (ug/L)	307 [213–454]
Phosphate (mmol/L)	1.45±0.39
Adjusted Calcium (mmol/L)	2.4±0.13
Albumin (g/L)	36±3.8
Parathyroid Hormone (ng/L)	240 [96–342]
hsCRP (mg/L)	1.32 [0.82–2.23]
IL-6 (pg/ml)	0.099 [0.086–0.115]

Data are mean±SD or median [IQR].
ERI, EPO Resistance Index, BP, Blood pressure; hsCRP, high sensitivity C Reactive Protein; IL-6, Interleukin 6.

assessed by maximum drop in systolic blood pressure over the HD treatment ($r = -0.270$, p = 0.063), as did ultrafiltration volume ($r = -0.270$, p = 0.058). Endotoxin levels were not significantly affected by the presence of diabetes mellitus (p = 0.61) or aspirin use (p = 0.56).

Ln ERI correlated significantly with ultrafiltration (UF) volume ($r = 0.332$, p = 0.026), a known driver of circulatory stress previously identified to be associated with increased intradialytic endotoxin translocation. Adjusting UF volume for body weight (L/kg), further strengthened this relationship ($r = 0.419$, p = 0.004). Ln ERI demonstrated a trend towards correlation with hsCRP ($r = 0.281$, p = 0.075) and inversely with BMI ($r = -0.259$, p = 0.082).

Ln ERI was not significantly affected by the presence of cardiovascular comorbidities (p = 0.28), diabetes mellitus (p = 0.78), or RAAS blockade (p = 0.41). EPO dose and Ln ERI did not demonstrate significant correlations with other parameters previously identified as linked to erythropoietin resistance, including ferritin, parathyroid hormone levels, ktV and serum albumin. This patient group were characterised by being well dialysed, iron replete with well controlled hyperparathyroidism. Univariable analysis is summarised in **Table 2**.

Multivariable analysis of factors contributing to EPO resistance revealed that serum endotoxin and ultrafiltration volume corrected for weight were independent variables associated with the natural logarithm of EPO resistance index in models adjusted for age, albumin, ferritin, PTH and Kt/V (see **Table 3**). In stepwise linear regression, the model predicting ln ERI comprised ultrafiltration volume corrected for body weight ($\beta = 0.472$, p = 0.001) and hsCRP ($\beta = 0.301$, p = 0.033) with a model fit of $R^2 = 0.297$ (Adjusted $R^2 = 0.260$).

Discussion

In this study, we demonstrated for the first time endotoxin as an independent determinant of EPO resistance. Significant endotoxaemia has been identified and described in the severe CKD and dialysis population [19,23] and these data confirm previous findings. Endotoxin levels seen in HD patients are extremely high, comparable with those reported in severe liver disease [24], post gut irradiation [25] and in severe decompensated congestive heart failure (CHF) [15]. Previous work in patients with acute heart failure showed ET to be systemically elevated, with higher levels in the hepatic vein compared to the left ventricle [26], identifying the gut as the source of ET. In CHF, bowel oedema and hypoperfusion have been identified as the two main factors influencing bowel wall permeability [27], and therefore ET translocation.

Factors involved in EPO resistance that can be modulated include iron deficiency, hyperparathyroidism, inadequate dialysis and malnutrition. Chronic inflammation, a common finding in CKD and dialysis patients, is strongly associated with EPO resistance [20]. Elevated circulating pro-inflammatory cytokines (PIC) including hsCRP, IL-6, and TNF-α demonstrate significant correlation with increasing levels of EPO hyporesponsiveness in

Table 2. Univariable associates of clinical and laboratory parameters with natural logarithm of EPO Resistance Index.

Parameter	R value	P value
Serum endotoxin (EU/ml)	0.311	0.04
Ultrafiltration volume (L)	0.332	0.026
UF volume/body weight (L/kg)	0.470	0.001
Age (years)	0.057	0.711
Body Mass Index (kg/m^2)	−0.259	0.082
Ferritin (ug/L)	0.08	0.6
Parathyroid Hormone (ng/L)	0.19	0.25
Kt/V$_{urea}$	−0.18	0.26
Albumin (g/L)	−0.70	0.67
hsCRP (mg/L)	0.280	0.07
IL-6 (ng/ml)	0.16	0.32

UF, ultrafiltration; hsCRP, high sensitivity C Reactive Protein; IL-6, Interleukin 6.

Table 3. Multivariable analysis model for natural logarithm of EPO Resistance Index (adjusted for age, albumin, ferritin, PTH and Kt/V).

	R^2	Adjusted R^2	Beta	SE	P value
UF volume/body weight (L/kg)	0.325	0.202	40.3	12.2	0.002
Serum endotoxin (EU/ml)	0.214	0.071	1.06	0.49	0.037

the dialysis population [20,28]. A variety of factors have been postulated as drivers of chronic inflammation in CKD, and endotoxin is a potential unifying feature of the interlinked malnutrition, inflammation and CV disease state in dialysis patients.

In this patient group, hsCRP demonstrated a trend towards correlation with ln ERI. This may be attributable to the narrow range of hsCRP values in this patient group, differences in immunoreactivity or insufficient patient numbers to achieve significance. Tachyphylactic response to endotoxin has been previously described, where further contact with, or incremental exposure to endotoxin can result in a diminishing physiological response. The use of native AV fistulae, ultrapure dialysis solution and absence of active intercurrent clinical events such as infection or vascular access issues will affect levels of inflammatory markers in the patient group. The complexities of the uraemic environment, dialysis related and patient specific factors will contribute towards variability in the individual's inflammatory response.

Exposure to ET results in release of a wide variety of PICs and binding via CD14 to systemic immune competent cells. Mechanisms of cytokine related anaemia include reduction of renal EPO production, inhibition of the proliferation and differentiation of erythroid progenitor cells in the bone marrow, impaired iron absorption and reduced iron delivery [29,30]. In animal models, induced endotoxaemia has been demonstrated to suppress ESA ability to stimulate erythropoiesis [31].

Endotoxin contamination of dialysis water has long been recognised as a cause of low grade inflammatory response and CV instability during dialysis [32]. Endotoxin exposure in suboptimally prepared dialysis water has been linked to increased EPO resistance [33], whereas transition to ultrapure dialysate can reduce systemic inflammation and EPO dose requirements [34]. Circulating serum ET levels of 0.69 EU/ml in our patient group were greatly elevated, above even the maximum current permitted levels of endotoxin in dialysate fluid of 0.25 EU/ml. Dialysis water in this study had undetectable levels of endotoxin during the study period, following dual pass water treatment. Circulating ET in these patients therefore originates from an alternate source, namely the gastrointestinal tract.

HD itself appears to be responsible for increasing exposure to translocated intestinal endotoxin, as evidenced by a large difference between patients with very severe CKD stage 5, but not yet started on dialysis, and those receiving dialysis [19]. HD, in combination with ultrafiltration, results in significant systemic haemodynamic perturbation and clinically significant reduction of regional perfusion in critical organs such as the heart and brain [35]. HD is well described as being capable of inducing recurrent cardiac ischaemic injury, associated with long term myocardial damage and increased mortality [36]. Previous work has demonstrated significant correlation between endotoxin and

severity of HD-induced cardiac stunning and relative hypotension [19].

Patients on long-term maintenance haemodialysis have evidence of mucosal ischaemia [37] and ultrafiltration causes a reduction in splanchnic blood volume [38] despite preserved blood pressure [39]. Mesenteric ischaemia results in disrupted gut mucosal structure and function, with increased gut permeability [40]. HD may result in recurrent regional hypoperfusion, particularly in the splanchnic vasculature. This can result in subclinical mesenteric ischaemia and injury, leading to altered membrane permeability and increased translocation of endotoxin.

Increasing ERI is associated with higher volumes of fluid removal during dialysis, and unsurprisingly this association increases when UF volume is corrected for body weight. Previous work has demonstrated significant correlation between endotoxaemia and dialysis induced haemodynamic stress, including severity of HD-induced cardiac stunning, markers of cardiac injury and relative hypotension [19]. Ultrafiltration volume is potentially a driver of both myocardial and splanchnic hypoperfusion, with end-organ injury resulting in system specific short-term injury and long-term damage, as well as a generalised inflammatory response.

Adding endotoxin into a simple linear regression model for ln ERI containing UF volume/weight and hsCRP strengthened the R^2 of the model (0.307), but both ET and hsCRP were no longer independent predictors within it. This is not unexpected, given the underlying pathophysiological processes linking these factors. The relationships between potential causes and consequences of endotoxaemia, may, in turn, influence EPO resistance. Multivariable analysis confirmed the independent association of serum endotoxin and of ultrafiltration volume corrected for weight with the natural logarithm of EPO resistance index, when adjusted for factors previously identified as influencing the response to EPO.

In terms of potential intervention, extended dialysis schedules are associated with marked reductions in UF requirements and intradialytic hypotension, lessening the haemodynamic insult [19], as well as improving Hb and lowering EPO requirements [41].

This study has potential limitations. Although this observational study was able to demonstrate a relationship between endotoxaemia and EPO resistance in HD patients, the sample size is inadequate to fully resolve factors relating to the degree of endotoxaemia or EPO hypo-responsiveness. Patients were not prevented from eating during HD, which could potentially influence gut perfusion and permeability, however the relatively high fibre and low fat meals provided are likely to have only limited impact on ET translocation. Areas of further work include longitudinal studies on ET, inflammatory response and EPO requirements, exploration of the effects of reduced endotoxin exposure on EPO requirements, and comparison of ET and ERI between different dialysis modalities.

Summary

This study suggests that endotoxaemia, either by direct interaction, or through its well documented effects on systemic inflammation, is a significant and potentially dominant factor in setting levels of EPO requirement. It raises the possibility that elevated EPO doses may in part merely be identifying patients subjected to significant haemodynamic perturbation, and suffering the myriad of negative biological consequences arising from sustained systemic exposure to endotoxin.

A greater understanding of the mechanism and factors influencing endotoxin translocation in the dialysis population is required. In addition, turning our attention to the dialysis procedure itself may yield additional benefits, both in terms of

EPO requirements, but also alleviating the haemodynamic impact of HD to improve long-term patient outcomes.

Acknowledgments

The authors gratefully acknowledge the time and commitment of patients and staff at Royal Derby Hospital.

Author Contributions

Conceived and designed the experiments: CWM JOB. Performed the experiments: JOB CCS PKT. Analyzed the data: LEAH JOB CCS PKT CWM. Contributed reagents/materials/analysis tools: LEAH JOB CCS PKL. Wrote the paper: LEAH JOB CCS PKL CWM.

References

1. Winearls CG, Oliver DO, Pippard MJ, Reid C, Downing MR, et al. (1986) Effect of human erythropoietin derived from recombinant DNA on the anaemia of patients maintained by chronic haemodialysis. Lancet 2: 1175–1178.
2. Ofsthun N, Labrecque J, Lacson E, Keen M, Lazarus JM (2003) The effects of higher hemoglobin levels on mortality and hospitalization in hemodialysis patients. Kidney Int 63: 1908–1914.
3. Macdougall IC, Tomson CR, Steenkamp M, Ansell D (2010) Relative risk of death in UK haemodialysis patients in relation to achieved haemoglobin from 1999 to 2005: an observational study using UK Renal Registry data incorporating 30,040 patient-years of follow-up. Nephrol Dial Transplant 25: 914–919.
4. Perlman RL, Finkelstein FO, Liu L, Roys E, Kiser M, et al. (2005) Quality of life in chronic kidney disease (CKD): a cross-sectional analysis in the Renal Research Institute-CKD study. Am J Kidney Dis 45: 658–666.
5. Pfeffer MA, Burdmann EA, Chen CY, Cooper ME, de Zeeuw D, et al. (2009) A trial of darbepoetin alfa in type 2 diabetes and chronic kidney disease. N Engl J Med 361: 2019–2032.
6. Singh AK, Szczech L, Tang KL, Barnhart H, Sapp S, et al. (2006) Correction of anemia with epoetin alfa in chronic kidney disease. N Engl J Med 355: 2085–2098.
7. Drueke TB, Locatelli F, Clyne N, Eckardt KU, Macdougall IC, et al. (2006) Normalization of hemoglobin level in patients with chronic kidney disease and anemia. N Engl J Med 355: 2071–2084.
8. Besarab A, Bolton WK, Browne JK, Egrie JC, Nissenson AR, et al. (1998) The effects of normal as compared with low hematocrit values in patients with cardiac disease who are receiving hemodialysis and epoetin. N Engl J Med 339: 584–590.
9. Badve SV, Hawley CM, Johnson DW (2011) Is the problem with the vehicle or the destination? Does high-dose ESA or high haemoglobin contribute to poor outcomes in CKD? Nephrology (Carlton) 16: 144–153.
10. Stivelman JC (1989) Resistance to recombinant human erythropoietin therapy: a real clinical entity? Semin Nephrol 9: 8–11.
11. Locatelli F, Aljama P, Barany P, Canaud B, Carrera F, et al. (2004) Revised European best practice guidelines for the management of anaemia in patients with chronic renal failure. Nephrol Dial Transplant 19 Suppl 2: ii1–47.
12. Regidor DL, Kopple JD, Kovesdy CP, Kilpatrick RD, McAllister CJ, et al. (2006) Associations between changes in hemoglobin and administered erythropoiesis-stimulating agent and survival in hemodialysis patients. J Am Soc Nephrol 17: 1181–1191.
13. Drueke T (2001) Hyporesponsiveness to recombinant human erythropoietin. Nephrol Dial Transplant 16 Suppl 7: 25–28.
14. Richardson D (2002) Clinical factors influencing sensitivity and response to epoetin. Nephrol Dial Transplant 17 Suppl 1: 53–59.
15. Anker SD, Egerer KR, Volk HD, Kox WJ, Poole-Wilson PA, et al. (1997) Elevated soluble CD14 receptors and altered cytokines in chronic heart failure. Am J Cardiol 79: 1426–1430.
16. Kotanko P, Carter M, Levin NW (2006) Intestinal bacterial microflora—a potential source of chronic inflammation in patients with chronic kidney disease. Nephrol Dial Transplant 21: 2057–2060.
17. Charalambous BM, Stephens RC, Feavers IM, Montgomery HE (2007) Role of bacterial endotoxin in chronic heart failure: the gut of the matter. Shock 28: 15–23.
18. Feng SY, Samarasinghe T, Phillips DJ, Alexiou T, Hollis JH, et al. (2010) Acute and chronic effects of endotoxin on cerebral circulation in lambs. Am J Physiol Regul Integr Comp Physiol 298: R760–766.
19. McIntyre CW, Harrison LE, Eldehni MT, Jefferies HJ, Szeto CC, et al. (2011) Circulating endotoxemia: a novel factor in systemic inflammation and cardiovascular disease in chronic kidney disease. Clin J Am Soc Nephrol 6: 133–141.
20. Gunnell J, Yeun JY, Depner TA, Kaysen GA (1999) Acute-phase response predicts erythropoietin resistance in hemodialysis and peritoneal dialysis patients. Am J Kidney Dis 33: 63–72.
21. Brenchley JM, Price DA, Schacker TW, Asher TE, Silvestri G, et al. (2006) Microbial translocation is a cause of systemic immune activation in chronic HIV infection. Nat Med 12: 1365–1371.
22. John SG, Owen PJ, Harrison LE, Szeto CC, Lai KB, et al. (2010) The impact of antihypertensive drug therapy on endotoxemia in elderly patients with chronic kidney disease. Clin J Am Soc Nephrol 6: 2389–2394.
23. Szeto CC, Kwan BC, Chow KM, Lai KB, Chung KY, et al. (2008) Endotoxemia is related to systemic inflammation and atherosclerosis in peritoneal dialysis patients. Clin J Am Soc Nephrol 3: 431–436.
24. Lumsden AB, Henderson JM, Kutner MH (1988) Endotoxin levels measured by a chromogenic assay in portal, hepatic and peripheral venous blood in patients with cirrhosis. Hepatology 8: 232–236.
25. Maxwell A, Gaffin SL, Wells MT (1986) Radiotherapy, endotoxaemia, and nausea. Lancet 1: 1148–1149.
26. Peschel T, Schonauer M, Thiele H, Anker SD, Schuler G, et al. (2003) Invasive assessment of bacterial endotoxin and inflammatory cytokines in patients with acute heart failure. Eur J Heart Fail 5: 609–614.
27. Krack A, Sharma R, Figulla HR, Anker SD (2005) The importance of the gastrointestinal system in the pathogenesis of heart failure. Eur Heart J 26: 2368–2374.
28. Kalantar-Zadeh K, McAllister CJ, Lehn RS, Lee GH, Nissenson AR, et al. (2003) Effect of malnutrition-inflammation complex syndrome on EPO hyporesponsiveness in maintenance hemodialysis patients. Am J Kidney Dis 42: 761–773.
29. Carrero JJ, Stenvinkel P (2010) Inflammation in end-stage renal disease–what have we learned in 10 years? Semin Dial 23: 498–509.
30. Weiss G, Goodnough LT (2005) Anemia of chronic disease. N Engl J Med 352: 1011–1023.
31. Brendt P, Horwat A, Schafer ST, Dreyer SC, Gothert J, et al. (2009) Lipopolysaccharide evokes resistance to erythropoiesis induced by the long-acting erythropoietin analogue darbepoetin alfa in rats. Anesth Analg 109: 705–711.
32. Raij L, Shapiro FL, Michael AF (1973) Endotoxemia in febrile reactions during hemodialysis. Kidney Int 4: 57–60.
33. Molina M, Navarro MJ, Palacios ME, de Gracia MC, Garcia Hernandez MA, et al. (2007) [Importance of ultrapure dialysis liquid in response to the treatment of renal anaemia with darbepoetin in patients receiving haemodialysis]. Nefrologia 27: 196–201.
34. Go AS, Chertow GM, Fan D, McCulloch CE, Hsu CY (2004) Chronic kidney disease and the risks of death, cardiovascular events, and hospitalization. N Engl J Med 351: 1296–1305.
35. McIntyre CW, Burton JO, Selby NM, Leccisotti L, Korsheed S, et al. (2008) Hemodialysis-induced cardiac dysfunction is associated with an acute reduction in global and segmental myocardial blood flow. Clin J Am Soc Nephrol 3: 19–26.
36. Burton JO, Jefferies HJ, Selby NM, McIntyre CW (2009) Hemodialysis-induced cardiac injury: determinants and associated outcomes. Clin J Am Soc Nephrol 4: 914–920.
37. Diebel L, Kozol R, Wilson RF, Mahajan S, Abu-Hamdan D, et al. (1993) Gastric intramucosal acidosis in patients with chronic kidney failure. Surgery 113: 520–526.
38. Mann JF, Gerstein HC, Pogue J, Bosch J, Yusuf S (2001) Renal insufficiency as a predictor of cardiovascular outcomes and the impact of ramipril: the HOPE randomized trial. Ann Intern Med 134: 629–636.
39. Jakob SM, Ruokonen E, Vuolteenaho O, Lampainen E, Takala J (2001) Splanchnic perfusion during hemodialysis: evidence for marginal tissue perfusion. Crit Care Med 29: 1393–1398.
40. Khanna A, Rossman JE, Fung HL, Caty MG (2001) Intestinal and hemodynamic impairment following mesenteric ischemia/reperfusion. J Surg Res 99: 114–119.
41. Chan CT, Floras JS, Miller JA, Richardson RM, Pierratos A (2002) Regression of left ventricular hypertrophy after conversion to nocturnal hemodialysis. Kidney Int 61: 2235–2239.

6

Should the Arteriovenous Fistula be Created before Starting Dialysis?: A Decision Analytic Approach

Swapnil Hiremath[1,2,3]*, Greg Knoll[1,2], Milton C. Weinstein[3]

1 Division of Nephrology, Kidney Research Center, Ottawa Hospital Research Institute, Ottawa, Ontario, Canada, 2 Clinical Epidemiology Program, Ottawa Hospital Research Institute, Ottawa, Ontario, Canada, 3 Department of Health Policy and Management, Harvard School of Public Health, Boston, Massachusetts, United States of America

Abstract

Background: An arteriovenous fistula (AVF) is considered the vascular access of choice, but uncertainty exists about the optimal time for its creation in pre-dialysis patients. The aim of this study was to determine the optimal vascular access referral strategy for stage 4 (glomerular filtration rate <30 ml/min/1.73 m^2) chronic kidney disease patients using a decision analytic framework.

Methods: A Markov model was created to compare two strategies: refer all stage 4 chronic kidney disease patients for an AVF versus wait until the patient starts dialysis. Data from published observational studies were used to estimate the probabilities used in the model. A Markov cohort analysis was used to determine the optimal strategy with life expectancy and quality adjusted life expectancy as the outcomes. Sensitivity analyses, including a probabilistic sensitivity analysis, were performed using Monte Carlo simulation.

Results: The wait strategy results in a higher life expectancy (66.6 versus 65.9 months) and quality adjusted life expectancy (38.9 versus 38.5 quality adjusted life months) than immediate AVF creation. It was robust across all the parameters except at higher rates of progression and lower rates of ischemic steal syndrome.

Conclusions: Early creation of an AVF, as recommended by most guidelines, may not be the preferred strategy in all pre-dialysis patients. Further research on cost implications and patient preferences for treatment options needs to be done before recommending early AVF creation.

Editor: Shree Ram Singh, National Cancer Institute, United States of America

Funding: The authors have no support or funding to report.

Competing Interests: The authors have declared that no competing interests exist.

* E-mail: shiremath@toh.on.ca

Introduction

The burden of chronic kidney disease (CKD) continues to increase, with 571,414 patients in the end-stage renal disease (ESRD) program in the United States in 2009 [1]. The majority of these patients, 398,861, are on hemodialysis. An even greater number of patients have advanced kidney failure with a glomerular filtration rate less than 30 ml/min/1.73 m^2 (Stage 4 CKD) [2]. In the United States alone, it is estimated that 0.35% of the adult population has stage 4 CKD, which translates into more than 800,000 people. In 2009, 116,395 CKD patients progressed to ESRD and started hemodialysis in the United States [1].

The arteriovenous fistula (AVF) has been identified as the optimal vascular access for hemodialysis patients based on improved survival and fewer complications as compared to arteriovenous grafts (AVG) and tunneled central venous catheters (CVC) [3]. Despite this, more than 80% of incident hemodialysis patients start with a CVC as their vascular access [1]. Timely creation of an AVF before the need for dialysis therapy may allow adequate time for the fistula to mature as well as provide sufficient time to perform another vascular access procedure if the first attempt fails, thus obviating the need for a CVC, though firm evidence for the same is lacking [4,5]. Hence, most guidelines recommend assessment of patients for access creation at the CKD 4 stage [5–9].

However, early AVF creation is not without problems. A small number of patients may develop ischemic steal syndrome from arterial ischemia in the distal limb or develop high output heart failure. Both of these complications usually require AVF ligation [10,11]. In addition, early AVF creation, prior to dialysis, will likely result in many patients undergoing unnecessary surgery since most stage 4 CKD patients are much more likely to die than to actually develop ESRD and require dialysis [12]. Lastly, greater than 25% of AVF may never mature enough to be used functionally [13].

Thus creation of an AVF when a patient has stage 4 CKD but is not yet on dialysis has both risks and potential benefits. There are no validated prediction models to determine which patients will progress to ESRD and thus should have an AVF created. Therefore, patients in stage 4 CKD have two options; they can either proceed with early AVF creation or start dialysis with a CVC and proceed with AVF later. We used a decision-analytic model to compare these two treatment options faced by patients with stage 4 CKD. The model estimated survival as well as quality-adjusted survival.

Methods

The Decision Model

We used a Markov model to compare two treatment strategies for stage 4 CKD patients: (1) AVF strategy and (2) Wait strategy. In the model, hypothetical cohorts of patients are followed for the remainder of their lifetimes [14]. With each monthly 'cycle' of the model, patients may move between several different health states (e.g. CKD stage 4 with no AVF, CKD stage 4 with AVF, Dialysis with CVC, Dialysis with AVF, death) according to the occurrence of clinical events (e.g. progression to dialysis, development of heart failure due to AVF, etc). The probabilities that each of these events occurs was determined using the best available data from the literature. Because some of the transition probabilities depend on the time since entering a state (such as mortality after starting dialysis), we created "tunnel" states which are essentially copies of a state that track the length of time spent in the state [15].

By simulating outcomes in large numbers of identical patients, the average accumulated survival time with the two treatment strategies may be estimated. For our base case analysis, we chose a 70-year-old patient with CKD stage 4, because the 65–74 year age group is the fastest growing segment in the dialysis population [1]. It also represents a cohort where clinical equipoise regarding the optimal strategy is the greatest [16].

Our decision model (Figure 1) evaluated the following two treatment strategies:

1. AVF Strategy: CKD stage 4 patients get referred for an AVF; and

2. Wait Strategy: CKD stage 4 patients are not referred for an AVF. When they reach the point of starting dialysis, they get a CVC as their vascular access and are then referred for AVF surgery.

During each cycle of the model (1 month in this analysis), hypothetical patients in any given health state are at risk of several events, which may result in transitions to other health states. For certain health states, we created "tunnel" states to force patients to remain in that state for a fixed number of cycles (e.g. to account for a three-month maturation period for AVF). Stage 4 CKD patients may progress to dialysis; CKD or dialysis patients with an AVF may develop heart failure or ischemic steal syndrome; patients with a CVC may develop central vein stenosis; death may occur while they are still in CKD stage 4 or while they are on dialysis.

Assumptions

The base case was that of a 70 year old man with CKD stage 4. We assumed that the only choice of renal replacement therapy

(RRT) for this patient was hemodialysis; peritoneal dialysis and renal transplantation were not considered in this analysis.

In the AVF strategy:

1. All patients with CKD stage 4 would be referred for an AVF; it would take 2 months to create an AVF and 3 months for it to mature and be functional.

2. If an AVF failed, another attempt to make an AVF would not be made.

3. If a patient with an AVF developed CHF or steal, the AVF would be ligated in the same month. Hence heart failure and steal syndrome were modeled as temporary health states.

In the wait strategy:

1. All CKD 4 patients progressing to need dialysis would start with a CVC.

2. Once on dialysis, they would all be referred to get an AVF, with the same waiting and maturation period as above.

3. During the 2 cycles of waiting to get AVF surgery, a proportion of patients would decide not to have an AVF and remain on dialysis with a CVC.

Probabilities

Estimates and plausible ranges of event probabilities were obtained from published articles and expert opinion (Table 1). Both deterministic threshold analyses and probabilistic sensitivity analyses were performed, as described below.

We identified 8 studies in the literature on mortality and progression to ESRD for stage 4 CKD patients [12,17–23] (Table 2). The rates of progression varied from a low of 4.27 per 100 person-years from a cardiac database [12] that likely had many patients with ischemic nephropathy, to a high of 14.3 per 100 person-years [20] from a nephrology database that had a significant proportion of proteinuric patients at high risk for progression. For our base case we used data from O'Hare et al [21] (9.31 per 100 person-years), since they provided data for patients aged 65 to 74 years. The lowest and highest rates of progression from the 8 studies were used in the sensitivity analyses. The mortality rate for stage 4 CKD patients ranged from a low of 4.5 per 100 person-years to a high of 33.45 per 100 person years in the same 2 studies [12,20]. As for progression, we used data from the O'Hare study [21], (mortality rate 11.68 per 100 person-years) with the extreme values used for sensitivity analyses.

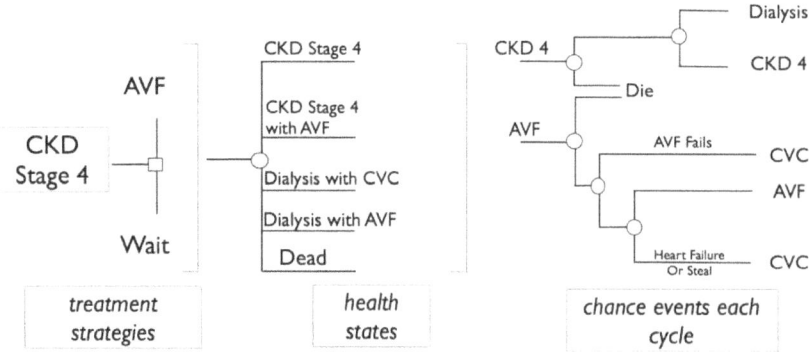

Figure 1. Schematic representation of the decision-analysis model.

Table 1. Probabilities and Utilities.

Variables	Best Estimate	Range (for sensitivity analysis)	Distribution	Reference
Rate of progression to ESRD	0.0076	0.00356–0.019	Lognormal	19
CKD stage 4 mortality	0.0097	0.00375–0.0279	Lognormal	19
Mortality on dialysis with CVC in first three months	0.042	0.0126–0.0503	Lognormal	27
Mortality on dialysis with CVC after three months	0.020	0.0126–0.0503	Lognormal	27
Mortality on dialysis with AVF in first three months	0.018	0.0061–0.0232	Lognormal	27
Mortality on dialysis with AVF after three months	0.013	0.0061–0.0232	Lognormal	27
Patient refusal for an AVF	0.0467	0.01–0.1	Beta	29
Central vein stenosis	0.017	0.001–0.05	Beta	29
Heart Failure due to AVF	0.0004	0.001–0.09	Lognormal	Expert opinion
Mortality due to heart failure	0.012	0.01–0.5	Beta	Expert Opinion
Surgical mortality	0.001	0.0001–0.005	Beta	Expert opinion
Ischemic steal syndrome	0.0504	0.001–0.09	Lognormal	29
AVF Failure: first three months	0.025	0–0.9	Lognormal	28
AVF Failure: after three months	0.016	0–0.9	Lognormal	28
AVF failure on dialysis	0.010	0–0.9	Lognormal	28
Utility of CKD stage 4 without AVF	0.62	0.40–0.84	Triangular	31
Utility of CKD stage 4 with AVF	0.62	0.40–0.84	Triangular	31
Utility of dialysis	0.51	0.20–0.82	Triangular	31

Six studies were identified which reported on mortality rates for patients starting dialysis with a CVC or fistula [24–29] (Table 3). The two studies in prevalent patients were published in 2001 and 2002, comprised younger patients (mean age <60 yrs), and had mortality rates of 7.29 to 13 per 100 person-years for patients with an AVF and 15.16 to 23 per 100 person-years for patients with CVC [25,27]. In contrast, the more recent studies included older, incident patients with higher mortality rates [24,26,28,29]. The mortality rate in patients with CVC, however, was approximately 1.5 to 2 times that of patients with an AVF in all the studies [24–29]. We used data from Xue et. al. for our base case, since that study provided separate mortality rates according to access type

for the first 90 days of dialysis and thereafter as well as included elderly patients in the 65–74 age range [29]. A tunnel state was created to account for the fact that the mortality rate is significantly higher in the first three months of dialysis before it levels off.

Rates of fistula failure were obtained from a Dutch prospective study [30]. Fistula failure rates due to the loss of fistula patency before cannulation were used to model failure rates in the CKD stage. Functional failure, which refers to loss of fistula patency after cannulation, was used to model failure rates in the dialysis states. We incorporated secondary fistula failure rates, which include intervening manipulations designed to re-establish or maintain the

Table 2. Summary of literature on mortality and progression to ESRD in CKD stage 4.

Study	Mean age (years)	GFR (ml/min)	Progression to ESRD	Mortality	Population
Keith (2001)	73.6±13.6	15–29	19.9%*	45.7%*	Large HMO
Go (2004)	70.1±14.5	15–29		11.36 per 100 PY‡	Large HMO
Patel (2005)	70.0±10.0	15–29	14.2 per 100 PY	20.1 per 100 PY	Veterans
O'Hare (2007)	65–74	15–29	9.31 per 100 PY	11.68 per 100 PY	Veterans
O'Hare (2007)	75–84	15–29	6.31 per 100 PY	15.39 per 100 PY	Veterans
Roderick (2009)	83.2±7.1	<30		19–29 per 100 PY	UK General Practice
Keough-Ryan (2008)	69.2±13.2	<30	4.27 per 100 PY	33.45 per 100 PY	Post acute cardiac event
Levin (2008)	66.8±14.5	<30	14.3 per 100 PY	4.5 per 100 PY	Referred population
Conway (2009)	Median 71.6	<30	3.8%†	10.4%†	Referred population

*crude data in percentages, over 66 months of follow up.
†crude 1 year data in percentages.
‡Age-Standardized Rates.
PY: patient-years.
HMO: Health Maintenance Oraganization.

Table 3. Summary of literature on difference in mortality with CVC and AVF.

Study	Mean age	Mortality with AVF (per 100 PY)	Mortality with CVC (per 100 PY)	Population
Dhingra (2001) Diabetes	59.2	13*	22*	Prevalent, DMMS Wave 1
Dhingra (2001) No Diabetes	59.2	11*	23*	Prevalent, DMMS Wave 1
Pastan (2002)	58.3±0.2	7.29	15.16	Prevalent ESRD Network 6
Xue (2003) First 90 days	~75	28.8	60.4	Incident Medicare
Xue (2003) Next 9 months	~75	21.6	52.8	Incident Medicare
Polkinghorne (2004)	61 (range 48–71)	8.6	26.1	Incident
Moist (2008)	68 (median)		HR 1.6†	Incident
Bradbury (2009)	62.5±15	9.96‡	53.62‡	Incident, DOPPS I & II

*Adapted from Adjusted patient survival data.
†Hazard ratio, compared to mortality with AVF.
‡Six month follow up data.
PY: patient-years.

functionality. Tunnel states were created to account for the high fistula failure rates in the first 3 months after creation which plateau thereafter. The probabilities of developing steal syndrome and central vein stenosis, and of refusing dialysis, were derived from a cross-sectional study [31]. Since there were only case reports and no summary estimates of the incidence rate of high output heart failure with AVF, it was assumed to be 5 per 1000 patient-months based on expert opinion (SH, GK). Since there were no data on operative mortality rate for an AVF creation or ligation surgery, it was similarly assumed to be 1 in 1000 based on expert opinion (SH, GK). Both of these subjective estimates were subjected to sensitivity analysis.

Outcomes

Life expectancy with each strategy was calculated based on the average accumulated survival time. Quality-adjusted life expectancy was calculated by weighting the time spent in each state with the preference-based utility of that state [32]. The utilities for the health states of CKD stage 4 and dialysis were obtained from a Canadian study that measured the Short Form-6D (SF-6D) and Health Utilities Index Mark 3 (HUI), the latter of which was used [33]. We assumed that an AVF would not result in a significant disutility for CKD stage 4 patients. We also assumed that utilities for dialysis patients with CVC and AVF would be the same; sensitivity analyses were performed to test these assumption. Utilities assigned to each month were the average of those for the patient's health state at the beginning and end of the month [34].

Analysis

The analysis was done using a Markov cohort method with 100,000 patients. Model verification (debugging) was done by building up the model from simple to more complex, checking each step visually, examining the state probabilities from the cohort analysis, exploring certain extreme values and doing a sensitivity analysis on all variables. The model was calibrated by comparing simulated events (mortality for dialysis patients in the model) to observed ones (from the USRDS report) [1]. A probabilistic sensitivity analysis was done by assigning probability distributions around model parameters and by using Monte Carlo simulation [35] (table 4). All analysis was done using TreeAge Pro 2008 software (version 1.3.1, Williamstown, MA) and JMP (version 8.0, SAS Inc., Cary, NC).

Results

Base Case Analysis

The results of the base case analysis showed that the wait strategy resulted in a slightly higher life expectancy (66.55 vs 65.9 months) and quality-adjusted life expectancy (QALE) (38.89 vs. 38.49 quality-adjusted life months) as compared to the AVF strategy (Table 5).

Table 4. Probability Distributions and parameter estimates used in the Probabilistic Sensitivity Analysis.

Variables	Distribution	Parameters
Rate of progression to ESRD	Lognormal	$\mu = -2.333; \sigma = 0.406$
CKD stage 4 mortality	Lognormal	$\mu = -2.577; \sigma = 0.415$
Mortality on dialysis with CVC in first three months	Lognormal	$\mu = -5.473; \sigma = 0.604$
Mortality on dialysis with CVC after three months	Lognormal	$\mu = -6.215; \sigma = 0.759$
Mortality on dialysis with AVF in first three months	Lognormal	$\mu = -6.320; \sigma = 0.901$
Mortality on dialysis with AVF after three months	Lognormal	$\mu = -6.645; \sigma = 0.724$
Patient refusal for an AVF	Beta	$r = 28; n = 599$
Central vein stenosis	Beta	$r = 10; n = 599$
Heart Failure due to AVF	Lognormal	$\mu = -9.210; \sigma = 0.601$
Mortality due to heart failure	Beta	$r = 5; n = 404$
Surgical mortality	Beta	$r = 1; n = 1000$
Ischemic steal syndrome	Lognormal	$\mu = -2.987; \sigma = 0.768$
AVF Failure: first three months	Lognormal	$\mu = -3.689; \sigma = 1.010$
AVF Failure: after three months	Lognormal	$\mu = -4.135; \sigma = 0.970$
AVF failure on dialysis	Lognormal	$\mu = -4.605; \sigma = 1.177$
Utility of CKD stage 4	Triangular	low = 0.40; most likely = 0.62; high = 0.84
Utility of dialysis	Triangular	low = 0.20; most Likely = 0.51; high = 0.82

Table 5. Results of base case analysis.

Strategy	Life expectancy (in months)	Gain in life expectancy	Quality adjusted life expectancy (in months)	Gain in quality adjusted life expectancy
Wait	66.55	0.65	38.89	0.50
AVF	65.90	-	38.49	-

Sensitivity Analysis

Multiple one-way sensitivity analyses were carried out for all the variables entered in the model. The optimal strategy changed at very high rates of progression of CKD to dialysis as well at lower rates of steal syndrome than used in the base case analysis. When the rate of progression was higher than 0.01126 (corresponding to 14.5 per 100 patient-years), the optimal strategy was to refer patients for AVF creation (Figure 2). The additional LE and QALE obtained at the highest rate of progression used in the sensitivity analysis were 0.05 and 0.03 months respectively. Similarly, the optimal strategy changed to AVF creation when the probability of steal syndrome was lower than 0.023. The additional LE and QALE obtained with the AVF strategy when there was no steal syndrome were 0.5 and 0.3 months respectively. If the utility of CKD stage 4 patients with an AVF was higher than 0.7 whilst maintaining the utility of CKD stage 4 patients without an AVF at 0.62, the optimal strategy reverted to the AVF strategy. When the fistula failure rates were changed to zero, the optimal strategy did not change. The optimal strategy is also otherwise robust across the range of probabilities tested for all other parameters (Table 1).

A two-way sensitivity analysis with respect to the probabilities of progression and steal syndrome is shown in Figure 3. It demonstrates that as the rate of progression to dialysis increases, the AVF strategy becomes optimal despite increasing probability of steal syndrome.

Incremental outcomes from the probabilistic sensitivity analysis, expressed as a difference of quality adjusted life expectancy obtained between the two strategies, were obtained using a Monte Carlo simulation. The probability that the wait strategy is optimal was 91.7% (Figure 4).

Discussion

In this decision analysis, we have shown that the wait strategy is the optimal strategy for our base case of a 70-year old patient with stage 4 CKD. However, the gains in life expectancy and quality-adjusted life expectancy are likely to be less than one month. The analysis was robust across the range of values for most variables in the model, with the possible exception of the rate of progression to ESRD and the rate of steal syndrome.

These results suggest that recommendations of the Fistula First Breakthrough Initiative and the various society guidelines, to

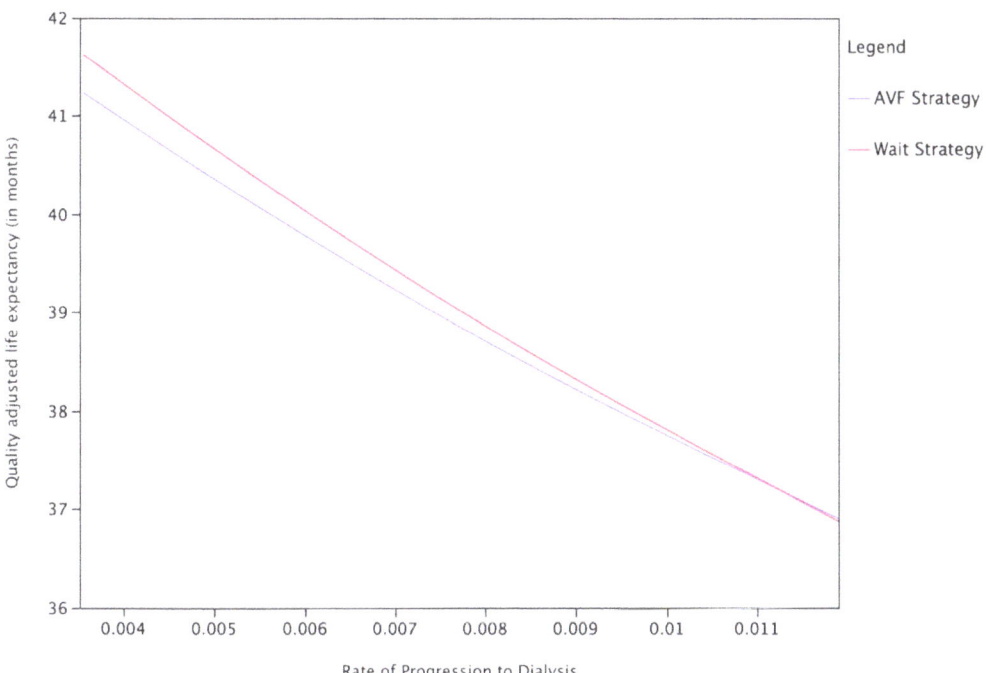

Figure 2. One way sensitivity analysis based on rate of progression of CKD stage 4 to dialysis: This demonstrates that the wait strategy results in a higher quality-adjusted life expectancy at lower rates of progression and the AVF strategy results in a higher quality adjusted life expectancy at higher rates of progression of CKD to dialysis.

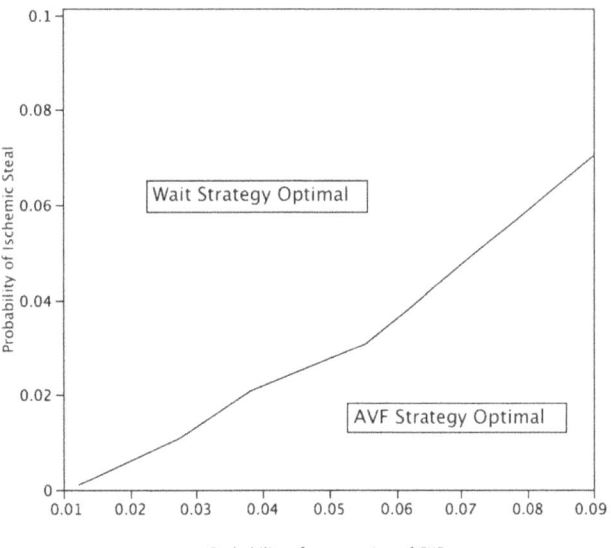

Figure 3. Two-way sensitivity analysis plotting rate of progression to dialysis and probability of steal: This demonstrates that the wait strategy results in a higher quality-adjusted life expectancy at lower rates of progression and lower probability of ischemic steal and the AVF strategy results in a higher quality adjusted life expectancy at higher rates of progression of CKD to dialysis and higher rates of ischemic steal.

consider early creation of AVF in the predialysis period, may not apply all patients. It might especially be prudent to wait in patients similar to our base case, who have a slow rate of progression and high rates of competing events. Indeed, it may not be optimal to wait in patients with a high rate of progression (such as proteinuric diabetic nephropathy) though the quality-adjusted life expectancy gained by early fistula creation in such patients is less than one month. Additionally, the assumption underlying these conclusions is that the patients who wait will get an AVF soon after initiation of dialysis, and will not be exposed to the deleterious effects of a CVC beyond 3 months. The strategy of initiating dialysis with a catheter in appropriate patients has been suggested before [36] and our study helps to quantify the benefit of such a decision. Also, conversion from a CVC to AVF has been reported to be associated with an improved survival [24] and hospitalization risk is also higher for patients who continue with a CVC compared to those who convert from a CVC to an AV access [37]. It could be argued that patients who start dialysis with a CVC may not want to have another surgery for AVF creation, but we incorporated that by inserting a parameter for higher patient refusal for AVF in the wait strategy.

In the present study, we are not suggesting that patients should start with and remain on a CVC, or that CVCs are superior to AVFs as vascular access. It has been suggested, however, that in the elderly population, and in octogenarians specifically, that an assessment of life expectancy and quality of life should be made while planning for vascular access [36,38].

The model construction itself had some limitations. We considered only hemodialysis as an option for our base case analysis. While this is the most common initial treatment modality for patients fitting our base case [39], some patients will indeed opt for peritoneal dialysis or kidney transplantation. This may limit the generalizability of our findings to all stage 4 CKD patients. We also assumed that only one attempt would be made to create an

AVF. This assumption resulted in most patients having a failed AVF by the time they started hemodialysis. In clinical practice, it could be argued that many of these patients would have had a second attempt at AVF creation. In our cross-sectional study, we found that a median of two attempts (range, 1 to 4) were made at AVF creation [31]. However, in sensitivity analysis, the wait strategy remained optimal despite an AVF failure rate of zero, suggesting that incorporating multiple attempts will not change the result. Lastly, we did not include AV grafts (AVG) as an option for vascular access. AVGs have been compared to AVFs in a decision analysis and were reported to have a lower median survival, albeit less than expected, by 2.6 months [40].

There were limitations related to the data sources used in the model. Since no randomized controlled trial has ever been done to compare outcomes between AVF and CVC in dialysis patients, we had to rely on data from administrative sources to obtain estimates of mortality rates in patients with CVC and AVF. However, many incident dialysis patients with a CVC in these databases may have been patients with acute renal failure in whom the mortality rate may be much higher than for patients with known renal disease and a planned start with a CVC. More accurate data reflecting lower mortality with CVC would, however, make the results favoring the wait strategy even stronger. We used post-intervention figures from a Dutch study in our estimates of fistula failure rates [30]. These figures might be optimistic in North American situations since European centers have a significantly higher prevalence of AVF compared to CVCs [41]; however lower fistula survival rates would make the wait strategy even more favorable. We chose wait times for access creation based on local data, however this may vary at other centres and novel approaches such as direct nephrologist selection for operation have resulted in shorter waiting times for access creation [42].

There were limitations related to the utilities in the model. We assumed that the utility for a patient with CKD stage 4 with an AVF would be the same as that of a patient with CKD stage 4 who did not have a fistula. Although the optimal strategy would change if having an AVF increased the utility for a CKD stage 4 patient, this is an unlikely scenario. In addition, we assumed that the utility of a dialysis patient with a CVC would be the same as for a dialysis patient with an AVF. Indeed, despite nephrologists' opinion of the AVF being the optimal access, interviews with patients who have refused an AVF suggest that they do not always focus on long-term mortality benefit, but rather day-to-day use and quality of life with a vascular access [43]. Although sensitivity analyses conducted on this parameter was robust, further studies are needed to correctly elucidate preference utilities in CKD and dialysis patients with different vascular access.

We did not assess the comparative costs of the two strategies, nor did we perform an incremental cost-effectiveness analysis. Because of the higher number of surgeries in the AVF strategy and the fact that the cost of an AVF surgery is higher than that of CVC insertion, it is likely that the cost would be higher in the AVF strategy, thus making the wait strategy dominant (more QALYs at lower cost) over the AVF strategy.

In summary, this analysis suggests that the optimal strategy in a typical elderly stage 4 CKD patients should be to wait and start with a CVC when required followed by AVF creation. This strategy was robust across most sensitivity analysis. However, it might not be optimal for patients with a very high probability of progression to dialysis, such as patients with proteinuric diabetic nephropathy. Further studies should be done to obtain more precise estimates of progression and develop prediction rules for progression of renal failure in CKD stage 4 which take competing events of death into account.

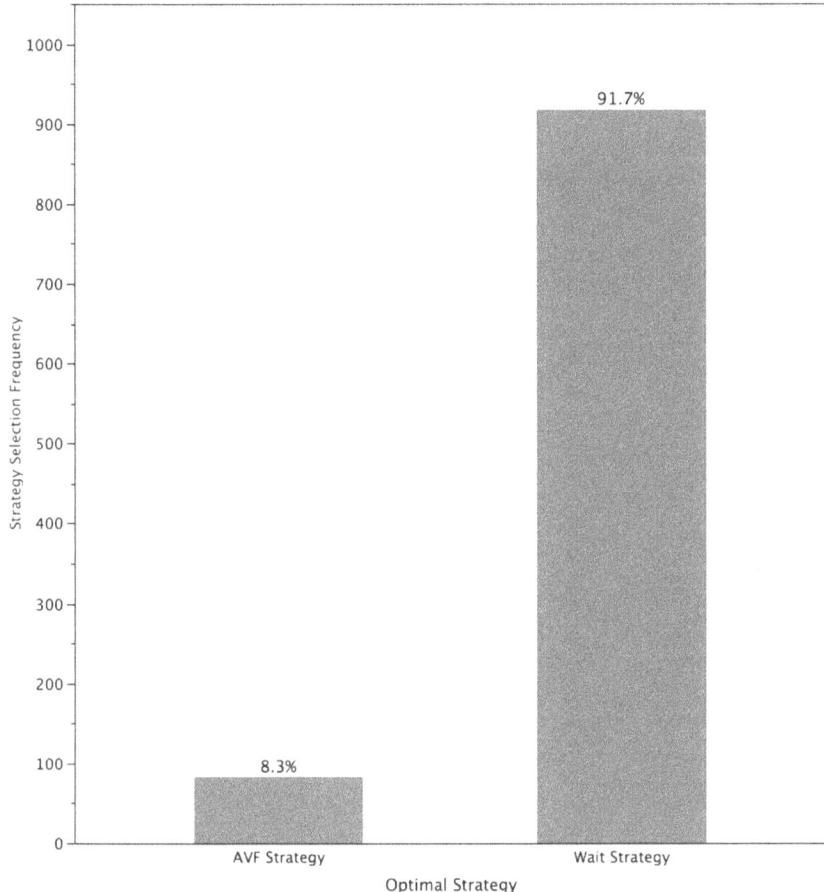

Figure 4. Incremental outcomes and strategy selection frequency with the probabilistic sensitivity analysis using a Monte Carlo simulation.

Acknowledgments

This project was developed initially during the course RDS 288 at the Harvard School of Public Health, course instructor Professor Myriam Hunink. It was also the practicum for the Masters of Public Health for one of the authors (SH) and the other 2 authors (GK and MCW) served as supervisors.

References

1. U.S.Renal Data System (2011) USRDS 2011 Annual Data Report: Atlas of Chronic Kidney Disease and End-Stage Renal Disease in the United States, National Institutes of Health, National Institute of Diabetes and Digestive and Kidney Diseases, Bethesda, MD, 2011. www.usrds.org. Accessed 2011 Oct 4.
2. K/DOQI Workgroup (2002) Part 4. Definition and classification of stages of chronic kidney disease. Am J Kidney Dis 39: S46–S75.
3. Besarab A (2008) Resolved: Fistulas are preferred to grafts as initial vascular access for dialysis. Pro J Am Soc Nephrol 19: 1629–1631.
4. Murad MH, Sidawy AN, Elamin MB, Rizvi AZ, Flynn DN, et al. (2008) Timing of referral for vascular access placement: a systematic review. J Vasc Surg 48: 31S–33S.
5. Luxton G (2010) The CARI guidelines. Timing of referral of chronic kidney disease patients to nephrology services (adult). Nephrology (Carlton) 15 Suppl 1: S2–11.
6. K/DOQI Workgroup (2006) Clinical practice guidelines for vascular access. Am J Kidney Dis 48 Suppl 1: S176–S247.
7. Besarab A, Brouwer D (2004) Improving arteriovenous fistula construction: Fistula first initiative. Hemodial Int 8: 199–206.
8. Jindal K, Chan CT, Deziel C, Hirsch D, Soroka SD, et al. (2006) Hemodialysis clinical practice guidelines for the Canadian Society of Nephrology. J Am Soc Nephrol 17: S1–27.
9. Tordoir J, Canaud B, Haage P, Konner K, Basci A, et al. (2007) EBPG on Vascular Access. Nephrol Dial Transplant 22 Suppl 2: ii88–117.
10. MacRae JM, Pandeya S, Humen DP, Krivitski N, Lindsay RM (2004) Arteriovenous fistula-associated high-output cardiac failure: a review of mechanisms. Am J Kidney Dis 43: e17–e22.
11. Scheltinga MR, van HF, Bruijninckx CM (2009) Time of onset in haemodialysis access-induced distal ischaemia (HAIDI) is related to the access type. Nephrol Dial Transplant.
12. Keough-Ryan TM, Kiberd BA, Cox JL, Thompson KJ, Clase CM (2008) Development of end stage renal disease following an acute cardiac event. Kidney Int 74: 356–363.
13. Patel ST, Hughes J, Mills JL, Sr (2003) Failure of arteriovenous fistula maturation: an unintended consequence of exceeding dialysis outcome quality Initiative guidelines for hemodialysis access. J Vasc Surg 38: 439–445.
14. Beck JR, Pauker SG (1983) The Markov process in medical prognosis. Med Decis Making 3: 419–458.
15. Hawkins N, Sculpher M, Epstein D (2005) Cost-effectiveness analysis of treatments for chronic disease: using R to incorporate time dependency of treatment response. Med Decis Making 25: 511–519.
16. O'Hare AM, Bertenthal D, Walter LC, Garg AX, Covinsky K, et al. (2007) When to refer patients with chronic kidney disease for vascular access surgery: should age be a consideration? Kidney Int 71: 555–561.
17. Conway B, Webster A, Ramsay G, Morgan N, Neary J, Whitworth C, Harty J (2009) Predicting mortality and uptake of renal replacement therapy in patients with stage 4 chronic kidney disease. Nephrol Dial Transplant 24: 1930–1937.

Author Contributions

Conceived and designed the experiments: SH GK MCW. Performed the experiments: SH. Analyzed the data: SH MCW GK. Contributed reagents/materials/analysis tools: SH MCW. Wrote the paper: SH MCW GK.

18. Go AS, Chertow GM, Fan D, McCulloch CE, Hsu CY (2004) Chronic kidney disease and the risks of death, cardiovascular events, and hospitalization. N Engl J Med 351: 1296–1305.
19. Keith DS, Nichols GA, Gullion CM, Brown JB, Smith DH (2004) Longitudinal follow-up and outcomes among a population with chronic kidney disease in a large managed care organization. Arch Intern Med 164: 659–663.
20. Levin A, Djurdjev O, Beaulieu M, Er L (2008) Variability and risk factors for kidney disease progression and death following attainment of stage 4 CKD in a referred cohort. Am J Kidney Dis 52: 661–671.
21. O'Hare AM, Choi AI, Bertenthal D, Bacchetti P, Garg AX, et al. (2007) Age affects outcomes in chronic kidney disease. J Am Soc Nephrol 18: 2758–2765.
22. Patel UD, Young EW, Ojo AO, Hayward RA (2005) CKD progression and mortality among older patients with diabetes. Am J Kidney Dis 46: 406–414.
23. Roderick PJ, Atkins RJ, Smeeth L, Mylne A, Nitsch DD, et al. (2009) CKD and mortality risk in older people: a community-based population study in the United Kingdom. Am J Kidney Dis 53: 950–960.
24. Bradbury BD, Chen F, Furniss A, Pisoni RL, Keen M, et al. (2009) Conversion of vascular access type among incident hemodialysis patients: description and association with mortality. Am J Kidney Dis 53: 804–814.
25. Dhingra RK, Young EW, Hulbert-Shearon TE, Leavey SF, Port FK (2001) Type of vascular access and mortality in U.S. hemodialysis patients. Kidney Int 60: 1443–1451.
26. Moist LM, Trpeski L, Na Y, Lok CE (2008) Increased hemodialysis catheter use in Canada and associated mortality risk: data from the Canadian Organ Replacement Registry 2001–2004. Clin J Am Soc Nephrol 3: 1726–1732.
27. Pastan S, Soucie JM, McClellan WM (2002) Vascular access and increased risk of death among hemodialysis patients. Kidney Int 62: 620–626.
28. Polkinghorne KR, McDonald SP, Atkins RC, Kerr PG (2004) Vascular access and all-cause mortality: a propensity score analysis. J Am Soc Nephrol 15: 477–486.
29. Xue JL, Dahl D, Ebben JP, Collins AJ (2003) The association of initial hemodialysis access type with mortality outcomes in elderly Medicare ESRD patients. Am J Kidney Dis 42: 1013–1019.
30. Huijbregts HJ, Bots ML, Wittens CH, Schrama YC, Moll FL, et al. (2008) Hemodialysis arteriovenous fistula patency revisited: results of a prospective, multicenter initiative. Clin J Am Soc Nephrol 3: 714–719.

31. Graham J, Hiremath S, Magner PO, Knoll GA, Burns KD (2008) Factors influencing the prevalence of central venous catheter use in a Canadian haemodialysis centre. Nephrol Dial Transplant 23: 3585–3591.
32. Johannesson M, Pliskin JS, Weinstein MC (1994) A note on QALYs, time tradeoff, and discounting. Med Decis Making 14: 188–193.
33. Davison SN, Jhangri GS, Feeny DH (2008) Comparing the Health Utilities Index Mark 3 (HUI3) with the Short Form-36 Preference-Based SF-6D in Chronic Kidney Disease. Value Health.
34. Naimark DM, Bott M, Krahn M (2008) The half-cycle correction explained: two alternative pedagogical approaches. Med Decis Making 28: 706–712.
35. Briggs AH (2004) Statistical approaches to handling uncertainty in health economic evaluation. Eur J Gastroenterol Hepatol 16: 551–561.
36. O'Hare AM, Allon M, Kaufman JS (2010) Whether and when to refer patients for predialysis AV fistula creation: complex decision making in the face of uncertainty. Semin Dial 23: 452–455.
37. Ng LJ, Chen F, Pisoni RL, Krishnan M, Mapes D, et al. (2011) Hospitalization risks related to vascular access type among incident US hemodialysis patients. Nephrol Dial Transplant 26: 3659–3666.
38. Vachharajani TJ, Moossavi S, Jordan JR, Vachharajani V, Freedman BI, et al. (2011) Re-evaluating the Fistula First Initiative in Octogenarians on Hemodialysis. Clin J Am Soc Nephrol 6: 1663–1667.
39. Canadian Institute for Health Information (2008) 2007 Annual Report—Treatment of End-Stage Organ Failure in Canada, 1996 to 2005 (Ottawa: CIHI, 2008).
40. Xue H, Lacson E, Jr., Wang W, Curhan GC, Brunelli SM (2010) Choice of vascular access among incident hemodialysis patients: a decision and cost-utility analysis. Clin J Am Soc Nephrol 5: 2289–2296.
41. Pisoni RL, Young EW, Dykstra DM, Greenwood RN, Hecking E, et al. (2002) Vascular access use in Europe and the United States: results from the DOPPS. Kidney Int 61: 305–316.
42. Barlow AD, Doughman TM, Warwick GL, Nicholson ML (2008) A successful scheme for reducing waiting times for arteriovenous fistula formation. J Vasc Access 9: 129–132.
43. Xi W, Harwood L, Diamant MJ, Brown JB, Gallo K, et al. (2011) Patient attitudes towards the arteriovenous fistula: a qualitative study on vascular access decision making. Nephrol Dial Transplant 26: 3302–3308.

7

Hepatitis C Virus in Vietnam: High Prevalence of Infection in Dialysis and Multi-Transfused Patients Involving Diverse and Novel Virus Variants

Linda Dunford[1,2], Michael J. Carr[1,2], Jonathan Dean[1,2], Allison Waters[1,2], Linh Thuy Nguyen[1,3], Thu Hong Ta Thi[1,3], Lan Anh Bui Thi[1,3], Huy Duong Do[1,3], Thu Thuy Duong Thi[1,3], Ha Thu Nguyen[1,3], Trinh Thi Diem Do[1,3], Quynh Phuong Luu[1,3], Jeff Connell[1,2], Suzie Coughlan[1,2], Hien Tran Nguyen[1,3], William W. Hall[1,2]*, Lan Anh Nguyen Thi[1,3]*

1 Ireland Vietnam Blood-Borne Virus Initiative (IVVI), Dublin, Ireland and Ha Noi Vietnam, 2 National Virus Reference Laboratory, University College Dublin, Dublin, Ireland, 3 Laboratory for Molecular Diagnostics, National Institute of Hygiene and Epidemiology, Ha Noi, Vietnam

Abstract

Hepatitis C virus (HCV) is a genetically diverse pathogen infecting approximately 2–3% of the world's population. Herein, we describe results of a large, multicentre serological and molecular epidemiological study cataloguing the prevalence and genetic diversity of HCV in five regions of Vietnam; Ha Noi, Hai Phong, Da Nang, Khanh Hoa and Can Tho. Individuals (n = 8654) with varying risk factors for infection were analysed for the presence of HCV Ab/Ag and, in a subset of positive specimens, for HCV RNA levels (n = 475) and genotype (n = 282). In lower risk individuals, including voluntary blood donors, military recruits and pregnant women, the prevalence of infection was 0.5% (n = 26/5250). Prevalence rates were significantly higher ($p<0.001$) in intravenous drug users (IDUs; 55.6%, n = 556/1000), dialysis patients (26.6%, n = 153/575) commercial sex workers (CSWs; 8.7%, n = 87/1000), and recipients of multiple blood transfusions (6.0%, n = 32/529). The prevalence of HCV in dialysis patients varied but remained high in all regions (11–43%) and was associated with the receipt of blood transfusions [OR: 2.08 (1.85–2.34), $p = 0.001$], time from first transfusion [OR: 1.07 (1.01–1.13), $p = 0.023$], duration of dialysis [OR: 1.31 (1.19–1.43), $p<0.001$] and male gender [OR: 1.60 (1.06–2.41), $p = 0.026$]. Phylogenetic analysis revealed high genetic diversity, particularly amongst dialysis and multi-transfused patients, identifying subtypes 1a (33%), 1b (27%), 2a (0.4%), 3a (0.7%), 3b (1.1%), 6a (18.8%), 6e (6.0%), 6h (4.6%) and 6l (6.4%) and 2 clusters of novel genotype 6 variants (2.1%). HCV genotype 1 predominated in Vietnam (60%, n = 169/282) but the proportion of infections attributable to genotype 1 varied between regions and risk groups and, in the Southern part of Vietnam, genotype 6 viruses dominated in dialysis and multi-transfused patients (73.9%). This study confirms a high prevalence of HCV infection in Vietnamese IDUs and, notably, reveals high levels of HCV infection associated with dialysis and blood transfusion.

Editor: Jason Blackard, University of Cincinnati College of Medicine, United States of America

Funding: The Ireland Vietnam Blood-Borne Virus Initiative is supported by Irish Aid, the Government of Ireland's programme of assistance to developing countries, and by the Atlantic Philanthropies. The funders had no role in study design, data collection and analysis, decision to publish, or preparation of the manuscript.

Competing Interests: The authors have declared that no competing interests exist.

* E-mail: William.hall@ucd.ie (WWH); lananh_2003@yahoo.com (LANT)

Introduction

Hepatitis C virus (HCV) has been estimated to infect approximately 2–3% of the world's population, with highest prevalence rates occurring in low and middle income regions including Africa and Southeast Asia [1–4]. Transmission of HCV involves direct exposure to contaminated blood and is associated with intravenous drug use, iatrogenic exposures, tattooing, body piercing and, less frequently, through vertical transmission and high risk sexual behaviour [1,4–8]. Iatrogenic routes of transmission implicated in HCV infection include blood transfusions, surgical and dental procedures, dialysis, acupuncture, needlestick injury and use of unsterilised needles [4,9–17]. The latter has been highlighted in Egypt where nationwide treatment for schistosomiasis under suboptimal hygiene conditions from 1960 to 1987 has resulted in national HCV seroprevalence rates of approximately 14% [12,18].

In industrialised countries, iatrogenic transmission of HCV is now rare and the burden of HCV infection is largely restricted to intravenous drug user (IDU) populations [18]. In contrast, iatrogenic transmission of HCV still occurs frequently in many resource-limited settings as a result of inadequate screening and failure to implement universal precautions [13,17,18]. Dialysis has been associated with transmission of HCV and prevalence rates as high as 18% in the Asia-Pacific region have been reported [17,19–21]. Transmission is more commonly associated with haemodialysis compared to peritoneal dialysis and has been shown to be increased following longer durations of dialysis and increased frequency of blood transfusion [10,11,17].

Chronic HCV infection is associated with high levels of morbidity and mortality and long term sequelae [22,23]. Studies have reported that up to 80% of infections may progress to chronic infection, of which 10–20% will result in the development fibrosis and cirrhosis, and up to 5% will develop hepatocellular carcinoma (HCC) [18,23]. Chronic HCV infection also has significant socio-economic implications, which are compounded by restrictions in access to expensive therapies and the lack of an effective vaccine. Co-morbidities associated with alcohol consumption and coinfection with other blood-borne viruses such as HBV and HIV are also associated with accelerated progression of liver disease [24–28].

HCV is a positive polarity, single-stranded RNA virus of the family *Flaviviridae*, genus *Hepacivirus* and is classified into six major groups (genotypes 1–6), each containing a variable number of more closely related distinct subtypes. Due to the absence of proof reading by the virally encoded RNA dependent RNA polymerase, the virus evolves rapidly and sequence diversity is extremely high, with 31–33% divergence between genotypes and 20–25% between subtypes [29]. Genotype 6 viruses are the most genetically diverse HCV genotype, with 23 subtypes currently recognised. New strains continue to be identified, with subtypes 6v and 6w recently described from China and Taiwan respectively [30,31]. Although some genotypes are widely distributed, there are clear epidemiological and geographical patterns associated with other genotypes such as the predominance of genotype 6 in Southeast Asia and Southern China [32].

There are limited studies regarding HCV infection in Vietnam and recently a call to action for nationwide screening of hepatitis viruses was published [33]. Prevalence rates in Vietnam appear to vary between regions and risk groups, ranging from 1–2.9% in the general population [33–35] to 46–87% in IDUs [16,33,36]. A broad distribution of HCV genotypes have been reported in Vietnam, with genotypes 1 and 6 predominating [37–39]. In the present study we have attempted to establish a catalogue of HCV infection in Vietnam by carrying out a large serological and molecular epidemiological study in different geographic regions and involving individuals with different risk factors for infection.

Materials and Methods

Ethics Statement

Ethical approval for the study was obtained from the National Institute of Hygiene and Epidemiology (NIHE) in Ha Noi. All specimens and survey information were obtained with informed, written consent and subsequently anonymised.

Study Group

This cross-sectional study serologically investigated 8654 specimens for HCV infection collected from eight different population groups including IDUs, commercial sex workers (CSWs), blood donors, military recruits, pregnant women, dialysis patients, elective surgery patients and recipients of multiple blood transfusions. Paired serum and plasma specimens were obtained during 2008 and 2009, along with detailed demographic information, from five sites in Vietnam: Ha Noi (n = 1750) and Hai Phong (n = 1750) in the North, Da Nang (n = 1750) in the Central region and Khanh Hoa (n = 1725) and Can Tho (n = 1679) in the South.

Viral Serology

All specimens were tested using a commercially available enzyme immunoassay (EIA) for HCV using the Monolisa Ag/Ab HCV Ultra (Bio-Rad Laboratories, CA, USA).

Quantitative RT-PCR

A representative subset of HCV Ab/Ag positive specimens (n = 475), which included all serological positives from dialysis and multi-transfused patients, were selected for molecular analysis.

Nucleic acid was extracted from 140 µl of plasma from HCV Ab/Ag positive specimens (n = 475), using the QIAamp Viral RNA minikit (Qiagen, Crawley, UK), as per the manufacturer's instructions. Brome mosaic virus (BMV) RNA (5 pg/specimen) was included during the extraction as an exogenous internal control to ensure sample addition and the absence of PCR inhibitors. HCV viral load (VL) was determined using a quantitative real-time reverse transcriptase polymerase chain reaction (qRT-PCR). BMV RNA was co-amplified as an internal control and serial dilutions of a plasmid-derived HCV RNA standard were used to prepare the standard curve. The PCR reaction was performed with previously published primers targeting the HCV 5′ untranslated region (UTR) [40]. Briefly, 5 µl of extracted RNA was reverse transcribed and amplified in qRT-PCR with 0.6 µM forward primer, 0.8 µM reverse primer and 0.4 µM probe in a 25 µl total reaction volume with the Superscript III One Step RT-PCR system with Platinum Taq DNA Polymerase (Invitrogen Life Technologies, Paisley, UK) on an ABI 7500 FAST real-time platform (Applied Biosystems, Warrington, UK) with the following cycling parameters: an initial 15 min incubation at $50°C$, followed by 2 min at $95°C$ and 45 cycles of $95°C$ for 15 s and $60°C$ for 34 s. The assay was calibrated against the WHO 3rd International Reference Standard for HCV RNA (NISBC Code 06/100) and validated with a limit of detection of 300 IU/ml plasma (2.48 $\log_{10}$ IU/ml) and a linear dynamic range of $3 \times 10^2 - 8 \times 10^7$ IU/ml (2.48–7.9 $\log_{10}$ IU/ml). The assay was optimised to ensure high concordance with a commercially available HCV Viral Load assay, giving an R^2 value of 0.95 when correlated with the Roche COBAS-Ampliprep COBAS-Taqman HCV Viral Load Assay. Inter-assay and intra-assay coefficients of variation ranged up to a maximum of 3.5% and 6.3%, respectively.

HCV Characterisation

For HCV genotyping, viral RNA from HCV RNA positive specimens were reverse transcribed using Superscript III RT kit and RNaseOUT (Invitrogen Life Technologies, Paisley, UK) as previously described [32]. cDNA was amplified with the Expand High Fidelity PCR system (Roche Applied Sciences, Mannheim, Germany) using 0.2 mM final concentration deoxynucleoside triphosphates (dNTPs) and 0.3 µM primers, as previously described [32,41]. A nested PCR targeting a 377 base pair (bp) region of the HCV *NS5B* gene was performed using previously published primers [32]. First and second round amplification of the *NS5B* gene were performed with a 2 min initial denaturation at $94°C$, followed by 28 cycles of $94°C$ for 15 s, $60°C$ for 30 s and $72°C$ for 45 s with a final extension step of 7 min at $72°C$ [32]. Single round amplification of a 494 bp region of the overlapping *core* and *E1* genes was performed with a 2 min initial denaturation at $94°C$, followed by 40 cycles of $94°C$ for 15 s, $60°C$ for 30 s and $72°C$ for 45 s and a final extension step of 7 min at $72°C$ using previously published primers [41]. Unincorporated primers and dNTPs were removed from HCV amplicon using Exo-SAP IT (Affymetrix, Cleveland, USA) and purified products were sequenced bidirectionally on an ABI 3730 sequencing platform. Contiguous assembly of sequences was performed by Lasergene version 8 (DNASTAR, Madison, WI, USA) [42]. Genbank accession numbers are JX102664 - JX103137.

Phylogenetic Analysis

Datasets comprising HCV *NS5B* and *core/E1* reference sequences, representing all currently assigned genotypes of HCV, were downloaded from the Los Alamos database (http://hcv.lanl.gov/content/sequence/HCV/ToolsOutline.html) and

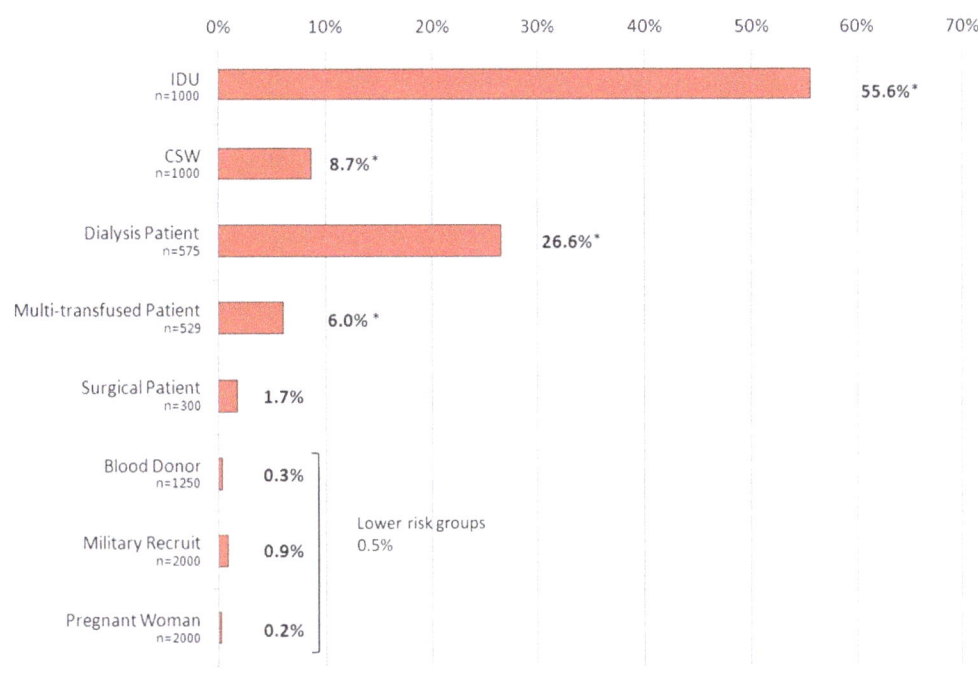

* Significantly higher prevalence compared to lower risk groups, p<0.0001

Figure 1. Seroepidemiology of HCV in 8 Different Vietnamese Risk Groups, n = 8654. The total percentage of HCV Ab/Ag positives in each population group is shown at the end of each bar. The number of samples tested from each group is listed below. 59.7% of CSWs testing positive for HCV also reported intravenous drug use.

aligned with the study sequences using Bioedit version 7.05 [43]. Phylogenetic trees for both the *NS5B* and *core/E1* sequences were constructed using the neighbour joining distance method under a Kimura-2-parameter model of evolution in PAUP* version 4.0 beta10 [44]. Phylogenies were heuristically searched using a subtree pruning and regrafting perturbation algorithm. Genotypes obtained by phylogenetic analysis were confirmed using the Los Alamos online database (http://hcv.lanl.gov/content/sequence/BASIC_BLAST/basic_blast.html). To further examine sequences from the epidemic in dialysis and multi-transfused patients, a midpoint rooted phylogenetic tree of the *NS5B* region was drawn with relevant reference and patient derived sequences. A neighbour joining tree was constructed in PAUP* based on the HKY85 model of evolution, a gamma distribution and a proportion of invariable sites using the tree bisection and reconnection (TBR) rearrangement scheme in a heuristic search. To further characterise novel sequences, maximum likelihood analyses were performed for both the *NS5B* and *core/E1* gene sequences using general time reversible (GTR) submodels, a gamma distribution and a proportion of invariable sites with a representative of each subtype of genotype 6. Statistical support for all tree topologies was evaluated with 1000 bootstrap replicates. Phylogenetic trees were visualised, annotated and coloured using Figtree v1.3 (http://tree.bio.ed.ac.uk/software/figtree).

Recombination analysis of all novel sequences identified was performed with the RDP3 software using six different programs – RDP, GENECONV, MaxChi, Bootscan, Chimaera and SiScan [45]. Analysis of pairwise nucleotide similarities was performed on both the *NS5B* and *core/E1* genes of novel sequences with representative genotype 6 reference sequences (6a–6w) using Bioedit version 7.05 [43].

Statistical Analysis

Data from the study is presented as the mean values ± standard deviation (SD) and ranges. Continuous variables, such as viral load, were compared between populations using the Student's t-test. Categorical data were analysed using the Chi-squared and odds ratio tests. Independent risk factors for HCV infection in dialysis patients were examined using logistic regression analysis and SPSS software version 18.0. p-values<0.05 were considered statistically significant.

Results

Prevalence of HCV Infection in Vietnam

In a sample of 5250 individuals considered to be at low risk for infection (voluntary blood donors, military recruits and pregnant women) the prevalence of HCV was 0.5%. Significantly higher HCV prevalence rates were identified in populations associated with higher risk activities, specifically IDUs (55.6%, n = 556/1000), dialysis patients (26.6%, n = 153/575), CSWs (8.7%, n = 87/1000) and multiply transfused patients (6.0%, n = 32/529; p<0.001; Figure 1). The prevalence of HCV in IDUs in Vietnam varied widely between the study sites; Ha Noi (59.5%, n = 119/200), Hai Phong (87%, n = 174/200), Da Nang (54%, n = 108/200), Khanh Hoa (20%, n = 40/200), Can Tho (57.5%, n = 115/200). Seventy-six percent (n = 166/218) of IDUs were viremic with a mean viral load of 5.25 ± 1.05 $\log_{10}$ IU/ml (range 2.1–7.3). HCV infection in the CSW cohort may also be associated with drug use practices as 59.7% of HCV positive CSWs reported previous injecting drug use. Sixty-five percent of HCV infected CSWs (n = 40/62) were viremic and these had a mean viral load of 5.21 ± 1.06 $\log_{10}$ IU/ml (2.78–7.6).

Risk Factors Associated with HCV in Dialysis and Multi-transfused Patients

Univariate odds ratio (OR) calculations revealed that dialysis and multi-transfused patients were significantly more likely to have been infected with HCV than lower risk groups, [multi-transfused 12.2 (6.98–21.32), $p<0.001$; dialysis 68.7 (43.06–109.59), $p<0.001$]. The prevalence of HCV in the multi-transfused patient group (6%, n = 32/529) also varied considerably between regions: Ha Noi (13%, n = 13/100), Hai Phong (1%, n = 1/100), Da Nang (4%, n = 4/100), Khanh Hoa (5.3%, n = 8/150) and Can Tho (7.6%, n = 6/79). In dialysis patients, the prevalence rates also varied between the study sites; Ha Noi (43%), Hai Phong (11%), Da Nang (32%), Khanh Hoa (33%) and Can Tho (17.3%; Table 1). The lowest prevalence of HCV in dialysis patients was in Hai Phong (11%) where patients reported no history of blood transfusion or prior surgery and also had a shorter mean duration of dialysis (Table 1). Conversely, the highest HCV prevalence identified in a dialysis group (Ha Noi, 43%) was associated with high levels of transfusion (90.7%) and longer duration of dialysis (mean 7.3 years; Table 1).

Overall, the prevalence of HCV in non-transfused dialysis patients was 17.4% (n = 30/172), whereas, in multi-transfused dialysis patients this was significantly higher (30.5%, n = 123/403; $p<0.001$). In fact, dialysis patients receiving blood transfusions were approximately twice as likely (OR: 2.08 (0.85–5.05), $p = 0.001$) to be infected with HCV compared to non-transfused dialysis patients. A multivariate regression analysis of the risk factors associated with HCV infection in dialysis patients confirmed that the duration of dialysis was strongly associated with HCV infection (Figure 2 and Table 2). Male gender and the number of years from first blood transfusion were also significantly associated with HCV infection (Table 2).

HCV Genetic Diversity in Vietnam

Phylogenetic analysis confirmed genetically diverse HCV populations and genotype analysis for both *NS5B* and *core/E1* regions were in agreement for all specimens tested. The distribution of genotypes and subtypes by risk group are summarised in Figure 3. Genotypes 1, 6, 3 and 2 were detected in 59.9% (n = 169), 37.9% (n = 107), 1.8% (n = 5) and 0.4% (n = 1) of subjects, respectively. Genotype 1 was the most prevalent HCV

genotype in our study, although this varied between regions as follows: Ha Noi (54%, n = 47/87), Hai Phong (72.1%, n = 31/43), Da Nang (81.4%, n = 35/43), Khanh Hoa (47.2, n = 25/53) and Can Tho (55.4%, n = 31/56).

Analysis of the different risk groups revealed that genotype 1 viruses accounted for a significantly higher proportion of HCV infections in both IDUs (70.1%, n = 87) and CSWs (63.7% n = 21), compared to dialysis (51%, n = 50) and multi-transfused (36.4% n = 8) patients, $p<0.001$ (Figure 3).

Genetic Diversity of HCV in Dialysis and Multi-transfused Patients

Genotypes 1, 2, 3 and 6 were identified in dialysis and multi-transfused individuals with nine recognised subtypes (1a, 1b, 2a, 3a, 3b, 6a, 6e, 6h, 6l) and two clusters of novel sequences (Figure 4). Genotype 1 viruses were dominant in dialysis and multi-transfused patients in the Northern and Central cities of Ha Noi (64%, n = 27/42), Hai Phong (83%, n = 5/6) and Da Nang (84%, n = 16/19). In contrast, genotype 6 was the predominant virus in the Southern regions of Khanh Hoa (71%, n = 20/28) and Can Tho (78%, n = 14/18). There is clear geographical clustering of some HCV variants and high levels of sequence identity within regions. For example, there are two distinct clades of 6h viruses from Ha Noi in the North and Can Tho in the South that cluster separately with high bootstrap support (Figure 4).

A monophyletic cluster of sequences from 16 dialysis patients from Khanh Hoa was observed, branching with a 6l reference strain originally identified in Vietnam in 1994. Seventy five percent (n = 12/16) of the 6l infected dialysis patients had also received multiple transfusions and there was an additional sequence clustering with the 6l clade from a multi-transfused individual not on dialysis. The mean duration of dialysis was 2.1 ± 1.2 years (range: 1–5) and at the time of specimen collection all patients were undergoing dialysis 2–3 times a week. Nine dialysis patients also reported a history of surgery. No other high risk factors for infection were reported and this cluster would therefore appear to be an example of HCV transmission within a dialysis unit. The specimens were all collected within a 4 week time period in 2009. In our study, subtype 6l was almost exclusively detected in Khanh Hoa and this subtype was detected in only one other individual: a military recruit from Da Nang

Table 1. Prevalence of HCV Infection in Dialysis Patients in Vietnam, n = 575.

	Ha Noi	Hai Phong	Da Nang	Khanh Hoa	Can Tho	Total
No. patients tested	100	100	100	125	150	575
HCV Ab/Ag pos	43.0% (43)	11.0% (11)	32.0% (32)	32.8% (41)	17.3% (26)	26.6% (153)
HCV RNA pos	90.7% (39)	54.5% (6)	68.8% (22)	73.1% (30)	61.5% (16)	73.9% (113)
Viral load $\log_{10}$ IU/ml	5.0 ± 1.0 (2.1–7.1)	3.4 ± 1.0 (2.4–4.6)	4.2 ± 1.2 (2.5–6.1)	4.6 ± 1.5 (2.1–6.9)	4.7 ± 1.2 (2.2–6.3)	4.6 ± 1.3 (2.1–7.1)
Variables in HCV positive patients						
Age, years	49.4 ± 13.3 (23–74)	25.2 ± 3.5 (21–30)	44.2 ± 12.9 (25–72)	46.4 ± 14.7 (24–77)	49.4 ± 15.0 (22–79)	45.7 ± 14.6 (21–79)
Gender, % Male	51.2% (22)	45.5% (5)	68.8% (22)	63.4% (26)	57.7% (15)	58.8% (90)
Years receiving dialysis	7.3 ± 3.1 (2–16)	1.8 ± 0.4 (1–2)	3.9 ± 2.0 (1–8)	2.8 ± 1.8 (1–8)	3.3 ± 2.4 (1–9)	4.4 ± 3.0 (1–16)
With history of transfusion	90.7% (39)	0% (0)	100% (32)	82.9% (34)	69.2% (18)	80.4% (123)
Years receiving transfusions	7.7 ± 4.5 (1–25)	n/a	4.2 ± 5.2 (<1–30)	3.7 ± 6.9 (<1–30)	3.5 ± 2.7 (<1–9)	5.2 ± 5.3 (<1–30)
With history of surgery	30.2% (13)	0% (0)	21.9% (7)	61.0% (25)	80.8% (21)	43.1% (66)

Data presented as mean ± SD (range) or % (number) as applicable.
No dialysis patients reported intravenous drug use or high risk sexual behaviour.
Pos - positive; n/a - not applicable.

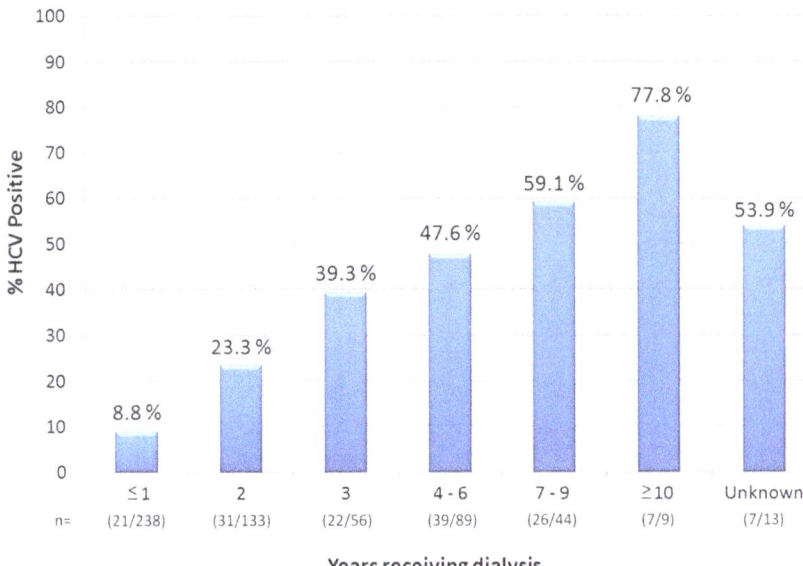

Figure 2. Seroepidemiology of HCV in Dialysis Patients. This figure depicts HCV prevalence in relation to duration of dialysis in years. Increased duration of dialysis is strongly associated with an increase in HCV infection ($p<0.001$).

(Figure 2). While the majority of sequences from Khanh Hoa dialysis patients were 6l (64%, n = 16/25), a number of other genotypes were also identified co-circulating in these patients including 1b, 2a, 3a and 6a, suggesting multiple introductions of HCV in dialysis centres.

Novel Variants of HCV

Novel HCV sequences forming two highly divergent clades within genotype 6 were identified with neighbour joining phylogenetic analyses (Figure 4). The two clusters of novel variants are annotated in Figures 4 and 5 as "unassigned group 1" and "unassigned group 2". Further analysis of these sequences using maximum likelihood methods, with a representative sequence from each currently recognised subtype within HCV genotype 6 (Figure 5), confirmed that the sequences do not cluster with any other subtypes of 6 and have full bootstrap support (>99%) for clustering within their own groups. Recombination analysis of the novel variants did not demonstrate any evidence of recombination in these sequences either in the *NS5B* or *core/E1* gene regions (data not shown).

A BLAST analysis against all available HCV sequences in the Los Alamos Database found the closest similarity for "unassigned group 1" sequences was 84% to another unclassified genotype 6

strain (GU049374) in the *NS5B* region and 77% similarity in the *core/E1* region to a Vietnamese subtype 6e strain (EU246931). A pairwise comparison of nucleotide sequence identity between each of the novel sequences showed 98.7–99.6% similarity to each other in the *NS5B* region and 98.9–99.7% similarity in the *core/E1* region. When compared to the 23 currently recognised HCV genotype 6 subtypes, group 1 sequences showed nucleotide similarities of 68.0–76.5% in the *NS5B* gene and 66.8–77.2% in the *core/E1* region. The four sequences that comprised "unassigned group 1" were amplified from samples collected from male dialysis patients in Can Tho. Two patients had been receiving blood transfusions over a 5–7 year period and the other two had not received any transfusions. All four reported a history of surgery. Other than iatrogenic exposures, no other high risk activities were reported.

The two sequences in "unassigned group 2" were 81–83% similar to 6t variants (EU246939 and EU632071) in the *NS5B* gene. Unassigned group 2 sequences had only 89.9% nucleotide sequence identity to each other but consistently grouped together with 100% bootstrap support. The group 2 sequences had 65.6–83.2% similarity over the *NS5B* gene with highest nucleotide identity to 6t viruses. "Unassigned group 2" sequences were identified in two male multi-transfused patients

Table 2. Factors Associated With HCV Infection among Dialysis Patients in Five Regions of Vietnam using Logistic Regression Analysis, n = 575.

Variable	OR	95% CI	p – value
Age	1.01	1.00–1.02	0.185
Male Gender	1.60	1.06–2.41	0.026*
Duration Receiving Transfusions (per 1 year increase)	1.07	1.01–1.13	0.023*
Duration Receiving Dialysis (per 1 year increase)	1.31	1.19–1.43	<0.001*
History of Surgery	0.98	0.64–1.50	0.936

*p values<0.05 deemed significant.

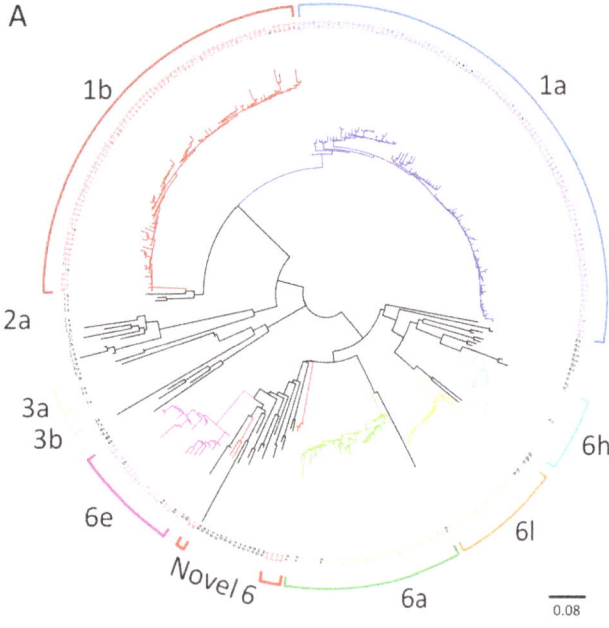

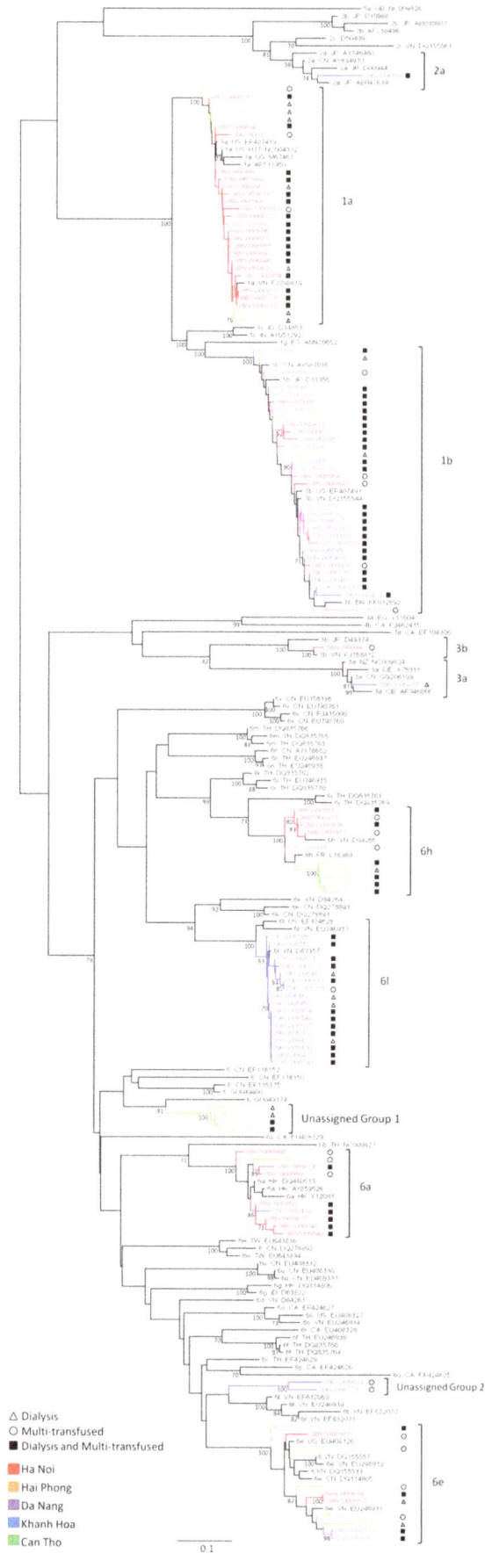

Genotype	Total (%)	IDU (%)	SW (%)	DIA (%)	MT (%)	Other (%)
☐ 1a	33.0	41.9	36.4	24.5	9.1	60.0
☐ 1b*	27.0	28.2	27.3	26.5	27.3	0.0
☐ 6a*	18.8	22.6	24.2	13.3	13.6	20.0
☐ 6l	6.4	0.0	0.0	16.3	4.5	20.0
☐ 6e	6.0	4.0	6.1	6.1	18.2	0.0
☐ 6h	4.6	1.6	3.0	7.1	13.6	0.0
☐ Novel 6	2.1	0.0	0.0	4.1	9.1	0.0
3b	1.1	0.8	3.0	0.0	4.5	0.0
3a	0.7	0.8	0.0	1.0	0.0	0.0
2a	0.4	0.0	0.0	1.0	0.0	0.0
	n=282	n=124	n=33	n=98	n=22	n=5

* 23 specimens included here were confirmed only with Core/E1 sequencing. 22 6a and 1 1b

Figure 3. Phylogenetic Analysis of the HCV *NS5B* Gene. Vietnamese HCV gene sequences from the present study (n = 259 *NS5B*) are presented with reference sequences (n = 74) downloaded from the Los Alamos database. Analysis was based on a 329-bp of the HCV *NS5B* gene (nucleotides 8282–8610 relative to H77 NC004102). "A" depicts a midpoint rooted radial phylogenetic tree constructed using the neighbour joining distance method under a Kimura-2-paramter model of evolution. Bootstrap values >70% were obtained for all major nodes separating the confirmed genotypes (not shown). The scale bar indicates an evolutionary distance of 0.08 nucleotide substitutions per site. Branches and annotations are colour coded for all HCV subtypes identified in this study, with reference sequences shown in black. Sequences are annotated by the study cohort from which they were obtained, namely: IDU, intravenous drug user; SW, commercial sex worker; DIA, dialysis patient; MT, multi-transfused patient; ES, elective surgery patient; MR, military recruit. Reference sequences are annotated by subtype name. "B" represents all obtained HCV genotypes/subtypes in the varying risk groups. In total, genotypes were identified for 282 specimens - 201 based on both the *NS5B* and *core/E1* regions, 58 from the *NS5B* region alone and 23 from the *core/E1* region only. Genbank accession numbers are JX102664–JX103137.

in Khanh Hoa in 2009. Neither had undergone dialysis but one reported having a surgical procedure with no other risks reported.

Figure 4. Molecular Characterisation of HCV Genotypes in Vietnamese Dialysis and Multi-transfused Patients. Analysis of HCV patient (n = 113) and reference sequences was performed on a 329-bp fragment of the HCV *NS5B* gene (nucleotides 8282–8610, numbering based on H77). A neighbour joining tree was constructed using the Kimura-2-parameter model of evolution with gamma distribution and a proportion of invariable sites. Bootstrap values over 70% are shown at the respective nodes. The scale bar indicates an evolutionary distance of 0.1 nucleotide substitutions per site. Reference sequences are annotated with their confirmed genotype and subtype, country of isolation where known and Genbank accession number. Sequences from dialysis and multi-transfused patients are represented in colour, differing by location - red for Ha Noi, orange for Hai Phong, purple for Da Nang, blue for Khanh Hoa and green for Can Tho. Open triangles are used to denote sequences from dialysis patients, open circles are used to denote sequences from multi-transfused patients and filled squares are used where a patient fits both of these criteria. Brackets select the subtypes in which sequences were identified in this study. Two unassigned groups of sequences were identified – a group of sequences obtained from four dialysis patients in Can Tho and sequences obtained from two multi transfused patients in Khanh Hoa and these are labelled as unclassified groups 1 and 2. For 6 additional specimens, 6a genotypes (5 Ha Noi and 1 Can Tho) were identified by *core/E1* sequencing.

Discussion

This study confirms a high prevalence of HCV infection in Vietnamese IDUs (55.6%) and also reveals high levels of HCV infection associated with dialysis (26.6%), particularly when compounded by a history of blood transfusion. The prevalence of HCV in IDUs varied significantly between regions, ranging from 20% in Khanh Hoa to over 80% in Hai Phong. Previous estimates of HCV infection in Vietnamese IDUs have been reported to range from 19–87%, again varying by region [16,36,37,46–48]. Indeed, a recent prospective study of IDUs in Ha Noi estimated that HCV prevalence in IDUs ranged from

30% to 70% depending on the length of time they had been injecting drugs [36].

In lower risk groups, including military recruits, voluntary blood donors and pregnant women, the prevalence of HCV was 0.5%, which is lower than in many previous reports which have ranged from 1–9% [16,35,46,47]. Sexual transmission of HCV is still relatively rare and, to date, HCV transmission within CSW cohorts in Vietnam has not been well studied. Although the prevalence described in CSWs in this study (8.7%) is higher than estimates from other Asian countries, this is likely confounded by the effect of injecting drug use practices as almost 60% of the HCV positive CSW cohort reported such activity. Evidence exists to support sexual transmission of HCV, although available data suggest the efficiency of transmission by the sexual route is low [49]. Despite this, a number of studies have reported a higher seroprevalence of HCV infection in CSWs compared to the general population. Seroprevalence studies from different geographical areas have reported a range of anti-HCV levels in female sex workers: including the Democratic Republic of Congo (6.6%), Thailand (2%), Afghanistan (1.9%) and South Korea (1.4%), although, only the latter excluded intravenous drug users from their study [50–53].

The prevalence of HCV infection we identified in dialysis patients (26.6%, range: 11–43%) was lower than a previous Vietnamese study which identified HCV in 54% of dialysis patients in Ho Chi Minh City in 1994 [16]. However, as seen in the IDU population, the HCV prevalence in dialysis patients varied significantly from region to region, ranging from 11% in Hai Phong to 43% in Ha Noi. In some regions, namely Ha Noi, Da Nang and Khanh Hoa, the HCV prevalence in dialysis patients was higher than that reported from neighbouring Asian countries in the last decade; 5.9% in Thailand, just below 10% in Taiwan and Hong Kong, 8.5–12.5% in Japan and 18% in Shanghai, China [17,54,55].

A - NS5B

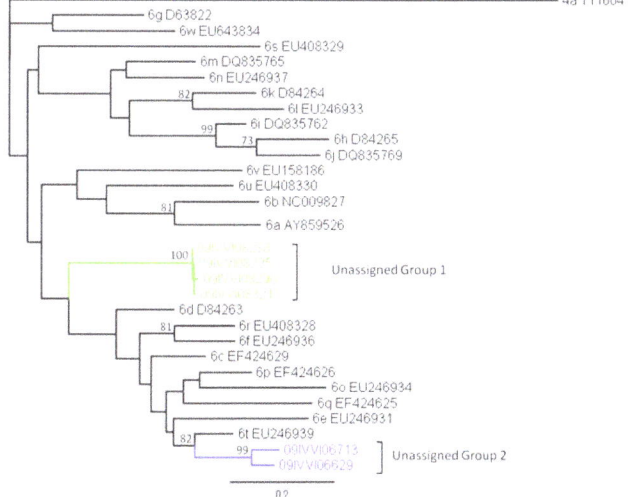

B - Core/E1

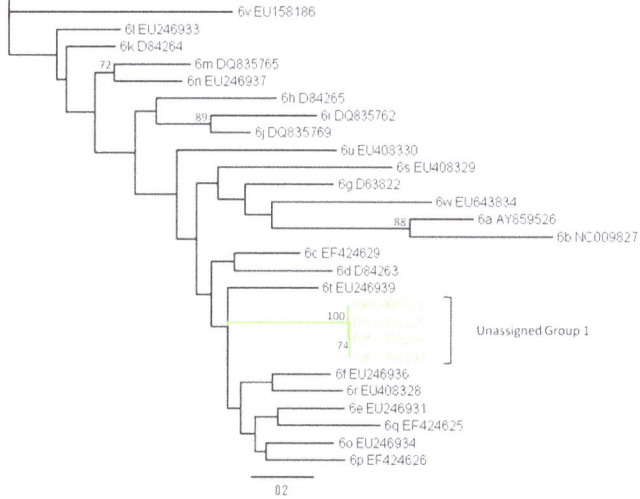

Figure 5. Maximum Likelihood Phylogenetic Analysis of Novel HCV Genotype 6 Sequences in both *NS5B* and *core/E1* Genes. HCV sequences identified in this study (coloured and marked by brackets) and reference sequences for all currently recognised subtypes of HCV genotype 6 are analysed with A) a 329-bp fragment of the HCV *NS5B* gene corresponding to nucleotides 8282 to 8610 of the H77 strain and B) a 446-bp fragment of the HCV *core* and *E1* genes corresponding to nucleotides 860 to 1305 of the H77 strain. Rooted trees were constructed using submodels of the general time reversible (GTR) model, a gamma distribution and a proportion of invariant sites. Bootstrap values over 70% are shown on the corresponding branches. Scale bar indicates an evolutionary distance of 0.2 substitutions per site. "Unassigned group 1" sequences were obtained from 4 dialysis patients in Can Tho and the sequences in unassigned group 2 were from multi-transfused patients in Khanh Hoa.

Blood transfusion remains a significant risk factor for HCV infection in Vietnam and our results demonstrated that 6% of multi-transfused patients were seropositive. Moreover, the high level of infection seen in the dialysis group was compounded by a history of transfusion in 70% of patients. Indeed, the prevalence of HCV was significantly higher in those dialysis patients who had received multiple blood transfusions than in those who had not (30.5% versus 17.4%; $p<0.001$), although this certainly could also have been influenced by the increased duration of dialysis (3.1 years versus 1.9 years). In recent years, Vietnam has reported a steady rise in voluntary unpaid blood donations and blood donor screening for HIV, HBV and HCV is now mandatory [56]. The high levels of HCV infection we detected in transfused individuals could possibly have been associated with a past practice of paid blood donation and a lack of rigorous blood donation screening for transfusion transmitted infections [16,47]. However, this remains to be established.

A significant association between increased HCV prevalence and longer duration of dialysis was established. Male gender and years from first transfusion were also seen to be independent risk factors for HCV infection in dialysis patients. These associations have been previously documented in dialysis centres in other countries [10,11,54]. Despite the association of HCV transmission with duration of dialysis, a high seroprevalence of 8.8% was also detected in dialysis patients that had been receiving treatment for one year or less.

Phylogenetic analysis identified high genetic diversity in circulating strains of HCV, confirming the polyphyletic nature of this virus in Vietnam. A wide variety of genotypes including 1a, 1b, 2a, 3a, 3b, 6a, 6e, 6h, 6l and novel variants were identified. Genotype 1 viruses (1a/1b) predominated throughout the country (60%) and also in the IDU (70.1%) and CSW (63.7%) cohorts. This is consistent with a recent report describing a predominance of genotype 1 in Hai Phong IDUs [37]. The high levels of genotype 1a and 1b in Vietnam are particularly significant as genotype 1-infected individuals are less likely to obtain a sustained virological response following treatment with pegylated interferon-α and ribavirin [57].

A different distribution of HCV genotypes was noted in the South of Vietnam (Khanh Hoa and Can Tho), where genotype 6 viruses were dominant in the dialysis and multi-transfused groups (73.9%). This is consistent with a recent report describing a predominance of genotype 6 in blood donors and patients with liver disease in Ho Chi Minh City [39]. Phylogenetic analysis revealed clear geographical clustering of some variants and identified a large monophyletic cluster of 6l viruses in dialysis and multi-transfused patients in Khanh Hoa. Previous reports have suggested that differences in HCV distribution between Northern and Southern regions of the country may be attributed to the fact that injecting drug use have been in widespread use for much longer in the South [58,59]. It would also appear that the high genetic diversity observed in dialysis patients indicates multiple introductions of HCV into Vietnamese dialysis units.

New subtypes of HCV, and indeed new genotypes, continue to be identified around the world [41]. In fact, many of the new subtypes of HCV recently recognised have been first described in Vietnam [41,60]. A proposal for a unified system of nomenclature

of HCV genotypes was published in 2005 along with guidelines to define what constitutes a new subtype and these have been adopted by the three international HCV databases, Los Alamos (United States), euHCVdb (France) and the Hepatitis Virus database in Japan [29]. Provisional designation of a new subtype requires at least 3 individuals to be independently infected with viruses that differ by a minimum of 15% at the nucleotide level in both the *core/E1* and *NS5B* region, but group together consistently when analysed by a variety of phylogenetic methods [29]. Here we describe two novel variants of HCV genotype 6 in Southern Vietnam. One variant (unclassified group 1), found in 4 dialysis patients in Can Tho, has less than 77% similarity within the *NS5B* and the *core/E1* regions to previously published strains of HCV, and the other variant (unclassified group 2), found in 2 multi-transfused patients in Khanh Hoa, had 83% identity to published strains in the *NS5B* region. These new variants, in particular group 1, meet the internationally accepted criteria for designation of a new subtype on the basis of nucleotide sequence divergence; however, confirmation of this will require the identification of further cases of infection elsewhere [29]. Further studies are also required to identify the geographical spread, if any, of these potential new HCV genotype 6 variants and to ascertain their frequency in the general population.

Overall, the results of our study clearly indicate that the burden of HCV infection remains high in IDUs, dialysis patients, CSWs and multi-transfused patients in Vietnam. As no effective vaccine for HCV exists, and treatment remains prohibitively expensive, the focus of public health interventions must be on preventative initiatives such as needle exchange programmes and providing integrated, cost-effective screening to enhance disease surveillance [61]. Encouraging results from needle and syringe programmes have been recently reported in Australia where HCV prevalence rates in IDUs declined from 62% to 50% from 2008 to 2009 [62]. Primary preventative measures, together with a safe supply of blood and reinforcement of universal precautions in the health care environment should help reduce the burden of infection over time.

Acknowledgments

This investigation is part of a larger epidemiological study of blood-borne viruses being performed by the Ireland Vietnam Blood-Borne Virus Initiative (IVVI), a collaborative partnership, between the National Virus Reference Laboratory (NVRL), Ireland and the National Institute of Hygiene and Epidemiology (NIHE), Vietnam. The goals of the IVVI are to develop capacity and infrastructure in clinical and diagnostic virology in Viet Nam.

The authors would like to acknowledge the excellent contributions from staff at the Laboratory for Molecular Diagnostics at NIHE in Ha Noi and at the National Virus Reference Laboratory in Dublin and all staff involved in specimen collection in Vietnam. The authors gratefully acknowledge Dr Ricardo Segurado and CSTAR in UCD for statistical assistance.

Author Contributions

Conceived and designed the experiments: LD Hien Tran Nguyen WWH LANT. Performed the experiments: LD JD LTN THTT Ha Thu Nguyen TTDD QPL LABT HDD TTDT. Analyzed the data: LD MC JD AW JC SC WWH LANT. Wrote the paper: LD MC JC SC WWH LANT.

References

1. Shepard CW, Finelli L, Alter MJ (2005) Global epidemiology of hepatitis C virus infection. The Lancet infectious diseases 5: 558–567.

2. Perz JFFL, Pecoraro C, Hutin YJF, Armstrong GL (2004) Estimated global prevalence of hepatitis C virus infection. 42nd Annual Meeting of the Infectious Disease Soceity of America; Boston, MA, USA Sept 30–Oct 3.

3. World Health Organisation (2000) Hepatitis C–global prevalence (update). Weekly epidemiological record/Health Section of the Secretariat of the League of Nations 75: 18–19.

4. Sievert W, Altraif I, Razavi HA, Abdo A, Ahmed EA, et al. (2011) A systematic review of hepatitis C virus epidemiology in Asia, Australia and Egypt. Liver

international : official journal of the International Association for the Study of the Liver 31 Suppl 2: 61–80.

5. Alter MJ (2011) HCV routes of transmission: what goes around comes around. Seminars in liver disease 31: 340–346.

6. Yan YX, Gao YQ, Sun X, Wang W, Huang XJ, et al. (2011) Prevalence of hepatitis C virus and hepatitis B virus infections in HIV-positive Chinese patients. Epidemiology and infection 139: 354–360.

7. Nelson PK, Mathers BM, Cowie B, Hagan H, Des Jarlais D, et al. (2011) Global epidemiology of hepatitis B and hepatitis C in people who inject drugs: results of systematic reviews. Lancet 378: 571–583.

8. Ferrero S, Lungaro P, Bruzzone BM, Gotta C, Bentivoglio G, et al. (2003) Prospective study of mother-to-infant transmission of hepatitis C virus: a 10-year survey (1990–2000). Acta obstetricia et gynecologica Scandinavica 82: 229–234.

9. Ali S, Ali I, Azam S, Ahmad B (2011) Frequency distribution of HCV genotypes among chronic hepatitis C patients of Khyber Pakhtunkhwa. Virology journal 8: 193.

10. El-kader YE-OA, Elmanama AA, Ayesh BM (2010) Prevalence and risk factors of hepatitis B and C viruses among haemodialysis patients in Gaza strip, Palestine. Virology journal 7: 210.

11. Gasim GI, Hamdan HZ, Hamdan SZ, Adam I (2012) Epidemiology of hepatitis B and hepatitis C virus infections among hemodialysis patients in Khartoum, Sudan. Journal of medical virology 84: 52–55.

12. Frank C, Mohamed MK, Strickland GT, Lavanchy D, Arthur RR, et al. (2000) The role of parenteral antischistosomal therapy in the spread of hepatitis C virus in Egypt. Lancet 355: 887–891.

13. WHO (2008) Global database on blood safety summary report 2004–2005.

14. Power JP, Lawlor E, Davidson F, Holmes EC, Yap PL, et al. (1995) Molecular epidemiology of an outbreak of infection with hepatitis C virus in recipients of anti-D immunoglobulin. Lancet 345: 1211–1213.

15. Chimparlee N, Oota S, Phikulsod S, Tangkijvanich P, Poovorawan Y (2011) Hepatitis B and hepatitis C virus in Thai blood donors. The Southeast Asian journal of tropical medicine and public health 42: 609–615.

16. Nakata S, Song P, Duc DD, Nguyen XQ, Murata K, et al. (1994) Hepatitis C and B virus infections in populations at low or high risk in Ho Chi Minh and Hanoi, Vietnam. Journal of Gastroenterology and Hepatology 9: 416–419.

17. Johnson DW, Dent H, Yao Q, Tranaeus A, Huang CC, et al. (2009) Frequencies of hepatitis B and C infections among haemodialysis and peritoneal dialysis patients in Asia-Pacific countries: analysis of registry data. Nephrology, dialysis, transplantation : official publication of the European Dialysis and Transplant Association - European Renal Association 24: 1598–1603.

18. Lavanchy D (2011) Evolving epidemiology of hepatitis C virus. Clinical microbiology and infection : the official publication of the European Society of Clinical Microbiology and Infectious Diseases 17: 107–115.

19. Fissell RB, Bragg-Gresham JL, Woods JD, Jadoul M, Gillespie B, et al. (2004) Patterns of hepatitis C prevalence and seroconversion in hemodialysis units from three continents: the DOPPS. Kidney international 65: 2335–2342.

20. Martin P, Fabrizi F (2008) Hepatitis C virus and kidney disease. Journal of hepatology 49: 613–624.

21. Jadoul M, Poignet JL, Geddes C, Locatelli F, Medin C, et al. (2004) The changing epidemiology of hepatitis C virus (HCV) infection in haemodialysis: European multicentre study. Nephrology, dialysis, transplantation : official publication of the European Dialysis and Transplant Association - European Renal Association 19: 904–909.

22. Group GBOHCW (2004) Global burden of disease (GBD) for hepatitis C. Journal of clinical pharmacology 44: 20–29.

23. Pawlotsky JM (2004) Pathophysiology of hepatitis C virus infection and related liver disease. Trends in microbiology 12: 96–102.

24. Zhou J, Dore GJ, Zhang F, Lim PL, Chen Y-MA (2007) Hepatitis B and C virus coinfection in The TREAT Asia HIV Observational Database. Journal of Gastroenterology and Hepatology 22: 1510–1518.

25. Alter MJ (2006) Epidemiology of viral hepatitis and HIV co-infection. Journal of hepatology 44: S6–9.

26. Kumar M, Kumar R, Hissar SS, Saraswat MK, Sharma BC, et al. (2007) Risk factors analysis for hepatocellular carcinoma in patients with and without cirrhosis: a case-control study of 213 hepatocellular carcinoma patients from India. Journal of Gastroenterology and Hepatology 22: 1104–1111.

27. Garcia-Garcia JA, Romero-Gomez M, Giron-Gonzalez JA, Rivera-Irigoin R, Torre-Cisneros J, et al. (2006) Incidence of and factors associated with hepatocellular carcinoma among hepatitis C virus and human immunodeficiency virus coinfected patients with decompensated cirrhosis. AIDS research and human retroviruses 22: 1236–1241.

28. Cho LY, Yang JJ, Ko KP, Park B, Shin A, et al. (2011) Coinfection of hepatitis B and C viruses and risk of hepatocellular carcinoma: systematic review and meta-analysis. International journal of cancer Journal international du cancer 128: 176–184.

29. Simmonds P, Bukh J, Combet C, Deleage G, Enomoto N, et al. (2005) Consensus proposals for a unified system of nomenclature of hepatitis C virus genotypes. Hepatology 42: 962–973.

30. Lee YM, Lin HJ, Chen YJ, Lee CM, Wang SF, et al. (2010) Molecular epidemiology of HCV genotypes among injection drug users in Taiwan: Full-length sequences of two new subtype 6w strains and a recombinant form_2b6w. Journal of medical virology 82: 57–68.

31. Wang Y, Xia X, Li C, Maneekarn N, Xia W, et al. (2009) A new HCV genotype 6 subtype designated 6v was confirmed with three complete genome sequences.

32. Journal of clinical virology : the official publication of the Pan American Society for Clinical Virology 44: 195–199.

33. Pybus OG, Barnes E, Taggart R, Lemey P, Markov PV, et al. (2009) Genetic history of hepatitis C virus in East Asia. Journal of virology 83: 1071–1082.

34. Gish RG, Bui TD, Nguyen CT, Nguyen DT, Tran HV, et al. (2012) Liver disease in Viet Nam: Screening, surveillance, management and education: A 5-year plan and call to action. Journal of Gastroenterology and Hepatology 27: 238–247.

35. Kallman JB, Tran S, Arsalla A, Haddad D, Stepanova M, et al. (2011) Vietnamese community screening for hepatitis B virus and hepatitis C virus. Journal of viral hepatitis 18: 70–76.

36. Nguyen VT, McLaws ML, Dore GJ (2007) Prevalence and risk factors for hepatitis C infection in rural north Vietnam. Hepatology international 1: 387–393.

37. Clatts MC, Colon-Lopez V, Giang le M, Goldsamt LA (2010) Prevalence and incidence of HCV infection among Vietnam heroin users with recent onset of injection. Journal of urban health : bulletin of the New York Academy of Medicine 87: 278–291.

38. Tanimoto T, Nguyen HC, Ishizaki A, Chung PT, Hoang TT, et al. (2010) Multiple routes of hepatitis C virus transmission among injection drug users in Hai Phong, Northern Vietnam. J Med Virol 82: 1355–1363.

39. Pham DA, Leuangwutiwong P, Jittmittraphap A, Luplertlop N, Bach HK, et al. (2009) High prevalence of Hepatitis C virus genotype 6 in Vietnam. Asian Pacific journal of allergy and immunology/launched by the Allergy and Immunology Society of Thailand 27: 153–160.

40. Pham VH, Nguyen HD, Ho PT, Banh DV, Pham HL, et al. (2011) Very high prevalence of hepatitis C virus genotype 6 variants in southern Vietnam: large-scale survey based on sequence determination. Japanese journal of infectious diseases 64: 537–539.

41. Daniel HD, Grant PR, Garson JA, Tedder RS, Chandy GM, et al. (2008) Quantitation of hepatitis C virus using an in-house real-time reverse transcriptase polymerase chain reaction in plasma samples. Diagnostic microbiology and infectious disease 61: 415–420.

42. Murphy DG, Willems B, Deschenes M, Hilzenrat N, Mousseau R, et al. (2007) Use of sequence analysis of the NS5B region for routine genotyping of hepatitis C virus with reference to C/E1 and 5' untranslated region sequences. Journal of clinical microbiology 45: 1102–1112.

43. Burland TG (2000) DNASTAR's Lasergene sequence analysis software. Methods in molecular biology 132: 71–91.

44. Hall TA (1999) BioEdit: a user-friendly biological sequence alignment editor and analysis program for Windows 95/98/NT. Nucleic Acids Symp Ser 41: 91–98.

45. Swofford DL (2003) PAUP*. Phylogenetic Analysis Using Parsimony (*and Other Methods). Version 4. Sinauer Associates, Sunderland, Massachusetts.

46. Martin DP, Lemey P, Lott M, Moulton V, Posada D, et al. (2010) RDP3: a flexible and fast computer program for analyzing recombination. Bioinformatics 26: 2462–2463.

47. Tran HT, Ushijima H, Quang VX, Phuong N, Li TC, et al. (2003) Prevalence of hepatitis virus types B through E and genotypic distribution of HBV and HCV in Ho Chi Minh City, Vietnam. Hepatology research : the official journal of the Japan Society of Hepatology 26: 275–280.

48. Kakumu S, Sato K, Morishita T, Trinh KA, Nguyen HB, et al. (1998) Prevalence of hepatitis B, hepatitis C, and GB virus C/hepatitis G virus infections in liver disease patients and inhabitants in Ho Chi Minh, Vietnam. Journal of medical virology 54: 243–248.

49. Quan VM, Go VF, Nam le V, Bergenstrom A, Thuoc NP, et al. (2009) Risks for HIV, HBV, and HCV infections among male injection drug users in northern Vietnam: a case-control study. AIDS care 21: 7–16.

50. Tahan V, Karaca C, Yildirim B, Bozbas A, Ozaras R, et al. (2005) Sexual transmission of HCV between spouses. The American journal of gastroenterology 100: 821–824.

51. Laurent C, Henzel D, Mulanga-Kabeya C, Maertens G, Larouze B, et al. (2001) Seroepidemiological survey of hepatitis C virus among commercial sex workers and pregnant women in Kinshasa, Democratic Republic of Congo. International journal of epidemiology 30: 872–877.

52. Taketa K, Ikeda S, Suganuma N, Phornphutkul K, Peerakome S, et al. (2003) Differential seroprevalences of hepatitis C virus, hepatitis B virus and human immunodeficiency virus among intravenous drug users, commercial sex workers and patients with sexually transmitted diseases in Chiang Mai, Thailand. Hepatology research : the official journal of the Japan Society of Hepatology 27: 6–12.

53. Todd CS, Nasir A, Stanekzai MR, Bautista CT, Botros BA, et al. (2010) HIV, hepatitis B, and hepatitis C prevalence and associated risk behaviors among female sex workers in three Afghan cities. AIDS 24 Suppl 2: S69–75.

54. Kweon SS, Shin MH, Song HJ, Jeon DY, Choi JS (2006) Seroprevalence and risk factors for hepatitis C virus infection among female commercial sex workers in South Korea who are not intravenous drug users. The American journal of tropical medicine and hygiene 74: 1117–1121.

55. Ohsawa M, Kato K, Itai K, Tanno K, Fujishima Y, et al. (2010) Standardized prevalence ratios for chronic hepatitis C virus infection among adult Japanese hemodialysis patients. Journal of epidemiology/Japan Epidemiological Association 20: 30–39.

55. Thanachartwet V, Phumratanaprapin W, Desakorn V, Sahassananda D, Wattanagoon Y, et al. (2007) Viral hepatitis infections among dialysis patients: Thailand registry report. Nephrology 12: 399–405.

56. World Health Organisation (2011) Blood Safety Fact Sheet No 279.

57. Zein NN (2000) Clinical significance of hepatitis C virus genotypes. Clinical microbiology reviews 13: 223–235.

58. Song P, Duc DD, Hien B, Nakata S, Chosa T, et al. (1994) Markers of hepatitis C and B virus infections among blood donors in Ho Chi Minh City and Hanoi, Vietnam. Clinical and diagnostic laboratory immunology 1: 413–418.

59. Nakano T, Lu L, Liu P, Pybus OG (2004) Viral gene sequences reveal the variable history of hepatitis C virus infection among countries. The Journal of infectious diseases 190: 1098–1108.

60. Lu L, Murphy D, Li C, Liu S, Xia X, et al. (2008) Complete genomes of three subtype 6t isolates and analysis of many novel hepatitis C virus variants within genotype 6. The Journal of general virology 89: 444–452.

61. World Health Organisation (2010) Viral Hepatitis.

62. Australia National Centre in HIV Epidemiology and Clinical Research (2010) Australia NSP Survey National Data Report 2005–2009: Prevalence of HIV, HCV and injecting and sexual behaviour among IDUs at needle and syringe programs. URL: http://www.med.unsw.edu.au/NCHECRweb.nsf/resources/NSP_Complete2/$file/ANSP.NDR.2005_2009.pdf Accessed 2012 June 26.

8

Hepcidin-25 in Chronic Hemodialysis Patients is Related to Residual Kidney Function and not to Treatment with Erythropoiesis Stimulating Agents

Neelke C. van der Weerd[1,2]*, **Muriel P. C. Grooteman**[1,3], **Michiel L. Bots**[4], **Marinus A. van den Dorpel**[5], **Claire H. den Hoedt**[5,6], **Albert H. A. Mazairac**[6], **Menso J. Nubé**[1,3], **E. Lars Penne**[1,6], **Carlo A. Gaillard**[1], **Jack F. M. Wetzels**[7], **Erwin T. Wiegerinck**[8,9], **Dorine W. Swinkels**[8,9], **Peter J. Blankestijn**[6], **Piet M. ter Wee**[1,3], **CONTRAST investigators**[¶]

1 Department of Nephrology, VU Medical Center, Amsterdam, The Netherlands, **2** Department of Nephrology, Academic Medical Center, University of Amsterdam, Amsterdam, The Netherlands, **3** Institute for Cardiovascular Research VU Medical Center (ICaR-VU), VU Medical Center, Amsterdam, The Netherlands, **4** Julius Center for Health Sciences and Primary Care, University Medical Center Utrecht, Utrecht, The Netherlands, **5** Department of Internal Medicine, Maasstad Hospital, Rotterdam, The Netherlands, **6** Department of Nephrology, University Medical Center Utrecht, Utrecht, The Netherlands, **7** Department of Nephrology, Radboud University Nijmegen Medical Center, Nijmegen, The Netherlands, **8** Department of Laboratory Medicine, Laboratory of Genetic, Endocrine and Metabolic Diseases, Radboud University Nijmegen Medical Center, Nijmegen, The Netherlands, **9** Hepcidinanalysis.com, Radboud University Nijmegen Medical Center, Nijmegen, The Netherlands

Abstract

Hepcidin-25, the bioactive form of hepcidin, is a key regulator of iron homeostasis as it induces internalization and degradation of ferroportin, a cellular iron exporter on enterocytes, macrophages and hepatocytes. Hepcidin levels are increased in chronic hemodialysis (HD) patients, but as of yet, limited information on factors associated with hepcidin-25 in these patients is available. In the current cross-sectional study, potential patient-, laboratory- and treatment-related determinants of serum hepcidin-20 and -25, were assessed in a large cohort of stable, prevalent HD patients. Baseline data from 405 patients (62% male; age 63.7±13.9 [mean SD]) enrolled in the CONvective TRAnsport STudy (CONTRAST; NCT00205556) were studied. Predialysis hepcidin concentrations were measured centrally with matrix-assisted laser desorption/ionization time-of-flight mass spectrometry. Patient-, laboratory- and treatment related characteristics were entered in a backward multivariable linear regression model. Hepcidin-25 levels were independently and positively associated with ferritin ($p<0.001$), hsCRP ($p<0.001$) and the presence of diabetes ($p=0.02$) and inversely with the estimated glomerular filtration rate ($p=0.01$), absolute reticulocyte count ($p=0.02$) and soluble transferrin receptor ($p<0.001$). Men had lower hepcidin-25 levels as compared to women ($p=0.03$). Hepcidin-25 was not associated with the maintenance dose of erythropoiesis stimulating agents (ESA) or iron therapy. In conclusion, in the currently studied cohort of chronic HD patients, hepcidin-25 was a marker for iron stores and erythropoiesis and was associated with inflammation. Furthermore, hepcidin-25 levels were influenced by residual kidney function. Hepcidin-25 did not reflect ESA or iron dose in chronic stable HD patients on maintenance therapy. These results suggest that hepcidin is involved in the pathophysiological pathway of renal anemia and iron availability in these patients, but challenges its function as a clinical parameter for ESA resistance.

Editor: Leighton R. James, University of Florida, United States of America

Funding: The Dutch CONvective TRAnsport STudy is financially supported by a grant from the Dutch Kidney Foundation (Nierstichting Nederland, grant C02.2019) and unrestricted grants from Fresenius Medical Care (The Netherlands) and Gambro Lundia AB (Sweden). Additional support for CONTRAST was received from the Dr. E.E. Twiss Fund, Roche Netherlands; the International Society of Nephrology/Baxter Extramural Grant Program; the Dutch Organization for Health Research and Development (ZonMW, grant 17088.2802); and for this particular study from Amgen BV Netherlands. The funders had no role in study design, data collection and analysis, decision to publish, or preparation of the manuscript.

Competing Interests: DWS is a co-founder and Medical Director of the "Hepcidinanalysis.com" initiative, which aims to serve the scientific and medical community with high-quality hepcidin-25 measurements (www.hepcidinanalysis.com). The other authors have declared that no competing interests exist. Furthermore, the main study was supported by funding from several commercial sources (Fresenius Medical Care, Gambro Lundia AB (Sweden), Roche Netherlands, Baxter Netherlands and Amgen BV Netherlands). This does not alter the authors adherence to all the PLoS ONE policies on sharing data and materials.

* E-mail: n.c.vanderweerd@amc.uva.nl

¶ Membership of the CONTRAST investigators is provided in the Acknowledgments.

Introduction

Hepcidin is a key regulator of iron homeostasis in humans. It induces internalization and degradation of ferroportin, which is a cellular iron exporter on enterocytes, macrophages and hepatocytes [1,2]. Hence, hepcidin reduces iron absorption from the gut and iron release from reticuloendothelial and hepatocyte stores. The bioactive form is hepcidin-25, a mainly protein-bound amino acid of 2.8 kD, whereas hepcidin-20 and hepcidin-22 are its isoforms with unknown biological function [2,3]. The expression of hepcidin is regulated in response to iron administration, erythropoietic demand, hypoxia and inflammatory signals [2,4].

Hepcidin is excreted with the urine. In patients with chronic kidney disease (CKD), serum levels of the active hepcidin-25 and its isoforms are increased [5,6]. In patients with end stage renal disease (ESRD) on dialysis, even higher levels of hepcidin have been observed [5,6]. Hepcidin is the intermediary between available iron stores on the one hand, and erythropoiesis on the other hand. Furthermore, it has been suggested that hepcidin is an important tool to predict the response to erythropoiesis stimulating agents (ESA) [7,8,9]. Therefore, hepcidin might be useful to assess the functional iron availability in patients with renal failure as high levels might indicate a blockade of iron release from its stores [10].

In several studies, patient-, laboratory- and treatment characteristics of CKD and ESRD patients have been related with hepcidin levels. Many studies have shown a relation between ferritin levels and hepcidin, both in CKD [5,6,9,11] and in hemodialysis (HD) patients [5,12,13,14,15]. Furthermore, studies in CKD and HD patients have shown associations with hepcidin and various other parameters such as residual kidney function (RKF) [6,11,16], ESA dose [11] and markers of inflammation including C-reactive protein (CRP), tumor necrosis factor α (TNF-α) and interleukin-6 (IL-6) [7,15]. In these studies, hepcidin has been measured with different techniques, mainly competitive immunoassays and mass spectrometry (MS) based methods, impeding direct comparisons [3,17,18]. Furthermore, most studies on hepcidin in HD patients included a limited number of patients, precluding multivariate statistics.

In the current study, patient-, laboratory- and treatment characteristics that are associated with hepcidin levels are evaluated with a state-of-the-art hepcidin assay in a prospective cohort of over 400 chronic HD patients, included in the CONvective TRAnsport STudy (CONTRAST).

Materials and Methods

Patients and Study Design

Baseline data from patients enrolled in the CONTRAST study (NCT00205556) were used. The rationale and the design of the CONTRAST study have been described before [19]. In short, prevalent HD patients were recruited from 2004 until 2010 and randomized to either continue treatment with low flux HD, or switch to treatment with post-dilution online hemodiafiltration, both with ultrapure dialysate, with a variable follow up until December 2010. Primary endpoint of the study is all cause mortality [20], and anemia management is a secondary endpoint. A total of 714 patients were recruited from 29 dialysis centers. In the design phase of CONTRAST, a protocol for blood sampling and storage was added, specifically for future studies on newly identified markers that would become potentially relevant and of interest. Hepcidin is an example of such a marker. In 17 of the 29 dialysis centers, in which blood sampling and storage was logistically feasible, predialysis blood samples from participating patients were drawn and stored at −80°C. The selection of centers participating in this sub-study was made prior to enrolment. The present analyses were based on a subset of patients from the main study, namely those participants (n = 405) from who additional blood samples were collected.

Patients were eligible for inclusion in the main study if they were treated two or three times per week with HD for at least two months. Exclusion criteria were age below 18 years, treatment with hemo(dia)filtration or high-flux HD in the six months prior to randomization, a life expectancy less than three months due to non-renal disease, participation in another clinical intervention trial evaluating cardiovascular outcomes and severe incompliance regarding frequency and/or duration of dialysis treatment.

The study was conducted in accordance with the Declaration of Helsinki and was approved by a central medical ethics committee and by all local medical ethics review boards. Written informed consent was obtained from all patients prior to enrolment (File S1). Patients provided informed consent for storage of blood samples for later analysis.

Treatment Protocol

Included patients were stable for at least two months with a minimum dialysis spKt/V$_{urea}$ of 1.2 per treatment and they were treated with either polysulfone (PS) or polyarylethersulfone (PAES) low-flux dialyzers with a UF coefficient varying between 10 and 21 ml/mmHg/h and a surface area from 1.3 to 2.2 m^2: F6HPS, F7HPS, F8HPS and F10HPS (Fresenius Medical Care, Bad Homburg, Germany) and Polyflux 14 L, 17 L and 21 L (Gambro Corporation AB, Lund, Sweden). Dialysis was performed with ultrapure dialysis fluids, containing less than 0.1 colony forming units per mL and less than 0.03 endotoxin units per mL.

Routine patient care and prescription of medication was practiced according to the opinion of the attending nephrologist and based on the Quality of Care Guidelines of the Dutch Federation of Nephrology. The Dutch Quality of Care Guideline on anemia management was derived from the European Best Practice Guidelines [21] and the KDOQI guidelines [22,23,24]. ESA and iron supplements were administered via the venous bloodline at the end of a dialysis session. Decisions on dose changes and the timing of these changes were made according to the opinion of the treating nephrologist.

Laboratory Protocol

Predialysis blood samples were drawn and routine laboratory assessments were analyzed in the local hospitals by standard laboratory techniques. The total iron-binding capacity (TIBC) was considered to represent serum transferrin level [25] and the transferrin saturation ratio (TSAT) was either provided by the local laboratory or calculated as serum iron divided by the TIBC. Hepcidin, soluble transferrin receptor (sTfR), hsCRP and IL-6 measurements were preformed centrally. For this purpose, predialysis blood samples were centrifuged at 1500 g and 4°C for 10 minutes and stored at −80°C.

Serum hepcidin-20 and -25 measurements were centrally performed by a validated combination of weak cation exchange (WCX) bead-based hepcidin enrichment followed by time-of-flight mass spectrometry (WCX-TOF-MS) [17]. For the quantification of hepcidin in serum, an internal standard (synthetic hepcidin-24, Peptide International Inc., Louisville, KY, USA) was used [26]. Peptide spectra were generated on a Microflex LT matrix-enhanced laser desorption/ionisation (MALDI-) TOF-MS platform (Bruker Daltonics GmbH, Bremen, Germany). Serum hepcidin-20 and -25 concentrations were expressed as nmol/L and the lower limit of detection of this method was 0.5 nmol/L. For hepcidin-25, the intra-assay coefficients of variation (CV) were 3.7% at 7.9 nmol/L, 2.3% at 13.4 nmol/L, and 2.2% at 3.1 nmol/L. The inter-assay CV were 9.1% at 7.8 nmol/L and 3.9% at 12.9 nmol/L [17]. This method enables the specific measurement of the hepcidin isoforms (hepcidin-25, hepcidin-22 and hepcidin-20) [17] and has been described before in CKD and HD patients [5]. It is an update of a previous method performed by the same laboratory [26,27]. sTfR (mg/L) was measured immunonephelometrically on a BN II System (Dade Behring Marburg GmbH, Marburg, Germany). hsCRP (mg/L) was measured with a particle-enhanced immunoturbidimetric assay on a Roche-Hitachi analyzer (Roche Diagnostics GmbH, Mannheim, Germany) with a lower quantification limit of 0.1 mg/L and

Table 1. Patient and treatment characteristics and laboratory parameters.[a]

	N = 405
Patient characteristics	
Male gender – no. (%)	252 (62)
Age (years)	63.7±13.9
Caucasian race – no. (%)	333 (82)
Dialysis vintage (years)	1.8 (0.9–3.6)
Cause of renal failure - no. (%)	
- vascular	131 (32)
- diabetes mellitus	63 (16)
- tubulointerstitial nephritis/glomerulo-nephritis/multisystem disease	96 (24)
- cystic disease	28 (7)
- other/unknown	87 (21)
Diabetes mellitus – no. (%)	85 (21)
History of cardiovascular disease – no. (%)	177 (44)
Current smoker – no. (%)	81 (20)
Body weight (kg)[b]	71.7±14.6
Systolic blood pressure (mmHg)[c]	142±18
Diastolic blood pressure (mmHg)[c]	73±11
BMI (kg/m²)	25.0±4.8
Residual diuresis – no. (%)[d]	230 (57)
eGFR (ml/min/1.73 m²)[e]	2.6 (1.2–5.1)
Treatment characteristics	
Treatment frequency 3x/week – no. (%)	375 (93)
Treatment time (min)	227±23
Bloodflow (mL/min)	298±39
Dialysis access – no. (%)	
- fistula	339 (84)
- graft	56 (14)
- central catheter	10 (2)
spKt/V (per dialysis)	1.39±0.20
Dialyzer – no. (%)	
- polysulfone	246 (61)
- polyarylethersulfone	147 (37)
- other	12 (3)
Prescription of ESA- no. (%)	364 (90)
Type of ESA – no. (%)	
- darbepoetin α	254 (70
- epoetin α/β	110 (30)
ESA dose (DDD/week)[f]	8.9 (6.0–15.4)
Use of iron replacement therapy – no. (%)	300 (74)
Irondose (mg/week)[g]	100 (50–100)
Prescription of RAS inhibitors – no. (%)	215 (53)
Prescription of statin – no. (%)	203 (50)
Laboratory parameters	
Hemoglobin (g/dL)	11.9±1.3
Hematocrit	0.36±0.04
MCV (fl)	94.9±6.2
Reticulocytes (x10⁹/L)	65.3±30.5
Ferritin (ng/mL)	378 (211–631)

Table 1. Cont.

	N = 405
TSAT (%)	24.3±12.4
sTfR (mg/L)[h]	1.58 (1.24–2.11)
Cholesterol (mg/dL)	143.1±38.7
Albumin (g/dL)	3.6±0.5
hsCRP (mg/L)	3.95 (1.38–10.41)
Il-6 (pg/mL)	2.06 (1.21–3.82)
Hepcidin-20 (nM)	6.3 (3.9–9.3)
Hepcidin-25 (nM)[i]	13.8 (6.6–22.5)

[a]Values represent mean ± SD, median (interquartile range) or proportion (%).
[b]Weight after dialysis (dry weight) defined as the mean of three consecutive values.
[c]Mean of pre- and post-dialysis blood pressure of three consecutive dialysis sessions.
[d]Defined as >100 mL per day.
[e]eGFR (estimated glomerular filtration rate) calculated as mean of creatinine and urea clearance in 24 h urine collection adjusted for body surface area, exclusively in patients with residual diuresis.
[f]In patients on ESA therapy.
[g]In patients on iron therapy.
[h]Reference value: 0.76–1.76 mg/L (Dade Behring Marburg GmbH, Marburg, Germany).
[i]Reference value (median [95% range]): men 65–69 years 5.3 (<0.05–13.9); women 65–69 years 4.9 (<0.05–14.2) [29].
Conversion factors for units: hemoglobin in g/dL to mmol/L, x 0.62; cholesterol in mg/dL to mmol/L, x 0.026; albumin in g/dL to g/L, x 10; no conversion necessary for ferritin in ng/mL to µg/L.
BMI = body mass index; ESA = erythropoiesis stimulating agents; RAS = renin angiotensin system; TSAT = transferrin saturation ratio; sTfR = soluble transferrin receptor; PTH = parathyroid hormone; hsCRP = high sensitive c-reactive protein; IL-6 = interleukin-6.

an intra-assay variation of 1.9% at the level of 0.57 mg/L and 0.3% at the level of 3.00 mg/L. The inter-assay variation was 1.9% at the level of 0.67 mg/L and 1.2% at the level of 3.64 mg/L. IL-6 (pg/mL) was measured with an immunometric assay (Sanquin, Amsterdam, The Netherlands). The intra-assay variation was 12% at the level of 1 pg/mL and 8% at the level of 3 pg/mL. The inter-assay variation was 19% at the level of 0.35 pg/mL (which was the lower quantification limit) and 12% at the level of 2.3 pg/mL.

Data Collection

Data on demography, cause of renal failure, history of cardiovascular disease (CVD), diabetes mellitus (DM), type of vascular access, dialysis vintage and treatment parameters were collected, as well as medication use. ESA was prescribed as epoetin α or β (Eprex® or Neorecormon® respectively, IU) or darbepoetin α (Aranesp®, µg) and expressed as a dose per week. To compare the different types of ESA, prescribed dosages were converted to daily defined doses (DDD), using conversion factors as provided by the World Health Organization (WHO) Drug Classification (http://www.whocc.no/atc_ddd_index/). For darbepoetin α (ATC code B03XA02), DDD is 4.5 µg and for epoetin α and β (ATC code B03XA01), DDD is 1000 IU. All patients on iron therapy used iron sucrose (Venofer®, mg/week).

RKF was defined as a urine production of >100 mL/d. In patients with RKF, the eGFR (estimated glomerular filtration rate) was calculated as the mean of creatinine and urea clearance in a 24 h urine collection, adjusted for body surface area [28].

Statistical Analysis

Variables were reported as proportions or means ± standard deviation (SD), or medians with 25th–75th percentiles when appropriate. The relation between hepcidin-20 and hepcidin-25 was evaluated with a Spearman's correlation test. All patient characteristics, laboratory parameters and treatment characteristics listed in table 1, were considered as possible determinants of hepcidin-25. First, relations between these determinants and hepcidin-25 were studied using a backward multivariable linear regression model with a p-value <0.15 as a cut-off level. Subsequently, the determinants that were related with Hepcidin-25 (with a p-value <0.15) were entered in a second multivariable regression model. In this second regression model, a double sided p-value <0.05 was considered statistically significant. The natural logarithm of hepcidin-25 (ln-hepcidin-25) was applied as the dependent variable in all regression models since the distribution of hepcidin-25 was positively skewed. The regression coefficients (B) were retransformed into percentages of change in hepcidin-25 by using the formula $(e^{B}-1) \times 100$, which means that for each increment in the determinant, hepcidin-25 changed with the specified percentage. Additionally, in a separate analysis, all regression models were adjusted for participating center to correct for local policies concerning anemia management and timing of ESA and iron administration and blood withdrawal.

To evaluate whether the relation between a determinant (e.g. hsCRP) and hepcidin-25 was modified by a second determinant (e.g. ferritin), the possibility of effect modification was explored by adding an interaction term (e.g. hsCRP x ferritin) to the multivariable regression model. If this interaction term turned out to be significant (p<0.05), the relation between the determinant and hepcidin-25 was analyzed separately in each stratum of the second determinant.

Statistical analyses were performed with PASW software (version 18.0, SPSS inc. Headquarters, Chicago, Illinois, US).

Results

Blood samples from 405 patients were available. All patient and treatment characteristics and laboratory parameters are listed in table 1 (baseline characteristics of the total CONTRAST cohort [n = 714] are listed in table S1). Mean (± SD) age of the patients was 63.7±13.9 years and 62% was male. Hepcidin-20 and hepcidin-25 were highly correlated (r = 0.76; p<0.001; figure 1). In this section, results for hepcidin-25 are presented. In analyses with hepcidin-20 as an outcome parameter, similar results were obtained (data not shown).

Multivariable Regression Analysis

In table 2, all determinants of hepcidin showing a p-value <0.15 in the backward multivariable linear regression model are listed. In the final model (R2 = 0.49), ferritin, hsCRP and the presence of diabetes mellitus showed a positive relation with hepcidin-25, whereas male gender, eGFR and sTfR had an inverse relation. Of note, no relation between hepcidin-25 and the weekly ESA dose and the administration of iron supplements was observed. Adjustment for participating center did not change the results (data not shown).

Interaction between Determinants

The relation between hsCRP and hepcidin-25 was modified by the ferritin level, as the interaction term (hsCRP x ferritin) was highly significant (p<0.001). This relation persisted after adjustment for other determinants of hepcidin-25. As depicted in figure 2, the relation between ferritin and hepcidin-25 was present

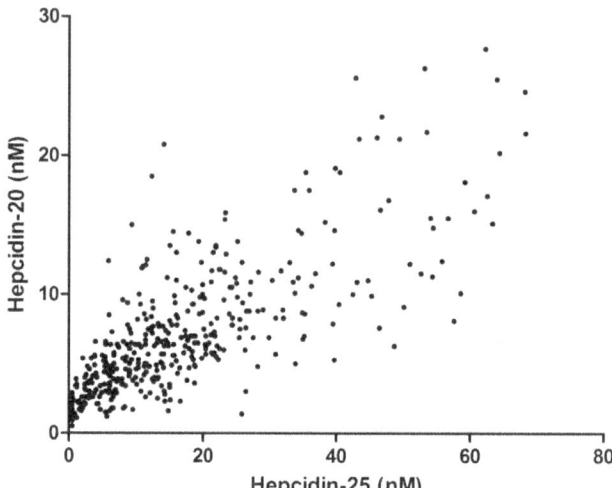

Figure 1. Correlation of Hepcidin-25 with its isoform hepcidin-20. Hepcidin-20 and -25 were measured with mass spectrometry (WCX-MALDI-TOF-MS, see section on laboratory protocol). r = 0.76; p-value <0.001.

irrespective of the level of inflammation (lowest hsCRP tertile: B = 0.020 per 10 ng/mL; 95%CI -0.015 to 0.026; p<0.001; middle hsCRP tertile: B = 0.014 per 10 ng/mL; 95%CI 0.010 to 0.018; p<0.001; highest hsCRP tertile: B = 0.015 per 10 ng/mL; 95%CI 0.010 to 0.020; p<0.001). In fact, the relation between hsCRP and hepcidin-25 was present in all three tertiles of ferritin (lowest tertile: B = 0.020 per mg/L; 95%CI −0.010 to 0.030; p<0.001; middle tertile: B = 0.009 per mg/L; 95%CI 0.000 to 0.018; p = 0.055; highest tertile: B = 0.007 per mg/L; 95%CI 0.001 to 0.013; p = 0.034).

No interaction between hemoglobin level and ESA dose on hepcidin-25 levels was observed as the interaction term (ESA dose X hemoglobin) was not statistically significant (p = 0.588). The absence of a relation between those parameters is readily apparent from figure 3.

Discussion

In this cross-sectional study in a cohort of stable prevalent HD patients, hepcidin-25 levels were shown to be independently and positively associated with iron stores (as reflected by ferritin levels), inflammation (hsCRP) and the presence of diabetes, and inversely with erythropoiesis (sTfR and reticulocyte count), residual kidney function (eGFR) and male gender. Of note, no relations between hepcidin-25 and either ESA dose or iron supplementation were observed.

In our study, ferritin was the strongest determinant of hepcidin, which has been well established before in healthy controls [29], CKD patients [5,6,9,11] and in patients with ESRD treated with HD and peritoneal dialysis [5,12,13,14,15]. Notably, the studies in HD patients included mostly low patient numbers. As can be seen from figure 2, the relation between hepcidin-25 and ferritin was present irrespective of the level of inflammation. However, whether hepcidin is upregulated in response to increased ferritin levels cannot be concluded from our study.

sTfR has proven to be a valuable tool to assess bone marrow erythropoietic activity and iron stores in HD patients treated with ESA [30,31]. However, it could not predict a response of intravenous iron administration on the hemoglobin level [32]. In our study, an inverse association between either sTfR and reticulocyte count, and hepcidin levels was observed, after

Table 2. Results from the multivariable regression analysis on hepcidin-25 levels.[a]

Determinant	Multivariable regression					
	B[b]	95% CI[b]	% change[c]	95% CI[c]	P-value
Gender (male)	−0.188	−0.361 to −0.016	−17.1	−30.3 to −1.6	0.032
Diabetes	0.246	0.034 to 0.458	27.9	3.5 to 58.1	0.023
Current smoker	−0.188	−0.390 to 0.014	−17.1	−32.3 to 1.4	0.067
Prescription of statins	−0.162	−0.332 to 0.009	−15.0	−28.3 to 0.9	0.063
Prescription of RAS inhibitors	0.113	−0.056 to 0.282	12.0	−5.4 to 28.7	0.053
eGFR (per mL/min/1.73 m^2)	−0.033	−0.057 to −0.008	−3.2	−5.5 to −0.5	0.008
Hemoglobin (per g/dL)	0.085	0.019 to 0.152	8.9	1.9 to 16.4	0.012
MCV	−0.011	−0.025 to 0.004	−1.1	−2.5 to 0.4	0.150
Reticulocytes (per 10 *10^9/L)	−0.034	−0.063 to −0.006	−3.3	−6.1 to −0.6	0.019
Ferritin (per 10 ng/mL)	0.016	0.013 to 0.018	1.6	1.3 to 1.8	<0.001
sTfR (per mg/L)	−0.409	−0.544 to −0.274	−33.6	−42.0 to −24.0	<0.001
hsCRP (per mg/L)	0.012	0.007 to 0.017	1.2	0.7 to 1.4	<0.001

[a]Regression analyses were performed with natural logarithm of hepcidin-25 as dependent variable. Potential determinants of hepcidin-25 were selected using a backward multivariable linear regression model with a p-value <0.15 used as a cut-off level in which all patient, treatment and laboratory characteristics as listed in table 1 were entered.
[b]The regression coefficient (B) denotes a natural logarithm. Positive values indicate an increase in hepcidin-25 and negative values a decrease with one unit increase of the determinant.
[c]Results of conversion of the regression coefficient (B) from natural logarithm to a percentage of change: for each increase in the determinant with one unit, hepcidin-25 changed with the percentage indicated in this column. Positive values indicate an increase in hepcidin-25 and negative values a decrease.
R^2 for multivariable regression model = 0.49. Further adjustment for participating center did not change the results (data not shown).

multivariable adjustments. Whether low hepcidin levels enhance erythropoiesis, or whether increased bone marrow erythropoietic activity suppresses expression of hepcidin, cannot be concluded from this cross-sectional study.

We showed a strong association between hepcidin-25 and hsCRP, but not with IL-6. Several studies have demonstrated a relation between CRP [5,7,15,33] or IL-6 [7,13] in small groups of chronic HD patients, whereas others did not [14]. The explana-

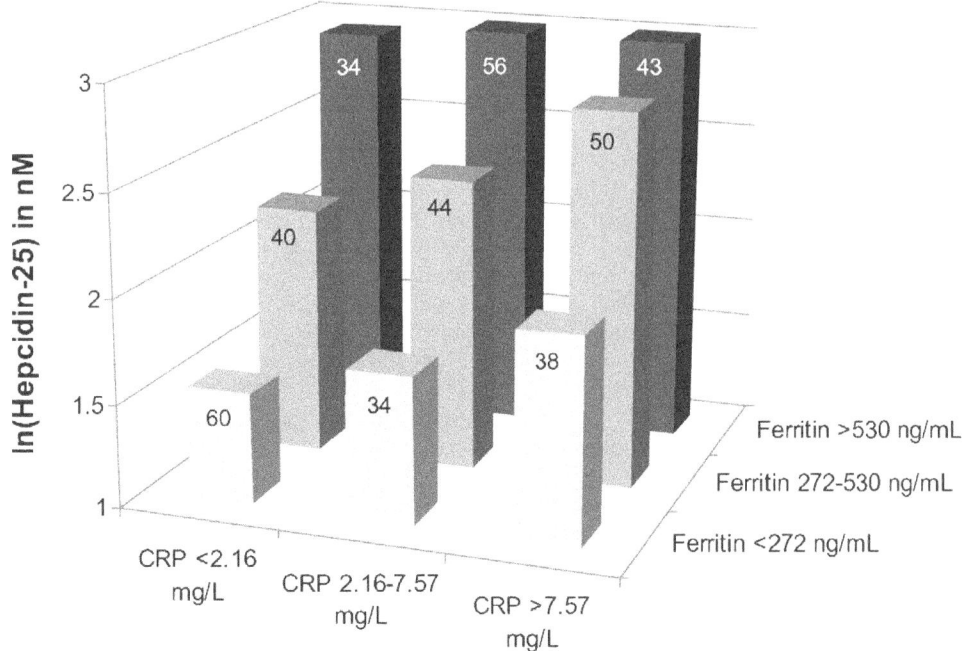

Figure 2. Relationship between ferritin, hsCRP and hepcidin-25. Hepcidin-25 was ln-transformed because of a positively skewed distribution. Values were adjusted for gender, diabetes, smoking status, prescription of statins and RAS inhibitors, eGFR, hemoglobin, MCV, absolute reticulocyte count and the level of soluble transferrin receptor. CRP and ferritin levels were divided in tertiles. Numbers in boxes represent number of patients per category. For 6 patients, ferritin and/or hsCRP levels were missing. P-value for interaction factor (hsCRP x ferritin) <0.001.

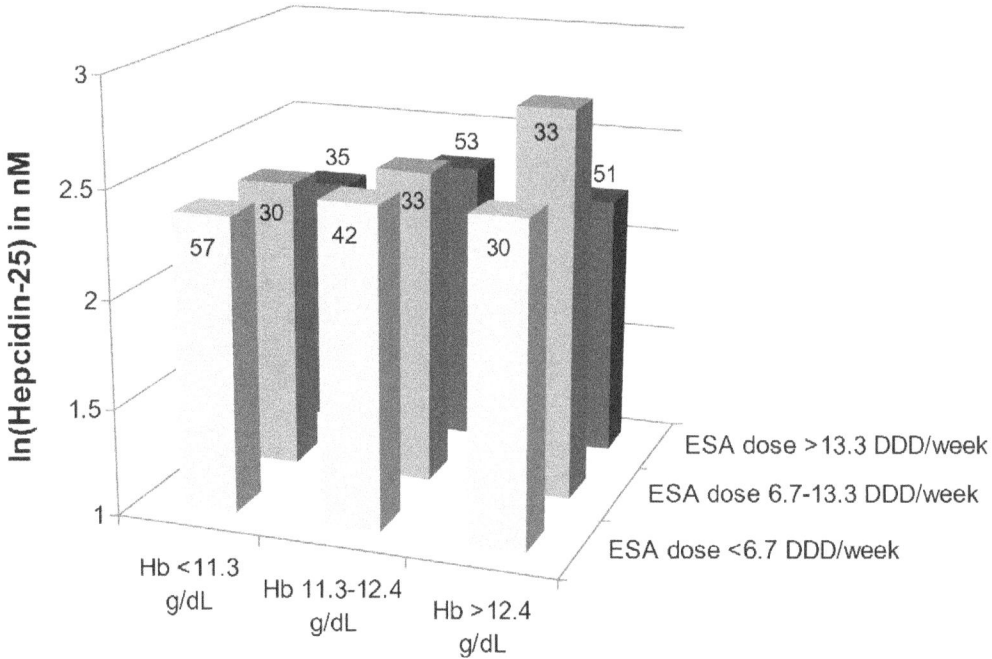

Figure 3. Relationship between ESA dose, hemoglobin and hepcidin-25. Hepcidin-25 was ln-transformed because of a positively skewed distribution. Values were adjusted for gender, diabetes, smoking status, prescription of statins RAS inhibitors, eGFR, MCV, absolute reticulocyte count, ferritin, hsCRP and soluble transferrin receptor. Only patients on ESA therapy are depicted (n = 364). Hemoglobin and ESA dose were divided in tertiles. Numbers in boxes represent number of patients per category. P-value for interaction factor (ESA dose x hemoglobin) NS.

tion for the association between hepcidin-25 and hsCRP, and not IL-6, is not readily apparent, especially as transcription of hepatic hepcidin is activated by binding of IL-6 to its receptor complex [1]. However, in a murine and human model investigating various factors associated with hepcidin expression, the role of IL-6 was limited [34]. Furthermore, the IL-6 assay used in our study showed a wide inter-assay variability, especially in the lower range. This could have resulted in less accurately measured values of IL-6 as compared to hsCRP, and hence less precision in the estimation.

We are the first to report an independent association between eGFR and both the active hepcidin-25 and the inactive isoform hepcidin-20 in HD patients. As we used a mass-spectrometry assay that specifically measures hepcidin-25, our results indicate that the observed association between eGFR and hepcidin-25 was not due to the concurrent measurement of inactive isoforms. To date, studies on the association between eGFR and hepcidin levels in CKD patients have been conflicting [5,6,11,35]. Low hepcidin levels (measured with a radioimmunoassay) were reported in HD and PD patients with residual diuresis [16], but RKF was not quantified in that study. Whether the high hepcidin levels in chronic HD patients were exclusively caused by decreased renal clearance, or whether other mechanisms are involved, cannot be concluded from our data.

In our study population, hepcidin-25 levels were significantly lower in men as compared to women. This can be explained by the fact that most women in our study will be post-menopausal, in whom higher hepcidin levels have been demonstrated [29]. Furthermore, we showed that diabetic patients had higher hepcidin levels. In one study, diabetic patients had higher levels of hepcidin than healthy age-matched controls, although this relation was not adjusted for possible confounders [36].

Interestingly, we did not observe an interaction between ESA dose and hemoglobin levels in relation to hepcidin-25 as has been demonstrated before by Ashby et al [11]. Therefore, it appears

that hepcidin, measured with a mass spectrometric assay in chronic HD patients on maintenance therapy with ESA, is not a marker of ESA resistance. Whether hepcidin-25 can predict an ESA response, as has been shown in patients with the cardio-renal syndrome [9], cannot be concluded from our cross-sectional data. Nevertheless, in a study in 24 HD patients, hepcidin levels of ESA responsive patients did not differ from those who were ESA resistant [12], which is in accordance with our results.

Concerning iron supplementation in HD patients, various effects of iron loading on hepcidin levels have been reported [14,37,38]. We did not observe a relationship between hepcidin and iron supplementation, which can be explained by the fact that patients in our study received maintenance iron therapy instead of a (single) loading dose. Recently, it was shown that hepcidin-25 levels did not predict a response to the administration of intravenous iron supplementation in HD patients on ESA maintenance therapy [38]. Hence, it appears that hepcidin is more a marker of iron stores than a predictor of the effect of iron therapy.

A number of studies showed that hepcidin levels could be lowered over a single HD session [13,15,39], although concentrations were back to baseline only one hour after the treatment [13]. Lowering of hepcidin by HD can be partly explained by appearance of (low) levels of hepcidin in the ultrafiltrate [5,16]. In addition, it has been shown that hepcidin can attach to the membrane of the dialyzer [5], which can be explained by the amphipathic and protein-bound structure of hepcidin [2]. Prospective research is needed to draw any conclusions on the effect of different dialyzers on hepcidin-levels.

Limitations and Strengths

Our study is limited by its cross-sectional design, which impedes assessing causal relationships. Furthermore, a specific treatment protocol for ESA and iron administration and timing of blood sampling was not provided. We tried to compensate for this by adjusting the regression models for participating center in an additional analysis, as the intervals between ESA and/or iron administration and blood sample withdrawal are supposed to be similar within a single treatment center. Since this did not change our results, we conclude that the dosing schedule was not a major confounder in our study. Another potential limitation of our study is the patient selection, based on centers where blood sampling and storage was logistically feasible. This might have introduced a selection bias of which the magnitude and direction cannot be estimated. As selective participation or non-participation must have occurred based on a logistical aspect, which is most probable not related to factors associated with hepcidin or determinants of hepcidin, selection bias seems unlikely.

The strength of our study is the large sample size and the prospective data collection. As far as we know, our study comprises the largest cohort of HD patients in which hepcidin measurements were performed, currently published. The large sample size facilitates multivariable statistics, which is an important method when examining the complex regulation of hepcidin [40]. Moreover, hepcidin measurements have been performed with a validated mass spectrometric technique, enabling specific quantification of the bioactive hepcidin-25.

Conclusions

In this cohort of chronic, stable HD patients, hepcidin-25 levels were independently associated with iron stores (as reflected by ferritin levels), erythropoiesis (reticulocyte count and sTfR), inflammation (hsCRP), eGFR, the presence of diabetes and gender. Hepcidin-25 was strongly correlated with its bio-inactive isoform hepcidin-20, and similar associations with hepcidin-20 were identified. Of note, hepcidin-25 was not associated with the maintenance dose of ESA or iron therapy.

Our findings confirm the role of hepcidin as a biomarker of iron stores and erythropoiesis in chronic HD patients and indicate that hepcidin is not a biomarker of ESA resistance in patients on ESA maintenance therapy. Furthermore, it underscores the potential important role of (limited) RKF in HD patients. However, whether low hepcidin levels in HD patients are associated with a favorable outcome in terms of morbidity and mortality is not clear yet. Furthermore, whether hepcidin measurements in HD patients provide additional information concerning anemia management compared to current available markers such as ferritin is questionable.

Acknowledgments

The authors are grateful to patients and nursing staff participating in this project.

Local Investigators:

The Netherlands: Academic Medical Center, Amsterdam – MG Koopman; Dianet Dialysis Centers, Utrecht – M Kooistra and B van Jaarsveld; Gelderse Vallei Hospital, Ede – GW Feith; Haga Hospital, The Hague – M van Buren; Jeroen Bosch Hospital, 's Hertogenbosch – EK Hoogeveen; Maasstad Hospital, Rotterdam – PJ van de Ven; Martini Hospital, Groningen – TK Kremer Hovinga; Medical Center Alkmaar, Alkmaar – WA Bax; Onze Lieve Vrouwe Gasthuis, Amsterdam – JO Groeneveld; Rijnstate Hospital, Arnhem – LJM Reichert; Slingeland Hospital, Doetinchem – J Huussen; University Medical Center St Radboud, Nijmegen – HW van Hamersvelt; University Medical Center Utrecht, Utrecht – WH Boer; VieCuri Medical Center, Venlo – WH van Kuijk; VU University Medical Center, Amsterdam – MG Vervloet; Zeeuws-Vlaanderen Hospital, Terneuzen – IMPMJ Wauters.

Norway: Haukeland University Hospital, Bergen – I Sekse.

Author Contributions

Conceived and designed the experiments: NCW MPCG MLB MAD CHH AHAM MJN ELP CAG JFMW DWS PJB PMW. Performed the experiments: NCW MPCG MLB CHH AHAM MJN ELP ETW DWS. Analyzed the data: NCW MPCG MLB CAG JFMW PMW. Contributed reagents/materials/analysis tools: NCW MPCG CHH ETW DWS. Wrote the paper: NCW MPCG MLB MAD CHH MJN ELP JFMW DWS PJB PMW.

References

1. Babitt JL, Lin HY (2010) Molecular mechanisms of hepcidin regulation: implications for the anemia of CKD. AmJKidney Dis 55: 726–741.
2. Kroot JJ, Tjalsma H, Fleming RE, Swinkels DW (2011) Hepcidin in human iron disorders: diagnostic implications. Clin Chem 57: 1650–1669.
3. Macdougall IC, Malyszko J, Hider RC, Bansal SS (2010) Current status of the measurement of blood hepcidin levels in chronic kidney disease. ClinJAmSocNephrol 5: 1681–1689.
4. Coyne DW (2011) Hepcidin: clinical utility as a diagnostic tool and therapeutic target. Kidney Int 80: 240–244.
5. Peters HPE, Laarakkers CMM, Swinkels DW, Wetzels JFM (2010) Serum hepcidin-25 levels in patients with chronic kidney disease are independent of glomerular filtration rate. NephrolDialTransplant 25: 848–853.
6. Zaritsky J, Young B, Wang HJ, Westerman M, Olbina G, et al. (2009) Hepcidin–a potential novel biomarker for iron status in chronic kidney disease. ClinJAmSocNephrol 4: 1051–1056.
7. Costa E, Swinkels DW, Laarakkers CM, Rocha-Pereira P, Rocha S, et al. (2009) Hepcidin serum levels and resistance to recombinant human erythropoietin therapy in haemodialysis patients. Acta Haematol 122: 226–229.
8. Swinkels DW, Wetzels JF (2008) Hepcidin: a new tool in the management of anaemia in patients with chronic kidney disease? NephrolDialTransplant 23: 2450–2453.
9. van der Putten K, Jie KE, van den Broek D, Kraaijenhagen RJ, Laarakkers C, et al. (2010) Hepcidin-25 is a marker of the response rather than resistance to exogenous erythropoietin in chronic kidney disease/chronic heart failure patients. EurJHeart Fail 12: 943–950.
10. Wish JB (2006) Assessing iron status: beyond serum ferritin and transferrin saturation. ClinJAmSocNephrol 1 Suppl 1: S4–S8.
11. Ashby DR, Gale DP, Busbridge M, Murphy KG, Duncan ND, et al. (2009) Plasma hepcidin levels are elevated but responsive to erythropoietin therapy in renal disease. Kidney Int 75: 976–981.
12. Kato A, Tsuji T, Luo J, Sakao Y, Yasuda H, et al. (2008) Association of prohepcidin and hepcidin-25 with erythropoietin response and ferritin in hemodialysis patients. AmJNephrol 28: 115–121.
13. Kuragano T, Shimonaka Y, Kida A, Furuta M, Nanami M, et al. (2010) Determinants of hepcidin in patients on maintenance hemodialysis: role of inflammation. AmJNephrol 31: 534–540.
14. Weiss G, Theurl I, Eder S, Koppelstaetter C, Kurz K, et al. (2009) Serum hepcidin concentration in chronic haemodialysis patients: associations and effects of dialysis, iron and erythropoietin therapy. EurJClinInvest 39: 883–890.
15. Zaritsky J, Young B, Gales B, Wang HJ, Rastogi A, et al. (2010) Reduction of serum hepcidin by hemodialysis in pediatric and adult patients. ClinJAmSocNephrol 5: 1010–1014.
16. Malyszko J, Malyszko JS, Kozminski P, Mysliwiec M (2009) Type of renal replacement therapy and residual renal function may affect prohepcidin and hepcidin. Ren Fail 31: 876–883.
17. Kroot JJ, Laarakkers CM, Geurts-Moespot AJ, Grebenchtchikov N, Pickkers P, et al. (2010) Immunochemical and mass-spectrometry-based serum hepcidin assays for iron metabolism disorders. Clin Chem 56: 1570–1579.
18. Kroot JJ, Kemna EH, Bansal SS, Busbridge M, Campostrini N, et al. (2009) Results of the first international round robin for the quantification of urinary and

plasma hepcidin assays: need for standardization. Haematologica 94: 1748–1752.

19. Penne EL, Blankestijn PJ, Bots ML, van den Dorpel MA, Grooteman MP, et al. (2005) Effect of increased convective clearance by on-line hemodiafiltration on all cause and cardiovascular mortality in chronic hemodialysis patients - the Dutch CONvective TRAnsport STudy (CONTRAST): rationale and design of a randomised controlled trial [ISRCTN38365125]. CurrControl Trials CardiovascMed 6: 8.

20. Grooteman MP, van den Dorpel MA, Bots ML, Penne EL, van der Weerd NC, et al. (2012) Effect of Online Hemodiafiltration on All-Cause Mortality and Cardiovascular Outcomes. J Am Soc Nephrol 23: 1087–1096.

21. Locatelli F, Aljama P, Barany P, Canaud B, Carrera F, et al. (2004) Revised European best practice guidelines for the management of anaemia in patients with chronic renal failure. NephrolDialTransplant 19 Suppl 2: ii1–47.

22. NKF-K/DOQI (2001) IV. NKF-K/DOQI Clinical Practice Guidelines for Anemia of Chronic Kidney Disease: update 2000. AmJKidney Dis 37: S182–S238.

23. NKF-K/DOQI (2006) KDOQI Clinical Practice Guidelines and Clinical Practice Recommendations for Anemia in Chronic Kidney Disease. AmJKidney Dis 47: S11–145.

24. NKF-K/DOQI (2007) KDOQI Clinical Practice Guideline and Clinical Practice Recommendations for anemia in chronic kidney disease: 2007 update of hemoglobin target. AmJKidney Dis 50: 471–530.

25. Gambino R, Desvarieux E, Orth M, Matan H, Ackattupathil T, et al. (1997) The relation between chemically measured total iron-binding capacity concentrations and immunologically measured transferrin concentrations in human serum. ClinChem 43: 2408–2412.

26. Swinkels DW, Girelli D, Laarakkers C, Kroot J, Campostrini N, et al. (2008) Advances in quantitative hepcidin measurements by time-of-flight mass spectrometry. PLoS One 3: e2706.

27. Kemna EH, Tjalsma H, Podust VN, Swinkels DW (2007) Mass spectrometry-based hepcidin measurements in serum and urine: analytical aspects and clinical implications. Clin Chem 53: 620–628.

28. Fouque D, Vennegoor M, ter WP, Wanner C, Basci A, et al. (2007) EBPG guideline on nutrition. NephrolDialTransplant 22 Suppl 2: ii45–ii87.

29. Galesloot TE, Vermeulen SH, Geurts-Moespot AJ, Klaver SM, Kroot JJ, et al. (2011) Serum hepcidin: reference ranges and biochemical correlates in the general population. Blood 117: e218–225.

30. Chiang WC, Tsai TJ, Chen YM, Lin SL, Hsieh BS (2002) Serum soluble transferrin receptor reflects erythropoiesis but not iron availability in erythropoietin-treated chronic hemodialysis patients. Clin Nephrol 58: 363–369.

31. Tarng DC, Huang TP (2002) Determinants of circulating soluble transferrin receptor level in chronic haemodialysis patients. Nephrol Dial Transplant 17: 1063–1069.

32. Singh AK, Coyne DW, Shapiro W, Rizkala AR (2007) Predictors of the response to treatment in anemic hemodialysis patients with high serum ferritin and low transferrin saturation. Kidney Int 71: 1163–1171.

33. Ford BA, Eby CS, Scott MG, Coyne DW (2010) Intra-individual variability in serum hepcidin precludes its use as a marker of iron status in hemodialysis patients. Kidney Int 78: 769–773.

34. Truksa J, Peng H, Lee P, Beutler E (2006) Bone morphogenetic proteins 2, 4, and 9 stimulate murine hepcidin 1 expression independently of Hfe, transferrin receptor 2 (Tfr2), and IL-6. Proc Natl Acad Sci U S A 103: 10289–10293.

35. Uehata T, Tomosugi N, Shoji T, Sakaguchi Y, Suzuki A, et al. (2012) Serum hepcidin-25 levels and anemia in non-dialysis chronic kidney disease patients: a cross-sectional study. Nephrol Dial Transplant 27: 1076–1083.

36. Jiang F, Sun ZZ, Tang YT, Xu C, Jiao XY (2011) Hepcidin expression and iron parameters change in Type 2 diabetic patients. Diabetes Res Clin Pract 93: 43–48.

37. Malyszko J, Malyszko JS, Mysliwiec M (2009) Serum prohepcidin and hepcidin in hemodialyzed patients undergoing iron therapy. Kidney Blood Press Res 32: 235–238.

38. Tessitore N, Girelli D, Campostrini N, Bedogna V, Pietro Solero G, et al. (2010) Hepcidin is not useful as a biomarker for iron needs in haemodialysis patients on maintenance erythropoiesis-stimulating agents. NephrolDialTransplant 25: 3996–4002.

39. Campostrini N, Castagna A, Zaninotto F, Bedogna V, Tessitore N, et al. (2010) Evaluation of hepcidin isoforms in hemodialysis patients by a proteomic approach based on SELDI-TOF MS. JBiomedBiotechnol 2010: 329646.

40. Zaritsky JJ, Young BY (2009) The utility of multivariate analysis in the study of hepcidin. Kidney Int 76: 912; author reply 912–913.

9

Determinants of Compliance Behaviours among Patients Undergoing Hemodialysis in Malaysia

Yoke Mun Chan[1,2]*, **Mohd Shariff Zalilah**[2], **Sing Ziunn Hii**[3]

1 Institute of Gerontology, University Putra Malaysia, Serdang, Malaysia, **2** Department of Nutrition and Dietetics, Faculty of Medicine and Health Sciences, University Putra Malaysia, Serdang, Malaysia, **3** Viva Life Science Private Limited, Petaling Jaya, Malaysia

Abstract

Background: Patients with end stage renal disease often fail to follow prescribed dietary and fluid regimen, leading to undesirable outcomes. This study aimed to examine and identify factors influencing dietary, fluid, medication and dialysis compliance behaviours in patients undergoing hemodialysis.

Methods: This was a cross-sectional study which employed purposive sampling design. A total of 188 respondents were recruited from 14 dialysis centres in Malaysia between 2008–2011. Self-reported compliance behaviours and biochemical measurements were used as evaluation tools.

Results: Compliance rates of dietary, fluid, medication and dialysis were 27.7%, 24.5%, 66.5% and 91.0%, respectively. Younger, male, working patients and those with longer duration on hemodialysis were found more likely to be non-compliant. Lacks of adequate knowledge, inadequate self-efficacy skills, forgetfulness and financial constraints were the major perceived barriers towards better compliance to fluid, dietary, medication and dialysis, respectively.

Conclusions: Healthcare professionals should recognise the factors hindering compliance from the patients' perspective while assisting them with appropriate skills in making necessary changes possible.

Editor: Emmanuel A. Burdmann, University of Sao Paulo Medical School, Brazil

Funding: The authors have no funding or support to report.

Competing Interests: One of the authors, SZH is YMC's spouse who has contributed significantly to the study, as clarified in the Author's Contributions of the Cover Letter. The company (Viva Life Science Private Limited) however had no role in the funding, study design, data collection and analysis, decision to publish, or preparation of the manuscript. This does not alter the authors' adherence to all the PLoS ONE policies on sharing data and materials.

* E-mail: yokemun@medic.upm.edu.my

Introduction

In Malaysia, there is consistent increase in the incidence of newly-diagnosed individuals with end-stage renal disease (ESRD) which requires renal replacement therapy each year, fuelled by the expansion of the aged population as well as the rapid emergence of diabetic nephropathy [1]. While peritoneal dialysis is the preferred treatment modality in Hong Kong [2] and Mexico [3], hemodialysis is still the predominant mode of treatment for ESRD patients in most countries [4–5] including Malaysia [1]. Peritoneal dialysis is grossly underutilized in Malaysia despite the conscious effort by the government to promote peritoneal dialysis as the dialysis modality of choice. This is largely attributed to the readily available hemodialysis centres provided by non-government organisations (NGOs) and private sectors besides better survival rate for hemodialysis patients [1]. Successful hemodialysis is highly dependent on the lifetime commitment of patients to four aspects of regimens, namely dietary guidelines, fluid restriction, medication and dialysis [6]. Although compliance to hemodialysis regimens is critical in the management of hemodialysis patients as failure to do so has been associated with increased risk of medical complications including higher risk of cardiac disease [7], poorer quality of life and decreased life expectancy [8–9],

nonadherence to one or more aspects of hemodialysis treatment regimen has been widely reported [10–11].

The reported prevalence of non-compliance rates among hemodialysis patients varies widely, ranging from 30–74%, 2–81%, 17–46% and 0–32% for compliance to fluid restrictions [12–14], diet restrictions [11–12,15], medication [14,16–17] and dialysis [17–19], respectively. These variations were partly attributed to the different population being studied and most likely the inconsistency in the measures used to define compliance rates. A number of variables have been identified to influence compliance rate among hemodialysis patients, with varying degrees of agreement between different studies. More consistent reported demographic correlates of non compliant were younger age [15,17,20] and male patients [12,15,21]. Other variables include education [15,22], employment status [22–23], duration on dialysis [24–26], health locus of control and social support [27].

In view of the rapidly increased of ESRD in Malaysia, there is a need to determine the compliance rate to therapeutic regimen among patients undergoing hemodialysis. Previous study identified non-compliance to fluid intake was prevalent among patients undergoing hemodialysis in a single centre in Malaysia [28]. Data on compliance to other treatment regimes (dietary, medication and dialysis attendance) is however not available. Hence this present study aimed to determine the overall compliance behaviour to therapeutic regimens among patients undergoing hemodialysis and to determine the factors contributing to compliance among these subjects.

Materials and Methods

This was a cross-sectional study with respondents recruited from 14 hemodialysis centres in Malaysia. A total of 346 subjects were screened, 217 were found meeting the selection criteria while eventually 188 respondents consented to participate, giving a response rate of 87%. The study employed purposive sampling as the selection of respondents was based on several eligible criteria. The inclusion criteria entailed receiving hemodialysis for four hour thrice weekly; attended routine hemodialysis treatment for a minimum of three months prior to the study; at least 18 years of age, suffers from no major acute diseases or major psychological disorders. The study protocol was approved by the Medical Research Ethics Committee of Faculty of Medicine and Health Sciences, Universiti Putra Malaysia, in accordance with current guidelines on Good Clinical Practice and the Declaration of Helsinki. Following ethics review board approval, the researchers explained the study to potential participants. Anonymity and confidentially were assured before signed individual consents were obtained from all subjects.

A set of structured questionnaire was developed to ascertain information on patients' demographic characteristics. Treatment conditions, medical history and proxy clinical measures include mean serum potassium and phosphorus levels for the last three measurements were retrospectively obtained from medical record. The modified Charlson's Comorbidity Index which has been validated in dialysis patients [29] was used to quantify subject's comorbidity score. Mean interdialytic weight gain (IDWG) which is defined as weight gain between two consecutive dialysis sessions for the past three months was obtained from subject's dialysis record. A 25-item dietary knowledge questionnaire, which was modified from Durose et al. (2004) [11], was used to assess subjects' knowledge on diet and fluid regimen including food sources for nutrients (e.g., chocolate is good food source for phosphorus), recommended dietary preparation/restriction (e.g., dark green leafy vegetables should be cut small before washing and immerse in water), and possible consequences of noncompliance to dietary recommendation (e.g., excessive intake of sodium and fluid is harmful to the heart). The answers were prepared in yes or no format with an additional "don't know" category to avoid bias attributable to guessing. Each correct response was given a score of one while zero score was given to incorrect or "don't know" response. The scores were weighted and converted to standardized normal distribution, giving a maximum score of 100 for the knowledge scale. The internal consistency (Cronbach's alpha) was 0.8, denoting a reasonable internal consistency of this instrument. A combination of objective and subjective measures was used to access the compliance rates in order to increase the reliability and validity of the compliance results [6].

Objective measures

Interdialytic weight gain (IDWG), serum potassium and phosphorus which have been widely used in many studies [12–13,30] were used as indicators of fluid and dietary compliance. In view of the absence of validated international cut-off values, the existing acceptable limits used in the dialysis units were applied to identify non-adherers. Subjects were considered as dietary compliant when both serum potassium and phosphorus were within the acceptable ranges. Fluid compliant of subject was defined when mean IDWG for the past three months were within

the acceptable range. Predialysis serum phosphate was selected as compliance indicator for medication [14,22]. Dialysis compliance was determined as the number of appointment or dialysis session skipped compared to the prescribed sessions in a given duration. The data was gathered retrospectively from the subjects' dialysis record books. Attendance to dialysis was classified arbitrarily as non-compliant if subjects skipped at least one dialysis treatment in the month before enrolment into the study.

Subjective Measures

To evaluate patients' compliance behaviour, a modified dialysis diet and fluid non-adherence questionnaire (DDFQ) [31] was used. There were eight subscales: two each (frequency and intensity) to measure the patients' compliance behaviour to dietary guidelines, fluid, prescribed phosphate binding medication and hemodialysis treatment, respectively. The frequency of non-compliance was assessed for the last 14 days while intensity of non-compliance was evaluated on a 5-point rating scale, where responses ranged from 0 as "very severe deviation" to 4 as "no deviation".

Data Analysis

Analyses were performed using the SPSS Windows Version 18 (Chicago, IL). Data were presented as mean standard deviation for continuous variables and percentages for categorical variables. Pearson's product moment correlation coefficients were computed to determine the associations between continuous variables. Stepwise multivariate linear regression analysis was performed to identify variables that predict the compliance indicators. Statistical significance was defined at $p < 0.05$.

Results

Subjects' characteristics are presented in Table 1. The mean age of subjects was 58 years old. There were 48.9% male and 51.1% female. A majority were married (80.3%) with more than half (51.1%) had at least completed secondary education. Approximately three-quarters were either retired or unemployed. Diabetes mellitus and glomerulonephritis were the two major known etiology of renal failure. The presence of co-morbidities was common in this sample, with hypertension being the most prevalent (67.0%) and followed by diabetes mellitus (46.3%).

As depicted in Table 2, while a total of 48.4% and 36.2% of the subjects perceived themselves as fluid or dietary compliant, approximately one-quarter of the subjects were actually adhered to dietary (27.7%) and fluid (24.5%) restrictions. Based on self-reported data, 16 subjects missed at least one dialysis session while the dialysis record book indicated 17 subjects actually skipped at least one dialysis session. This gave a high consistency in dialysis compliance rates between self-reported data and data retrieved from patients' dialysis record. On the other hand, self-reported compliance to medication was 50.5%, while clinically determined rate using serum phosphorus was 66.5%. The percentage of self-reported non-compliance (mild to very severe) to prescribed dialysis, medication, fluid and dietary recommendation were 8.5%, 49.5, 51.6 and 63.8%, respectively (Table 3). According to the degree of deviation, majority of the subjects deviated either mildly or moderately from the recommended regimens. There were however a total of 19.7% and 11.7% of the subjects reported severe and very severe degrees of deviation from dietary and medication recommendation, respectively.

Perceived barriers contributing to non-complaint to treatment regimens were identified and are shown in Table 4. A total of 86.2% of the subjects admitted compliant to fluid prescription was

Table 1. Demographics and clinical characteristics of subjects.

Characteristics		Mean (SD)	Range	%
Age (years)		58.2 (10.5)	23 – 75	
Sex	Male			48.9
	Female			51.1
Marital status	Single			12.8
	Married			80.3
	Divorced/Widowed			6.9
Education	No formal education			10.6
	Primary school			38.3
	Secondary school and above			51.1
Employment	Employed			25.5
	Unemployed			66.0
	Retired			8.5
Primary diagnosis of renal failure	Diabetes mellitus			25.5
	Glomerulonephritis			8.5
	Unknown cause			29.8
	Others			37.1
Duration of dialysis (months)		63.2 (39.3)	5 – 162	
Presence of co-morbidity	Hypertension			67.0
	Diabetes mellitus			46.3
	Ischaemic heart disease			14.9
Dry weight (kg)		56.8 (14.0)		
Interdialytic weight gain (kg)		2.8 (0.7)		

the most difficult and challenging aspect, especially during hot weather while 72.9% reported difficulty following their dietary prescription. This was followed by 52.1% who reported had difficulty taking medications as prescribed. The need to change eating habits and inability to resist favourite foods (88.1%) and the highly complexity of dietary recommendation (87.0%) were the major factors cited for dietary non-compliance, superimposed the knowledge factor (74.7%). On the other hand, lacking of knowledge or information pertaining to fluid management was the major factor cited for fluid non-compliance (92.8%) followed

Table 2. Comparison between clinically determined and self-reported compliance rates.

Compliance Indicator	Clinically Determined compliance rates (%)	Self-reported compliance rates (%)
Dietary	27.7[1]	36.2
Fluid	24.5[2]	48.4
Medication	66.5[3]	50.5
Attendance to dialysis	91.0[4]	91.5

[1]Both serum potassium and phosphorus achieved compliance criteria.
[2]IDWG achieved compliance criteria.
[3]Serum phosphorus achieved compliance criteria.
[4]17 subjects skipped at least one dialysis session (data derived from dialysis record).
[5]16 patients self-reported missing at least one dialysis session.

by the complexity of fluid management. Forgetfulness, associated side effects/complications and complexity of the prescribed medications treatment were the three major factors perceived by patients contributing to non-compliance to medications. A majority (70.6%) of the subjects reported they had difficulty adhering to phosphate binder *per se* due to its associated side effects such as constipation and the unpleasant experience to take large quantities with meals. Large tablet burden was reported as barrier to compliance for 60.6% of the subjects. There were 12.2% of the subjects admitted having difficulty to comply with dialysis attendance attributed by financial constraint and lacks of transportation facility.

As shown in Table 5, there were positive correlations between age and compliance on dietary ($r = 0.186$, $p < 0.05$), fluid ($r = 0.385$, $p < 0.01$) and medication ($r = 0.271$, $p < 0.01$), respectively, indicating younger subjects were more non-compliant to the therapeutic regimen compared to their older age counterparts. Female subjects were statistically more compliant to dietary ($r = 0.252$, $p < 0.05$) and fluid restriction ($r = 0.310$, $p < 0.01$). There was however no significant different between male and female subjects on medication compliance ($r = 0.172$, $p > 0.05$). Employment status was found to be inversely related to dietary ($r = -0.355$, $p < 0.01$) and fluid ($r = -0.441$, $p < 0.01$) compliances. These results suggested that subjects who were employed were more likely to be non-compliant to dietary and fluid restrictions. Longer hemodialysis vintage was associated with poorer compliances on fluid ($r = -0.410$, $p < 0.01$) and medication ($r = -0.368$, $p < 0.01$), implying that patients who had longer lengths of time on dialysis were more likely to have hyperphosphatemia and gained more IDWG. Knowledge scores on potassium and phosphorus

Table 3. Self-reported of intensity of treatment compliance.

Deviation of Regimen	Degree of deviation	Mean Compliance Score	Frequency	%
Dietary		2.73		
	No deviation		68	36.2
	With deviation		120	63.8
	Mild		50	26.6
	Moderate		33	17.5
	Severe		25	13.3
	Very Severe		12	6.4
Fluid*		3.06		
	No deviation		90	48.4
	With deviation		96	51.6
	Mild		34	18.3
	Moderate		50	26.9
	Severe		8	4.3
	Very Severe		4	2.1
Medication		3.03		
	No deviation		95	50.5
	With deviation		93	49.5
	Mild		34	18.1
	Moderate		37	19.7
	Severe		14	7.4
	Very Severe		8	4.3
Dialysis		3.91		
	No deviation		172	91.5
	With deviation		16	8.5
	Mild		16	8.5
	Moderate		0	0
	Severe		0	0
	Very Severe		0	0

*Two subjects refused to disclosure information.

were negatively correlated with compliance on dietary ($r = -0.345$, $p < 0.01$) and medication ($r = -0.278$, $p < 0.05$), respectively. On the other hand, there were no significant correlations between knowledge scores on fluid or sodium with dietary, fluid or medication compliance. These findings suggest that higher knowledge on dietary aspects may not associated with better compliance rates.

Self-reported dietary compliance score was positively correlated with compliance on dietary ($r = 0.236$, $p < 0.05$) and medication ($r = 0.197$, $p < 0.05$), while self-reported medication compliance score was correlated with compliance on medication ($r = 0.412$, $p < 0.01$). There were also significant correlations between fluid compliance with self-reported compliance score on fluid ($r = 0.342$, $p < 0.05$) and dialysis ($r = 0.213$, $p < 0.05$). These data may suggest that the self-reported data can be used to determine the compliance behaviors of hemodialysis patients, in the absence of clinical measures. On the other hand, there were no significant associations between compliance indicators and education level or family income.

Stepwise multivariate linear regression analyses were performed to identify variables that predict the compliance behaviours. As displayed in Table 6, higher fluid compliant was predicted by female gender ($\beta = 0.207$, $p < 0.05$), older age ($\beta = 0.195$, $p < 0.05$), higher self-reported fluid compliance score ($\beta = 0.168$, $p < 0.05$), shorterhemodialysis vintage ($\beta = -0.155$, $p < 0.01$) and being not employed ($\beta = -0.125$, $p < 0.05$). Meanwhile, higher dietary compliance was predicted by higher self-reported dietary compliance score ($\beta = 0.250$, $p < 0.05$), female gender ($\beta = 0.162$, $p < 0.05$), older age ($\beta = 0.147$, $p < 0.05$) and no employment ($\beta = -0.142$, $p < 0.05$) while higher medication compliance was significantly predicted by higher self-reported medications compliance score ($\beta = 0.353$, $p < 0.01$), shorter hemodialysis vintage ($\beta = -0.224$, $p < 0.05$) and older age ($\beta = 0.181$, $p < 0.05$). The variation for these three models ranged from 21.5–39.2%.

Discussion

Diabetes mellitus accounted for the primary renal disease in this cohort of study, which is also a characteristic reported by the national renal registry of Malaysia [1]. A high proportion of hemodialysis patients in Malaysia had difficulty in following diet and fluid restriction. This finding is consistent with the range of compliance behaviours reported in other studies among dialysis patients [12–13,28]. Compared to a recent study conducted in Hong Kong [26], our compliance rates on dietary and dialysis

Table 4. Perceived barriers contributing to non-compliance on treatment regimens.

		Dietary (%)	Fluid (%)	Medication (%)	Dialysis Attendance (%)
Non-compliance Rate[1]		63.8	51.6	49.5	8.5
Difficult to comply [2]		72.9	86.2	52.1	12.2
Perceived barriers	Lacks of knowledge or information[3]	74.7	92.8	55.4	NA
	Affects food preference	88.1	64.2	36.1	NA
	Alters lifestyle[4]	69.2	56.8	54.7	NA
	Complexity[5]	87.0	75.4	75.8	NA
	Side effects/Complications	NA	NA	78.3	NA
	Forgetfulness	NA	NA	80.6	NA
	Large tablet burden	NA	NA	60.6	NA
	Financial constraint and lacks of transportation facility	NA	NA	NA	100

[1]Data derived from Table 2.
[2]Percentage of subjects who admitted having difficulty adhering to the treatment regimens (multiple responses were possible).
[3]Lacks of knowledge (e.g. water allowance for different weather conditions, type of foods to be consumed or restricted).
[4]Alters lifestyle (e.g. the need to consume mega dosage of supplements and medicines).
[5]Complexity (e.g. Nutrient composition of different foods; when and how to consume phosphate binders).

were comparable, but the compliance rates on fluid and medication were 24% and 39% lower. We compared with another study in United States [24] and found that their compliance rates of diet, fluid and medication were 26–47% higher than those reported in our study. A recent publication on the diabetes control also revealed that there was poor compliance on diet, exercise and self-monitoring blood glucose among type 2 diabetics in Malaysia [32]. Although evidence is still lacking to

generalise whether Malaysians are less likely to adhere to medical regimes than other populations, the available data suggest that extra efforts and appropriate strategies are needed to assist our hemodialysis patients to achieve the desirable recommendations, especially on fluid and medication.

The findings that our subjects perceived themselves as more compliant to dialysis than medication prescription, dietary or fluid restrictions are similar to earlier studies [24,26,33]. This may be attributed by the need for higher willpower, more appropriate knowledge and skill to achieve dietary and fluid recommendations. The mean self-reported compliance rates for fluid and dietary

Table 5. Correlation between compliance behaviors and variables.

Variables		Dietary Compliance	Fluid Compliance	Medication Compliance
Age		0.186*	0.385**	0.271**
Sex[1]		0.252*	0.310**	0.172
Education level		−0.124	−0.102	−0.108
Employment Status		−0.355**	−0.441**	−0.187
Family income		−0.129	−0.138	−0.115
Vintage on hemodialysis		−0.152	−0.410**	−0.368**
Knowledge scores on	Potassium	−0.345**	0.167	0.109
	Phosphorus	0.162	0.134	−0.278*
	Fluid	0.087	0.123	−0.153
	Sodium	0.113	−0.162	0.144
Self-reported Compliance score	Dietary	0.236*	0.166	0.197*
	Fluid	−0.174	0.342*	−0.156
	Medication	−0.151	−0.152	0.412**
	Dialysis	0.137	0.213*	0.102

[1]Female is a reference group in sex.
*p<0.05.
**p<0.01.

Table 6. Standardized coefficients of the linear regression model predicting compliance.

Compliance Behaviors	Variables	Standardized coefficients (β)	Adjusted R²
Fluid	Age	0.207	0.392
	Sex[1]	0.195	
	Fluid compliance score	0.168	
	Hemodialysis vintage	−0.155	
	Employment[2]	−0.125	
Dietary	Dietary compliance score	0.250	0.341
	Age	0.162	
	Sex[1]	0.147	
	Employment[2]	−0.142	
Medication	Medications compliance score	0.353	0.215
	Hemodialysis vintage	−0.224	
	Age	0.181	

[1]Female is a reference group in sex.
[2]Job engagement is a reference group in employment.

were 9% and 19% higher than the clinically determined rates. Other studies have also reported that hemodialysis patients consistently overestimated their compliance to fluid and dietary recommendations [13,27,34]. There is no clear explanation for this, but it is likely that the long duration of dependence on dialysis (length of time on dialysis) may cause hemodialysis patients to accustom to the restrictions imposed by the disease and perceived themselves as having better compliance than they actually did. Secondly, the use of clinical data for example serum potassium and phosphorus as the direct measures of dietary compliance could be misleading as these clinical data may also be affected by factors such as dialysis adequacy, medication and other factors yet to be identified. On the other hand, self-reported medication compliance was found to be underestimated by 16% as compared to clinically measured compliance indicator. Tomasello et al. (2004) [35] reported a similar finding where non-compliance to treatment was 58% and 31% when assessed using clinical and self-report measures, respectively. This may provide an impetus that using a single indicator to document the overall medication compliance rate could be insufficient and thus more comprehensive assessment tool is therefore needed.

Older age appeared to be the most important predictor among all predictor variables, explaining variance in all three compliance behaviours. Other studies have also reported that older age was associated with higher compliances to fluid restriction and medication prescription [24,36–37]. Possible explanations are older patients may have more structured lifestyle that accommodates the demands of the treatment regimen while younger patients may perceive themselves as less vulnerable to negative health outcomes [38], confirming the existence of an "intentional noncompliance" [39]. The finding that younger patients were more likely to be non-compliant to treatment recommendation may lead to the future poorer quality of life and higher rates of mortality among these dialysis patients. The dialysis patients in Malaysia are perceived as relatively young [40]. In view of the younger cohort of dialysis patients together with the higher tendency of these patients to be non-compliant to treatment, it is highly recommended that action plans need to be formulated to address the projected higher mortality rates and poorer quality of life among our dialysis population. We shared that women were more compliant to diet and fluid restriction than men and this findings are similar to other studies [12,26,31]. Female hemodialsysis patients had consistently reported to have a lower adjusted hazard ratio for mortality compared to their male counterparts in Malaysia [1]. It is likely that women are more health conscious than men. How gender differences in compliance may benefit patients concerning health outcomes in the long run however deserves for longitudinal research.

The correlations between higher self-reported compliance to medication and dietary compliance with lower phosphorus levels are of particular importance. Cardiovascular events are the leading cause of death in dialysis patients. The increased incidence of cardiovascular event in dialysis patients is associated with hyperphosphatemia [30], making phosphate control an important goal of treatment. While dialysis *per se* cannot remove the significant quantities of phosphate from the body, the appropriate restriction in dietary phosphorus intake and use of phosphate binder are therefore critically important to manage hyperphosphatemia. It is then necessary for hemodialysis patients to comply with *both* the dietary phosphorus intake and phosphate binding medication in reducing the risk of adverse clinical outcomes.

We demonstrated that higher knowledge scores were not associated with better compliance rates, which suggest that knowledge is not the sole factor related to compliance rate. This finding is congruent with other studies [11–12,37]. While Zrinyi et al. (2003) [23] showed that employment may improve the dietary compliance and it is associated with better patient-staff relationships, we found that hemodialysis patients who were employed were more likely to be non-compliant to diet and fluid restriction. This concurs with other study [13]. Working dialysis subjects may consume more outside foods that contain generally higher amount of sodium and potassium, which could lead to a higher challenge in handling thirst stimulus and subsequent increased in serum potassium level.

We found that subjects with longer duration on hemodialysis were more non-compliant. This finding concurs with other studies [13,25,41]. It is postulated that end stage renal disease patients may be more eager to change their dietary habits to meet the requirement of a newly-received life-saving hemodialysis treatment. However as time passes, these patients may feel bored and easily get frustrated with the need to comply with long lists of dietary and fluid restrictions [26]. Patients new to dialysis treatment may also receive more social support and were therefore higher degree of compliant is expected [26]. However, over the long run, it may be difficult for patients to resist the wide variety of food available. In view of this, healthcare providers should identified the individual's perceived barrier, explore patients' willingness and readiness to make changes to their dietary habits to achieve the optimum effect of compliance.

In conclusion, the majority of our subjects were compliant to dialysis prescription. However, compliance to other regimens especially for fluid and diet restriction remains poor. Younger male, working patients and those with long experience with dialysis warrant increased scrutiny and deserve for special attention and support. Besides knowledge, lacking of appropriate self-efficacy skills and regimen complexity were the perceived barriers hindering better compliance from the patients' perspective. Healthcare professionals should recognize that the perceived barriers to compliance vary according to types of treatment. For example, while adequate knowledge and information are needed to improve fluid compliance, appropriate self-efficacy skills and coping strategies are needed to enable hemodialysis patients to achieve the optimum effect of dietary compliance. Messages deliver by the healthcare professional should be "simple and practical", allowing the patients to understand and practice the messages within their capabilities. Reinforcement of messages together with more frequent counseling encounters may promote a better understanding of the prescriptions subsequently a higher compliance rates among the patients.

Our study design was cross-sectional in nature and the sample size was relatively small which could limit the cause-effect interpretation and generalisation of finding. Selection bias is also possible where only patients who were generally healthier or more health conscious were more likely to participate in the study. Despite these limitations, the study highlighted several important findings that require further investigations using stronger research design and larger sample size.

Author Contributions

Conceived and designed the experiments: YMC MSZ SZH. Performed the experiments: YMC SZH. Analyzed the data: YMC. Contributed reagents/materials/analysis tools: YMC MSZ SZH. Wrote the paper: YMC. Critically reviewed the paper for important intellectual content and provided technical support: MSZ SZH.

References

1. Lim YN, Ong LM, Goh BL (2011) 18th Report of the Malaysian Dialysis and Transplant Registry 2010. Retrieved from Clinical Research Centre of Ministry of Health Malaysia: http://www.msn.org.my/nrr/documents/nrr_report2011/contents.pdf. Accessed 2012 April 5.

2. Yu AW, Chau KF, Ho YW, Li PK (2007) Development of the "peritoneal dialysis first" model in Hong Kong. Perit Dial Int 27 (Suppl 2): S53–S55.

3. Cueto-Manzano AM, Rojas-Campos E (2007) Status of renal replacement therapy and peritoneal dialysis in Mexico. Perit Dial Int 27(2): 142–148.

4. Tan CC, Chan CM, Ho CK, Wong KS, Lee EJ, et al. (2005) Health economics of renal replacement therapy: perspectives from Singapore. Kidney Int 67 (Suppl 94): S19–S22.

5. United States Renal Data System (USRDS), 2009. USRDS annual data report. Accessed from http://www.usrds.org/adr.html. Accessed 2012 March 18.

6. Wolcott DL, Maida CA, Diamond R, Nissenson AR (1986) Treatment compliance in end-stage renal disease patients on dialysis. Am J Nephrol 6 (5), 329–338.

7. Karamanidou C, Clatworthy J, Weinman J, Horne R (2008) A systematic review of the prevalence and determinants of nonadherence to phosphate binding medication in patients with end-stage renal disease. BMC Nephrology 9: 2.

8. Baines LS, Jindal RM (2000) Non-compliance in patients receiving haemodialysis: an in-depth review. Nephron 85(1): 1–7.

9. Hoover H (1989) Compliance in patients on hemodialysis: a review of the literature. J Am Diet Assoc 89(7): 957–959.

10. Denhaerynck K, Manhaeve D, Dobbels F, Garzoni D, Nolte C, et al. (2007) Prevalence and consequences of nonadherence to hemodialysis regimens. Am J Crit Care 16(3): 222–236.

11. Durose CL, Holdsworth M, Watson V, Przygrodzka F (2004) Knowledge of dietary restrictions and the medical consequences of noncompliance by patients on hemodialysis are not predictive of dietary compliance. J Am Diet Assoc 104(1): 35–41.

12. Kugler C, Vlaminck H, Haverich A, Maes B (2005) Nonadherence with diet and fluid restrictions among adults having hemodialysis. J Nurs Scholarsh 37(1): 25–29.

13. Lee SH, Molassiotis A (2002) Dietary and fluid compliance in Chinese hemodialysis patients. Int J Nurs Stud 39(7): 695–704.

14. Lin CC, Liang CC (1997) The relationship between health locus of control and compliance of hemodialysis patients. Kaohsiung J Med Sci 13(4): 243–254.

15. Bame SI, Petersen N, Wray NP (1993) Variation in hemodialysis patient compliance according to demographic characteristics. Soc Sci Med 37(8): 1035–1043.

16. Betts DK, Crotty GD (1988) Response to illness and compliance of long-term hemodialysis patients. J Am Nephrol Nurses Assoc 15(2): 96–100.

17. Leggat JE, Orzol SM, Hulbert-Shearon TE, Golper TA, Jones CA, et al. (1998) Noncompliance in hemodialysis: predictors and survival analysis. Am J Kidney Dis 32(1): 139–145.

18. Bleyer AJ, Hylander B, Sudo H, Nomoto Y, de la Torre E, et al. (1999) An international study of patient compliance with hemodialysis. JAMA 281(13): 1211–1213.

19. Sherman RA, Cody RP, Matera JJ, Rogers ME, Solanchick JC (1994) Deficiencies in delivered hemodialysis therapy due to missed and shortened treatments. Am J Kidney Dis 24(6): 921–923.

20. Kimmel PL, Peterson RA, Weihs KL, Simmens SJ, Boyle DH, et al. (1995) Behavioral compliance with dialysis prescription in hemodialysis patients. J Am Soc Nephrol 5(10): 1826–1834.

21. Everett KD, Sletten C, Carmach C, Brantley PJ, Jones GN, et al. (1993) Predicting noncompliance to fluid restrictions in hemodialysis patients. Dialysis Transplant 22: 614–620.

22. Curtin RB, Svarstad BL, Keller TH (1999) Hemodialysis patients' noncompliance with oral medications. J Am Nephrol Nurses Assoc 26(3): 307–316.

23. Zrinyi M, Juhasz M, Balla J, Katona E, Ben T, et al. (2003) Dietary self-efficacy: determinant of compliance behaviours and biochemical outcomes in haemodialysis patients. Nephrol Dial Transplant 18(9): 1869–1873.

24. Kim Y, Evangelista LS (2010) Relationship between illness perceptions, treatment adherence, and clinical outcomes in patients on maintenance hemodialysis. Nephrol Nurs J 37(3): 271–280.

25. Kimmel PL, Varela MP, Peterson RA, Weihs KL, Simmens SJ, et al. (2000) Interdialytic weight gain and survival in hemodialysis patients: effects of duration of ESRD and diabetes mellitus. Kidney Int 57(5): 1141–1151.

26. Lam LW, Twinn SF, Chan SW (2010) Self-reported adherence to therapeutic regimen among patients undergoing continuous ambulatory peritoneal dialysis. J Adv Nurs 66(4): 763–773.

27. Brown J, Fitzpatrick R (1988) Factors influencing compliance with dietary restrictions in dialysis patients. J Psychosom Res 32(2): 191–196.

28. Barnett T, Tang LY, Pinikahana J, Tan SY (2008) Fluid compliance among patients having haemodialysis: can an educational programme make a difference? J Adv Nurs 61(3): 300–306.

29. Beddhu S, Bruns FJ, Saul M, Seddon P, Zeidel ML (2000) A simple comorbidity scale predicts clinical outcomes and costs in dialysis patients. Am J Med 108:609–613.

30. Block GA, Hulbert-Shearon TE, Levin NW, Port FK (1998) Association of serum phosphorus and calcium x phosphate product with mortality risk in chronic hemodialysis patients: a national study. Am J Kidney Dis 31(4): 607–617.

31. Vlaminck H, Maes B, Jacobs A, Reyntjens S, Evers G (2001) The dialysis diet and fluid non-adherence questionnaire: validity testing of a self-report instrument for clinical practice. J Clin Nurs 10(5): 707–715.

32. Mafauzy M, Hussein Z, Chan SP (2011) The status of diabetes control in Malaysia: Results of DiabCare 2008. Med J Malaysia 66(3): 175–181.

33. Mok E, Tam B (2001) Stressors and coping methods among chronic haemodialysis patients in Hong Kong. J Clin Nurs 10(4): 503–511.

34. Cummings KM, Becker MH, Kirscht JP, Levin NW (1982) Psychosocial factors affecting adherence to medical regiments in a group of hemodialysis patients. Med Care 20(6): 567–580.

35. Tomasello S, Dhupar S, Sherman RA (2004) Phosphate binders, K/DOQI guidelines, and compliance: the unfortunate reality. Dialysis Transplant 33(5): 236–242.

36. Kara B, Caglar K, Kilic S (2007) Nonadherence with diet and fluid restrictions and perceived social support in patients receiving hemodialysis. J Nurs Scholarsh 39(3): 243–248.

37. Park KA, Choi KS, Sim YM, Kim SB (2008) Comparison of dietary compliance and dietary knowledge between older and younger Korean hemodialysis patients. J Ren Nutr 18(5): 415–423.

38. Kutner NG (2001) Improving compliance in dialysis patients: does anything work? Semin Dial 14(5): 324–327.

39. Hussey LC, Gilliland K (1989) Compliance, low literacy, and locus of control. Nurs Clin N Am 24(3): 605–611.

40. Schober-Halstenberg HJ (2009) End-stage renal disease in aging societies: a global perspective. J Ren Nutr 19(5 Suppl): S3–S4.

41. Oka M, Chaboyer W (1999) Dietary behaviors and sources of support in hemodialysis patients. Clin Nurs Res 8(4): 302–314.

10

Hemodialysis Removes Uremic Toxins that Alter the Biological Actions of Endothelial Cells

Kalliopi Zafeiropoulou[1], Theodora Bita[2⁹], Apostolos Polykratis[1⁹], Stella Karabina[1], John Vlachojannis[2¶], Panagiotis Katsoris[1*¶]

1 Department of Biology, University of Patras, Patras, Achaia, Greece, 2 Department of Internal Medicine-Nephrology, University Hospital of Patras, Patras, Achaia, Greece

Abstract

Chronic kidney disease is linked to systemic inflammation and to an increased risk of ischemic heart disease and atherosclerosis. Endothelial dysfunction associates with hypertension and vascular disease in the presence of chronic kidney disease but the mechanisms that regulate the activation of the endothelium at the early stages of the disease, before systemic inflammation is established remain obscure. In the present study we investigated the effect of serum derived from patients with chronic kidney disease either before or after hemodialysis on the activation of human endothelial cells in vitro, as an attempt to define the overall effect of uremic toxins at the early stages of endothelial dysfunction. Our results argue that uremic toxins alter the biological actions of endothelial cells and the remodelling of the extracellular matrix before signs of systemic inflammatory responses are observed. This study further elucidates the early events of endothelial dysfunction during toxic uremia conditions allowing more complete understanding of the molecular events as well as their sequence during progressive renal failure.

Editor: Timothy W. Secomb, University of Arizona, United States of America

Funding: The authors have no support or funding to report.

Competing Interests: The authors have declared that no competing interests exist.

* E-mail: katsopan@upatras.gr

⁹ These authors contributed equally to this work.

¶ These authors also contributed equally to this work.

Introduction

Chronic kidney disease (CKD) is due to a progressive loss of renal function that may lead to complications such as cardiovascular disease or pericarditis. To fully investigate the underlying cause of kidney damage, various forms of medical imaging, blood tests or renal biopsy are employed to find out if there is a reversible cause for the kidney malfunction. Established CKD or chronic renal failure (CRF) are terms that describe the late stage of kidney damage, when the disease is considered irreversible. Current therapy strategies aim the delay of the clinical manifestations to the final stages of the disease. Generally, agents targeting the functional control of the endothelium, such as angiotensin converting enzyme inhibitors (ACEIs) or angiotensin-II receptor antagonists (ARBs) are used, as they have been found to delay the clinical manifestations of the CKD [1,2,3,4]. Nevertheless, even under treatment with ACEIs or ARBs, patients progressively lose proper renal function. For these reasons understanding the primary responses of the endothelium to each stages of the kidney disease is of major importance for the design of efficient therapeutic strategies.

The endothelium is the major site of control of vascular functions [5]. Under physiological conditions the vascular endothelium regulates processes that include vascular tone, vascular permeability to nutrients, macromolecules and leukocytes recruitment (and thus inflammation), platelet adhesion and aggregation, activation of the coagulation cascade and fibrinolysis [6,7,8,9,10,11]. Endothelial dysfunction reflects the combination of altered endothelial properties resulting to improper

preservation of organ function. Endothelial dysfunction might be characterized by altered basement membrane synthesis, increased vascular tone and permeability -which contributes to increased blood pressure and atherogenesis- and loss of antithrombotic and profibrinolytic properties. Such alterations do not necessarily occur simultaneously and may differ according to the nature of the injury and the intrinsic site-specific properties of endothelium.

CKD leads to altered properties and responses of the endothelium [12,13,14]. However, the mechanisms by which increased uremia might influence endothelial cells, and especially the early responses of endothelial cells to the stimuli present in the serum of patients with CKD, are still not well understood. Systemic exposure of the vasculature to uremic toxins may lead to endothelial activation [15] and to features associated with systemic inflammation like hypertension and atherosclerosis. Hemodialysis (HD) or nephrectomy are generally used as approaches for the treatment of the sort-term effects of renal disease [16], nevertheless patients under long term HD treatment do not have reduced risk of vascular disease [17,18,19,20].

The present study was designed to investigate the short-term in vitro effect of serum from patients with CKD on endothelial cells and the relative effect of HD on endothelial cell activation and function. We focused on the early responses of the endothelial cells to the uremic toxins, before the inflammatory activation of the endothelial cells (expression of adhesion molecules, secretion of chemokines) is established. For this purpose sera from patients either before or after the HD procedure were collected and their relative effect on the activation of human umbilical vein endothelial cells was investigated. This experimental approach enabled us to clearly use the best internal controls available since the sera from the same patients were used. Our results clearly demonstrate that the initial response of endothelial cells to uremic toxins involves a rearrangement of the local micro-environment and extracellular matrix, a response that was up to date not appreciated.

Materials and Methods

Serum samples from CRF patients

Ten adult (men) patients on chronic maintenance HD, middle-aged 45 ± 5 years old, who were clinically stable and free of active infection, autoimmune diseases or other traditional factors implicated to endothelial dysfunction (diabetes mellitus, hypertension, hyperlipidemia, smoking) and had no signs or symptoms of cardiovascular disease, participated in the study. None of the patients received antihypertensive drugs, immunosuppressive treatment, lipid-lowering agents, non-steroidal anti-inflammatory drugs or antioxidants such as vitamin E, C or allopurinol in the preceding 4 weeks. End stage kidney disease was attributed to glomerulonephritis in 3 cases, interstitial nephritis in 2 and polycystic kidney disease in 3 and was undetermined in 2 cases. The patients were routinely haemodialyzed three times weekly for 4.0 h with DCEA polysulfone membranes - surface $1.7~mm^2$, bicarbonate dialysate and low molecular weight heparin-enoxaparin as anticoagulation. The dialysate was endotoxin-free (Coatest Kabi Vitrum). Dialysis prescription was guided by the goal of achieving a value of $Kt/V\geq1.3$. They were on erythropoietin therapy and the mean dosage was 90.5 (range 30.2–162) U/kg body weight/week. Body mass index (BMI) was calculated by dividing the weight in kilograms by the square of the height in meters.

For this study, we obtained ethics approval from the ethics committee of University of Patras.

Endothelial cell culture

Primary human umbilical vein endothelial cells (HUVEC) were isolated from umbilical cord vein by collagenase digestion as previously described [21] and used at passages 2–4. The cells were grown as monolayers in M199 medium supplemented with 15% fetal bovine serum (FBS), 150 µg/ml endothelial cell growth supplement, 5 U/ml heparin sodium, 100 U/ml penicillin-streptomycin and 50 µg/ml gentamycin. Cultures were maintained at $37°C$, 5% CO_2 and 100% humidity.

Migration assay

Migration assays were performed as previously described [22] in 24-well microchemotaxis chambers (Costar, Avon, France), using uncoated polycarbonate membranes with 8 µm pores. Briefly, HUVEC were harvested and resuspended at a concentration of 10^5 cells/0.1 ml in medium containing 0.25% BSA. The bottom chamber was filled with 0.6 ml of medium containing 0.25% BSA and pre- or post-HD serum at dilutions ranging from 5% to 20% v/v. The upper chamber was loaded with 10^5 cells and incubated for 4 h at $37°C$. After completion of the incubation, the filters were fixed with saline-buffered formalin and stained with 0.33% toluidine blue solution. The cells that migrated through the filter were quantified by counting the entire area of each filter, using a grid and an Optech microscope at a $20\times$ magnification.

Cell proliferation assay

Cell number was assessed using the 3-[4,5-dimethylthiazol-2-yl]-2,5- dimethyltetrazolium bromide (MTT) assay [23]. HUVEC were seeded at 5×10^4 cells/well in 24-well tissue culture plates in the corresponding culture medium. Cells were incubated in the absence of serum for 4 h. Pre- or post- HD serum was added to the medium of the cells at dilutions ranging from 5% to 20% v/v and the number of cells was measured after 48 h. MTT stock (5 mg/ml in PBS) at a volume equal to 1/10 of the medium was added and plates were incubated at $37°C$ for 2 h. The medium was then removed, the cells were washed with PBS pH 7.4 and 100 ml acidified isopropanol (0.33 ml HCl in 100 ml isopropanol) was added to all wells and agitated thoroughly to solubilize the dark blue formazan crystals. The solution was transferred to a 96-well plate and immediately read on a microplate reader (Biorad) at a wavelength of 490 nm.

Cell number was also determined by crystal violet assay: Adherent cells were fixed with methanol and stained with 0.5% crystal violet in 20% methanol for 20 min. After gentle rinsing with water, the retained dye was extracted with 30% acetic acid and the absorbance was measured at 590 nm.

Annexin-V Binding Staining

The Annexin V-FITC Detection Kit I (PharMingen, San Diego, CA) was used according to the manufacturer's instructions. Cells were serum-starved for 4 h and pre- or post-HD serum was added to the medium of the cells at 20% v/v dilution. Cells were collected after 12 or 24 h incubation. Samples were analyzed in a FACScan flow cytometer (Becton Dickinson). For each sample, 10,000 ungated events were acquired.

In vitro endothelial cell wound healing assay

HUVEC were grown in 6-well plates as confluent monolayers. The monolayers were incubated in the absence of serum for 4 h and wounded in a line across the well with a 200-µl standard pipette tip. Cells were washed twice with serum-free media and incubated with 20% v/v pre- or post-HD serum for 24 h. The area of the initial wound was photographed using a charge-coupled device camera connected to an inverted microscope (Axiovert 35; Zeiss, Thornwood, NY). The wound healing effect was calculated compared with the area of the initial wound.

Gelatin Zymography

The activity of MMP-2 and MMP-9 was examined by zymography as previously described [24]. Endothelial cells were cultured in 6-well plates as confluent monolayer. HUVEC were serum-starved for 4 h and then incubated with culture medium supplemented with 20% pre- or post- HD serum. 4 h later the medium was replaced by minimal medium. 8 or 20 h later the media were collected, centrifuged, and aliquots of the supernatants were loaded with a non-reducing sample buffer onto a 10% sodium dodecyl sulfate (SDS)-polyacrylamide gel containing 1 mg/mL gelatin and electrophoresed. Gels were washed twice with 2.5% Triton X-100 solution for 30 min and once with 10 mM Tris-HCl buffer (pH 8.0) for 30 min. Gels were further incubated in 50 mM Tris-HCl (pH 8.0) containing 0.5 mM $CaCl_2$ and 0.1 mM $ZnCl_2$ at $37°C$ for 24 h. The gels were stained with 1% Coomassie Blue R-250 in 10% methanol and 5% acetic acid and subsequently destained with 10% methanol and 5% acetic acid. The relative amounts of MMP-9 and MMP-2 were quantified by NIH Image Analysis software and normalized to the total number of cells of each well (using Crystal violet method).

Immunoblot analysis

Endothelial cells were cultured in 6-well plates as confluent monolayer. HUVEC were serum-starved for 4 h and then incubated with culture medium supplemented with 20% pre- or post- HD serum. 4 h later the medium was replaced by minimal medium. 8 or 20 h later the media were collected, centrifuged, and aliquots of the supernatants were analyzed by SDS-PAGE and proteins were blotted onto PVDF membranes (Millipore, Bedford, MA). Blocking was performed in a 5% fat-free dry milk in 0.2% Tween-20 in PBS and membranes were further incubated with primary antibodies for 1 h (1:2000 dilution in TBS containing 0.1% Tween 20 (TBS-T) and 1% BSA), washed with 0.1% Tween- 20 in PBS, and then incubated with anti-mouse peroxidase-conjugated secondary antibody (1:2000 in TBS containing 0.1% Tween 20 (TBS-T) and 3% fat free dry milk). Visualization of immunoreactive proteins was performed with enhanced chemiluminescence reagents (ECL kit; Amersham Pharmacia Biotech). The normalization was based on the number of cells of each well that was estimated using Crystal violet method.

RNA isolation and reverse transcriptase-polymerase chain reaction analysis of MMP-2,-9 and TIMP-1, -2 mRNA

Total RNA was isolated from HUVEC cultured with 20% pre- or post-HD serum for 6, 12 or 24 h using Nucleospin® RNA II (Macherey-Nagel) according to manufacturer's instructions. Reverse transcriptase-PCRs were performed using the Access Reverse Transcriptase-PCR system (Promega). The sequences of the primers used in our studies are the following: GAPDH: 5'-TCT AGA CGG CAG GTC AGG TCC ACC-3' and 5'-CCA CCC ATG GCA AAT TCC ATG GCA- 3', MMP-2: 5'-ACA GTC CGC CAA ATG AAC C- 3' and 5'-CCT GGG CAA CAA ATA TGA G- 3', **MMP-9:** 5'-GCC TTG GAA GAT GAA TGG AA - 3' and 5'- CAT CGT CAT CCA GTT TGG TG- 3', **TIMP-1:** 5'-TGC AGT TTT CCA GCA ATG AG - 3' and 5'-CTG TTG TTG CTG TGG CTG AT - 3', **TIMP-2:** 5'-TTT GAG TTG CTT GCA GGA TG - 3' and 5'-ATT TGA CCC AGA GTG GAA CG -3', **COLLAGEN IV:** 5'-TTT CCA GGG TAG CCA GAT GCT C - 3' and 5'-GGG GTT ACA AGG TGT CAT TGG G - 3', **ELASTIN:** 5'-CCA TAC TTG GCT GCC TTA GC - 3' and 5'-CAC TGG GGT ATC CCA TCA AG - 3'.

Statistical analysis

Comparison of mean values among groups was done using ANOVA and the unpaired Student t-test. Homogeneity of variance was tested by Levene's test. Each experiment included at least triplicate measurements for each condition tested. All results are expressed as the mean ± SD of at least three independent experiments. Values of p less than 0.05 were taken to be significant (*p<0.05, **p<0.01, ***p<0.001).

Results

Uremic toxins present in the serum of patients with CKD alter endothelial cell properties *in vitro*

Although CKD is positively associated with dysfunction of the endothelium, the effect of the uremic toxins of patients on the immediate responses of endothelial cells is not clearly demonstrated. To study the above mentioned effect, we isolated sera from patients with CKD right before or after HD, an approach that was not followed or appreciated in previous studies. At first we investigated the role of uremic toxins in the sera of our patients on the proliferation of endothelial cells. We incubated HUVEC with three different concentrations of sera. As shown in Figure 1A, incubation of HUVEC with increased concentrations of pre-HD serum resulted in reduced proliferation of endothelial cells compared to the relative concentrations of post-HD serum.

Increased concentrations of serum resulted in increased proliferation in both pre- and post-HD sera, nevertheless in all the concentrations tested in our experiments the effect on proliferation was enhanced in the samples stimulated with post-HD serum. The stimulatory effect of the uremic toxins-free serum (post-HD serum) on the proliferation of HUVEC reached 30% compared to the pre-HD serum, when a concentration of 20% was used in the medium. These results indicate that the differential concentration mainly of uremic toxins present in the serum of patients with CKD before and after HD affects proliferation of primary endothelial cells in vitro.

Basal apoptosis can be observed in cultured cells under normal conditions. Furthermore, since post-HD serum is not believed to be completely free of uremic toxins, we investigated the effect of either pre- or post-HD serum on the apoptosis of HUVEC *in vitro*. We used the concentration of 20% of serum in the cultured medium where the effect on HUVEC proliferation was more pronounced. As shown in Figure 1B, incubation of endothelial cells with either pre- or post-HD sera leads to a time dependent increase in the percentage of apoptotic cells. This effect is more pronounced when cells are cultured with pre- HD serum and reaches an 80% increase in the number of apoptotic cells compared to cells cultures with post-HD sera after 72 hours. Nevertheless, the percentage of apoptotic cells in culture even under these conditions cannot be the soul reason for the decreased total number in our proliferation assays (Figure 1A), arguing for a combined effect of uremic-toxins on both the proliferation and cell survival of endothelial cells.

It is known that systemic inflammation affects the migration of endothelial cells, inhibiting the healing processes *in vivo* [25]. To study the effect of uremic toxins on migration, we incubated HUVEC with increasing concentrations of either pre-HD or post-HD serum. As shown in Figure 1C, pre-HD serum has a realtivelly small positive effect on the migration of endothelial cells in the different concentrations used. On the contrary, when post-HD serum was used, a dose-dependent induction on the migration of endothelial cells was observed that reached almost 70% induction at serum concentration of 20**%**.

The combination of endothelial cells proliferation/survival and migration *in vivo* might have an impact in wound healing processes. The effect of the concentration of uremic toxins before and after the HD in the healing responses of endothelial cells *in vitro* has not been so far addressed. To investigate this we used the widely used scratch assay. Wound repair was assessed 24 h after incubation with 20% pre- or post-HD serum. As shown in Figure 1D, endothelial wound repair in monolayers exposed to pre-HD serum was significantly lower than in cells exposed to post-HD serum.

Uremic toxins present in the sera of patients with CKD promote the expression and activity of ECM-degrading proteinases

So far our results indicate that the uremic toxins alter the biological activities of endothelial cells *in vitro*, and are in accordance with previously published data [26,27,28,29,30]. Nevertheless, previous studies have been focused on the response of endothelial cell (*in vitro*) after long term stimulation with inflammatory stimuli or of the endothelium (*in vivo*) under conditions of systemic inflammation. We decided to focus on the early responses of endothelial cells upon stimulation with uremic toxins sera. At first we tested if the serum from the same patients before or after the HD could affect the deposition of extracellular matrix. We stimulated HUVEC with the above-mentioned sera and assessed for the activation of metalloproteinases (MMPs) either at the protein level by zymography on the medium of the

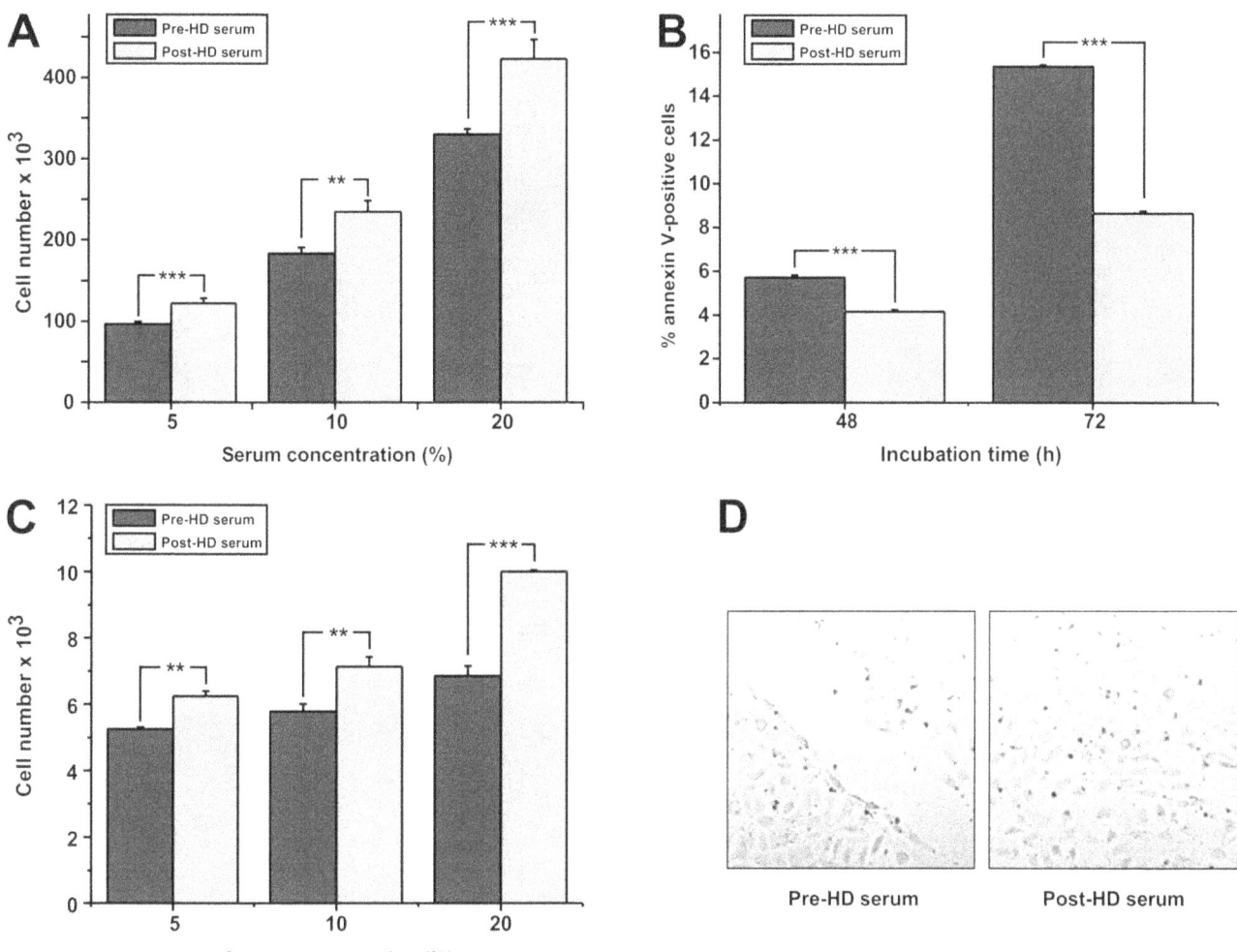

Figure 1. Effect of pre- or post-HD serum on proliferation, apoptosis, migration and wound healing activities of HUVEC. (A): HUVEC were incubated in medium supplemented with 5%, 10%, 20% pre- or post-HD serum and 48 h later their number was estimated by crystal violet. (B): HUVEC were incubated in medium supplemented with 20% pre- or post-HD serum and 48 or 72 h later the number of apoptotic cells was measured by FACS. (C): HUVEC were incubated in microchemotaxis chambers in culture medium supplemented with 5%, 10%, 20% pre- or post-HD serum and 4 h later the number of cells that migrated through the filter was quantified. (D) Endothelial monolayers were scratched, incubated in culture medium supplemented with 20% pre- or post-HD serum and 24 h later representative images of the plates were taken. Data are expressed as mean ± SEM of three independent experiments. *, ** and *** represent p<0.05, p<0.01 and p<0.001 respectively.

cells or at the mRNA level by RT-PCR. As shown in Figure 2A, the pre-HD serum induces a dose dependent increase in both MMP-2 and MMP-9 protein levels in the medium of HUVEC as compared to the relevant samples where post-HD serum was used. Since the difference was more pronounced when 20% of either pre- or post-HD serum was added to the culture medium, we performed all following experiments using this serum concentration. As shown in Figure 2B, incubation of HUVEC with pre-HD serum led to increased MMP-9 activity in the cell supernatant after 12 and 24 hours, while it also increases MMP-2 protein levels after 24 hours as compared to the effect of the post-HD serum. Furthermore incubation of HUVEC with pre- or post- HD serum at the concentration of 20% induces MMP-2 and MMP-9 expression levels in a statistically significant manner reaching a maximum at 6 and 12 hours respectively (Figure 2C).

Since both *in vitro* and *in vivo*, activity of MMPs is counterbalanced by the expression of naturally expressed inhibitors (tissue inhibitors of metalloproteinases, TIMPs), we assessed the expression levels of TIMP-1 and TIMP-2 protein levels on supernatants

from HUVEC that were stimulated with sera at the concentration of 20%. As shown in Figure 3A, we observed a statistically significant increase of TIMP-1 and TIMP-2 protein levels when HUVEC were incubated with post-HD serum, compared to pre-HD serum. This increased accumulation of TIMP-1 and -2 proteins in the medium of cells cultured with uremic-free sera can be attributed to increased expression of the relative genes, as shown in Figure 3B.

Uremic toxins present in the sera of patients with CKD inhibit the expression of extracellular matrix proteins

To investigate the effect of uremic toxins in the sera from patients with CKD on the expression of extracellular matrix components by endothelial cells we analyzed the expression levels of collagen IV and elastin. As shown in Figure 4, incubation of endothelial cells with either pre- or post-HD sera induces the expression of both collagen IV and elastin. This increase is more pronounced when endothelial cells are incubated with the post-HD serum. These data suggest that uremic toxins could inhibit the

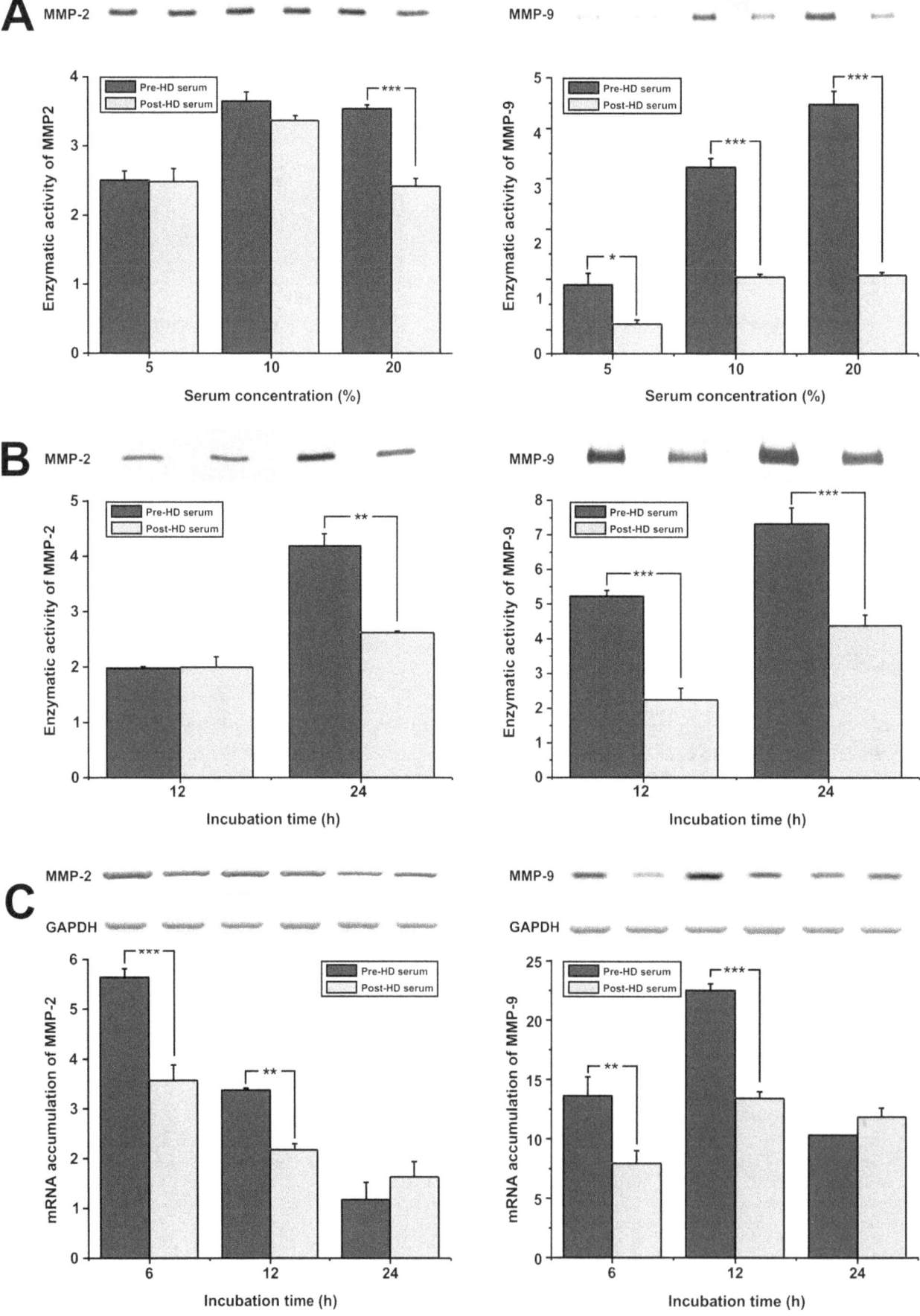

Figure 2. Effect of pre- or post-HD serum on MMP-2, -9 expression. (A): HUVEC were incubated in medium supplemented with 5%, 10%, 20% pre- or post- HD serum. 4 h later the medium was replaced by minimal medium and 20 h later the supernatants were analyzed for MMP-2 and MMP-9 activity by zymography. (B): HUVEC were incubated with culture medium supplemented with 20% pre- or post- HD serum. 4 h later the medium was replaced by minimal medium and 8 or 20 h later the supernatants were analyzed for MMP-2 and MMP-9 activity by zymography. (C): HUVEC were incubated in culture medium supplemented with 20% pre- or post- HD serum. 6, 12, or 24 h later total RNA was extracted from the cells, RT-PCR reactions were performed using specific primers for MMP-2, MMP-9 or GAPDH mRNAs, the PCR products were analyzed in agarose gels and quantified. Data are expressed as mean $\pm$ SEM of three independent experiments.. *, ** and *** represent $p < 0.05$, $p < 0.01$ and $p < 0.001$ respectively.

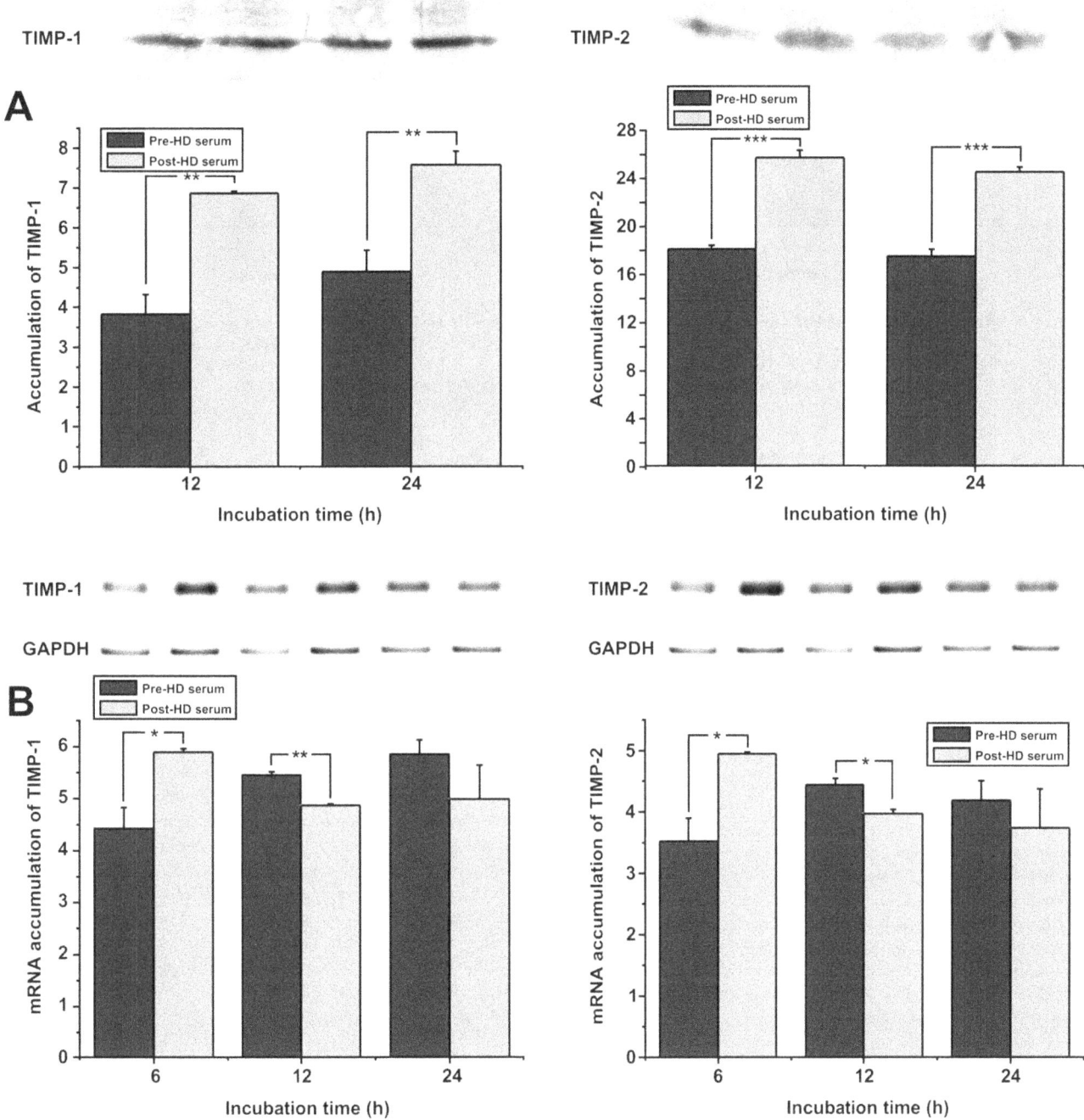

Figure 3. Effect of pre- or post-HD serum on the expression of TIMP-1 and TIMP-2. (A): HUVEC were incubated in culture medium supplemented with 20% pre- or post- HD serum. 4 h later the medium was replaced by minimal medium and 8 or 20 h later the supernatants were analyzed for TIMP-1 and TIMP-2 proteins by SDS-PAGE. (B): HUVEC were incubated with culture medium supplemented with 20% pre- or post- HD serum. 6, 12, or 24 h later total RNA was extracted from the cells, RT-PCR reactions were performed using specific primers for TIMP-1, TIMP-2 or GAPDH mRNAs, the PCR products were analyzed in agarose gels and quantified. Data are expressed as mean $\pm$ SEM of three independent experiments. * and ** represent $p < 0.05$ and $p < 0.01$ respectively.

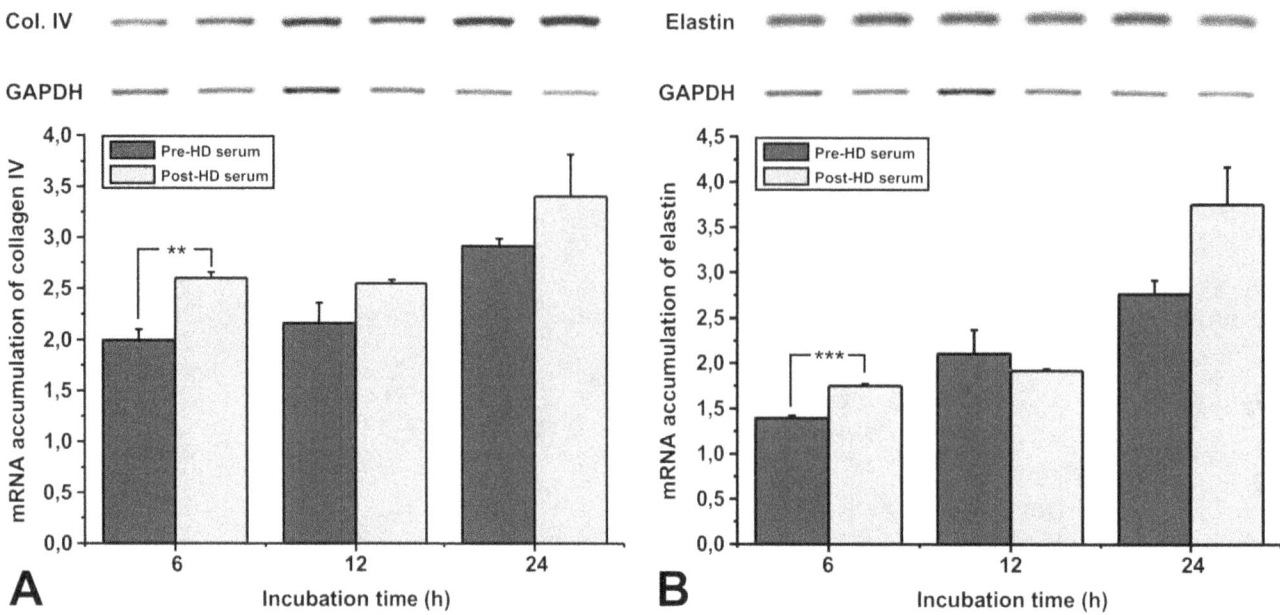

Figure 4. Effect of pre- or post-HD serum on the expression of collagen-IV and elastin. HUVEC were incubated with culture medium supplemented with 20% pre- or post- HD serum. 6, 12, or 24 h later total RNA was extracted from the cells, RT-PCR reactions were performed using specific primers for Collagen IV, Elastin or GAPDH mRNAs, the PCR products were analyzed in agarose gels and quantified. Data are expressed as mean ± SEM of three independent experiments. *, ** and *** represent p<0.05, p<0.01 and p<0.001 respectively.

immediate healing response of endothelial cells *in vivo* after injury or local endothelial loss due to apoptosis.

Discussion

Uremic toxins contribute to endothelial dysfunction in CKD. In renal failure, endothelial dysfunction and cardiovascular complications are closely linked [14,31–35]. Endothelial cell damage correlates with thrombosis, hypertension and may be also responsible for accelerated atherosclerosis in patients with CKD. Traditional risk factors cannot explain the high incidence of cardiovascular disease in patients with CKD therefore several studies focus on other parameters such as endothelial dysfunction or insulin resistance. In this paper, we focused on the mechanism of endothelial dysfunction induced by uremic toxins, including the remodelling of the extracellular matrix.

Our results demonstrate that uremic toxins modulate primary responses of endothelial cells that correlate with the function of endothelium *in vivo*. Endothelial loss, due to apoptosis leads to vascular complications like thrombosis, increased inflammatory infiltration to the intimal area of the arteries and impaired NO production that lead to hypertension and atherosclerosis. Our results demonstrate that uremic toxins induce apoptosis of endothelial cells *in vitro*. This result is in line with previous reports that link increased endothelial cell apoptosis and renal failure, an effect that was mainly attributed to increased levels of AGEs [34,36]. *In vivo* loss of the endothelial monolayer leads to the formation of a thrombus but it might also be compensated by the increased proliferation of endothelial cells neighboring the damaged area or from direct recruitment of endothelial cell precursors from the bone marrow or circulation [37]. Our results indicate that in parallel to the increased apoptosis that is observed in endothelial cells when they are incubated with media containing uremic toxins, a decreased proliferation and migration capacity of the endothelial cells is observed. These results might also explain the thrombophilia that is observed in patients with renal failure

that often leads to vascular clotting, heart attacks and strokes. The fact that increased apoptosis, reduced proliferation and inhibition of migration were dependent on the concentration of the serum as well as the fact these effects were reversed by HD, indicate that the primary response of endothelial cells to ingredients of the sera in patients with CKD is to the uremic toxins. This result is of particular interest since in a previous study low levels of AGEs were not linked to a better survival rate in HD patients [38]. Our results indicate thought that HD significantly improves endothelial biological functions *in vitro* indicating that the primary endothelial damage is related most probably to uremic toxins.

Several studies indicated the role of disturbed extracellular matrix metabolism in defective myocardial and vascular remodelling [39–52]. Therefore MMPs as well as their tissue inhibitors have been proposed as a group of factors that add to the pathogenesis of atherosclerosis. Animal models and *in vitro* investigations have shown their multifaceted actions, varying from protective and anti-atherogenic in the case of TIMP-2, through neutral of TIMP-1 or ambiguous of MMP-9, to pro-atherogenic of MMP-2 [52–57]. Moreover, gelatinases A and B (MMP-2 and MMP-9) constitute risk factors for myocardial infarction [58] whereas their tissue inhibitors TIMPs have an impact on postmyocardial infarction remodelling [59,60] and correlate positively with left ventricular mass and wall thickness [61]. The role of MMPs in CKD has been studied extensively [62–65], and especially the impact on ischemic acute renal injury and scarring in the course of glomerulopathies [66–68].

Our data demonstrate that uremic toxins modulate the expression of MMP production by endothelial cells *in vitro* as well as their enzymatic activity. Interestingly, our data clearly demonstrate an opposite effect of uremic toxins on the production of MMPs and TIMPs. When the protein levels were evaluated a clear reduction in the production of TIMP-1 and -2 was observed in endothelial cells that were cultured with pre-HD serum. Relative expression levels of TIMP RNA supported these results.

The initial strong induction of TIMP-1 and -2 expression levels when endothelial cells were cultured with post-HD serum were followed by a moderate increased production of TIMPs at prolonged periods of incubation of endothelial cells with pre-HD serum. This response of the cells to uremic sera can only be explained by a time-dependent and well-orchestrated response of endothelial cells in "danger signals" *in vivo* [69–72]. The original response of endothelial cells to uremic toxins leads to the activation of MMPs without affecting the initial levels of TIMPs. Further exposure of the endothelium might initiate the activation of inhibitory pathways that aim the resolution of the inflammation produced by the uremic toxins. In the absence of obvious uremia (like in the case of post-HD serum) the relative production of MMPs versus TIMPs seems to be more balanced which most probably reflects the response of a functional endothelium *in vivo*. Such an endothelial response to uremic toxins *in vivo* might lead to degradation of the extracellular matrix and the basal membrane of the endothelial cells, leading to increased endothelial loss due to anoikis *in vivo*. One could speculate that the expression of MMPs might potentiate the ability of the endothelial cells to modulate the extracellular matrix locally and induce wound healing. Though, this is most probably not the case since our experiments clearly demonstrate a decreased ability of endothelial cells to migrate and cover damaged regions *in vitro*. The increased MMP production seems to correlate more with the increased thrombotic incidence and atherosclerosis observed in patients with kidney disease. Increased MMP activity correlates with atherosclerosis development and plaque rupture. Plaque vulnerability especially is linked to intimal thickening, loss of the collagen fibrous cap surrounding mostly necrotic areas of atherosclerotic lesions, or increased angiogenesis and hemorrhage within the atherosclerotic lesions. Our results suggest that uremic toxins, by modulating the expression and activity of MMPs might be major regulators of the thrombogenic incidents observed in patients with CKD.

Our results demonstrate that endothelial cells contribute at the early response to uremic toxins to the overall systemic inflammation observed in patients with CKD. This response resembles the procedure of the activation of the endothelium during atherosclerosis. During the early stages of atherosclerosis progression endothelial cells express adhesion molecules (e.g. VCAM-1,

ICAM-1, E-selectin) as well as chemokines (e.g. MCP-1, MCP-3, Fractalkine) [25,69,73,74] upon activation of the nuclear factor-kappa B [75]. This response leads to the recruitment of immune cells (namely monocytes) into the intima of the large arteries. At latter stages the disease does not depend on the endothelial response but mainly to the cells of the immune system either resolve the initial inflammation or activate an adaptive immune response [76–78]. We would like to propose a similar process during the development and establishment of CKD At the early stages the accumulation of uremic toxins in the plasma of patients could lead to altered functions of the endothelium, reorganization of the extracellular matrix of the large arteries and an inflammatory response. At latter stages, the presence of uremic toxins might have no effect on the activation of specific molecular response in endothelial cells, though it could contribute to increased apoptosis and reduced wound healing. The practical significance of this hypothesis, and the stage where the progression of the disease is still endothelial-dependent definitively deserves further investigation.

The advantage of this study relies on the fact that we used pre-HD and post-HD sera from the same patients. To our understanding our approach provided the best internal controls to study the direct effect of uremic toxins present in patients with CKD on endothelial cells. This approach prevented us from using sera from healthy patients since HD could not be applied. Nevertheless this was not the aim of this study that aimed on the net effect or uremic toxins on endothelial cells and not the overall effect of sera from patients with CKD compared to normal sera on endothelial cells (an approach that was used extensively in the past). Our results demonstrate that uremic toxins contribute to a great extend to deregulation of endothelial cells, most probably at the early stages of the development of kidney disease. Further studies are ongoing regarding the clinical evaluation and significance of our results.

Author Contributions

Conceived and designed the experiments: PK JV AP. Performed the experiments: KZ TB SK. Analyzed the data: PK JV AP. Contributed reagents/materials/analysis tools: PK JV. Wrote the paper: PK JV AP.

References

1. Kitagawa S, Yamaguchi Y, Kunitomo M, Sameshima E, Fujiwara M (1994) NG-nitro-L-arginine-resistant endothelium-dependent relaxation induced by acetylcholine in the rabbit renal artery. Life Sci 55: 491–498.
2. Matsuda H, Hayashi K, Wakino S, Kubota E, Honda M, et al. (2004) Role of endothelium-derived hyperpolarizing factor in ACE inhibitor-induced renal vasodilation in vivo. Hypertension 43: 603–609.
3. Ruilope LM, Redon J, Schmieder R (2007) Cardiovascular risk reduction by reversing endothelial dysfunction: ARBs, ACE inhibitors, or both? Expectations from the ONTARGET Trial Programme. Vasc Health Risk Manag 3: 1–9.
4. Sahin G, Yalcin AU, Akcar N (2007) Effect of N-acetylcysteine on endothelial dysfunction in dialysis patients. Blood Purif 25: 309–315.
5. Chappey O, Wautier MP, Wautier JL (1997) Structure and functions of the endothelium. Rev Prat 47: 2223–2226.
6. Anggard EE (1992) The regulatory functions of the endothelium. Jpn J Pharmacol 58 Suppl 2: 200P–206P.
7. Fleming I, Bauersachs J, Busse R (1996) Paracrine functions of the coronary vascular endothelium. Mol Cell Biochem 157: 137–145.
8. Kharbanda RK, Deanfield JE (2001) Functions of the healthy endothelium. Coron Artery Dis 12: 485–491.
9. Ryan JW, Ryan US (1982) Metabolic functions of the pulmonary vascular endothelium. Adv Vet Sci Comp Med 26: 79–98.
10. van Hinsbergh VW (1992) Regulatory functions of the coronary endothelium. Mol Cell Biochem 116: 163–169.
11. Vane JR, Anggard EE, Botting RM (1990) Regulatory functions of the vascular endothelium. N Engl J Med 323: 27–36.
12. Hayakawa H, Raij L (1999) Relationship between hypercholesterolaemia, endothelial dysfunction and hypertension. J Hypertens 17: 611–619.
13. Ishikawa M, Namiki A, Kubota T, Fukazawa M, Joki N, et al. (2001) Effect of hyperhomocysteinemia on endothelial activation and dysfunction in patients with end-stage renal disease. Am J Cardiol 88: 1203–1205.
14. Kunz K, Petitjean P, Lisri M, Chantrel F, Koehl C, et al. (1999) Cardiovascular morbidity and endothelial dysfunction in chronic haemodialysis patients: is homocyst(e)ine the missing link? Nephrol Dial Transplant 14: 1934–1942.
15. Takagi M, Wada H, Mukai K, Kihira H, Yano S, et al. (1994) Increased vascular endothelial cell markers in patients with chronic renal failure on maintenance haemodialysis. Blood Coagul Fibrinolysis 5: 713–717.
16. Lazarus JM, Hampers C, Merrill JP (1974) Hypertension in chronic renal failure. Treatment with hemodialysis and nephrectomy. Arch Intern Med 133: 1059–1066.
17. Baradaran A, Nasri H (2005) Correlation of serum parathormone with hypertension in chronic renal failure patients treated with hemodialysis. Saudi J Kidney Dis Transpl 16: 288–292.
18. Jacobson SH, Egberg N, Hylander B, Lundahl J (2002) Correlation between soluble markers of endothelial dysfunction in patients with renal failure. Am J Nephrol 22: 42–47.
19. Kornerup HJ (1976) Hypertension in end-stage renal disease. The relationship between blood pressure, plasma renin, plasma renin substrate and exchangeable sodium in chronic hemodialysis patients. Acta Med Scand 200: 257–261.
20. Szczepanska M, Szprynger K, Adamczyk P, Trembecka-Dubel E, Oswiecimska J (2005) Arterial hypertension in children with end-stage renal failure treated with hemodialysis. Pol Merkur Lekarski 18: 17–21.
21. Jaffe EA, Nachman RL, Becker CG, Minick CR (1973) Culture of human endothelial cells derived from umbilical veins. Identification by morphologic and immunologic criteria. J Clin Invest 52: 2745–2756.

22. Polykratis A, Katsoris P, Courty J, Papadimitriou E (2005) Characterization of heparin affin regulatory peptide signaling in human endothelial cells. J Biol Chem 280: 22454–22461.

23. Mosmann T (1983) Rapid colorimetric assay for cellular growth and survival: application to proliferation and cytotoxicity assays. J Immunol Methods 65: 55–63.

24. Chung TW, Kim JR, Suh JI, Lee YC, Chang YC, et al. (2004) Correlation between plasma levels of matrix metalloproteinase (MMP)-9/MMP-2 ratio and alpha-fetoproteins in chronic hepatitis carrying hepatitis B virus. J Gastroenterol Hepatol 19: 565–571.

25. Libby P (2002) Inflammation in atherosclerosis. Nature 420: 868–874.

26. Brodsky SV, Yamamoto T, Tada T, Kim B, Chen J, et al. (2002) Endothelial dysfunction in ischemic acute renal failure: rescue by transplanted endothelial cells. Am J Physiol Renal Physiol 282: F1140–1149.

27. Caramelo C, Espinosa G, Manzarbeitia F, Cernadas MR, Perez Tejerizo G, et al. (1996) Role of endothelium-related mechanisms in the pathophysiology of renal ischemia/reperfusion in normal rabbits. Circ Res 79: 1031–1038.

28. Costa-Hong V, Bortolotto LA, Jorgetti V, Consolim-Colombo F, Krieger EM, et al. (2009) Oxidative stress and endothelial dysfunction in chronic kidney disease. Arq Bras Cardiol 92: 381–386.

29. Cross J (2002) Endothelial dysfunction in uraemia. Blood Purif 20: 459–461.

30. Karbowska A, Boratynska M, Kusztal M, Klinger M (2009) Hyperuricemia is a mediator of endothelial dysfunction and inflammation in renal allograft recipients. Transplant Proc 41: 3052–3055.

31. Annuk M, Zilmer M, Fellstrom B (2003) Endothelium-dependent vasodilation and oxidative stress in chronic renal failure: impact on cardiovascular disease. Kidney Int Suppl: S50–53.

32. Bolton CH, Downs LG, Victory JG, Dwight JF, Tomson CR, et al. (2001) Endothelial dysfunction in chronic renal failure: roles of lipoprotein oxidation and pro-inflammatory cytokines. Nephrol Dial Transplant 16: 1189–1197.

33. Guerra RJ, Brotherton AF, Goodwin PJ, Clark CR, Armstrong ML, et al. (1989) Mechanisms of abnormal endothelium-dependent vascular relaxation in atherosclerosis: implications for altered autocrine and paracrine functions of EDRF. Blood Vessels 26: 300–314.

34. Linden E, Cai W, He JC, Xue C, Li Z, et al. (2008) Endothelial dysfunction in patients with chronic kidney disease results from advanced glycation end products (AGE)-mediated inhibition of endothelial nitric oxide synthase through RAGE activation. Clin J Am Soc Nephrol 3: 691–698.

35. Zoccali C, Maio R, Tripepi G, Mallamaci F, Perticone F (2006) Inflammation as a mediator of the link between mild to moderate renal insufficiency and endothelial dysfunction in essential hypertension. J Am Soc Nephrol 17: S64–68.

36. Nin JW, Ferreira I, Schalkwijk CG, Prins MH, Chaturvedi N, et al. (2009) Levels of soluble receptor for AGE are cross-sectionally associated with cardiovascular disease in type 1 diabetes, and this association is partially mediated by endothelial and renal dysfunction and by low-grade inflammation: the EURODIAB Prospective Complications Study. Diabetologia 52: 705–714.

37. Song G, Nguyen DT, Pietramaggiori G, Scherer S, Chen B, et al. (2010) Use of the parabiotic model in studies of cutaneous wound healing to define the participation of circulating cells. Wound Repair Regen 18: 426–432.

38. Schwedler SB, Metzger T, Schinzel R, Wanner C (2002) Advanced glycation end products and mortality in hemodialysis patients. Kidney Int 62: 301–310.

39. Chen H, Li D, Saldeen T, Mehta JL (2003) TGF-beta 1 attenuates myocardial ischemia-reperfusion injury via inhibition of upregulation of MMP-1. Am J Physiol Heart Circ Physiol 284: H1612–1617.

40. Djuric T, Zivkovic M, Radak D, Jekic D, Radak S, et al. (2008) Association of MMP-3 5A/6A gene polymorphism with susceptibility to carotid atherosclerosis. Clin Biochem 41: 1326–1329.

41. Hayashidani S, Tsutsui H, Ikeuchi M, Shiomi T, Matsusaka H, et al. (2003) Targeted deletion of MMP-2 attenuates early LV rupture and late remodeling after experimental myocardial infarction. Am J Physiol Heart Circ Physiol 285: H1229–1235.

42. Kelly D, Khan S, Cockerill G, Ng LL, Thompson M, et al. (2008) Circulating stromelysin-1 (MMP-3): a novel predictor of LV dysfunction, remodelling and all-cause mortality after acute myocardial infarction. Eur J Heart Fail 10: 133–139.

43. Lee WY, Wei HJ, Lin WW, Yeh YC, Hwang SM, et al. (2011) Enhancement of cell retention and functional benefits in myocardial infarction using human amniotic-fluid stem-cell bodies enriched with endogenous ECM. Biomaterials 32: 5558–5567.

44. Lehrke M, Greif M, Broedl UC, Lebherz C, Laubender RP, et al. (2009) MMP-1 serum levels predict coronary atherosclerosis in humans. Cardiovasc Diabetol 8: 50.

45. Lindsey ML (2004) MMP induction and inhibition in myocardial infarction. Heart Fail Rev 9: 7–19.

46. Matsumura S, Iwanaga S, Mochizuki S, Okamoto H, Ogawa S, et al. (2005) Targeted deletion or pharmacological inhibition of MMP-2 prevents cardiac rupture after myocardial infarction in mice. J Clin Invest 115: 599–609.

47. Matsusaka H, Ikeuchi M, Matsushima S, Ide T, Kubota T, et al. (2005) Selective disruption of MMP-2 gene exacerbates myocardial inflammation and dysfunction in mice with cytokine-induced cardiomyopathy. Am J Physiol Heart Circ Physiol 289: H1858–1864.

48. Napoli C (2002) MMP inhibition and the development of cerebrovascular atherosclerosis: The road ahead. Stroke 33: 2864–2865.

49. Pradhan-Palikhe P, Vikatmaa P, Lajunen T, Palikhe A, Lepantalo M, et al. (2010) Elevated MMP-8 and decreased myeloperoxidase concentrations associate significantly with the risk for peripheral atherosclerosis disease and abdominal aortic aneurysm. Scand J Immunol 72: 150–157.

50. Tarin C, Gomez M, Calvo E, Lopez JA, Zaragoza C (2009) Endothelial nitric oxide deficiency reduces MMP-13-mediated cleavage of ICAM-1 in vascular endothelium: a role in atherosclerosis. Arterioscler Thromb Vasc Biol 29: 27–32.

51. Wakatsuki S, Suzuki J, Ogawa M, Masumura M, Muto S, et al. (2008) A novel IKK inhibitor suppresses heart failure and chronic remodeling after myocardial ischemia via MMP alteration. Expert Opin Ther Targets 12: 1469–1476.

52. Zureik M, Beaudeux JL, Courbon D, Benetos A, Ducimetiere P (2005) Serum tissue inhibitors of metalloproteinases 1 (TIMP-1) and carotid atherosclerosis and aortic arterial stiffness. J Hypertens 23: 2263–2268.

53. de Nooijer R, Verkleij CJ, von der Thusen JH, Jukema JW, van der Wall EE, et al. (2006) Lesional overexpression of matrix metalloproteinase-9 promotes intraplaque hemorrhage in advanced lesions but not at earlier stages of atherogenesis. Arterioscler Thromb Vasc Biol 26: 340–346.

54. Florys B, Glowinska B, Urban M, Peczynska J (2006) Metalloproteinases MMP-2 and MMP-9 and their inhibitors TIMP-1 and TIMP-2 levels in children and adolescents with type 1 diabetes. Endokrynol Diabetol Chor Przemiany Materii Wieku Rozw 12: 184–189.

55. Ho FM, Liu SH, Lin WW, Liau CS (2007) Opposite effects of high glucose on MMP-2 and TIMP-2 in human endothelial cells. J Cell Biochem 101: 442–450.

56. Luttun A, Lutgens E, Manderveld A, Maris K, Collen D, et al. (2004) Loss of matrix metalloproteinase-9 or matrix metalloproteinase-12 protects apolipoprotein E-deficient mice against atherosclerotic media destruction but differentially affects plaque growth. Circulation 109: 1408–1414.

57. Wang CQ, Wang S, Tang DM, Lin X, Ding HY, et al. (2005) Effects of TIMP-2 gene transfer on atherosclerotic plaque in rabbits. Zhonghua Xin Xue Guan Bing Za Zhi 33: 405–410.

58. Jefferis BJ, Whincup P, Welsh P, Wannamethee G, Rumley A, et al. (2010) Prospective study of matrix metalloproteinase-9 and risk of myocardial infarction and stroke in older men and women. Atherosclerosis 208: 557–563.

59. Kandalam V, Basu R, Abraham T, Wang X, Awad A, et al. (2010) Early activation of matrix metalloproteinases underlies the exacerbated systolic and diastolic dysfunction in mice lacking TIMP3 following myocardial infarction. Am J Physiol Heart Circ Physiol 299: H1012–1023.

60. Kandalam V, Basu R, Abraham T, Wang X, Soloway PD, et al. (2010) TIMP2 deficiency accelerates adverse post-myocardial infarction remodeling because of enhanced MT1-MMP activity despite lack of MMP2 activation. Circ Res 106: 796–808.

61. Hansson J, Lind L, Hulthe J, Sundstrom J (2009) Relations of serum MMP-9 and TIMP-1 levels to left ventricular measures and cardiovascular risk factors: a population-based study. Eur J Cardiovasc Prev Rehabil 16: 297–303.

62. Andrews KL, Betsuyaku T, Rogers S, Shipley JM, Senior RM, et al. (2000) Gelatinase B (MMP-9) is not essential in the normal kidney and does not influence progression of renal disease in a mouse model of Alport syndrome. Am J Pathol 157: 303–311.

63. Musial K, Zwolinska D (2011) Matrix metalloproteinases (MMP-2,9) and their tissue inhibitors (TIMP-1,2) as novel markers of stress response and atherogenesis in children with chronic kidney disease (CKD) on conservative treatment. Cell Stress Chaperones 16: 97–103.

64. Pawlak K, Mysliwiec M, Pawlak D (2011) Peripheral blood level alterations of MMP-2 and MMP-9 in patients with chronic kidney disease on conservative treatment and on hemodialysis. Clin Biochem 44: 838–843.

65. Schaefer L, Han X, Gretz N, Hafner C, Meier K, et al. (1996) Tubular gelatinase A (MMP-2) and its tissue inhibitors in polycystic kidney disease in the Han:SPRD rat. Kidney Int 49: 75–81.

66. Caron A, Desrosiers RR, Langlois S, Beliveau R (2005) Ischemia-reperfusion injury stimulates gelatinase expression and activity in kidney glomeruli. Can J Physiol Pharmacol 83: 287–300.

67. Cheng S, Pollock AS, Mahimkar R, Olson JL, Lovett DH (2006) Matrix metalloproteinase 2 and basement membrane integrity: a unifying mechanism for progressive renal injury. FASEB J 20: 1898–1900.

68. Johnson TS, Haylor JL, Thomas GL, Fisher M, El Nahas AM (2002) Matrix metalloproteinases and their inhibitions in experimental renal scarring. Exp Nephrol 10: 182–195.

69. Hansson G (1997) Vascular immune reactions in arteritis and atherosclerosis. Receptors for endothelial adhesion. Lakartidningen 94: 852–854.

70. Hansson GK, Bondjers G (1987) Endothelial dysfunction and injury in atherosclerosis. Acta Med Scand Suppl 715: 11–17.

71. Maier JA, Malpuech-Brugere C, Zimowska W, Rayssiguier Y, Mazur A (2004) Low magnesium promotes endothelial cell dysfunction: implications for atherosclerosis, inflammation and thrombosis. Biochim Biophys Acta 1689: 13–21.

72. Mysliwiec M, Borawski J, Naumnik B, Rydzewska-Rosolowska A (2004) Endothelial dysfunction, atherosclerosis and thrombosis in uremia–possibilities of intervention. Rocz Akad Med Bialymst 49: 151–156.

73. Hansson GK, Libby P (2006) The immune response in atherosclerosis: a double-edged sword. Nat Rev Immunol 6: 508–519.

74. Libby P, Aikawa M, Jain MK (2006) Vascular endothelium and atherosclerosis. Handb Exp Pharmacol 176 Pt 2: 285–306.

11

Preoperative Proteinuria is Associated with Long-Term Progression to Chronic Dialysis and Mortality after Coronary Artery Bypass Grafting Surgery

Vin-Cent Wu[1,9], Tao-Min Huang[2,9], Pei-Chen Wu[3], Wei-Jie Wang[4], Chia-Ter Chao[1], Shao-Yu Yang[1], Chih-Chung Shiao[6], Fu-Chang Hu[7], Chun-Fu Lai[1], Yu-Feng Lin[8], Yin-Yi Han[8], Yih-Sharng Chen[5], Ron-Bin Hsu[5], Guang-Huar Young[5], Shoei-Shen Wang[5], Pi-Ru Tsai[5], Yung-Ming Chen[1], Ting-Ting Chao[9*], Wen-Je Ko[5,8*], Kwan-Dun Wu[1], the NSARF Group[¶]

1 Division of Nephrology, Department of Internal Medicine, National Taiwan University Hospital, Taipei, Taiwan, 2 Division of Nephrology, Department of Internal Medicine, Yun-Lin Branch, National Taiwan University Hospital, Douliou, Taiwan, 3 Division of Nephrology, Department of Internal Medicine, Da Chien General Hospital, Miaoli, Taiwan, 4 Department of Internal Medicine, Taoyuan General Hospital, Department of Health, Executive Yuan, Taoyuan, Taiwan, 5 Department of Surgery, National Taiwan University Hospital, Taipei, Taiwan, 6 Division of Nephrology, Department of Internal Medicine, Saint Mary's Hospital, and Saint Mary's Medicine, Nursing, and Management College, Luodong, Yilan, 7 International Harvard Statistical Consulting Company, Taipei, Taiwan, 8 Department of Raumatology, National Taiwan University Hospital, Taipei, Taiwan, 9 Medical Research Center, Cardinal Tien Hospital, Fu Jen Catholic University College of Medicine, Taipei, Taiwan

Abstract

Aims: Preoperative proteinuria is associated with post-operative acute kidney injury (AKI), but whether it is also associated with increased long- term mortality and end -stage renal disease (ESRD) is unknown.

Methods and Results: We studied 925 consecutive patients undergoing CABG. Demographic and clinical data were collected prospectively, and patients were followed for a median of 4.71 years after surgery. Proteinuria, according to dipstick tests, was defined as mild (trace to 1+) or heavy (2+ to 4+) according to the results of the dipstick test. A total of 276 (29.8%) patients had mild proteinuria before surgery and 119 (12.9%) patients had heavy proteinuria. During the follow-up, the Cox proportional hazards model demonstrated that heavy proteinuria (hazard ratio [HR], 27.17) was an independent predictor of long-term ESRD. There was a progressive increased risk for mild proteinuria ([HR], 1.88) and heavy proteinuria ([HR], 2.28) to predict all–cause mortality compared to no proteinuria. Mild ([HR], 2.57) and heavy proteinuria ([HR], 2.70) exhibited a stepwise increased ratio compared to patients without proteinuria for long–term composite catastrophic outcomes (mortality and ESRD), which were independent of the baseline GFR and postoperative acute kidney injury (AKI).

Conclusion: Our study demonstrated that proteinuria is a powerful independent risk factor of long-term all-cause mortality and ESRD after CABG in addition to preoperative GFR and postoperative AKI. Our study demonstrated that proteinuria should be integrated into clinical risk prediction models for long-term outcomes after CABG. These results provide a high priority for future renal protective strategies and methods for post-operative CABG patients.

Editor: Shahab A. Akhter, University of Chicago, United States of America

Funding: This study was supported by The Ta-Tung Kidney Foundation, Taiwan National Science Council (grant NSC 96-2314-B-002-164, NSC 96-2314-B-002-033-MY3, NSC 97-2314-B-002-155-MY2, NSC 98-2314-B-002-155-MY4) and National Taiwan University Hospital grant, NTUH.098-001177, NTUH 100-001667. The funders had no role in study design, data collection and analysis, decision to publish, or preparation of the manuscript.

Competing Interests: The authors have declared that no competing interests exist.

* E-mail: q91421028@ntu.edu.tw (TTC); kowj@ntu.edu.tw (WJK)

9 These authors contributed equally to this work.

¶ For a list of the members of The National Taiwan University Study Group on Acute Renal Failure please see the Acknowledgments section.

Introduction

Although coronary artery bypass grafting (CABG) surgery can result in improved quality and prolongation of life in selected patients, several factors have been identified as independent predictors of poor outcomes [1]. The pre-operative estimated glomerular filtration rate (eGFR) is one of the most powerful predictors of CABG outcome [2,3]. In addition, even a mild elevation of serum creatinine after surgery carries a significant risk of adverse outcomes [4].

Based on experience with chronic kidney disease (CKD), proteinuria (detected either by dipstick tests or the albumin-creatinine ratio [ACR]) has been shown to be strongly associated with adverse outcomes, including incident acute kidney injury (AKI), renal disease progression, cardiovascular events, and long-term mortality in the general population [5–8]. Recent reports from large epidemiologic studies have shown that patients with proteinuria have a higher risk of adverse outcomes than those without proteinuria at the same stage of CKD [9,10]. It has been suggested that GFR and proteinuria should be used together to identify patients at risk [5,9–11]. Screening for proteinuria is a better strategy than relying on a low eGFR to identify individuals who are at risk for accelerated GFR loss in population screening [12]. Furthermore, the episode of AKI could provide further long-term prognostic information in addition to eGFR and proteinuria [11]. We previously reported that pre-operative proteinuria, independent of pre-operative eGFR and other co-morbidities, could predict AKI in patients undergoing CABG [13]. No study has shown pre-operative proteinuria to be an independent risk factor of long-term mortality and dialysis dependence in post-CABG patients with a high mortality rate.

The objective of this study was to estimate the post-discharge, long-term mortality, and ESRD risk associated with pre-operative proteinuria, while adjusting for pre-operative eGFR with post-operative AKI and other co-morbidities in post-CABG patients.

Results

Among the 1136 adult patients who underwent CABG during the period from January 2003 to December 2006, 50 patients had undergone dialysis before surgery, 30 patients were CKD stage 5 before surgery, and 76 patients did not have urinalysis measurements before surgery. During the hospital admission, 55 patients expired. Therefore, only 925 patients were included in the final analysis (Figure S1).

Patients with impaired renal function (low eGFR or proteinuria; Table 1, 2)

Three hundred nineteen patients (34.5%) were classified as CKD stage 3, while 52 (5.6%) patients were classified as stage 4 pre-operatively. The patients with higher CKD stages (stages 3 and 4) were older and had higher Charlson scores, lower pre-operative Hb levels, required more tracheostomies, had more post-cardiac surgery AKI than patients with preserved kidney function. Patients with stage 4 CKD were more likely to have PAD, undergo CPB, and required post-operative RRT than patients with preserved kidney function.

A total of 276 (29.8%) patients had mild proteinuria before surgery and 119 (12.9%) patients had heavy proteinuria. Those with proteinuria were more likely to have DM, impaired left ventricular contractility, CHF, and post-operative AKI. These patients also had significantly lower eGFRs, higher Charlson scores, and lower pre-operative hemoglobin (Hb) levels than non-proteinuric patients. Patients with heavy proteinuria were more likely to have PAD, CVA, tracheostomies, receive CPB, and require post-operative RRT.

In patients with preserved eGFR, 147 (15.9%) patients had mild proteinuria and 34 (3.7%) patients had heavy proteinuria. In stage 3 CKD patients, 11 (15.6%) had mild proteinuria and 65 (18.1%) had heavy proteinuria, and in stage 4 patients, 12 (4.3%) had mild proteinuria and 27 (22.7%) had heavy proteinuria (Table S1).

Long-term adverse outcomes were stratified by CKD stage and the severity of proteinuria (Table 3). Patients with preserved eGFR and without proteinuria had the lowest rates of post-operative RRT (0.3%), mortality (5.6%), and composite outcomes (5.9%). The severity of proteinuria showed a dose response-type increased risk for adverse long-term outcomes in patients with preserved eGFR, and CKD stage 3, but not in patients with CKD stage 4.

ESRD after CABG (Table 4, Fig. 1)

During follow-up, the total incidence of ESRD was 0.2, 1.1, and 5.5 per 100 person–years among surviving hospital patients with

pre-operative normal, mild, and heavy proteinuria, respectively. We included the variables listed in Table 1, 2 into regression analysis to identify significant factors associated with post-operative ESRD. CKD stages were representative of pre-operative renal function, as stated in the Methods. The Cox proportional hazards model demonstrated heavy proteinuria (HR, 27.17) and CKD stage 4 (HR, 91.21) as independent predictors of long-term ESRD (Table S2). The interaction term between CKD and proteinuria (p<0.001) was inverse related to long-term ESRD. The magnitude of the increases associated with ESRD grew progressively with heavier baseline proteinuria. (HR = 5.282, p<0.001 for trend)

All-cause mortality after CABG (Table 4, Fig. 2)

The incidence for all-cause mortality was 1.9, 5.1, and 8.0 per 100 person–years among patients with normal, mild, and strong proteinuria, respectively.

We also put all the variables listed in Table 1, 2 into regression analysis for identifying important risk factors of post-operative mortality. In the final model, there was a progressive increased risk of mild proteinuria (HR, 1.88) and heavy proteinuria (HR, 2.28) to predict all–cause mortality in addition to CKD stages and postoperative AKI. (Table S3). The other significant factors of long-term mortality were older age, low LVEF, a history of CAD, absence of HTN, and post-operative RRT requirements.

The interaction term between CKD and proteinuria was not significant (p>0.05). (Table S3). The test for linear trend across proteinuria categories was significant. (HR = 1.542 , p<0.001).

Post-operative long-term composite outcomes

HRs for long–term composite outcomes associated with the CKD and proteinuria categories are shown in Fig. 3. Patients with mild (HR, 2.57) and heavy proteinuria (HR, 2.70) and patients with CKD stage 3 (HR, 2.24) and stage 4 (HR, 3.52) had a stepwise increased ratio compared to patients without proteinuria or patients with preserved eGFR stages (Table S4).

HRs were obtained using Cox proportional hazards regression for categorical analysis and adjusted for factors listed in Table 1, 2 with CKD stages as representative of pre-operative kidney function (Fig. 4). Figure 4a showed survival curves for proteinuria categories across eGFR categories. The HRs for long-term composite outcome increased with the severity of proteinuria (Figure S2), and also increased with CKD stages. Both CKD stages and postoperative AKI modified the frequency and consequences of proteinuria status. (Figure 4b) The HR for composite outcome was the highest with heavy proteinuria strata within stage 4 CKD (HR, 11.58; 95% CI, 5.20–26.70; p<0.001). The risk for composite outcome was magnified further when mild proteinuria was present in those with baseline stage 4 CKD (HR, 9.9; 95% CI, 4.83–20.30; p<0.001) compared to patients with a preserved CKD stage without proteinuria. The magnitude of the increases associated with composite outcome grew progressively with heavier baseline proteinuria. (HR = 1.649 , p<0.001 for trend).

Several sensitivity analyses were undertaken. We compared the characteristics of the 76 patients without pre-operative urinalysis with the patients included in the data analysis. Similar results were noted with respect to age (p = 0.870), gender (p = 0.799), CKD stages (p = 0.786), DM (p = 0.250), long-term ESRD (p = 0.999), long-term mortality (p = 0.327), and long-tem composite outcome (p = 0.647). DM had an additive interaction with CKD stages in predicting long-term mortality. Because of this, we repeated our logistic regression model stratified by diabetes status. Heavy proteinuria was associated with an even greater risk of mortality

Table 1. Patients' demographics, classified by CKD stages or proteinuria.

	All (n = 925)	CKD Stage			Proteinuria on dipstick		
		Preserved eGFR	Stage 3	Stage 4	Normal	Mild	Heavy
		(n = 554)	(n = 319)	(n = 52)	(n = 530)	(n = 276)	(n = 119)
Patient characteristics							
Gender (male)	75.9%	82.3%	69.6%***	46.2%***	79.2%	75.7%	61.3%***
Age (years)	65.9±10.9	63.5±11.3	69.6±8.6***	69.0±10.9***	65.1±11.4	67.3±9.9*	66.2±10.1
Body mass index (kg/m^2)	25.0±3.7	25.1±3.3	25.1±4.2	24.3±3.8	25.1±3.4	25.4±4.2	24.2±3.5
Charlson score	1.8±1.8	1.5±1.5	2.2±2.0***	3.3±1.6***	1.5±1.5***	2.0±1.9***	3.0±2.2***
LVEF<60%	46.9%	42.1%	49.8%*	80.8%***	40.8%	51.1%**	64.7%***
Hypertension	69.2%	65.9%	74.6%**	71.2%	68.1%	69.9%	72.3%
DM	43.4%	38.4%	48.6%**	63.5%***	34.9%	44.6%**	78.2%***
PAD	9.0%	6.9%	9.4%	28.8%***	6.4%	8.3%	21.8%***
CVA	9.9%	8.8%	11.0%	15.4%*	7.9%	11.6%	15.1%*
CHF	15.9%	11.2%	19.4%***	44.2%***	10.4%	19.2%***	32.8%***
COPD	8.1%	7.6%	9.4%	5.8%	7.2%	11.2%	5.0%
Recent MI	26.3%	24.0%	28.5%	36.5%	23.4%	32.2%**	25.2%
Af	6.6%	5.4%	9.4%*	1.9%	5.1%	8.7%	8.4%
Peri-operative condition							
Vasopressor dependence	3.6%	2.7%	4.2%*	9.7%**	2.2%	5.7%**	5.1%
Tracheostomy	2.2%	1.1%	3.4%*	5.8%*	0.9%	2.5%	6.7%***
Non-elective surgery	10.5%	9.4%	11.7%	13.5%	6.8%	15.4%***	15.1%**
Cardiopulmonary bypass	13.6%	12.5%	14.1%	23.1%*	11.3%	15.9%	18.5%*
AKI	15.1%	9.9%	20.4%***	38.5%***	9.6%	19.6%***	29.4%***
RRT	3.6%	2.0%	3.5%	22.4%***	1.5%	2.2%	16.4%***

among patients with diabetes (HR, 3.34) than among those without (HR, 1.88) diabetes.

Discussion

We have found that proteinuria is potentially a risk factor of postoperative adverse outcome; however, this simple test is usually neglected in current practice. These findings should make clinicians more concerned about the presence of low quantities of protein in the urine. Our study is the first report to show a marked impact of proteinuria at the time of CABG on long-term mortality and ESRD prediction in post-CABG patients. The National Kidney Foundation staging system for CKD incorporates proteinuria only in the preserved eGFR stages (CKD stages 1 and 2). An association between proteinuria and long- term mortality or ESRD after cardiac surgery has not yet been validated. We showed that proteinuria is associated with a higher risk of long-term ESRD and mortality; even mild proteinuria could predict long- term adverse outcomes. This association was essentially unaltered despite extensive statistical adjustment for traditional CABG risk factors, including chronic kidney disease, AKI, or diabetes mellitus. This adds weight to the growing body of evidence that proteinuria should be considered a high risk condition and that this risk is in addition to any risk attributable to reduced eGFR [5].

The results clearly demonstrated that pre-operative proteinuria is an important, yet neglected predictor for long-term composite outcomes after cardiac surgery. However, the current widely used prognostic scoring systems do not use proteinuria [14]. Preventive interventions have been most studied in patients at high risk because high-risk patients benefit more from such interventions than low-risk patients [15]. Thus, it is very important to develop an inclusive and accurate staging system, especially for patients who are undergoing a procedure associated with significant risks, such as cardiac surgery. Also, this is the first report to systemically investigate the relationship between proteinuria and post-operative long –term renal outcomes and demonstrate the strong association with adverse renal outcomes.

Risk for ESRD according to severity of proteinuria

We have previously reported heavy proteinuria, regardless of baseline eGFR or other co-morbidities, to be independently associated with severe AKI requiring RRT after cardiac surgery [13]. Proteinuria reflects a size-selective dysfunction of the glomerular barrier usually associated with a decline in the GFR that may result in ESRD [16]. There is some evidence that overt albuminuria might be associated with tubulointerstitial damage. Patients with documented proteinuria have less physiologic adaptability and are less able to tolerate kidney hemodynamic changes and other nephrotoxic insults [17].

In a previous population-based cohort study, macroalbuminuria is a better risk marker than low eGFR to identify population screening of individuals who are at risk for accelerated GFR loss [12]. In fact, our CABG patients with preserved kidney function and positive dipstick proteinuria have a greater risk for having a composite outcome than patients with stage 3 CKD and without proteinuria detected by dipstick.

Table 2. Operative characteristics and renal function, classified by CKD stages or proteinuria.

	All (n = 925)	CKD Stage			Proteinuria on dipstick		
		Preserved eGFR	Stage 3	Stage 4	Normal	Mild	Heavy
		(n = 554)	(n = 319)	(n = 52)	(n = 530)	(n = 276)	(n = 119)
CABG parameters							
Aortic cross clamp time(min),(n)	103± 41 (31)	82± 36 (15)	101± 58 (13)	102± 23 (3)	105± 65 (12)	108±36 (14)	97± 25 (5)
Cardiopulmonary bypass(min),(n)	125± 53 (130)	127±51 (75)	123± 71 (42)	127± 41 (13)	125± 60 (60)	128± 63 (48)	120± 32 (22)
Triple vessel disease	93.4%	81.2%	86.2%	88.5%	81.7%	87.0%	92.4%
Left main diseases	37.8%	38.8%	35.4%	42.3%	37.5%	42.0%	29.4%
IABP	9.1%	7.8%	11.0%	11.5%	7.7%	10.9%	10.9%
Preoperative IABP	7.4%	6.1%	9.4%	7.7%	5.5%	9.4%	10.9%
ECMO	1.2%	0.9%	1.3%	3.8%	0.6%	2.2%	1.7%
Mitral insufficiency							
Mild	18.9%	19.9%	17.2%	19.2%	19.1%	20.7%	14.3%
Moderate/severe	8.6%	7.6%	8.2%	23.1%***	5.8%	9.4%	19.3%
Pre-operative laboratory data							
Creatinine (mg/dL)	1.3±0.5	1.0±0.2	1.5±0.3***	2.6±0.55***	1.12±0.4	1.3±0.4**	1.7±0.7***
eGFR(ml/min/1.73 m^2)	64.4±21.1	77.6±14.6	48.12±8.4***	23.22±4.02***	69.±18.7	62.3±21.2***	48.10±22.0***
Hemoglobin (g/dL)	12.9±1.9	13.4±1.6	12.5±2.06***	10.9±1.8***	13.2±1.8	12.8±1.9*	11.9±1.9***

Comparison with patients with preserved estimated GFR ($\geq$60 ml/min/1.73 m^2) or no proteinuria: *$p < 0.05$; **$p < 0.01$; and ***$p < 0.001$.
Abbreviations; CABG: coronary artery bypass grafting surgery; CKD: chronic kidney disease; eGFR: estimated glomerular filtrating rate; ESRD: end stage renal disease.

Risk for mortality according to severity of proteinuria

We found the association between eGFR and mortality differed by severity of proteinuria. Decreased eGFR and increased proteinuria independently contributed to the cumulative probability of all-cause mortality and the risk persisted after full multivariable adjustments, including post-operative AKI. Previous studies have demonstrated that AKI is associated with increased long-term mortality after cardiothoracic surgery, even with a small change in serum creatinine [18]. Further, pre-operative proteinuria and CKD stages, independent of post-operative AKI, are associated with an increased risk of long–term mortality.

When the analysis focused on post-operative composite outcome, patients with impaired eGFR and proteinuria were found to have a greater risk than those without proteinuria. Even mild proteinuria (trace to 1+) increased the risk of a patient with stage 3 CKD to the same risk as stage 4 CKD (Figs. 4). Most strikingly, patients with preserved GFR ($\geq$60 mL/min/1.73 m^2) had a risk comparable to stage 3 CKD, if mild proteinuria (trace to 1+) was present (Fig. 4). These categories of patients have previously been neglected, even though they made up 32.7% (181 of 554 patients) of our cohort. This means that one-third of patients undergoing CABG surgery, who are at an increased risk of long-term mortality and ESRD, are not identified by the current risk scoring systems based only on sCr or GFR measurements. On the other hand, the absence of an interaction effect of CKD and proteinuria in the prediction of long-term mortality was notable because a very small amount of protein

Table 3. Adverse outcomes in 925 CABG patients with various CKD stages and degrees of proteinuria.

Outcomes	ESRD (n = 41)			p^b	Mortality (n = 138)			p^b	Composite outcome (n = 164)			p^b
Proteinuria												
CKD Stages	Normal	Mild	Heavy		Normal	Mild	Heavy		Normal	Mild	Heavy	
Preserved eGFR (n = 554)	0.3%	1.4%	11.8%	<0.001	5.6%	15.6%	14.7%	0.001	5.9%	17.0%	26.5%	<0.001
Stage 3 (n = 319)	1.4%	2.6%	17.2%	<0.001	15.3%	24.8%	34.5%	0.009	16.7%	26.5%	43.1%	<0.001
Stage 4 (n = 51)	23.1%	58.3%	38.5%	0.195	30.8%	41.7%	48.1%	0.580	46.2%	75.0%	66.7%	0.288
p^a	<0.001	<0.001	0.028		<0.001	0.035	0.018		<0.001	<0.001	0.007	

Abbreviations; CABG: coronary artery bypass grafting surgery; CKD: chronic kidney disease; eGFR: estimated glomerular filtrating rate; ESRD: end stage renal disease.
p: The tests for linear trend across CKD categories (p^a) and across proteinuria categories (p^b). Composite outcome: composite outcome of end stage renal disease and mortality. To be noted, 15 patients of them received chronic dialysis before mortality.

Table 4. Factors associated with long- term adverse outcomes (N = 925).

Hazard Ratio(95% CI)	ESRD		all cause mortality		composite outcome	
Covariate	Unadjusted	adjusted	Unadjusted	adjusted	Unadjusted	adjusted
Proteinuria						
No proteinuria	1	—	—	—	—	—
	(reference)					
Mild proteinuria	3.93	2.83	2.29	1.88	2.42	2.70
	(1.48–10.40)**	(1.01–7.99)*	(1.55–3.39) ***	(1.27–2.80)*	(1.67–3.49) ***	(1.69–4.33)***
Heavy proteinuria	10.10	27.17	2.65	2.28	3.36	2.57
	(3.98–25.73)***	(8.77–84.15)**	(1.68–4.18)***	(1.42–3.66)**	(2.23–5.06) ***	(1.68–3.91)***
CKD Stage						
Preserved CKD stage	1	—	—	—	—	—
	(reference)					
Stage 3	3.29	10.71	2.35	1.53	2.33	2.24
	(1.32–8.15)*	(0.93–123.2)	(1.62–3.41) ***	(1.20–2.28)*	(1.64–3.30) ***	(1.40–3.57)***
Stage 4	35.52	91.21	4.85	1.88	7.35	3.52
	(14.25–88.52)***	(31.05–267.94)***	(2.83–8.33) ***	(1.03–3.43)*	(4.65–11.63)***	(2.09–5.94)***

Abbreviations: CI: confidence interval; CKD: chronic kidney disease.
The long- term adverse outcome uses the Cox's proportional hazard model adjusted for age, genders, admission conditions including CKD stage, postoperative acute kidney injury, renal replacement therapy, co-morbidities (hypertension, liver cirrhosis, congestive heart failure, diabetic mellitus, chronic obstructive pulmonary disease , coronary artery disease, hepatitis, cancer, atrial fibrillation), Carlson score, intervention (extracorporeal membrane oxygenation, Ventilator, intra-aortic balloon pumping, use intra-cerebral pressure monitor, Mitral insufficiency, temporary cardiac pacemaker, Swan- Ganz catheter, Sengstaken-Blakemore tube).
*$p<0.05$;
**$p<0.01$; and
***$p<0.001$.

in urine was associated with a significant risk of mortality in the CKD patients [19]. These findings should motivate clinicians to become more concerned about the presence of low quantities of protein in the urine.

A previous small study about CABG showed proteinuria is factor to affect long-term cardiovascular death [20]. However, CKD was not a risk factor in their study. Bouts of evidence show the pre-operative estimated glomerular filtration rate (eGFR) is

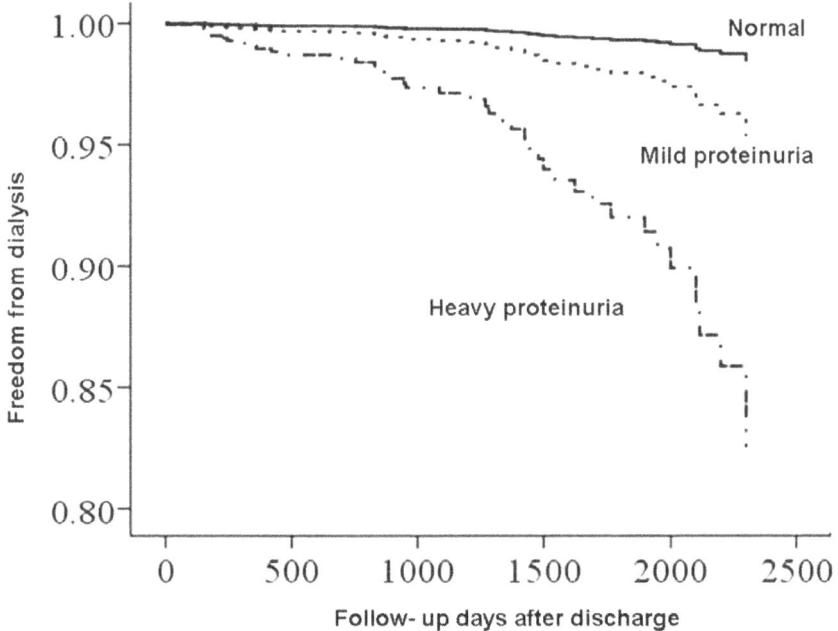

Figure 1. Proportion of freedom from long- term dialysis dependence, stratified by different severities of proteinuria defined by preoperative dipstick. (Mild proteinuria, p = 0.166; Heavy proteinuria, p = 0.001; No proteinuria was the reference calculated by multivariable Cox proportional hazard analyses).

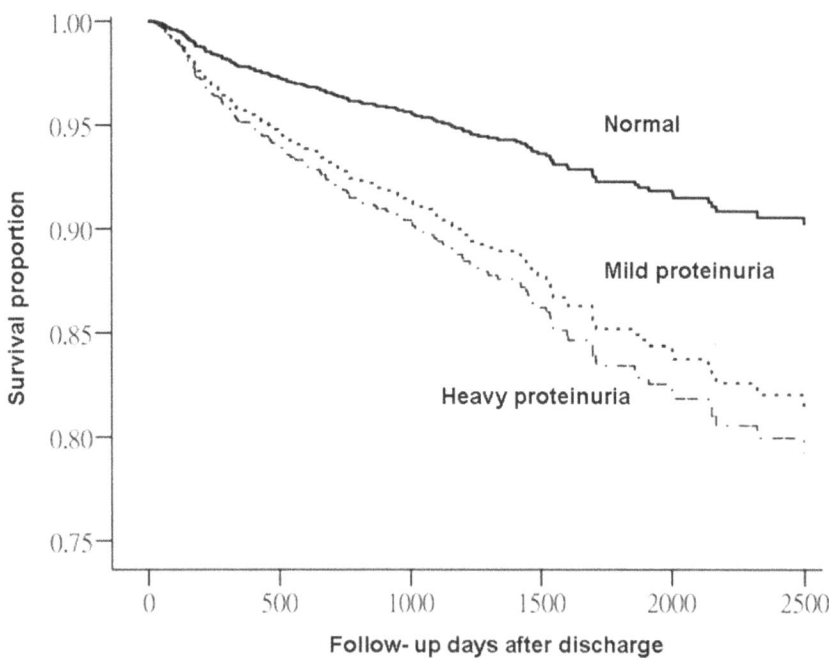

Figure 2. Adjusted risk for long- term all- cause mortality after hospital discharge stratified by different severities of proteinuria defined by preoperative dipstick. (Mild porteinuria, p = 0.005; Heavy proteinuria, p = 0.008; no proteinuria was the reference calculated by multivariable Cox proportional hazard analyses).

one of the most powerful predictors of CABG outcome [2,3]. In addition, we report that proteinuria is a powerful independent risk factor of long-term all-cause mortality and ESRD after CABG in addition to preoperative GFR.

The association between higher CKD stages and higher long-term cumulative composite outcomes increased significantly with an increased severity of proteinuria. In linear trend analysis, the severity of proteinuria showed a dose response-type increasing risk for long-term outcomes in patients with preserved eGFR, and CKD stage 3, but not for stage 4. (please see table 3). However, in multivariable model the HRs for long-term composite outcome increased with the severity of proteinuria (Figure S2), and also

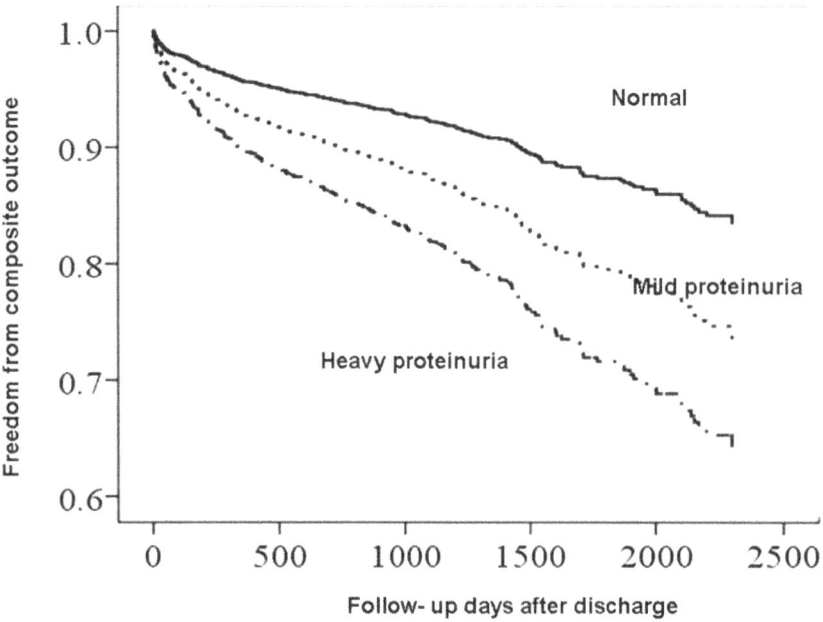

Figure 3. Proportion of freedom from long- term composite outcome after hospital discharge, composite outcome of ESRD and mortality, stratified by different severities of proteinuria defined by preoperative dipstick. (Mild proteinuria, p<0.001; Heavy proteinuria, p<0.001; No proteinuria was the reference calculated by multivariable Cox proportional hazard analyses).

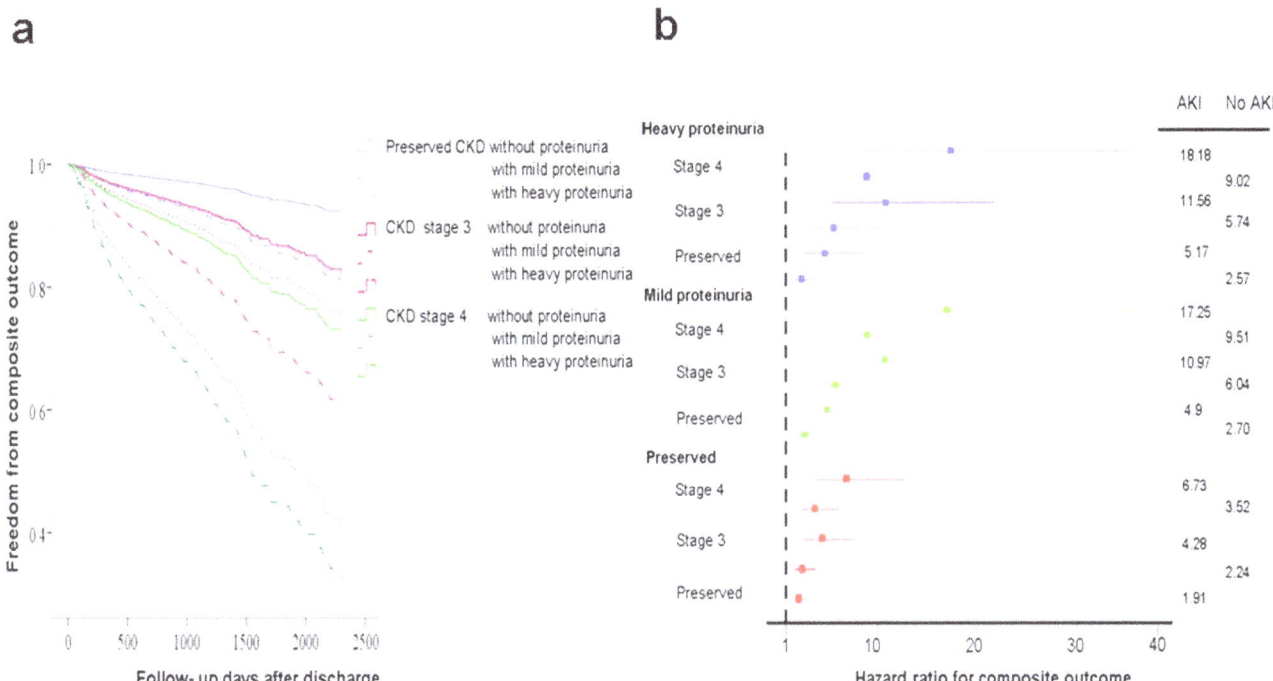

Figure 4. The composite outcome after hospital discharge (long- term end-stage renal disease or mortality) for urinary proteinuric categories across chronic kidney disease (CKD) categories using Cox proportional hazards regression (a) plot of freedom from composite outcome, *p<0.05; **p<0.01; and ***p<0.001 compared to patients with preserved eGFR and normal proteinuria. (b) Hazard ratio (HRs) stratified by proteinuria, baseline kidney function, and postoperative acute kidney injury (AKI) adjusted for factors listed in Table 1. The horizontal bars represent 95% CIs for HRs of participants who had proteinuria for various values of CKD stages and AKI.

increased with CKD stages. This association was observed in participants with and without a history of DM in sensitivity analysis and this result could enhance the joint effects of proteinuria and CKD stages.

Pre-operative proteinuria is not only a marker of chronic renal insults, but may also serve as a surrogate of organ damage. Patients with more severe proteinuria had higher Charlson scores. In our analysis, patients with more severe proteinuria had poor cardiac contractility, DM, PAOD, and CHF, which implies that these patients actually have renal damage and proteinuria secondary to other extra-renal insults. Proteinuria may not just be a marker for adverse outcomes. *In vitro* studies have demonstrated that exposure of renal proximal tubule cells to albumin induced an inflammatory cytokine cascade [21,22]. These events ultimately lead to tubulointerstitial inflammation and fibrosis in long-standing proteinuric nephropathy. The strong predictive effects of proteinuria within 2 days before surgery and the simplicity of its measurements suggest that periodic measurement of proteinuria along with other major CVD risk factors should be considered in long-term follow-up of post CABG patients. Whether or not medications that decrease proteinuria might also be associated with a decrease in mortality in persons undergoing CABG is an important question to be addressed in future studies.

In a large community –based cohort of adults, the risk of long – term mortality composite renal outcome increased substantially with the presence and severity of proteinuria, in addition to reduced eGFR [11]. Similarly, outcomes associated with post CABG AKI have focused on definitions incorporating in proteinuria, magnitude of increase in serum creatinine [13]. Our CABG patients also provide a useful demonstration of the burden of post-operative AKI. (fig. 4b) This disorder was more likely to prognosis to mortality and

composite outcomes during long-term follow-up and was substantially more common at low GFR and with heavy proteinuria.

Study strengths and limitations

The strength of this study was that it assessed the outcomes in a large cohort of patients undergoing CABG in multiple centers. Therefore, the results are likely to be widely applicable. The study population of CABG patients without severe CKD provided a well-defined and homogenous study population in the present study.

There were some limitations to the current study that should be considered. First, detection of proteinuria was performed with dipsticks. In addition, the differences between the dipstick test and ACR in risk assessment of long-term outcomes were not examined in the current study. The epidemiologic studies on this topic either used a dipstick test for proteinuria [11] or quantitatively measured albuminuria. Of note, the urine dipstick examination is inexpensive and readily performed and interpreted. These two tests were well-correlated [23] and the dipstick test is useful for risk stratification despite being a less precise measure of albuminuria in general population cohorts [24,25]. Second, the absence of data on the specific cause of mortality, such as myocardial infarction and heart failure could be a limitation, thus we used all-cause mortality as the primary end point, which is entirely objective [26]. Finally, we assumed that the baseline covariates persisted throughout the follow-up period. Additional assessments would be desirable, especially to evaluate risks that vary over time. Increased numbers of outcome events, including cause-specific mortality and incident ESRD, will buttress the conclusions presented herein.

The present study demonstrated that proteinuria, detected by urine dipstick test, is a powerful independent risk factor for long-term composite outcomes (all-cause mortality and ESRD) in post–

CABG patients. The association between CKD stages and long-term composite outcomes differed significantly across severity of proteinuria. A further strength was that pre-operative proteinuria in addition to pre-operative CKD stages and post-operative AKI is associated with increased long–term mortality risk. A substantial proportion of patients undergoing cardiac surgery have an elevated risk of adverse outcomes that are not apparent from the current risk scoring systems. This is an important insight for physicians who care post-CABG patients, and further studies will be needed to determine the optimal post-discharge follow-up of renal function for patients with pre-operative proteinuria.

Methods

Study population

This is a secondary analysis of a prospectively-collected database. Patients undergoing CABG surgery at the National Taiwan University Hospital (NTUH) and its two branches between January 2003 and December 2006 were enrolled [27]. Inclusion criteria were age ≥18 years and first-time cardiac surgery. The exclusion criteria were a history of pre-operative renal replacement therapy (RRT) with any modality and an estimated GFR<15 mL/min. Patients with no urinalysis reports within 48 hours prior to surgery were also excluded. Patient data collected from the NSARF database included basic demographic characteristics, peri-operative laboratory investigations, type and timing of surgery, and post-operative renal outcome [27,28]. The goals of this study were to evaluate the post-CABG long-term outcomes associated with proteinuria. Patients undergoing pre-operative chronic dialysis, stage 5 CKD, or death during the index hospital admission were excluded. This study was approved by the Institutional Review Board of National Taiwan University Hospital (NTUH) (No. 31MD03). The informed consent was waived by the ethics committee because there was no breach of privacy and it did not interfere with clinical decisions related to patient care.

Clinical assessment of study patients

Pre-operative variables, such as age, gender, left ventricular ejection fraction (LVEF) measured by ventriculography or angiography, hypertension (HTN; blood pressure ≥140/90 mmHg or using anti-hypertensive medications), diabetes mellitus (DM; using oral hypoglycemic agents or insulin), peripheral artery disease (PAD) determined by clinical diagnosis or imaging results, previous cerebral vascular accident (CVA; ischemic or hemorrhagic), New York Heart Association (NYHA) functional class III or IV congestive heart failure (CHF), chronic obstructive pulmonary disease (COPD) requiring long-term bronchodilators or steroids, recent myocardial infarction (MI), i.e., <30 days before surgery, and pre-operative laboratory data were all collected. Coronary artery disease (CAD) was defined as the diagnosis of ischemic heart disease before admission and positive electrocardiographic findings. Patients with associated diseases were assessed using the Charlson co-morbidity score [29]. Peri-operative vasopressor (adrenaline, dopamine, dobutamine, norepinephrine, or isoproterenol) dependence and use of extra-corporeal membrane oxygenation (ECMO) or an intra-aortic balloon pump (IABP) were noted. Patients who underwent emergent or urgent surgical procedures were considered non-elective surgery. Utilization of cardiopulmonary bypass (CPB) and CPB duration during surgery was also recorded.

Pre-operative GFR and proteinuria

The following 3 parameters were used to represent pre-operative GFR: serum creatinine, eGFR, and CKD stage (preserved eGFR, stage 3 or 4, according to eGFR). The baseline serum creatinine (sCr) was the datum obtained at hospital discharge from the previous admission in those who had more than one admission within 1 year before the index admission [30], or a pre-operative creatinine obtained in pre-operative testing excluding the measurements that were performed in the emergency department [18,31,32]. The eGFR in each patient was calculated using the 4-variable MDRD equation [33]. CKD stages were determined using the NKF definition, as follows: $15 \text{ mL/min/m}^2 \leq \text{eGFR} < 30 \text{ mL/min/m}^2$ was classified as stage 4; and $30 \text{ mL/min/m}^2 \leq \text{eGFR} < 60 \text{ mL/min/m}^2$ was classified as stage 3. Patients with an $\text{eGFR} \geq 60 \text{ mL/min/m}^2$ had preserved GFR.

Proteinuria was measured using a dipstick within 2 days before surgery. To classify the severity of proteinuria, we defined negative as "no proteinuria," trace to 1+ as "mild proteinuria," and 2+ to 4+ as "heavy proteinuria." The test strips were measured by an automatic dipstick autoanalyzer (AUTION MAX, AX-4030; ARKRAY, Inc., Kyoto, Japan) with automatic correction of the specific gravity using a pH test pad in a routine laboratory environment. This classification was adopted in a large epidemiologic study in Alberta, Canada [10]. Although ACR is favored for detection of proteinuria, dipstick examination remains the most convenient and inexpensive choice for screening [10]. If there were more than one measurement in 2 days prior to surgery, we chose the most severe result for analysis.

AKI and RRT

The definition of AKI was based on the Acute Kidney Injury Network (AKIN) criteria, and has been well-validated in cardiac surgery patients for in-hospital mortality prediction [34]. In the NSARF database, sCr values were recorded daily after surgery. Urine output was recorded every hour in the critical care setting.

Long-term mortality and dialysis dependence

The long-term outcomes for this analysis were mortality, ESRD, and composite outcome (long–term ESRD or mortality) after discharge. Patient survival after discharge was determined through the databank of the National Health Insurance Research Database (NHIRD) in January 2009 [35]. All-cause mortality was documented by matching unique identity numbers with the NHIRD.

The NHIRD contains health care data from >99% of the entire population of 23.74 million in Taiwan, and it covers all inpatient and outpatient medical benefit claims. We also cross–linked our study population with the nationally comprehensive TAIWAN Society Nephrology registry, which recorded all dialysis patients in the island every 3 months.

Statistical analysis

Statistical analyses were performed with SPSS for Windows (version 15.0; SPSS, Inc., Chicago, IL, USA). A two-sided p value≤0.05 was considered statistically significant. Continuous variables were presented as the mean and standard deviation (mean ± SD). Categorical variables were summarized as the frequency and percentage. A group difference in demographic characteristics was examined between each renal dysfunction group (CKD stages or proteinuria) and the preserved renal function group by two-sample t-test or chi-square test as appropriate.

The long-term outcomes were based on Cox's proportional hazard model adjusted for age, gender, admission categories, CKD stage, post-operative AKI, RRT, co-morbidities (HTN, liver cirrhosis, CHF, DM, COPD, CAD, hepatitis, cancer, and atrial fibrillation (Af), Carlson score, intervention (ECMO, mechanical ventilation, IABP, intra-cerebral pressure monitor (ICP), temporary cardiac pacemaker (TCP), a Swan- Ganz catheter, PiCCO, and a Sengstaken-Blakemore tube) and censored on 1 January 2009. Survival curves for all-cause mortality or freedom from dialysis were generated from adjusted Cox models. Survival models were initiated at the time of hospital discharge and followed until death or last follow-up time. There was high collinearity among sCr, estimated GFR (MDRD), and CKD stage, so we adjusted the input variable of the CKD stage to be representative of kidney function to emphasize the effect of preoperative kidney stage. Yet, there is a significant positive relationship between the level of proteinuria and CKD stage (p<0.001) and the risk of AKI might be different in patients with and without DM [36]. Thus, the interaction effects between proteinuria, CKD stages, postoperative AKI, and diabetics on adverse outcomes were also considered.

For the long-term dialysis, an individual who survived at index discharge was censored at death or at the end of the study period. Hazard ratios (HRs) and 95% confidence intervals (CIs) were derived from the Cox proportional hazard model. The incidence of chronic dialysis and all-cause mortality were stratified for participants with different severities of proteinuria. To help visualize the analysis results, we investigated the relationship between the effects of the level of CKD stages and severity of proteinuria by adding interaction terms and plotted by fitting the basic Cox regression analyses separately for the strata of the level of dipsticks.

Finally, sensitivity analyses were conducted. We compared the basic demography and outcomes of the 76 patients without preoperative urinalysis with the study patients. A two-sided P value<0.05 was considered to indicate statistical significance.

Supporting Information

Figure S1 Flow diagram of the study population. (AKI, acute kidney injury; CABG, coronary artery bypass grafting; CKD, chronic kidney disease; ESRD, end stage renal disease; ICU, intensive care unit).

Figure S2 Hazard ratio (HRs) for the compo site outcome after hospital discharge (long- term end-stage renal disease or mortality)

for urinary proteinuric categories across chronic kidney disease (CKD) categories. (adjusted for factors listed in Table 1. $^{*}p<0.05$; $^{**}p<0.01$; and $^{***}p<0.001$ compared to patients with preserved eGFR and normal proteinuria).

Table S1 Percentage of patients in groups stratified by chronic kidney disease (CKD) stage and proteinuria.

Table S2 Factors associated with long- term end stage renal disease (N = 925).

Table S3 Factors associated with long- term all- cause mortality (N = 925).

Table S4 Factors associated with long- term composite outcome (N = 925).

Acknowledgments

The authors would like to thank the staff of the Second and Seven Core Lab of the Department of Medical Research in National Taiwan University Hospital for technical assistance.

We express our sincere gratitude to all participants of the NSARF.

The National Taiwan University Hospital study group for Acute Renal Failure (NSARF) includes: Wen-Je Ko, MD, PhD, Vin-Cent Wu, MD, Yu-Feng Lin, MD, Yih-Sharng Chen, MD, PhD, Yung-Ming Chen, MD, Chih-Chung Shiao, MD, Chun-Fu Lai, MD, Wei-Jie Wang, MD, Pei-Chen Wu, MD, Chia-Ter Chao, MD, Cheng-Yi Wang, MD, Yung-Wei Chen, MD, Pi-Ru Tsai, RN, Wen-Yi Li, MD, Yu-Chang Yeh, MD, Tao-Min Huang, MD, Fu-Chang Hu, MS, ScD, and Kwan-Dun Wu, MD, PhD.

Author Contributions

Conceived and designed the experiments: VCW TMH PCW. Performed the experiments: WJW CTC SYY SSW PRT TTC. Analyzed the data: YYH CCS FCH YMC TTC WJK KDW. Contributed reagents/materials/analysis tools: CFL YFL YYH YSC RBH GHY SSW. Wrote the paper: VCW.

References

1. Eagle KA, Guyton RA, Davidoff R, Ewy GA, Fonger J, et al. (1999) ACC/AHA Guidelines for Coronary Artery Bypass Graft Surgery: A Report of the American College of Cardiology/American Heart Association Task Force on Practice Guidelines (Committee to Revise the 1991 Guidelines for Coronary Artery Bypass Graft Surgery). American College of Cardiology/American Heart Association. J Am Coll Cardiol 34: 1262–1347.
2. Cooper WA, O'Brien SM, Thourani VH, Guyton RA, Bridges CR, et al. (2006) Impact of renal dysfunction on outcomes of coronary artery bypass surgery: results from the Society of Thoracic Surgeons National Adult Cardiac Database. Circulation 113: 1063–1070.
3. Hillis GS, Croal BL, Buchan KG, El-Shafei H, Gibson G, et al. (2006) Renal function and outcome from coronary artery bypass grafting: impact on mortality after a 2.3-year follow-up. Circulation 113: 1056–1062.
4. Lassnigg A, Schmidlin D, Mouhieddine M, Bachmann LM, Druml W, et al. (2004) Minimal changes of serum creatinine predict prognosis in patients after cardiothoracic surgery: a prospective cohort study. J Am Soc Nephrol 15: 1597–1605.
5. Grams ME, Astor BC, Bash LD, Matsushita K, Wang Y, et al. (2010) Albuminuria and Estimated Glomerular Filtration Rate Independently Associate with Acute Kidney Injury. J Am Soc Nephrol 21: 1757–1764.
6. Klausen K, Borch-Johnsen K, Feldt-Rasmussen B, Jensen G, Clausen P, et al. (2004) Very low levels of microalbuminuria are associated with increased risk of coronary heart disease and death independently of renal function, hypertension, and diabetes. Circulation 110: 32–35.
7. Mann JF, Gerstein HC, Pogue J, Bosch J, Yusuf S (2001) Renal insufficiency as a predictor of cardiovascular outcomes and the impact of ramipril: the HOPE randomized trial. Ann Intern Med 134: 629–636.
8. Hillege HL, Fidler V, Diercks GF, van Gilst WH, de Zeeuw D, et al. (2002) Urinary albumin excretion predicts cardiovascular and noncardiovascular mortality in general population. Circulation 106: 1777–1782.

9. Hallan SI, Ritz E, Lydersen S, Romundstad S, Kvenild K, et al. (2009) Combining GFR and albuminuria to classify CKD improves prediction of ESRD. J Am Soc Nephrol 20: 1069–1077.
10. Hemmelgarn BR, Manns BJ, Lloyd A, James MT, Klarenbach S, et al. (2010) Relation between kidney function, proteinuria, and adverse outcomes. JAMA 303: 423–429.
11. James MT, Hemmelgarn BR, Wiebe N, Pannu N, Manns BJ, et al. (2011) Glomerular filtration rate, proteinuria, and the incidence and consequences of acute kidney injury: a cohort study. Lancet 376: 2096–2103.
12. Halbesma N, Kuiken DS, Brantsma AH, Bakker SJ, Wetzels JF, et al. (2006) Macroalbuminuria is a better risk marker than low estimated GFR to identify individuals at risk for accelerated GFR loss in population screening. J Am Soc Nephrol 17: 2582–2590.
13. Huang TM, Wu VC, Young GH, Lin YF, Shiao CC, et al. (2011) Preoperative Proteinuria Predicts Adverse Renal Outcomes after Coronary Artery Bypass Grafting. J Am Soc Nephrol 22: 156–163.
14. DeRose JJ, Jr., Toumpoulis IK, Balaram SK, Ioannidis JP, Belsley S, et al. (2005) Preoperative prediction of long-term survival after coronary artery bypass grafting in patients with low left ventricular ejection fraction. J Thorac Cardiovasc Surg 129: 314–321.
15. Bove T, Landoni G, Calabro MG, Aletti G, Marino G, et al. (2005) Renoprotective action of fenoldopam in high-risk patients undergoing cardiac surgery: a prospective, double-blind, randomized clinical trial. Circulation 111: 3230–3235.
16. Ruggenenti P, Remuzzi G (2006) Time to abandon microalbuminuria? Kidney Int 70: 1214–1222.
17. Hsu CY, Ordonez JD, Chertow GM, Fan D, McCulloch CE, et al. (2008) The risk of acute renal failure in patients with chronic kidney disease. Kidney Int 74: 101–107.

18. Hobson CE, Yavas S, Segal MS, Schold JD, Tribble CG, et al. (2009) Acute kidney injury is associated with increased long-term mortality after cardiothoracic surgery. Circulation 119: 2444–2453.

19. Wen CP, Cheng TY, Tsai MK, Chang YC, Chan HT, et al. (2008) All-cause mortality attributable to chronic kidney disease: a prospective cohort study based on 462 293 adults in Taiwan. Lancet 371: 2173–2182.

20. Orii K, Hioki M, Iedokoro Y, Shimizu K Prognostic factors affecting clinical outcomes after coronary artery bypass surgery: analysis of patients with chronic kidney disease after 5.9 years of follow-up. J Nihon Med Sch 78: 156–165.

21. Donadelli R, Abbate M, Zanchi C, Corna D, Tomasoni S, et al. (2000) Protein traffic activates NF-kB gene signaling and promotes MCP-1-dependent interstitial inflammation. Am J Kidney Dis 36: 1226–1241.

22. Abbate M, Zoja C, Remuzzi G (2006) How does proteinuria cause progressive renal damage? J Am Soc Nephrol 17: 2974–2984.

23. Konta T, Hao Z, Takasaki S, Abiko H, Ishikawa M, et al. (2007) Clinical utility of trace proteinuria for microalbuminuria screening in the general population. Clin Exp Nephrol 11: 51–55.

24. James MT, Hemmelgarn BR, Wiebe N, Pannu N, Manns BJ, et al. (2010) Glomerular filtration rate, proteinuria, and the incidence and consequences of acute kidney injury: a cohort study. Lancet 376: 2096–2103.

25. Matsushita K, van der Velde M, Astor BC, Woodward M, Levey AS, et al. (2010) Association of estimated glomerular filtration rate and albuminuria with all-cause and cardiovascular mortality in general population cohorts: a collaborative meta-analysis. Lancet 375: 2073–2081.

26. Lauer MS, Blackstone EH, Young JB, Topol EJ (1999) Cause of death in clinical research: time for a reassessment? J Am Coll Cardiol 34: 618–620.

27. Wu VC, Ko WJ, Chang HW, Chen YS, Chen YW, et al. (2007) Early renal replacement therapy in patients with postoperative acute liver failure associated with acute renal failure: effect on postoperative outcomes. J Am Coll Surg 205: 266–276.

28. Wu VC, Ko WJ, Chang HW, Chen YW, Lin YF, et al. (2008) Risk factors of early redialysis after weaning from postoperative acute renal replacement therapy. Intensive Care Med 34: 101–108.

29. Charlson ME, Pompei P, Ales KL, MacKenzie CR (1987) A new method of classifying prognostic comorbidity in longitudinal studies: development and validation. J Chronic Dis 40: 373–383.

30. Uchino S, Bellomo R, Goldsmith D, Bates S, Ronco C (2006) An assessment of the RIFLE criteria for acute renal failure in hospitalized patients. Crit Care Med 34: 1913–1917.

31. Wu VC, Huang DM, Ko WJ, Wu KD (2011) Acute-on-chronic kidney injury predicted long-term dialysis and mortality in critical patients after discharge. Kidney Int: in press.

32. Palevsky PM, Zhang JH, O'Connor TZ, Chertow GM, Crowley ST, et al. (2008) Intensity of renal support in critically ill patients with acute kidney injury. N Engl J Med 359: 7–20.

33. Levey AS, Bosch JP, Lewis JB, Greene T, Rogers N, et al. (1999) A more accurate method to estimate glomerular filtration rate from serum creatinine: a new prediction equation. Modification of Diet in Renal Disease Study Group. Ann Intern Med 130: 461–470.

34. Haase M, Bellomo R, Matalanis G, Calzavacca P, Dragun D, et al. (2009) A comparison of the RIFLE and Acute Kidney Injury Network classifications for cardiac surgery-associated acute kidney injury: a prospective cohort study. J Thorac Cardiovasc Surg 138: 1370–1376.

35. Insurance BoNH (2007) National Health Insurance in Taiwan. Available at wwwnhigovtw/english/indexasp accessed 20 August 2009.

36. Parfrey PS, Griffiths SM, Barrett BJ, Paul MD, Genge M, et al. (1989) Contrast material-induced renal failure in patients with diabetes mellitus, renal insufficiency, or both. A prospective controlled study. N Engl J Med 320: 143–149.

12

Ankle-Brachial Index: A Simple Way to Predict Mortality among Patients on Hemodialysis

Zaida Noemy Cabrera Jimenez, Benedito Jorge Pereira, João Egidio Romão Jr, Sonia Cristina da Silva Makida, Hugo Abensur, Rosa Maria Affonso Moyses, Rosilene Motta Elias*

Renal Division, Internal Medicine, Hospital das Clínicas, University of São Paulo School of Medicine, São Paulo, Brazil

Abstract

Background: Ankle-brachial index (ABI) can access peripheral artery disease and predict mortality in prevalent patients on hemodialysis. However, ABI has not yet been tested in incident patients, who present significant mortality. Typically, ABI is measured by Doppler, which is not always available, limiting its use in most patients. We therefore hypothesized that ABI, evaluated by a simplified method, can predict mortality in an incident hemodialysis population.

Methodology/Principal Findings: We studied 119 patients with ESRD who had started hemodialysis three times weekly. ABI was calculated by using two oscillometric blood pressure devices simultaneously. Patients were followed until death or the end of the study. ABI was categorized in two groups normal (0.9–1.3) or abnormal (<0.9 and >1.3). There were 33 deaths during a median follow-up of 12 months (from 3 to 24 months). Age (1 year) (hazard of ratio, 1.026; p = 0.014) and ABI abnormal (hazard ratio, 3.664; p = 0.001) were independently related to mortality in a multiple regression analysis.

Conclusions: An easy and inexpensive technique to measure ABI was tested and showed to be significant in predicting mortality. Both low and high ABI were associated to mortality in incident patients on hemodialysis. This technique allows nephrologists to identify high-risk patients and gives the opportunity of early intervention that could alter the natural progression of this population.

Editor: Emmanuel A. Burdmann, University of Sao Paulo Medical School, Brazil

Funding: Zaida Noemy Cabrera Jimenez was supported by Conselho Nacional de Desenvolvimento Científico e Tecnológico (CNPQ), Brazil. The funders had no role in study design, data collection and analysis, decision to publish, or preparation of the manuscript.

Competing Interests: The authors have declared that no competing interests exist.

* E-mail: rosilenemotta@hotmail.com

Introduction

Despite significant technological advances, mortality among patients on hemodialysis remains inexcusably high, particularly in the first year of therapy [1].

One way to potentially reduce mortality is to alert medical staff to patients at increased risk of death in order to facilitate timely diagnostic and therapeutic interventions.

Hemodialysis patients are at an increased risk for atherosclerotic disorders, including peripheral arterial disease (PAD) [2]. PAD is a strong predictor for all-cause and cardiovascular mortality in hemodialysis patients [3,4].

Ankle-brachial index (ABI) is a simple, noninvasive, and reliable test for PAD screening. Usually ABI is classified as low (<0.9), normal (0.9–1.3) and high (>1.3). Both low and high ABI are correlated to high mortality in patients on hemodialysis [5]. Low ABI is related to PAD, and high ABI is caused by no compressible arteries and vascular calcification. Therefore, an abnormal ABI value is a significant predictor of mortality among patients on hemodialysis [4,6].

ABI was already identified as a predictor of mortality among prevalent patients on hemodialysis. Incident patients on hemodialysis are even at higher risk. The annual number of patients beginning dialysis has grown, mostly because of the growing prevalence of hypertension and diabetes, the main underlying cause of kidney disease [7,8]. Most analyses of survival on dialysis exclude the first 90-day period. There have been minimal improvements in mortality rate during the first year, over the past decade, even without including the initial 90 days [1,7]. ABI could be an easy way to identify patients at the highest risk.

We recently tested measuring ABI by using two oscillometric blood pressure devices simultaneously [9], simulating an ABI-form device.

The results demonstrated good reproducibility and low intra-observer variability. The ABI was extensively tested in three consecutive dialysis sessions, as well as pre and post dialysis. The question that remained was if this technique could be significant in predicting mortality.

We therefore tested the general hypothesis that ABI measured by two oscillometric blood pressure devices can predict mortality in an incident hemodialysis population.

Methods

Subjects

Patients were enrolled from January 2008 to January 2010. Inclusion criteria were patients with end-stage renal disease (ESRD) at least 18 years of age undergoing their first month of

Table 1. Characteristics of the study population.

Variables	N = 119
Age, years	53.1 ± 18.8
Male, n (%)	82 (68.9)
Etiology of ESRD, n (%)	
Hypertension	35 (29.4)
Diabetes	44 (37.0)
Glomerulonephritis	18 (15.1)
Others	22 (18.5)
Hypertension, n (%)	118 (99.1)
Diabetes mellitus, n (%)	49 (47.2)
Family history of CV disease, n (%)	62 (52.1)
Smoking, ever vs. never, n (%)	36 (30.2)
Sedentary habits, n (%)	92 (77.3)
Ankle-brachial index	1.16 ± 0.23
Systolic Blood Pressure, mmHg	149.4 ± 23.8
Diastolic Blood Pressure, mmHg	85.9 ± 17.2
Albumin level, g/dl	3.4 ± 0.7
Phosphorus level, mg/dl	5.8 ± 2.2
Calcium corrected, mg/dl	9.0 ± 1.1
Calcium x Phosphorus, mg/dl	48.3 ± 18.3
Total cholesterol, mg/dl	167.9 ± 44.9
Hemoglobin, g/dl	9.3 ± 1.7
C-reactive protein, mg/L	35.9 ± 48.9
Parathyroid hormone, pg/ml	372.7 ± 484.2

CV, cardiovascular; Calcium corrected = calcium + (4-albumin) ×0.8.
Values are expressed as mean ± SD or n (percentage).

conventional hemodialysis three times weekly in the University of Sao Paulo School of Medicine's Hospital das Clinicas. This was a prospective observational study.

We excluded anyone who had been treated for infection, had bilateral amputation, bilateral fistula or had atrial fibrillation. Prior to ABI measurement, demographic characteristics, and medical history were recorded. Biochemical data were measured within 2 weeks of ABI measurement and dialysis initiation.

ABI Measurement

The measurements were done by using two oscillometric devices (Omron Corp 705 CP Corp, Tokyo, Japan) simultaneously to measure blood pressure in the upper and lower extremities. The pre dialysis ABI was used in this new technique which was already intra-observer validated and described [9]. Briefly, measurements were done pre dialysis, with the patient at rest in the supine position, after 5 minutes of the beginning of the session. The protocol was performed by the same examiner in all situations. During the study, only raw blood pressure values were recorded, and stored on a database for later ABI calculation. Our technique showed that ABI can be measured by two oscillometric devices at the same time, with good reproductibility and low intra-observer variation.

Follow-up

The outcome of this study was all-cause mortality. Patients were censored in case of renal transplantation or recovery of renal function. Vital status was ascertained by telephone contact. The censor date was 31st January 2010. Date of death was verified by contacting relatives and/or the staff of the dialysis clinic. Survival time was defined as the time of the baseline (first day of ABI measurement) to the date of death or end of follow-up.

Ethic Statements

The protocol was approved by the Research Ethics Boards of the University of Sao Paulo School of Medicine, and all subjects provided written informed consent before participation.

Data Analysis

Differences between continuous variables and categorical variables were calculated using Student t test for normally distributed continuous variables and by Mann-Whitney U test for abnormally distributed variables. The $\chi 2$ or Fisher exact test was used to compare nominal variables. To compare the 3 groups according to ABI <0.9, from 0.9 to 1.3 and >1.3, one-way analysis of variance was applied, with Tukey post-hoc test.

Mortality was the outcome of the follow-up. The relation of ABI categories and all-cause mortality was analyzed by Kaplan-Meier survival plots and log-rank test. A stepwise multivariate cox regression was undertaken to identify the relative risk of all-cause mortality (entry threshold, $P<0.05$; removal threshold, $P<0.10$) with the significant candidate variables (age, diabetes, calcium x phosphorus product, parathyroid hormone and C-reactive protein). A lower level of the −2 log-likelihood indicates a better model fit. Data are presented as means ±SD unless indicated otherwise. A P-value <0.05 was considered significant. Analyses were performed with the use of SPSS 17.0.1 (SPSS Inc., Chicago, Ill).

Results

Subjects

Out of 123 consecutive ESRD patients, 4 lost the follow-up. Therefore, 119 patients were studied (82 men and 37 women), whose baseline characteristics were shown in Table 1. Diabetes, hypertension and glomerulonephritis accounted for 80% of the underlying causes of renal disease. The majority of the patients had a family history of cardiovascular disease (51.2%), 30.2% were smokers, 47.2% had diabetes, hypertension was found in almost 100% of the patients, and 77.3% presented sedentary behavior, which configure in a high cardiovascular risk population. Anemia, altered bone mineral metabolism, and inflammation (expressed by C-reactive protein) were also observed.

Characteristics of the study population regarding ABI categories (normal 0.9–1.3, low <0.9, and high >1.3 are presented in Table 2. Distribution of observed ABI at the baseline is shown in Figure 1. The significant differences between these 3 groups were age (p = 0.011), albumin (p = 0.040) and hemoglobin (p = 0.010). Cardiovascular risk factors observed at the baseline were well distributed among the three groups.

During the study there were 33 deaths on a median follow-up of 12 months (from 3 to 24 months). Table 3 shows the differences in basal characteristics between the group of patients who died and the group that survived. Patients who died were more likely to be older (p = 0.003), and with lower PTH (p = 0.044). Gender, diabetes, family history of cardiovascular disease, smoking and sedentary habitus, blood pressure, and biochemical variables did not distinguish survivors and non-survivors. The ABI as a continuous variable was virtually identical in survivors and non-survivors (p = 0.998). However, abnormal ABI was more frequent among patients who died than in patients who survived (63.6% vs. 13.9%, p<0.0001).

Table 2. Characteristics of the study population according to ABI.

Variable	ABI			
	<0.9 N = 12	0.9–1.3 N = 73	>1.3 N = 34	p
Age, years	68.8 ± 16.6*	53.7 ± 17.9	42.3 ± 18.2	0.001
Male sex, n (%)	7 (58.3)	49 (67.1)	26 (76.5)	0.440
Diabetes mellitus, n (%)	5 (41.7)	29 (39.7)	15 (44.1)	0.911
Family history of CV disease, n (%)	6 (50)	41 (56.2)	15 (44.1)	0.503
Smoking, ever vs. never, n (%)	4 (33)	23 (31.5)	9 (26.5)	0.844
ABI	0.68 ± 0.16*	1.13 ± 0.11	1.40 ± 0.08*	0.0001
Albumin level, g/dl	3.4 ± 0.9	3.5 ± 0.6	3.1 ± 0.8*	0.040
Calcium x Phosphorus, mg²/dl²	47.7 ± 22.0	49.7 ± 18.6	45.6 ± 16.6	0.564
Total cholesterol, mg/dl	162.4 ± 36.8	168.3 ± 46.9	169.1 ± 43.9	0.903
Hemoglobin, g/dl	9.9 ± 2,1	9.5 ± 1.6	8.6 ± 1.5*	0.010
C-reactive protein, mg/l	55.0 ± 69.8	31.0 ± 41.3	39.6 ± 54.9	0.260
Parathyroid hormone, pg/ml	463.6 ± 302.1	397.7 ± 555.7	286.2 ± 360.4	0.448

CV, cardiovascular; ABI, ankle-brachial index; Corrected Calcium = calcium + (4-albumin) ×0.8.
Values are expressed as Mean ± SD. *p<0.05 by post-test, comparing to ABI 0.9–1.3.

Figure 2 shows an unadjusted Kaplan-Meier survival curve analysis demonstrating that abnormal ABI was associated with greater all-cause mortality. The mean survival time and 95% confidence interval was 21.1±0.8 months (19.6–22.6) for normal ABI, and 16.2±1.2 months (13.8–18.7) for abnormal ABI; log-rank test p = 0.0001.

Upon multivariable Cox regression analyses of all-cause mortality by forward stepwise, the association between abnormal ABI and mortality remained. The HR associated with abnormal ABI was 3.664 times higher than normal ABI (p = 0.001, 95% CI, 1.708–7.861) (Table 4).

Discussion

Our study has given rise to important findings that provide novel possibilities into the diagnostic and interventions in an incident population on hemodialysis. We found that abnormal baseline ABI can predict mortality in hemodialysis patients. In addition, we accessed ABI by a simple and easy method. These findings suggest that ABI may be measured at patient's entry on hemodialysis therapy, even in centers without Doppler or an ABI-form device.

Our study population was representative of the total dialysis population in Brazil, according to the Brazilian Society of Nephrology [10,11] in terms of age, gender distribution and cause

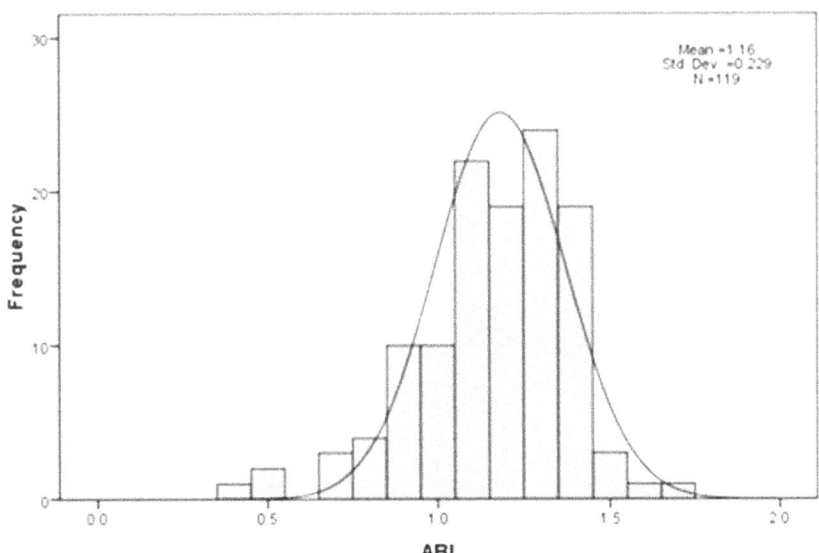

Figure 1. Frequency distribution of baseline ankle-brachial index (ABI).

Table 3. Survivors and non-survivors.

Variable	Survivors N = 86	Non-survivors N = 33	p
Age, years	50.0±18.3	61.2±17.8	0.003
Male sex, n (%)	58 (67.4)	27 (81.8)	0.671
Diabetes mellitus, n (%)	31 (36.0)	19 (57.6)	0.161
Family history of CV disease, n (%)	44 (51.2)	19 (57.6)	1
Smoking, ever vs. never, n (%)	26 (30.2)	10 (30.3)	0.830
Sedentary habitus, n (%)	68 (79.1)	26 (78.8)	0.355
ABI	1.16±0.18	1.15±0.32	0.998
Abnormal ABI, %	13.9	63.3	<0.0001
Systolic BP, mmHg	150.5±25.4	148.7±24.0	0.735
Diastolic BP, mmHg	86.9±19.9	81.0±16.9	0.146
Albumin level, g/dl	3.5±0.6	3.2±0.8	0.104
Calcium x Phosphorus, mg^2/dl^2	50.2±19.2	43.5±15.1	0.195
Total cholesterol, mg/dl	168.5±40.5	166.3±55.3	0.810
Hemoglobin, g/dl	9.2±1.8	9.4±13	0.612
C-reactive protein, mg/l	29.5±39.6	52.8±65.5	0.071
Parathyroid hormone, pg/ml	412.0±549.1	266.5±203.5	0.044

CV, cardiovascular disease; ABI, ankle-brachial index.
Values are expressed as Mean ± SD.

of ESRD. The prevalence of diabetes is also similar to the American and European reports [7,12,13]. However, all these data refer to the prevalent population and we studied an incident population. This specific population has an even higher risk of mortality. Some reported annual rate of mortality simply does not take into account the first 3 months of hemodialysis. The lack of information in the literature regarding diagnostic and possible therapeutic interventions in this selected population calls for new studies.

The incidence of patients in hemodialysis has increased in Brazil. The estimated number of patients starting treatment in 2010 was 18,972 (incidence rate: 99.5/million) [11].

We demonstrated that our sample size of incident patients on hemodialysis is at a high risk of mortality, with a family history of cardiovascular events, sedentary and smoking habits, presence almost universal of hypertension, diabetes and all dialysis-related biochemical abnormalities also associated to the high mortality risk. Indeed, we observed that 27.7% of the entire population had died after a 2-year period of follow-up.

The present data build on the previous findings showing that ABI is a good tool to detect high risk patients on hemodialysis. However, a mainly prevalent population on hemodialysis was studied, showing that both low and high ABI were associated to high overall and cardiovascular mortality [4,5,14,15].

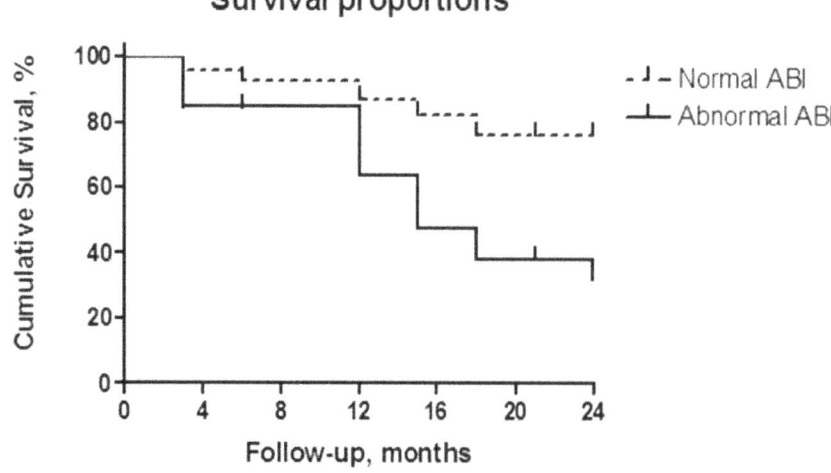

Figure 2. Kaplan-Meier survival curves according to ABI categories: normal (0.9–1.3) or abnormal (<0.9 and >1.3). A lower risk of mortality was observed for normal ABI [superior dashed line]; A higher risk of mortality was observed for abnormal ABI [continuous line]. Log-rank p = 0.0003;

Table 4. Cox regression Survival Analyses of All-cause Mortality, by Forward Stepwise (Likelihood ratio).

Variable	Hazard Ratio (95% Confidence interval)	P
Model 1		0.001 (entire model)
Abnormal ABI	3.564 (1.663–7.638)	0.001
Model 2		0.0001 (entire model)
Age (1 year)	1.026 (1.005–1.048)	0.014
Abnormal ABI	3.664 (1.708–7.861)	0.001

Initial Log Likelihood function −2 Log likelihood: 255.798.
Variables in the model: age, ABI as categorical (normal and abnormal), diabetes, C-reactive protein, albumin, hemoglobin, and PTH.

We could demonstrate similar results of previous studies by using a modified method in measuring ABI. It is important, however, to emphasize that we had previously tested the intra-observer reproducibility. Based on this, we may suggest the use of this simple technique but we not guarantee applicability to other dialysis population. Different from previous studies, we accessed patients within their first month of dialysis. This approach allows us early recognition of patients at high risk of mortality.

The critical question is if the use of our simple technique in detecting abnormal ABI can eventually improve outcomes. There is no indication whether or not knowing the prognosis will improve outcomes. Possibly, we can at least alert medical staff to implement therapeutic interventions in those patients with abnormal ABI. Nevertheless, the clinical utility of our technique has to be studied rigorously in further studies. These studies should enrol larger sample sizes and evaluate different examiners measuring ABI.

Our study is subject to some limitations. First, it only shows associations between abnormal ABI and mortality in one selected dialysis population; this may not be applicable to all hemodialysis population. Second, the sample size was small. Third, we did not compare our technique to the gold-standard method, Doppler, in order to prove they can be interchangeable, although this was not an objective of the present data. Forth, we had no access to

medication in use and dose of dialysis during the follow-up period. Finally, we could not distinguish between overall and cardiovascular cause of mortality, because the lack of accurate information relevant to the deaths of the patients within the study population.

However, our method was extensively tested and validated previously, and although we examined a small sample size, a direct relationship between abnormal ABI and mortality was found.

In conclusion, these data suggest that abnormal ABI was associated with increased mortality among incident patients on hemodialysis. The ABI could be measured by using at the same time two oscillometric blood pressure devices and then, making an easier and more largely applicable method in detecting patients with the highest risk of mortality. Our results also suggest the need for randomized trials to determine whether more aggressive interventions will change the outcomes.

Author Contributions

Conceived and designed the experiments: ZCNJ BJP SCSM JER RME. Performed the experiments: ZCNJ SCSM. Analyzed the data: ZCNJ SCSM BJP JER HA RMAM RME. Contributed reagents/materials/analysis tools: ZCNJ. Wrote the paper: ZCNJ BJP HA RMAM RME.

References

1. Himmelfarb J, Ikizler TA (2010) Hemodialysis. N Engl J Med 363: 1833–1845.
2. Cheung AK, Sarnak MJ, Yan G, Dwyer JT, Heyka RJ, et al. (2000) Atherosclerotic cardiovascular disease risks in chronic hemodialysis patients. Kidney Int 58: 353–362.
3. Newman AB, Shemanski L, Manolio TA, Cushman M, Mittelmark M, et al. (1999) Ankle-arm index as a predictor of cardiovascular disease and mortality in the Cardiovascular Health Study. The Cardiovascular Health Study Group. Arterioscler Thromb Vasc Biol 19: 538–545.
4. Ono K, Tsuchida A, Kawai H, Matsuo H, Wakamatsu R, et al. (2003) Ankle-brachial blood pressure index predicts all-cause and cardiovascular mortality in hemodialysis patients. J Am Soc Nephrol 14: 1591–1598.
5. Chen SC, Chang JM, Hwang SJ, Tsai JC, Liu WC, et al. (2010) Ankle brachial index as a predictor for mortality in patients with chronic kidney disease and undergoing haemodialysis. Nephrology (Carlton) 15: 294–299.
6. Kitahara T, Ono K, Tsuchida A, Kawai H, Shinohara M, et al. (2005) Impact of brachial-ankle pulse wave velocity and ankle-brachial blood pressure index on mortality in hemodialysis patients. Am J Kidney Dis 46: 688–696.
7. Collins AJ, Foley RN, Chavers B, Gilbertson D, Herzog C, et al. (2012) United States Renal Data System 2011 Annual Data Report: Atlas of chronic kidney disease & end-stage renal disease in the United States. Am J Kidney Dis 59: A7, e1–420.
8. Chan KE, Maddux FW, Tolkoff-Rubin N, Karumanchi SA, Thadhani R, et al. (2011) Early outcomes among those initiating chronic dialysis in the United States. Clin J Am Soc Nephrol 6: 2642–2649.
9. Jimenez ZN, de Castro I, Pereira BJ, de Oliveira RB, Romao JE, Jr., et al. (2012) When Is the Best Moment to Assess the Ankle Brachial Index: Pre- or Post-Hemodialysis? Kidney Blood Press Res 35: 242–246.
10. Censos Sociedade Brasileira de Nefrologia website. Available at http://www.sbn.org.br/leigos/index.php?censo Accessed 2011 Sep 10
11. Sesso RC, Lopes AA, Thome FS, Lugon JR, Santos DR (2011) 2010 report of the Brazilian dialysis census. J Bras Nefrol 33: 442–447.
12. Collins AJ, Foley RN, Herzog C, Chavers B, Gilbertson D, et al. (2009) United States Renal Data System 2008 Annual Data Report. Am J Kidney Dis 53: S1–374.
13. Zoccali C, Kramer A, Jager K (2009) The databases: renal replacement therapy since 1989-the European Renal Association and European Dialysis and Transplant Association (ERA-EDTA). Clin J Am Soc Nephrol 4 Suppl 1: S18–22.
14. Tanaka M, Ishii H, Aoyama T, Takahashi H, Toriyama T, et al. (2011) Ankle brachial pressure index but not brachial-ankle pulse wave velocity is a strong predictor of systemic atherosclerotic morbidity and mortality in patients on maintenance hemodialysis. Atherosclerosis 219: 643–647.
15. Adragao T, Pires A, Branco P, Castro R, Oliveira A, et al. (2012) Ankle-brachial index, vascular calcifications and mortality in dialysis patients. Nephrol Dial Transplant 27: 318–325.

13

Electrocardiographic Left Ventricular Hypertrophy and Outcome in Hemodialysis Patients

Seung Jun Kim[1], Hyung Jung Oh[1], Dong Eun Yoo[1], Dong Ho Shin[1], Mi Jung Lee[1], Hyoung Rae Kim[1], Jung Tak Park[1], Seung Hyeok Han[1], Tae-Hyun Yoo[1], Kyu Hun Choi[1], Shin-Wook Kang[1,2]*

1 Department of Internal Medicine, College of Medicine, Yonsei University, Seoul, Korea, 2 Severance Biomedical Science Institute, Brain Korea 21, Yonsei University, Seoul, Korea

Abstract

Background and Aims: Electrocardiography (ECG) is the most widely used initial screening test for the assessment of left ventricular hypertrophy (LVH), an independent predictor of cardiovascular mortality in patients with end-stage renal disease (ESRD). However, traditional ECG criteria based only on voltage to detect LVH have limited clinical utility for the detection of LVH because of their poor sensitivity.

Methods: This prospective observational study was undertaken to compare the prognostic significance of commonly used ECG criteria for LVH, namely Sokolow-Lyon voltage (SV) or voltage-duration product (SP) and Cornell voltage (CV) or voltage-duration product (CP) criteria, and to investigate the association between echocardiographic LV mass index (LVMI) and ECG-LVH criteria in ESRD patients, who consecutively started maintenance hemodialysis (HD) between January 2006 and December 2008.

Results: A total of 317 patients, who underwent both ECG and echocardiography, were included. Compared to SV and CV criteria, SP and CP criteria, respectively, correlated more closely with LVMI. In addition, CP criteria provided the highest positive predictive value for echocardiographic LVH. The 5-year cardiovascular survival rates were significantly lower in patients with ECG-LVH by each criterion. In multivariate analyses, echocardiographic LVH [adjusted hazard ratio (HR): 11.71; 95% confidence interval (CI): 1.57–87.18; P = 0.016] and ECG-LVH by SP (HR: 3.43; 95% CI: 1.32–8.92; P = 0.011) and CP (HR: 3.07; 95% CI: 1.16–8.11; P = 0.024) criteria, but not SV and CV criteria, were significantly associated with cardiovascular mortality.

Conclusions: The product of QRS voltage and duration is helpful in identifying the presence of LVH and predicting cardiovascular mortality in incident HD patients.

Editor: Giuseppe Schillaci, University of Perugia, Italy

Funding: This work was supported by the Brain Korea 21 Project for Medical Science, Yonsei University, by the National Research Foundation of Korea (NRF) grant funded by the Korea government (MEST) (No. 2011-0030711), and by a grant of the Korea Healthcare Technology R&D Project, Ministry of Health and Welfare, Republic of Korea (A102065). The funders had no role in study design, data collection and analysis, decision to publish, or preparation of the manuscript.

Competing Interests: The authors have declared that no competing interests exist.

* E-mail: kswkidney@yuhs.ac

Introduction

Cardiovascular disease is prevalent and the most common cause of morbidity and mortality in patients with end-stage renal disease (ESRD) [1]. Even though coronary artery disease and arrhythmia are not uncommon, left ventricular hypertrophy (LVH) is the most frequent cardiovascular manifestation in these patients [2,3]. LVH is known to be present in more than 70% of incident ESRD patients and increases the risk for cardiac ischemia and congestive heart failure in patients on dialysis [4,5]. In addition, LVH is a very strong independent predictor of cardiovascular mortality not only among patients with hypertension but also among ESRD patients [6–9].

LVH in ESRD patients is mainly attributed to hypertension and anemia [10,11]. However, accumulating evidence shows that volume overload, arteriovenous fistula, hyperparathyroidism, and oxidative stress also play a role in the pathogenesis of LVH in

dialysis patients [12–15]. Moreover, LVH regression by modifying these risk factors is associated with improved all-cause and cardiovascular survival [7], while progression of LVH has independent prognostic value for cardiovascular events in dialysis patients [8]. Therefore, early identification of LVH and aggressive treatment to regress LVH should become an important part of management for ESRD patients.

To date, several imaging modalities, such as echocardiography, magnetic resonance imaging (MRI), and computerized tomography, have been performed to detect LVH [16–18]. In general, however, electrocardiography (ECG) is more widely used for the assessment of LVH [19]. ECG is a noninvasive, convenient, inexpensive, and easily reproducible test, but the clinical utility of traditional, purely voltage-based ECG criteria for the detection of LVH is limited due to poor sensitivity [20]. Therefore, criteria based on the combination of voltage and QRS duration have been developed and have improved the sensitivity for LVH in the hypertensive population [21,22]. In addition, several studies elucidated the relationship between LVH based on different electrocardiographic criteria and echocardiographic LVH [23]. Moreover, a very recent study demonstrated the impact of LVH determined by different ECG criteria on clinical outcome in chronic kidney disease [24]. However, little is known about the association between electrocardiographic and echocardiographic LVH in patients with CKD and ESRD. Furthermore, no study has explored whether the prognostic power of ECG varies in ESRD patients based on the diagnostic criteria for LVH. In this prospective study, therefore, we compared commonly used ECG criteria for LVH to ascertain their prognostic significance and investigated the association between echocardiographic LV mass and ECG-LVH criteria in incident hemodialysis (HD) patients.

Methods

Ethics statement

The study was carried out in accordance with the Declaration of Helsinki and approved by the Institutional Review Board of Yonsei University Health System Clinical Trial Center. We obtained informed written consent from all participants involved in our study.

Patients

For this prospective observational study, we initially recruited a total of 603 patients who consecutively started maintenance HD at Yonsei University Health System, Seoul, Korea, between January 2006 and December 2008 and were regularly followed-up at the outpatient clinic. Echocardiography was not performed in 35 patients due to noncompliance or other personal reasons, and in 44 patients it was undergone before the initiation of HD. Of these patients, 207 patients were also excluded for the following reasons: age <18 years (n = 4) or >75 years (n = 11), previous history of peritoneal dialysis or kidney transplantation before HD (n = 139), severe systolic dysfunction (ejection fraction <30%, n = 7), severe valvular heart disease (n = 11), underlying malignancy (n = 21), decompensated liver cirrhosis (n = 3), complete bundle branch block (n = 9), and pacemaker insertion (n = 2). Thus, a total of 317 patients were included in the final analysis.

Data collection

Demographic and clinical data at the time of HD initiation, including age, gender, and comorbidities, were recorded. The results of the following laboratory tests performed at the same time were also collected: hemoglobin, serum albumin, total cholesterol, calcium, phosphate, and high-sensitivity C-reactive protein levels. The single-pool Kt/V in HD patients was measured with standard Gotch equations on the mid-dialysis day near at the time of discharge [25].

ECG

Upon admission, a standard 12-lead electrocardiogram was recorded using a MAC 5500 machine (GE Medical system, Milwaukee, WI, USA). All of the patients underwent an additional ECG on a nondialysis day, within 24 hours after the last HD and near the time of discharge, and this follow-up ECG was used for analysis. The output from the MAC 5500 provided QRS duration, PR interval, QT interval, and axes in an automated fashion, but not QRS voltage of every lead. Thus, two independent technicians measured the voltage and discrepancies of >2 mm were resolved by a third reader. The cut-off point for LVH by Sokolow-Lyon voltage (RV5/6+SV1) was ≥35 mm and by Cornell voltage (RaVL+SV3) was ≥28 mm in men and ≥20 mm in women [21].

Products of QRS duration multiplied by the Cornell voltage combination (with 6 mm added in women) ≥2440 mm•msec and by the Sokolow-Lyon voltage combination ≥3674 mm•msec in men and ≥3224 mm•msec in women were used to determine LVH [22]. The QTc interval was calculated based on Bazett's formula: QTc interval = $QT/\sqrt{RR}$, and the following criteria were used to determine QTc interval prolongation: QTc≥460 msec in women; QTc≥450 msec in men [26].

Echocardiography

Echocardiography was performed at the time of follow-up ECG based on the imaging protocol recommended by the American Society of Echocardiography using a SONOS 7500 (Philips Ultrasound, Bothell, WA, USA). LV systolic function was defined by LV ejection fraction (LVEF) using a modified biplane Simpson's method from the apical two- and four-chamber views. LV mass (LVM) was determined using the method described by Devereux and Reichek [27], and LV mass index (LVMI) was calculated by dividing LVM by body surface area (BSA). Echocardiographic LVH was defined as a LVMI>131 g/m^2 for men and >100 g/m^2 for women [28]. Hypertrophy was considered concentric if LV relative wall thickness was >0.43, and patients with normal LV mass were considered to have normal LV geometry if relative wall thickness was ≤0.43 or to have concentric remodeling if relative wall thickness was increased [23]. Left atrial volume was assessed by the biplane area-length method from the apical two- and four-chamber views and was indexed for BSA. Mitral inflow was assessed with Doppler echocardiography from the apical four-chamber view, and pulse-wave tissue Doppler imaging of the septal mitral annulus was also obtained from the apical four-chamber view. Systolic RV pressure was calculated using the modified Bernoulli equation [4×(tricuspid systolic jet)^2+10 mmHg].

Outcome measures

All the patients included in this study were followed-up every 3 months at the outpatient clinic, and all deaths and hospitalizations were recorded in the serious adverse events database. For this study, the mortality events were retrieved from the database and carefully reviewed. Cardiovascular mortality, the primary study endpoint, was considered to be death from myocardial infarction or ischemia, congestive heart failure, pulmonary edema, and cerebral hemorrhage or vascular disorder.

Statistical analysis

Statistical analysis was performed using SPSS version 18.0 (SPSS Inc, Chicago, IL, USA). Continuous variables were expressed as mean ± SD, and categorical variables as percentages. To determine differences between the two groups, Student's t-test or Mann-Whitney U test was used for continuous variables and the chi-square test was used for categorical variables. Pearson's correlation analysis was performed to estimate the association between LVMI and ECG criteria measurements. Cumulative survival curves were generated by the Kaplan-Meier method, and between-group survival was compared by a log-rank test. The independent prognostic values of electrocardiographic and echocardiographic LVH for cardiovascular mortality were ascertained by Cox proportional hazards regression analysis, which included only the significant variables in univariate analysis. Factors of specific interest were also included in another multivariate analysis. However, each ECG-LVH or echocardiographic criterion was entered separately because there was a

Table 1. Clinical and biochemical characteristics according to the presence or absence of electrocardiographic LVH.

	Sokolow-Lyon voltage LVH			Sokolow-Lyon product LVH			Cornell voltage LVH			Cornell product LVH		
	No (n = 257)	Yes (n = 60)	P	No (n = 274)	Yes (n = 43)	P	No (n = 279)	Yes (n = 38)	P	No (n = 274)	Yes (n = 43)	P
Age (years)	56.4±14.3	58.3±13.8	0.36	56.0±14.2	61.5±13.0	0.018	56.6±14.4	58.0±12.1	0.57	56.5±14.4	58.4±12.6	0.42
Male gender	130 (51%)	40 (67%)	0.024	144 (53%)	26 (61%)	0.33	152 (54%)	22 (58%)	0.40	144 (53%)	26 (61%)	0.33
Diabetes	143 (56%)	31 (52%)	0.58	149 (54%)	25 (58%)	0.65	151 (54%)	23 (61%)	0.46	148 (54%)	26 (61%)	0.43
Hypertension	227 (88%)	54 (90%)	0.71	239 (87%)	42 (98%)	0.045	245 (88%)	36 (95%)	0.21	240 (88%)	41 (95%)	0.14
Coronary artery disease	39 (15%)	15 (25%)	0.07	44 (16%)	10 (23%)	0.24	46 (17%)	8 (21%)	0.48	41 (15%)	13 (30%)	0.01
History of smoking	36 (14%)	12 (20%)	0.24	40 (15%)	8 (19%)	0.50	43 (15%)	5 (13%)	0.72	40 (15%)	8 (19%)	0.50
Primary renal disease			0.54			0.77			0.88			0.52
Diabetes	143 (56%)	30 (50%)		149 (54%)	24 (56%)		150 (54%)	23 (61%)		147 (54%)	26 (61%)	
Glomerulonephritis	24 (9%)	4 (7%)		26 (10%)	2 (5%)		25 (9%)	3 (8%)		24 (9%)	4 (9%)	
ADPKD	7 (3%)	1 (2%)		7 (3%)	1 (2%)		7 (3%)	1 (3%)		6 (2%)	2 (5%)	
Others	83 (32%)	25 (42%)		92 (34%)	16 (37%)		97 (35%)	11 (29%)		97 (35%)	11 (26%)	
Body mass index (kg/m^2)	23.8±3.4	22.5±3.1	0.008	23.7±3.4	22.8±3.2	0.11	23.7±3.5	22.8±2.5	0.12	23.6±3.4	22.9±3.4	0.20
MBP (mmHg)	99.0±14.2	100.5±14.4	0.48	99.1±14.3	100.8±13.9	0.47	98.8±14.0	103.2±15.3	0.08	99.3±14.1	99.4±14.9	0.97
Heart rate (bpm)	73.5±13.5	75.0±13.5	0.44	74.1±13.6	72.4±12.8	0.46	73.7±13.7	75.0±12.6	0.58	74.1±13.4	72.3±14.1	0.42
Blood urea nitrogen (mg/dl)	93.7±32.1	93.4±28.8	0.95	93.3±31.2	95.7±33.3	0.64	94.3±32.2	88.9±25.8	0.32	93.1±31.4	97.2±32.3	0.42
Creatinine (mg/dl)	9.8±4.7	9.9±4.2	0.86	9.8±4.6	9.7±4.3	0.92	9.9±4.7	9.1±3.5	0.32	9.7±4.7	10.2±4.1	0.55
eGFR (ml/min/1.73 m^2)	6.5±3.0	6.3±2.4	0.71	6.5±3.0	6.3±2.5	0.73	6.5±2.9	6.4±2.7	0.82	6.5±3.0	6.1±2.6	0.37
Calcium (mg/dl)	7.8±1.1	8.0±1.1	0.18	7.8±1.1	8.0±1.1	0.18	7.8±1.1	8.1±0.9	0.07	7.8±1.1	7.9±1.2	0.56
Phosphate (mg/dl)	6.2±1.9	6.3±1.7	0.85	6.2±1.9	6.3±1.8	0.78	6.2±1.9	6.1±1.9	0.80	6.2±1.8	6.5±2.1	0.32
Albumin (g/dl)	3.5±0.7	3.6±0.6	0.33	3.5±0.7	3.6±0.5	0.33	3.5±0.7	3.4±0.6	0.26	3.5±0.7	3.5±0.6	0.95
Cholesterol (mg/dl)	161.9±50.0	155.3±41.2	0.34	161.3±49.3	157.0±43.1	0.60	159.0±48.2	173.0±48.8	0.10	160.1±49.0	164.2±45.1	0.61
Hemoglobin (g/dl)	8.4±1.6	8.6±1.3	0.56	8.4±1.6	8.7±1.4	0.34	8.4±1.6	8.8±1.5	0.16	8.4±1.6	8.6±1.6	0.55
C-reactive protein (mg/l)	0.8±0.9	1.1±1.5	0.18	0.8±1.1	0.8±1.0	0.91	0.8±1.1	0.8±0.9	0.88	0.8±1.1	1.0±1.2	0.40
Single-pool Kt/V	1.3±0.3	1.2±0.3	0.76	1.1±0.4	1.2±0.3	0.79	1.2±0.4	1.3±0.3	0.71	1.2±0.3	1.3±0.3	0.81
No of antihypertensive drugs	2.1±1.2	2.2±1.2	0.55	2.1±1.2	2.1±1.1	0.89	2.1±1.2	2.4±1.1	0.13	2.1±1.2	2.2±1.0	0.79
Antihypertensive drugs												
β-blockers	144 (56%)	30 (50%)	0.40	151 (55%)	23 (54%)	0.84	152 (55%)	22 (58%)	0.69	152 (56%)	22 (51%)	0.60
ACE inhibitors or ARBs	148 (58%)	39 (65%)	0.29	160 (58%)	27 (63%)	0.59	158 (57%)	29 (76%)	0.02	159 (58%)	28 (65%)	0.38
Calcium channel blockers	191 (74%)	47 (78%)	0.52	205 (75%)	33 (77%)	0.79	206 (74%)	32 (84%)	0.17	203 (74%)	35 (81%)	0.30
Statin use	74 (29%)	17 (28%)	0.94	74 (27%)	17 (40%)	0.09	77 (28%)	14 (37%)	0.24	72 (26%)	19 (44%)	0.02
Coronary revasculization	31 (12%)	16 (27%)	0.004	31 (11%)	16 (37%)	<0.001	37 (13%)	10 (26%)	0.03	33 (12%)	14 (33%)	<0.001
Stroke	16 (6%)	7 (12%)	0.14	20 (7%)	3 (7%)	0.94	19 (7%)	4 (11%)	0.41	19 (7%)	4 (9%)	0.58

ADPKD, autosomal dominant polycystic kidney disease; MBP, mean arterial blood pressure; BPM, beat per minute; eGFR, estimated glomerular filtration rate; No, number; ACE, angiotensin converting enzyme; ARB, angiotensin II receptor blocker; LVH, left ventricular hypertrophy.
Data are presented as n (%) or mean ± SD.

significant interaction with each other. The hazard ratios (HRs) and 95% confidence intervals (CIs) were calculated using the estimated regression coefficients and standard errors. The positive predictive values for echocardiographic LVH and cardiovascular mortality were also analyzed by receiver operating characteristic (ROC) curve analysis with calculated area under the ROC curve (AUC). The correlation coefficients between LVMI and each ECG criterion measurements and the AUC of each ECG-LVH criterion for echocardiographic LVH and cardiovascular mortality were compared using a two-tailed Z-score. P-values less than 0.05 were considered statistically significant.

Results

Clinical and biochemical characteristics

The baseline patient characteristics according to the presence ECG-LVH are shown in Table 1. The mean age was 56.7±14.2 years (range: 18–75 years), and 53.6% were male. Of the 317 patients, LVH was present in 60 patients (18.9%) by Sokolow-Lyon voltage (SV), 43 (13.6%) by Sokolow-Lyon voltage-duration product (SP), 38 (12.0%) by Cornell voltage (CV), and 43 (13.6%) by Cornell voltage-duration product (CP) criteria. The proportion of male patients was significantly higher in the ECG-LVH group

Table 2. Echocardiographic and electrocardiographic parameters according to the presence or absence of echocardiographic LVH.

	Sokolow-Lyon voltage LVH			Sokolow-Lyon product LVH			Cornell voltage LVH			Cornell product LVH		
	No (n=257)	Yes (n=60)	P	No (n=274)	Yes (n=43)	P	No (n=279)	Yes (n=38)	P	No (n=274)	Yes (n=43)	P
Echocardiography												
Ejection fraction (%)	62.2±10.1	57.8±10.5	0.003	62.0±10.0	57.0±11.6	0.003	61.8±10.0	58.4±12.1	0.05	62.3±9.7	55.7±12.1	0.001
LVEDD (mm)	51.5±5.2	53.5±5.5	0.011	51.5±5.0	54.4±6.3	0.001	51.8±5.0	52.9±7.2	0.34	51.5±5.0	54.3±6.7	0.01
IVS thickness (mm)	10.7±1.8	11.6±1.7	<0.001	10.8±1.8	11.7±1.6	0.001	10.8±1.7	11.9±2.2	<0.001	10.7±1.7	12.0±2.1	<0.001
PW thickness (mm)	10.6±1.6	11.5±1.6	0.001	10.7±1.7	11.5±1.5	0.004	10.7±1.6	11.7±1.6	0.001	10.6±1.6	11.8±1.4	<0.001
LV mass index (g/m²)	127.3±27.7	145.0±26.3	<0.001	127.7±27.2	149.7±27.9	<0.001	128.1±27.5	149.5±26.9	<0.001	127.2±27.0	152.6±26.7	<0.001
LA volume index (ml/m²)	34.6±12.2	40.8±12.7	<0.001	34.6±12.0	43.6±13.0	<0.001	35.2±12.4	39.8±12.5	0.032	34.9±12.2	41.2±13.0	0.002
RV pressure (mmHg)	31.7±10.6	33.4±11.2	0.28	31.7±10.4	34.0±12.2	0.22	31.8±10.8	33.8±10.1	0.31	31.6±10.4	34.5±12.1	0.12
E/E'ratio	16.6±7.1	18.1±8.0	0.17	16.5±6.9	19.6±9.1	0.046	16.3±6.9	21.1±8.1	<0.001	16.4±6.7	19.8±9.6	0.033
Echocardiographic LVH	169 (54%)	49 (60%)	0.017	181 (53%)	37 (65%)	0.009	184 (53%)	34 (69%)	0.003	181 (53%)	37 (70%)	0.009
Relative wall thickness	0.42±0.08	0.43±0.07	0.18	0.42±0.08	0.43±0.07	0.59	0.42±0.07	0.45±0.10	0.12	0.42±0.08	0.44±0.08	0.05
Concentric remodeling/LVH	105 (41%)	31 (52%)	0.13	113 (41%)	23 (53%)	0.13	113 (41%)	23 (61%)	0.019	112 (41%)	24 (56%)	0.07
Electrocardiography												
PR interval (msec)	168.5±30.6	163.8±25.4	0.28	167.4±30.1	169.2±27.3	0.73	168.7±30.1	160.3±25.6	0.11	167.0±28.9	171.9±34.3	0.33
QRS duration (msec)	93.0±14.7	94.0±11.2	0.63	91.4±11.9	104.7±20.4	<0.001	93.0±14.2	94.6±13.2	0.50	91.3±13.4	105.1±12.6	<0.001
QTc interval (msec)	458.0±35.6	467.0±40.8	0.12	457.3±35.7	475.1±39.7	0.003	458.8±35.2	466.6±46.1	0.22	457.1±33.3	476.5±50.9	0.019
ST-T abnormalities	17 (7%)	13 (22%)	<0.001	16 (6%)	14 (33%)	<0.001	15 (5%)	15 (40%)	<0.001	12 (4%)	18 (42%)	<0.001
Sokolow-Lyon voltage (mm)	23.8±6.3	41.3±5.4	<0.001	24.8±7.1	42.0±6.8	<0.001	26.3±8.6	33.3±11.0	0.001	26.0±8.5	34.3±10.6	<0.001
Sokolow-Lyon voltage LVH	-	-	-	24 (9%)	36 (84%)	<0.001	42 (15%)	18 (47%)	<0.001	40 (15%)	20 (47%)	<0.001
Sokolow-Lyon product	2225±743	3888±759	<0.001	2260±694	4322±695	<0.001	2450±914	3194±1264	0.001	2376±862	3583±1121	<0.001
Sokolow-Lyon product LVH	7 (3%)	36 (60%)	<0.001	-	-	-	28 (10%)	15 (40%)	<0.001	23 (8%)	20 (47%)	<0.001
Cornell voltage (mm)	15.0±5.5	21.9±7.1	<0.001	15.4±5.6	21.6±8.5	<0.001	14.8±5.1	26.9±5.2	<0.001	14.6±4.8	26.8±5.3	<0.001
Cornell voltage LVH	20 (8%)	18 (30%)	<0.001	23 (8%)	15 (35%)	<0.001	-	-	-	13 (5%)	25 (58%)	<0.001
Cornell product	1660±553	2270±848	<0.001	1668±531	2458±960	<0.001	1618±480	2931±679	<0.001	1577±423	3036±510	<0.001
Cornell product LVH	23 (9%)	20 (33%)	<0.001	23 (8%)	20 (47%)	<0.001	18 (7%)	25 (66%)	<0.001	-	-	-

LV, left ventricle; IVS, interventricular septum; PW, posterior wall; LA, left atrium; RV, right ventricle; E/E', ratio of early mitral inflow velocity to peak mitral annulus velocity; LVH, left ventricular hypertrophy.
Data are presented as mean ± SD.

by SV criteria, whereas the proportion of patients with hypertension was significantly higher in the ECG-LVH group by SP criteria (P<0.05). In addition, there was a significant difference in body mass index (BMI) between patients with and without ECG-LVH only by SV criteria (22.5±3.1 vs. 23.8±3.4 kg/m², P=0.008). Moreover, patients with ECG-LVH by CP criteria showed a significantly higher prevalence of coronary artery disease (P<0.05). A history of coronary revascularization was significantly more prevalent in patients with ECG-LVH by each criterion than in those without ECG-LVH (P<0.05). Blood urea nitrogen, creatinine, albumin, and cholesterol concentrations and Kt/V were also comparable between patients with and without ECG-LVH by each criterion.

Echocardiographic and electrocardiographic findings

As shown in Table 2, LV mass index (LVMI) and left atrial volume index were significantly higher, while LV ejection fraction was significantly lower in patients with LVH by each criterion compared to those without ECG-LVH. In addition, the early mitral inflow velocity to peak mitral annulus velocity (E/E') ratio was significantly higher only in patients with ECG-LVH by QRS

voltage-duration product criteria. On the other hand, QT interval was significantly prolonged in patients with ECG-LVH based on SP and CP criteria than in those without ECG-LVH by these criteria.

Pearson's correlation analysis revealed that SP (r=0.357, P<0.001) and CP (r=0.410, P<0.001) criteria seemed to correlate more closely with LVMI compared to SV (r=0.319, P<0.001) and CV (r=0.388, P<0.001) criteria, respectively, but the differences did not reach statistical significance (SP vs. SV, Z statistic=0.542, P=0.59; CP vs. CV, Z statistic=0.172, P=0.86) (Figure 1). The positive predictive values of SP (86.0%) and CP (89.5%) for echocardiographic LVH were also higher relative to those of SV (81.7%) and CV (86.0%). Among the four ECG criteria, moreover, the CP criteria provided the highest predictive value for echocardiographic LVH in ROC curve analysis (AUC=0.657, P<0.001) (Figure 2). Furthermore, the AUC of the CP criteria was significantly greater than those of the other three ECG-LVH criteria (CP vs. CV, Z statistic=4.793, P<0.001; CP vs. SP, Z statistic=2.707, P=0.007; CP vs. SV, Z statistic=2.146, P=0.032).

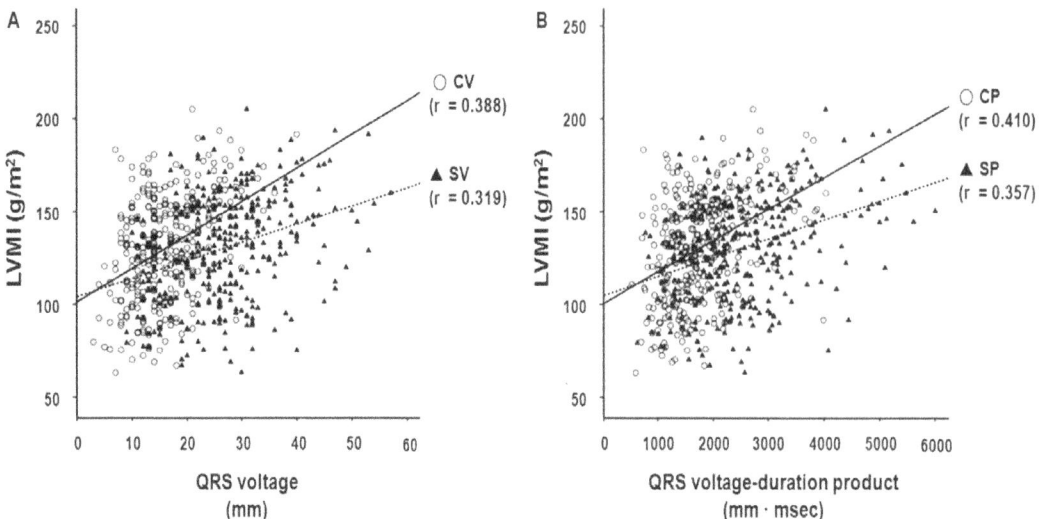

Figure 1. Correlation between electrocardiographic LVH and left ventricular mass index (LVMI). (A) Sokolow-Lyon voltage (SV), Cornell voltage (CV), (B) Sokolow-Lyon voltage-duration product (SP), and Cornell voltage-duration product (CP) correlated significantly with LVMI. Data are correlation coefficients (r).

Clinical outcomes

During the mean follow-up duration of 27.4±17.2 months (3.0–64.0 months), 41 patients (12.9%) died over 725 patient-years of cumulative follow-up, yielding a crude mortality rate of 5.66/100 patient-years. Among them, 25 patients (7.9%) died from cardiovascular causes. Patients with echocardiographic LVH had a significantly lower cardiovascular mortality-free survival than those without echocardiographic LVH (72.2% vs. 98.0%, P = 0.003). In addition, the 5-year cardiovascular survival rates

were significantly lower in patients with ECG-LVH by SV (60.7% vs. 88.1%, P = 0.026), SP (50.6% vs. 87.6%, P = 0.001), CV (56.2% vs. 87.0%, P = 0.017), and CP criteria (55.7% vs. 87.7%, P = 0.001) (Figure 3). Moreover, patients with ST-T wave abnormalities secondary to LVH, including a horizontal or downsloping ST segment and T wave inversion, showed significantly lower cardiovascular survival rates compared to those without these findings (39.5% vs. 87.3%, P = 0.005). However, there was no significant difference in cardiovascular mortality between patients with concentric and eccentric LVH and between patients with and without QTc interval prolongation. The overall mortality was also comparable between patients with and without echocardiographic LVH or ECG-LVH.

Table 3 shows the hazard ratios (HRs) for cardiovascular mortality according to the presence of echocardiographic or electrocardiographic LVH. In an unadjusted Cox regression model, there was a significant increased risk for cardiovascular mortality in patients with echocardiographic LVH and ECG-LVH by each criterion. In multivariate analysis adjusted for age, diabetes, and coronary artery disease, which were revealed as significant independent predictors of cardiovascular mortality in univariate analysis, echocardiographic LVH and ECG-LVH based on QRS voltage-duration product were still significantly associated with cardiovascular mortality, but the significant association between ECG-LVH by purely voltage-based criteria and cardiovascular mortality in the unadjusted model disappeared (Model 1). Moreover, even when factors of specific interest, such as ejection fraction, ST-T wave changes, and QTc interval, were included in a multivariate model, echocardiographic LVH (HR: 11.71; 95% CI: 1.57–87.18; P = 0.016) and ECG-LVH by SP (HR: 3.43; 95% CI: 1.32–8.92; P = 0.011) and CP (HR: 3.07; 95% CI: 1.16–8.11; P = 0.024) criteria, but not SV and CV criteria, were significantly associated with cardiovascular mortality (Model 2). In ROC curve analysis, CP criteria provided the highest predictive value for cardiovascular mortality (AUC = 0.720, P<0.001), but there were no statistical differences in the AUC among the four ECG-LVH criteria (Figure 4).

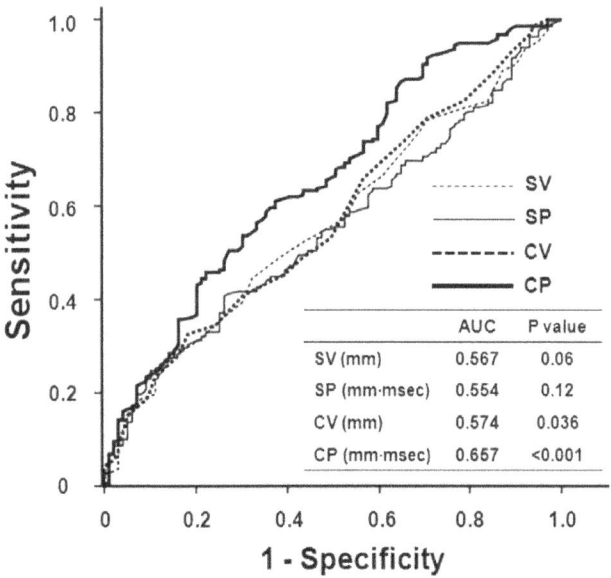

Figure 2. ROC curve analysis for echocardiographic LVH. The ROC curve was constructed by plotting the sensitivity (true positive rate) vs. 1-specificity (false positive rate) for each ECG-LVH criterion. At the highest predicted probability, sensitivities of Sokolow-Lyon voltage (SV), Sokolow-Lyon voltage-duration product (SP), Cornell voltage (CV), and Cornell voltage-duration product (CP) were 27.1%, 40.8%, 32.6%, and 45.9%, respectively.

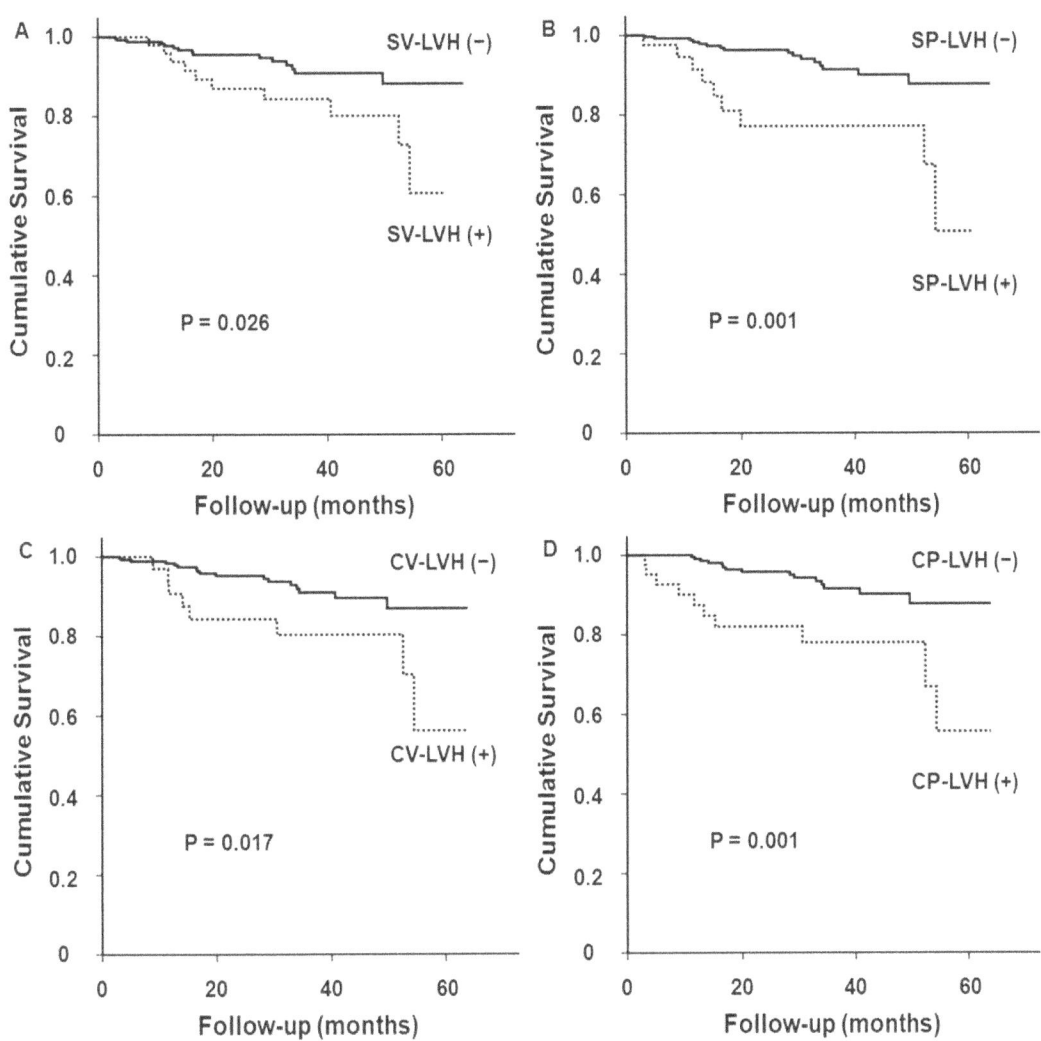

Figure 3. Kaplan-Meier curves for cardiovascular survival. Compared to patients without electrocardiographic LVH, the 5-year cardiovascular survival rates were significantly lower in patients with electrocardiographic LVH based on (A) Sokolow-Lyon voltage (SV), (B) Sokolow-Lyon voltage-duration product (SP), (C) Cornell voltage (CV), and (D) Cornell voltage-duration product criteria (CP).

Discussion

In ESRD patients, LVH detected by ECG or echocardiography is the most common manifestation of cardiovascular disease and strongly predicts cardiovascular morbidity and mortality [2,3,7–9]. In this study, we demonstrate that SP and CP criteria correlated more closely with LVMI determined by echocardiography compared to SV and CV criteria, respectively, and that CP criteria provide the highest predictive value for identification of LVH. In addition, LVH based on QRS voltage-duration product is an independent predictor of cardiovascular mortality in incident HD patients, whereas LVH by QRS voltage-based criteria is not.

Prevalence of LVH

LVH is prevalent in patients with CKD and its prevalence is known to increase as eGFR decreases [4,5,29,30]. However, previous studies show wide variation in the prevalence of LVH in CKD and ESRD patients. A very recent study revealed that the prevalence of ECG-LVH by the Sokolow-Lyon criteria was 10% and by Cornell criteria was 14% in patients with CKD [24]. However, in a Spanish multicenter study on hypertensive patients,

more than 20% of the subjects with CKD had ECG-LVH by Cornell criteria [22]. Meanwhile, Foley et al. demonstrated that LVH by echocardiography was present in 74% of ESRD patients at the start of dialysis [4], whereas Levin et al. found the overall prevalence of echocardiographic LVH to be 36% of ESRD patients [5]. In the 4D study, even though all patients were ESRD patients on hemodialysis and had type 2 diabetes, only 12.4% had EKG-LVH by Sokolow-Lyon criteria [31]. The results of the present study also revealed wide variation in the prevalence of LVH: 18.9% by SV, 13.6% by SP, 12.0% by CV, 13.6% by CP criteria, and 68.8% by echocardiography. We surmise that these discrepancies in the prevalence of LVH can be attributed to differences in patient age, gender, ethnicity, BMI, hemoglobin levels, and residual renal function and the proportion of patients with hypertension. Particularly, obesity has been shown to decrease the sensitivity of precordial lead ECG criteria, especially SV criteria, for the identification of LVH because QRS amplitudes are attenuated by interposed tissue, which increases the distance of exploring electrodes from LV [32]. In our study, the prevalence of ECG-LVH by SV criteria might in part be influenced by a relatively low BMI of the subjects, and the

Table 3. Cox regression models for cardiovascular mortality.

	unadjusted		Model 1		Model 2	
	HR (95% CI)	P-value	HR (95% CI)	P-value	HR (95% CI)	P-value
Echocardiographic LVH	10.88 (1.47–80.43)	0.019	9.11 (1.22–67.82)	0.031	11.71 (1.57–87.18)	0.016
Sokolow-Lyon voltage LVH	2.42 (1.08–5.42)	0.031	1.68 (0.71–3.97)	0.24	2.00 (0.86–4.68)	0.11
Sokolow-Lyon product LVH	3.75 (1.64–8.53)	0.002	2.80 (1.19–6.54)	0.018	3.43 (1.32–8.92)	0.011
Cornell voltage LVH	2.70 (1.16–6.31)	0.022	2.25 (0.95–5.30)	0.06	1.84 (0.68–4.97)	0.23
Cornell product LVH	3.69 (1.65–8.25)	0.001	2.64 (1.14–6.13)	0.024	3.07 (1.16–8.11)	0.024

Data are reported as hazard ratio (HR) and 95% confidence interval (CI).
Model 1: Adjusted for age, diabetes, and coronary artery disease.
Model 2: Adjusted for ejection fraction, ST-T wave abnormalities, and QTc interval.

accuracy of SV criteria might be lessened because they were not gender-based. Whether LVH was assessed by echocardiography or ECG and which ECG criteria were used to define LVH may contribute to this wide variation in the prevalence of LVH.

LVH and cardiovascular outcomes

Mounting evidence indicates that LVH is a powerful independent predictor of cardiovascular mortality in patients with CKD and ESRD [9]. Moreover, the change in LVH has been demonstrated as a strong prognostic factor in these patients. A previous prospective study on prevalent HD patients revealed that the rates of LVMI increase were significantly higher in patients with incident cardiovascular events than in those without such events, and that cardiovascular event-free survival in patients with changes in LVMI below the 25th percentile was significantly higher than in those with changes above the 75th percentile [8]. Similarly, in a cohort study of 153 incident ESRD patients

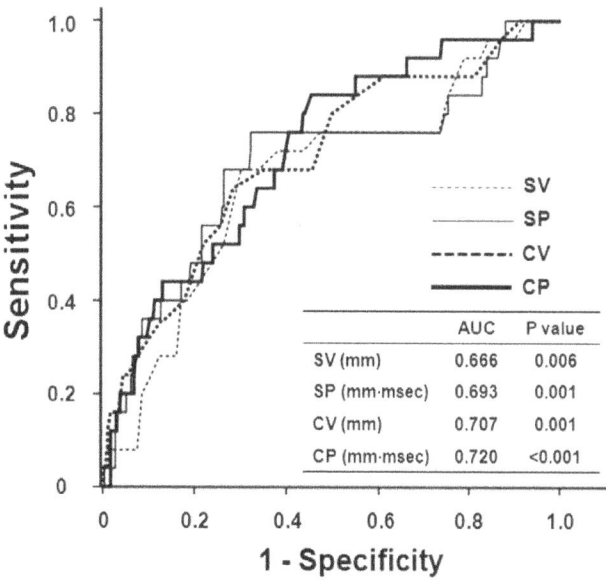

Figure 4. ROC curve analysis for cardiovascular mortality. The ROC curve was constructed by plotting the sensitivity (true positive rate) vs. 1-specificity (false positive rate) for each ECG-LVH criterion. At the highest predicted probability, sensitivities of Sokolow-Lyon voltage (SV), Sokolow-Lyon voltage-duration product (SP), Cornell voltage (CV), and Cornell voltage-duration product (CP) were 68.1%, 72.3%, 64.2%, and 76.0%, respectively.

receiving HD, a 10% reduction in LVM during a mean follow-up duration of 54 months resulted in a 22% decrease in all-cause mortality and a 28% decrease in cardiovascular mortality [7]. Furthermore, in that study, LVM regression was independently associated with improved patient survival even after adjustment for age, gender, diabetes, history of cardiovascular disease, and all nonspecific cardiovascular risk factors. While these two studies used echocardiography to assess LVMI or LVM as an indicator of LVH, similar results were observed in hypertensive patients with ECG-LVH [33,34]. With a median interval of 23 days, persistent ECG-LVH at baseline and follow-up identified patients with greater LVM and a higher prevalence of echocardiographic LVH, suggesting that these patients may be at higher risk for subsequent morbidity and mortality [23]. We did not clarify the impact of the changes in LVM or LVMI by echocardiography, newly developed ECG-LVH, and the regression or persistence of ECG-LVH on patients' outcome. Nevertheless, consistent with most previous studies, the baseline echocardiographic LVH at the time of HD initiation was found to be significantly associated with worse cardiovascular survival in incident ESRD patients.

ECG for the detection of LVH

ECG is a simple tool for the detection of LVH and is widely used in clinical setting [19]. According to the Kidney Disease Outcome Quality Initiative (K/DOQI) practice guidelines, recording of an ECG is recommended in every patient at the initiation of renal replacement therapy and yearly thereafter [35]. Due to the relatively low sensitivity of traditional ECG criteria for the detection of LVH, however, the clinical utility of ECG is limited [20]. On the other hand, prolongation of QRS duration is often observed in patients with LVH [36]. In addition, QRS duration was demonstrated to correlate with LVM [21]. Even though the mechanism for QRS prolongation in LVH has not been clearly determined, it may be related to a longer time required to activate myocardium, decreased conduction velocity in hypertrophic myocardium, and changes in activation sequence or in the relative conductivity of fibrotic intracellular and extracellular spaces [21]. In fact, the VIPE study, which evaluated the effect of candesartan-based treatment on LVH in hypertensive patients, demonstrated that candesartan treatment for 6 months not only reduced LVM, but also shortened the QRS duration [37]. Nevertheless, QRS duration alone has been proven to be poorly sensitive at clinically relevant levels of specificity [36]. For these reasons, there have been many attempts to increase the sensitivity of ECG for the identification of LVH by combining the voltage criteria with QRS duration, and these efforts have modestly improved the performance of ECG for detecting LVH in the general population and hypertensive patients [22]. However, most previous studies on CKD or ESRD patients used voltage criteria to determine ECG-LVH and did not validate ECG-LVH criteria for clinical outcomes [31]. Moreover, few studies have explored the relationship between electrocardiographic and echocardiographic LVH. In this study, we tried to elucidate the correlation between commonly used criteria of ECG-LVH and echocardiographic LVH, and found that SP and CP criteria correlated more closely with LVMI determined by echocardiography than SV and CV criteria, respectively and that CP criteria provided the highest predictive value for echocardiographic LVH. Furthermore, besides echocardiographic LVH, ECG-LVH only by SP and CP criteria was an independent risk factor for cardiovascular mortality in incident HD patients. These findings suggest that the considering QRS duration in addition to voltage may not only improve the identification of LVH but also serve as a more significant predictor of cardiovascular outcome in ESRD patients.

Echocardiography for the detection of LVH

Echocardiography is a noninvasive procedure and provides an accurate assessment of ventricular size, geometry, and function. However, in ESRD patients, echocardiographic measurements, particularly of LVM, are highly dependent on the timing of echocardiography in relationship to dialysis sessions and to intravascular volume [38]. In addition, compared to MRI, echocardiography is known to significantly overestimate LVM in HD patients when LVH and dilation are present [17]. Moreover, the intra-observer and inter-observer variability of echocardiography are significantly higher than those of MRI. Nevertheless, MRI is not routinely performed because it is not widely available, is expensive, and cannot be used in patients with cardiac implantable devices. Consistent with most clinical and research studies, we used LVMI by echocardiography to determine LVH. Furthermore, since the ability to detect LVH in HD patients is improved by performing echocardiography on a nondialysis day, preferably between 12 and 18 hours after the last dialysis session, patients included in the present study underwent echocardiography on a nondialysis day, within 24 hours after the last dialysis, and near the time of discharge to minimize the volume effect on echocardiographic parameters.

Limitations

Our study has several limitations. First, since the study subjects were all Korean ESRD patients on HD, the association between

EKG-LVH criteria and clinical outcomes may not be generalizable to other populations. In addition, even though the number of patients was small (18 patients), patients with severe systolic dysfunction and severe valvular heart disease were excluded in this study because we inferred that these cardiac conditions *per se* could not only strongly affect the patient survival but also influence QRS voltage and duration. Nevertheless, we could not completely affirm that there was no selection bias. Second, the 5-year mortality rates in the present study were relatively lower compared to those of previous studies on Western ESRD patients [8,30,31], but they were comparable to those of Japanese patients on HD [29]. Moreover, a small number of events limited the power of the statistical analysis in identifying independent predictors of cardiovascular mortality. Therefore, only 3 factors could be evaluated at a time in the multivariate analysis to maintain the statistical power. Third, we analyzed only the ECG taken at the time of echocardiography. Thus, the possibility of intra-individual variability could not be completely excluded. However, the lower day-to-day variability that has been demonstrated for the measurement of QRS duration could enhance the general use of voltage-duration product criteria to lessen the influence of day-to-day variability [39]. Fourth, LVMI by echocardiography was regarded as the differentiating indicator of LVH in this study. As mentioned earlier, even though MRI is considered to be the "gold standard" technique for the assessment of LVM [17], we were unable to routinely perform MRI in all incident ESRD patients mainly due to its cost. Finally, follow-up ECG and echocardiography were not included for analysis in the present study. It would be worthwhile to investigate the impact of changes in ECG-LVH by different criteria on patient outcomes.

Conclusions

This study shows that ECG-LVH based on QRS voltage-duration product predicts adverse cardiovascular outcomes better than ECG-LVH by QRS voltage-based criteria in incident HD patients. Our findings suggest that standard ECG itself may be of help in risk stratification and in providing therapeutic direction for the management of these patients.

Author Contributions

Analyzed the data: HJO DEY. Wrote the paper: SJK SWK. Carried out data collection: DHS MJL HRK JTP. Participated in the interpretation of data: SHH THY KHC.

References

1. Foley RN, Parfrey PS, Sarnak MJ (1998) Clinical epidemiology of cardiovascular disease in chronic renal disease. Am J Kidney Dis 32: S112–119.
2. Middleton RJ, Parfrey PS, Foley RN (2001) Left ventricular hypertrophy in the renal patient. J Am Soc Nephrol 12: 1079–1084.
3. Levin A, Djurdjev O, Thompson C, Barrett B, Ethier J, et al. (2005) Canadian randomized trial of hemoglobin maintenance to prevent or delay left ventricular mass growth in patients with CKD. Am J Kidney Dis 46: 799–811.
4. Foley RN, Parfrey PS, Harnett JD, Kent GM, Martin CJ, et al. (1995) Clinical and echocardiographic disease in patients starting end-stage renal disease therapy. Kidney Int 47: 186–192.
5. Levin A, Thompson CR, Ethier J, Carlisle EJ, Tobe S, et al. (1999) Left ventricular mass index increase in early renal disease: impact of decline in hemoglobin. Am J Kidney Dis 34: 125–134.
6. Silberberg JS, Barre PE, Prichard SS, Sniderman AD (1989) Impact of left ventricular hypertrophy on survival in end-stage renal disease. Kidney Int 36: 286–290.
7. London GM, Pannier B, Guerin AP, Blacher J, Marchais SJ, et al. (2001) Alterations of left ventricular hypertrophy in and survival of patients receiving hemodialysis: follow-up of an interventional study. J Am Soc Nephrol 12: 2759–2767.
8. Zoccali C, Benedetto FA, Mallamaci F, Tripepi G, Giacone G, et al. (2004) Left ventricular mass monitoring in the follow-up of dialysis patients: prognostic value of left ventricular hypertrophy progression. Kidney Int 65: 1492–1498.
9. Shlipak MG, Fried LF, Cushman M, Manolio TA, Peterson D, et al. (2005) Cardiovascular mortality risk in chronic kidney disease: comparison of traditional and novel risk factors. JAMA 293: 1737–1745.
10. Glassock RJ, Pecoits-Filho R, Barberato SH (2009) Left ventricular mass in chronic kidney disease and ESRD. Clin J Am Soc Nephrol 4 Suppl 1: S79–91.
11. Naito Y, Tsujino T, Matsumoto M, Sakoda T, Ohyanagi M, et al. (2009) Adaptive response of the heart to long-term anemia induced by iron deficiency. Am J Physiol Heart Circ Physiol 296: H585–593.
12. Martin LC, Franco RJ, Gavras I, Matsubara BB, Garcia S, et al. (2004) Association between hypervolemia and ventricular hypertrophy in hemodialysis patients. Am J Hypertens 17: 1163–1169.
13. MacRae JM, Levin A, Belenkie I (2006) The cardiovascular effects of arteriovenous fistulas in chronic kidney disease: a cause for concern? Semin Dial 19: 349–352.
14. Fujii H, Kim JI, Abe T, Umezu M, Fukagawa M (2007) Relationship between parathyroid hormone and cardiac abnormalities in chronic dialysis patients. Intern Med 46: 1507–1512.

15. Gross ML, Ritz E (2008) Hypertrophy and fibrosis in the cardiomyopathy of uremia–beyond coronary heart disease. Semin Dial 21: 308–318.

16. Levy D, Garrison RJ, Savage DD, Kannel WB, Castelli WP (1990) Prognostic implications of echocardiographically determined left ventricular mass in the Framingham Heart Study. N Engl J Med 322: 1561–1566.

17. Stewart GA, Foster J, Cowan M, Rooney E, McDonagh T, et al. (1999) Echocardiography overestimates left ventricular mass in hemodialysis patients relative to magnetic resonance imaging. Kidney Int 56: 2248–2253.

18. Truong QA, Ptaszek LM, Charipar EM, Taylor C, Fontes JD, et al. (2010) Performance of electrocardiographic criteria for left ventricular hypertrophy as compared with cardiac computed tomography: from the Rule Out Myocardial Infarction Using Computer Assisted Tomography trial. J Hypertens 28: 1959–1967.

19. Casale PN, Devereux RB, Kligfield P, Eisenberg RR, Miller DH, et al. (1985) Electrocardiographic detection of left ventricular hypertrophy: development and prospective validation of improved criteria. J Am Coll Cardiol 6: 572–580.

20. Levy D, Labib SB, Anderson KM, Christiansen JC, Kannel WB, et al. (1990) Determinants of sensitivity and specificity of electrocardiographic criteria for left ventricular hypertrophy. Circulation 81: 815–820.

21. Okin PM, Roman MJ, Devereux RB, Kligfield P (1995) Electrocardiographic identification of increased left ventricular mass by simple voltage-duration products. J Am Coll Cardiol 25: 417–423.

22. Calderon A, Barrios V, Escobar C, Ferrer E, Barrios S, et al. (2010) Detection of left ventricular hypertrophy by different electrocardiographic criteria in clinical practice. Findings from the Sara study. Clin Exp Hypertens 32: 145–153.

23. Okin PM, Devereux RB, Jern S, Julius S, Kjeldsen SE, et al. (2001) Relation of echocardiographic left ventricular mass and hypertrophy to persistent electrocardiographic left ventricular hypertrophy in hypertensive patients: the LIFE Study. Am J Hypertens 14: 775–782.

24. Agarwal R, Light RP (2011) Determinants and prognostic significance of electrocardiographic left ventricular hypertrophy criteria in chronic kidney disease. Clin J Am Soc Nephrol 6: 528–536.

25. Gotch FA, Sargent JA (1985) A mechanistic analysis of the National Cooperative Dialysis Study (NCDS). Kidney Int 28: 526–534.

26. Rautaharju PM, Surawicz B, Gettes LS, Bailey JJ, Childers R, et al. (2009) AHA/ACCF/HRS recommendations for the standardization and interpretation of the electrocardiogram: part IV: the ST segment, T and U waves, and the QT interval: a scientific statement from the American Heart Association Electrocardiography and Arrhythmias Committee, Council on Clinical Cardiology; the American College of Cardiology Foundation; and the Heart Rhythm Society. Endorsed by the International Society for Computerized Electrocardiology. J Am Coll Cardiol 53: 982–991.

27. Devereux RB, Alonso DR, Lutas EM, Gottlieb GJ, Campo E, et al. (1986) Echocardiographic assessment of left ventricular hypertrophy: comparison to necropsy findings. Am J Cardiol 57: 450–458.

28. Liao Y, Cooper RS, Durazo-Arvizu R, Mensah GA, Ghali JK (1997) Prediction of mortality risk by different methods of indexation for left ventricular mass. J Am Coll Cardiol 29: 641–647.

29. Goodkin DA, Bragg-Gresham JL, Koenig KG, Wolfe RA, Akiba T, et al. (2003) Association of comorbid conditions and mortality in hemodialysis patients in Europe, Japan, and the United States: the Dialysis Outcomes and Practice Patterns Study (DOPPS). J Am Soc Nephrol 14: 3270–3277.

30. Cheung AK, Sarnak MJ, Yan G, Berkoben M, Heyka R, et al. (2004) Cardiac diseases in maintenance hemodialysis patients: results of the HEMO Study. Kidney Int 65: 2380–2389.

31. Krane V, Heinrich F, Meesmann M, Olschewski M, Lilienthal J, et al. (2009) Electrocardiography and outcome in patients with diabetes mellitus on maintenance hemodialysis. Clin J Am Soc Nephrol 4: 394–400.

32. Okin PM, Jern S, Devereux RB, Kjeldsen SE, Dahlof B (2000) Effect of obesity on electrocardiographic left ventricular hypertrophy in hypertensive patients : the losartan intervention for endpoint (LIFE) reduction in hypertension study. Hypertension 35: 13–18.

33. Mathew J, Sleight P, Lonn E, Johnstone D, Pogue J, et al. (2001) Reduction of cardiovascular risk by regression of electrocardiographic markers of left ventricular hypertrophy by the angiotensin-converting enzyme inhibitor ramipril. Circulation 104: 1615–1621.

34. Okin PM, Devereux RB, Jern S, Kjeldsen SE, Julius S, et al. (2004) Regression of electrocardiographic left ventricular hypertrophy during antihypertensive treatment and the prediction of major cardiovascular events. JAMA 292: 2343–2349.

35. (2005) K/DOQI clinical practice guidelines for cardiovascular disease in dialysis patients. Am J Kidney Dis 45: S1–153.

36. Molloy TJ, Okin PM, Devereux RB, Kligfield P (1992) Electrocardiographic detection of left ventricular hypertrophy by the simple QRS voltage-duration product. J Am Coll Cardiol 20: 1180–1186.

37. Barrios V, Escobar C, Calderon A, Tomas JP, Ruiz S, et al. (2006) Regression of left ventricular hypertrophy by a candesartan-based regimen in clinical practice. The VIPE study. J Renin Angiotensin Aldosterone Syst 7: 236–242.

38. Harnett JD, Murphy B, Collingwood P, Purchase L, Kent G, et al. (1993) The reliability and validity of echocardiographic measurement of left ventricular mass index in hemodialysis patients. Nephron 65: 212–214.

39. Willems JL, Poblete PF, Pipberger HV (1972) Day-to-day variation of the normal orthogonal electrocardiogram and vectorcardiogram. Circulation 45: 1057–1064.

14

Comparative Survival and Economic Benefits of Deceased Donor Kidney Transplantation and Dialysis in People with Varying Ages and Co-Morbidities

Germaine Wong[1,2,3]*, **Kirsten Howard**[2], **Jeremy R. Chapman**[3], **Steven Chadban**[4], **Nicholas Cross**[5], **Allison Tong**[1], **Angela C. Webster**[1,2,3], **Jonathan C. Craig**[1,2]

1 Centre for Kidney Research, Children's Hospital at Westmead, Westmead, Australia, **2** School of Public Health, University of Sydney, Sydney, Australia, **3** Centre for Transplant and Renal Research, Westmead Hospital, Sydney, Australia, **4** Central Clinical School, University of Sydney, Sydney, Australia, **5** Department of Nephrology, Christchurch Hospital, Christchurch, New Zealand

Abstract

Background: Deceased donor kidneys for transplantation are in most countries allocated preferentially to recipients who have limited co-morbidities. Little is known about the incremental health and economic gain from transplanting those with co-morbidities compared to remaining on dialysis. The aim of our study is to estimate the average and incremental survival benefits and health care costs of listing and transplantation compared to dialysis among individuals with varying co-morbidities.

Methods: A probabilistic Markov model was constructed, using current outcomes for patients with defined co-morbidities treated with either dialysis or transplantation, to compare the health and economic benefits of listing and transplantation with dialysis.

Findings: Using the current waiting time for deceased donor transplantation, transplanting a potential recipient, with or without co-morbidities achieves survival gains of between 6 months and more than three life years compared to remaining on dialysis, with an average incremental cost-effectiveness ratio (ICER) of less than $50,000/LYS, even among those with advanced age. Age at listing and the waiting time for transplantation are the most influential variables within the model. If there were an unlimited supply of organs and no waiting time, transplanting the younger and healthier individuals saves the most number of life years and is cost-saving, whereas transplanting the middle-age to older patients still achieves substantial incremental gains in life expectancy compared to being on dialysis.

Conclusions: Our modelled analyses suggest transplanting the younger and healthier individuals with end-stage kidney disease maximises survival gains and saves money. Listing and transplanting those with considerable co-morbidities is also cost-effective and achieves substantial survival gains compared with the dialysis alternative. Preferentially excluding the older and sicker individuals cannot be justified on utilitarian grounds.

Editor: Pieter H. M. van Baal, Erasmus University Rotterdam, The Netherlands

Funding: GW is the recipient of the Don and Lorraine Jacquot Fellowship, and is also partially funded by the Screening and Diagnostic Test Evaluation Program (STEP) and the Health Economics Research, Modelling and Evaluation in Sydney (HERMES) Capacity Building Grant. The funders had no role in study design, data collection and analysis, decision to publish, or preparation of the manuscript.

Competing Interests: The authors have declared that no competing interests exist.

* E-mail: germaine.wong@health.nsw.gov.au

Introduction

End-stage kidney disease (ESKD) is a global health problem, with currently over one million people worldwide living on some form of renal replacement therapy [1]. Kidney transplantation is the treatment of choice for most patients with ESKD because of improved duration and quality of life compared with dialysis, however demand for kidneys exceeds supply in all parts of the world [2–4]. Despite the concerted international effort by transplant authorities to increase the number of living donor kidneys, through introduction of the paired kidney exchange and ABO incompatible programs [5–9], many suitable potential recipients are unable to find a suitable live donor. Deceased donor transplantation is the only other alternative for people on dialysis, but the availability of deceased donor organs is limited, with a very small proportion of the prevalent dialysis population (less than 30%, 25% and 10% in the United States, Europe and Australia, respectively) receiving a deceased donor organ each year [2–4].

Being on the deceased donor waiting list is a necessary step to receiving a deceased donor transplant, but the listing or de-listing criteria vary between countries and between transplant units [10]. Patient selection for listing is clinician and centre dependent, which may lead to apparent disparity in decision-making according to co-morbid status, age and socio-economic status. For example, compared to patients without diabetes, the likelihood of a diabetic being listed on the active waiting list is reduced by at least 2-fold, perhaps or fear of poor outcomes after transplantation [11]. Fewer than 5% of those on the transplant waiting list in Australia are greater than 65 years old [2–4,12]. Minority groups such as Indigenous populations have fewer referrals to transplant centres, fewer complete transplant assessment and a much smaller proportion become candidates for transplantation compared to non-Indigenous populations [12–14]. Gender bias also exists in many countries, with recent studies reporting a consistent and significant negative association between being female and being active on the transplant waiting list [15–18].

Although policy-makers and transplant authorities have attempted to incorporate the principle of equity during the process of rationing scarce organ resources, such as integrating the recipients' waiting time on dialysis and recipients' immune sensitisation status in allocation algorithms [2,3,19], allocation policies have generally sought to maximise absolute graft and recipient survival by limiting the high-risk groups (such as diabetic patients or those with known cardiac disease), to transplantation [20–23]. It is these same groups of patients who have the bleakest prognosis on dialysis and may thereby achieve the greatest incremental gains from transplantation. The potential gains in life expectancy and health expenditure achieved by wait-listing people with co-morbidities compared to non-waitlisting are largely unknown. In this study, we aim to estimate the average and incremental survival benefits and health care costs of being listed on the deceased kidney donor waiting list compared to non waitlisting among individuals on dialysis, to allow better and informed decision-making around patient selection for listing.

Methods

From a third-party payer perspective, a probabilistic model was developed to simulate the natural history of a hypothetical group of potential candidates (n = 10,000), stratified according to their underlying co-morbid states: history of cardiovascular disease, diabetes mellitus, cerebrovascular disease, obesity, current smoking and varying ages at listing and transplantation. These variables were chosen because of the reduced patient and graft survival associated with these co-morbidities [24].

Structure of the model

The simplified structure of the model is outlined in figure 1. The cost-effectiveness model was constructed with two arms to compare the health benefits (in life-years gains) and costs of listing and transplanting potential candidates (with and without co-morbidities) with the health benefits and costs if they were to remain on dialysis. The progression of each individual through the model was depended on the age-specific transition probabilities through mutually exclusive health states of kidney transplantation and dialysis. The entire lifetime of an individual was modelled, whereby each transplant recipient was at risk of allograft failure and subsequent return to dialysis at the end of each annual cycle. The models assumed all transplant recipients were transplanted only once: all failed transplant recipients were subsequently managed on dialysis until death, and are represented by the black arrows in Figure 1. The model terminated when all potential recipients were deceased. We had set *a priori* the current Australian rate of deceased donor transplantation and did not account for the effects of variations in living donor transplantation.

We assumed the current average age of transplant (age = 45) [2–4,12], the current waiting time and the annual probability of receiving a deceased donor kidney on the transplant waiting list in Australia. The risk of non-fatal cardiovascular events, and all-

cause mortality, and for transplant recipients, the risk of post-transplant complications and events such as delayed graft function and wound infections, were dependent upon their underlying co-morbid health states. The model assumed a small proportion of patients with ESKD chose not to proceed with any form of renal replacement therapy. It also assumed a proportion of patients on dialysis would withdraw from dialysis each year (and opt for palliative and conservative management) and die during the concurrent year. Among those who remained on dialysis, we assumed an exponential relationship between the risk of dying from cardiac and non-cardiac causes, and the total time spent on dialysis.

Sensitivity analysis

Assumptions were tested over a range of plausible values to assess the robustness of the uncertainties in the model's parameter estimates using sensitivity analyses. Using one-way sensitivity analyses, we identified all the influential variables within the model. Probabilistic sensitivity analysis was also undertaken. Instead of just using point estimates for parameter values, this approach assigns a distribution to each model parameter, and samples from that distribution using Monte Carlo simulation [25,26] to estimate the expected value of each option. We used the log-normal distributions for relative risks and gamma distributions for costs, and randomly sampled over 10,000 iterations for each variable of interest. Scenario analyses were also conducted to assess the overall costs and benefits of deceased donor organ transplantation compared to being on dialysis if there were unlimited supply of deceased donor organs (i.e. no waiting time) for all individuals with varying co-morbidities.

Ethics

Ethics approval for this study was not required as no new participants were recruited for this study. Clinical parameter estimates for the model were sourced from published literature and from de-identified data from existing data registry.

Input parameter estimates for the model

Clinical data: A comprehensive literature search was conducted to identify the best available data on the clinical events that occurred before and after transplantation for recipients of kidney transplants and patients on dialysis. Age-specific probabilities for the following variables for transplant and dialysis patients were sourced from de-identified data from the Australian and New Zealand Dialysis and Transplant registry (ANZDATA) [27] and the National Organ Matching Service (NOMS): probability of receiving a deceased donor kidney transplant, graft failure and return to dialysis, experiencing a non-fatal cardiac event, and all-cause mortality. Other relevant data such as the probability of experiencing a transplant-associated complication including delayed graft function, acute rejection, re-hospitalisation or death was sourced from published literature. The ANZDATA Registry holds the records of all patients on renal replacement therapy in Australia and New Zealand since 1963 [27]. It contains comprehensive information such as the incidence, prevalence and outcomes data for all patients for whom indefinite renal replacement therapy is anticipated and the data is updated regularly by surveying all renal units 6 monthly before 2004, and annually since then. Multivariate Cox proportional hazard models were conducted to assess the association between cardiovascular disease, cerebrovascular disease, diabetes mellitus, smoking status, recipient age and obesity, and all-cause mortality among the listed dialysis and transplant recipients. The adjusted hazard ratios for deaths associated with the co-existing co-morbidities in transplant

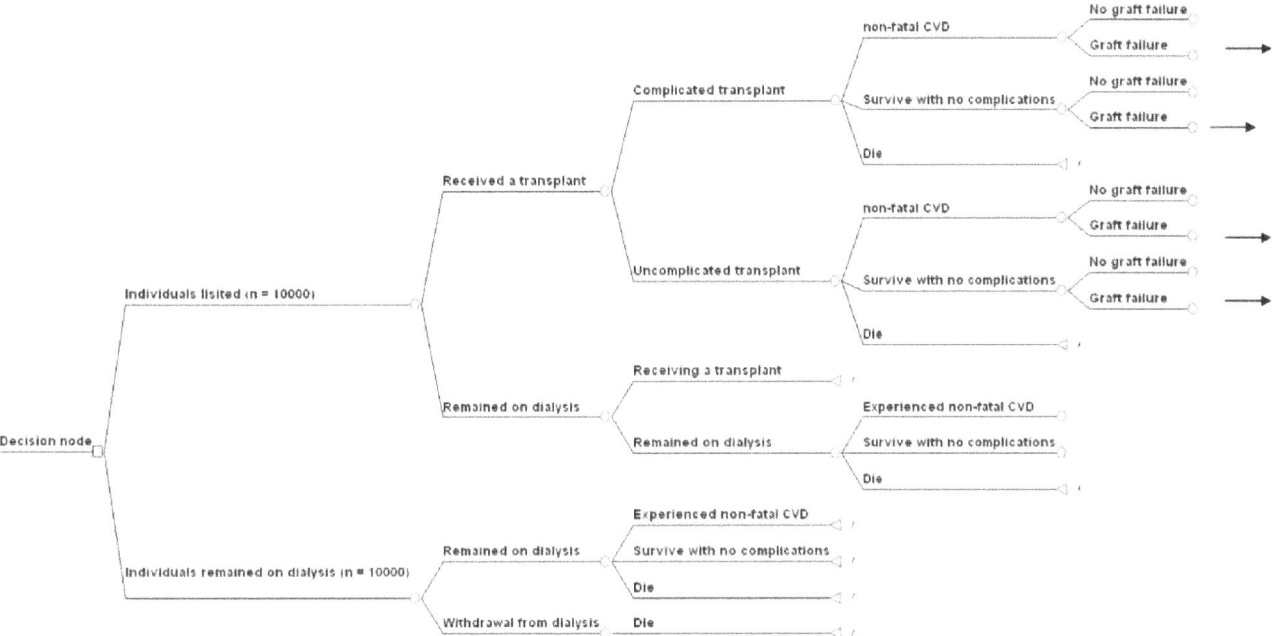

Figure 1. Simplified structure of the model.

recipients and listed patients on dialysis were estimated using data from the ANZDATA Registry between 2004 and 2008. The adjusted hazard ratios for deaths associated with the co-existing co-morbidities in transplant recipients and patients on dialysis, and other relevant clinical data for the model are shown in Appendix S1.

Cost data: Appendix S2 shows all the cost inputs of the model. Unit costs for initial and maintenance dialysis, initial (complicated and uncomplicated), annual resources use for individuals with and without co-morbidities such as diabetes and cardiovascular disease, and maintenance costs for kidney transplantation were obtained from the Australian Refined Diagnosis Related Groups [28], the Medicare Benefits Schedule of Australia [29–32] and the published literature. All foreign currencies were converted to the 2008 Australian dollar using the Purchasing Power Parities [33] and the Medicare component of the Consumer Price Index (CPI).

Model outcomes

The model outcomes included the total costs and health outcomes (expressed in life years gain) of dialysis and receiving a deceased donor kidney transplant, and the incremental costs and health benefits (in life years gains) of receiving a deceased donor kidney transplant compared to remaining on dialysis. The incremental cost-effectiveness ratio (ICER) of receiving a deceased donor kidney compared to being on dialysis was calculated for both case scenarios using the following formula:

$$ICER = (CostNew - CostComparator)/$$

$$(EffectivenessNew - EffectivenessComparator)$$

Future costs and benefits were discounted using a discount rate of 5% per annum and half-cycle corrections were employed. We used TreeAge Pro Suite 2009 (TreeAge software, Williamstown, MA, USA) [34] and Microsoft® Excel to develop and analyse the model.

Results

Table 1 shows the total and incremental health benefits (in life years), and the total and incremental costs of waitlisting compared to non-waitlisting among individuals with ESKD and varying co-morbidities. The average gains in life years associated with listing in 45-year old potential recipient with no underlying co-morbidities compared to remaining unlisted and on dialysis were 2.41 life years, with an incremental cost-effectiveness ratio (ICER) of less than $15,000/LYS.

Among those with underlying co-morbidities, the incremental benefits of being listed varied between 0.50 life years in a 60-year old with diabetes mellitus to 1.93 life years in a 45-year old with cardiovascular disease. Compared to non-listing, listing an average 45-year old individual with ESKD, with and without co-morbidities on the transplant waiting list is cost-effective, and the ICERs are substantially below the accepted cost-effectiveness threshold of $50,000 per life year saved (LYS) [35].

The cumulative incremental gains in life years from listing and transplanting individuals with varying co-morbidities are shown in Figure 2. Assuming the current waiting time on the decreased donor list, the benefits of transplantation are not evident until 4–5 years after waitlisting. A 25-year old with no co-morbidities, continues to gain survival benefits from being listed on the deceased donor list over time. This compares with listing an older recipient who is a diabetic, has a history of stroke or is a current smoker who achieve modest gains in life years (plateaus to a maximum of 0.7 to one life year gain) compared to non-waitlisting.

Sensitivity analysis

Scenario analysis. Age at the time of listing and the waiting-time on the deceased donor transplant list are the most influential variables within the model. The extent of the variability associated with the age of listing and the waiting time on dialysis on the incremental health outcomes of listing compared with non-listing is shown in Figure 3. Assuming the median time to deceased donor

Table 1. Incremental costs and health benefits associated with listing compared to non-waitlisting among individuals with varying co-morbidities.

Characteristics of the potential recipients	Strategies	Total health benefits (LYS)	Total healthcare costs ($)	Incremental benefits (LYG)	Incremental costs ($)	ICER ($/LYS)
A 25-year old without co-morbidities	Listing	13.12	590,551	3.84	−16,272	-
	Not listing	9.28	606,823			
A 45-year old without co-morbidities	Listing	9.57	504,908	2.41	28,269	11,730
	Not listing	7.16	476,639			
A 45-year old with cardiovascular disease	Listing	7.59	479,363	1.93	27,783	14,395
	Not listing	5.66	451,580			
An obese 45 year old	Listing	8.65	556,462.	1.57	23,282	14,829
	Not listing	6.75	533,180			
A 45-year old with diabetes mellitus	Listing	6.01	360,172	1.48	13,268	8,965
	Not listing	4.52	346,904			
A 45-year old who had a stroke	Listing	8.42	539,750	1.92	24,340	12,677
	Not listing	6.50	515,410			
A 45-year old current smoker	Listing	8.81	573,295	1.81	19,690	10,878
	Not listing	7.00	553,605			
A 60-year old without co-morbidities	Listing	7.78	509,423	1.38	49,667	35,902
	Not listing	6.39	495,394			
A 60-year old with cardiovascular disease	Listing	5.86	430,074	0.88	30,350	34,489
	Not listing	4.98	399,724			
An obese 60-year old	Listing	6.67	490,699	0.62	10,954	17,668
	Not listing	6.05	479,745			
A 60-year old with diabetes mellitus	Listing	4.55	336,340	0.50	10,753	21,506
	Not listing	4.05	312,852			
A 60-year old who had a stroke	Listing	6.74	497,109	0.95	35,264	37,120
	Not listing	5.79	461,845			
A 60-year old smoker	Listing	7.26	539,394	0.96	39,278	40,915
	Not listing	6.30	500,116			

kidney transplant is approximately 4–5 years in Australia, the incremental benefits of listing a 25-year old with no co-morbidities compared to non-waitlisting are 3.84 life years, with savings of over $16,000. The incremental health outcomes substantially decrease to less than 1.5 life years, with incremental costs of over $80,000 in a 65-yr old. If the waiting time of transplantation were to decrease, the maximal gains in life expectancy from transplantation compared to maintenance dialysis in a 25-year old with no co-morbidities are over 5 life years, with savings over $60,000.

Compared with maintenance dialysis, the incremental benefits associated with transplanting a 65-year old with no co-morbidities are gains of two extra life years, but with savings over $100,000. The greatest change in the incremental gains in life expectancy occurred in the "middle-age" population, varying between gains of 2 extra life years under the current waiting-time and availability of deceased organs, to over 5 extra life years if there were perfect supply of resources and no waiting time for decreased donor kidneys.

Probabilistic sensitivity analyses. The scatter plots shown in Figure 4 illustrate the mean incremental costs and health outcomes, and the uncertainties surrounding the mean parameter estimates associated with listing a 45- and a 60-year old potential

recipient with diabetes compared to no listing. The x-axis represents the incremental gains in life years, and the y-axis represents the incremental costs of listing compared with non-waitlisting [25]. The two scattered plots are located on the northeast (NE) quadrant of the cost-effectiveness plane, with positive incremental costs and effects, indicating that listing and transplantation is both more effective but more costly than dialysis in a 45- and a 60-year old with diabetes mellitus. Compared to non-waitlisting, listing a 45-year old diabetic achieves on average, a gain of 1.5 (±0.5) extra life years compared to non-waitlisting. Listing an older person with diabetes achieves a gain of 0.62 life years, but varies between 0.45 to 0.80 life years compared with non-waitlisting.

Discussion

Decision analytical modelling based upon current Australian outcomes of dialysis and transplantation, waitlisting and transplanting patients with ESRD, even in the presence of identified co-morbidities, is cost-effective and can be expected to achieve substantial gains of between 0.5 to more than three extra life years compared to non-waitlisting and maintenance dialysis. Given the current waiting time for decreased donor transplantation, the

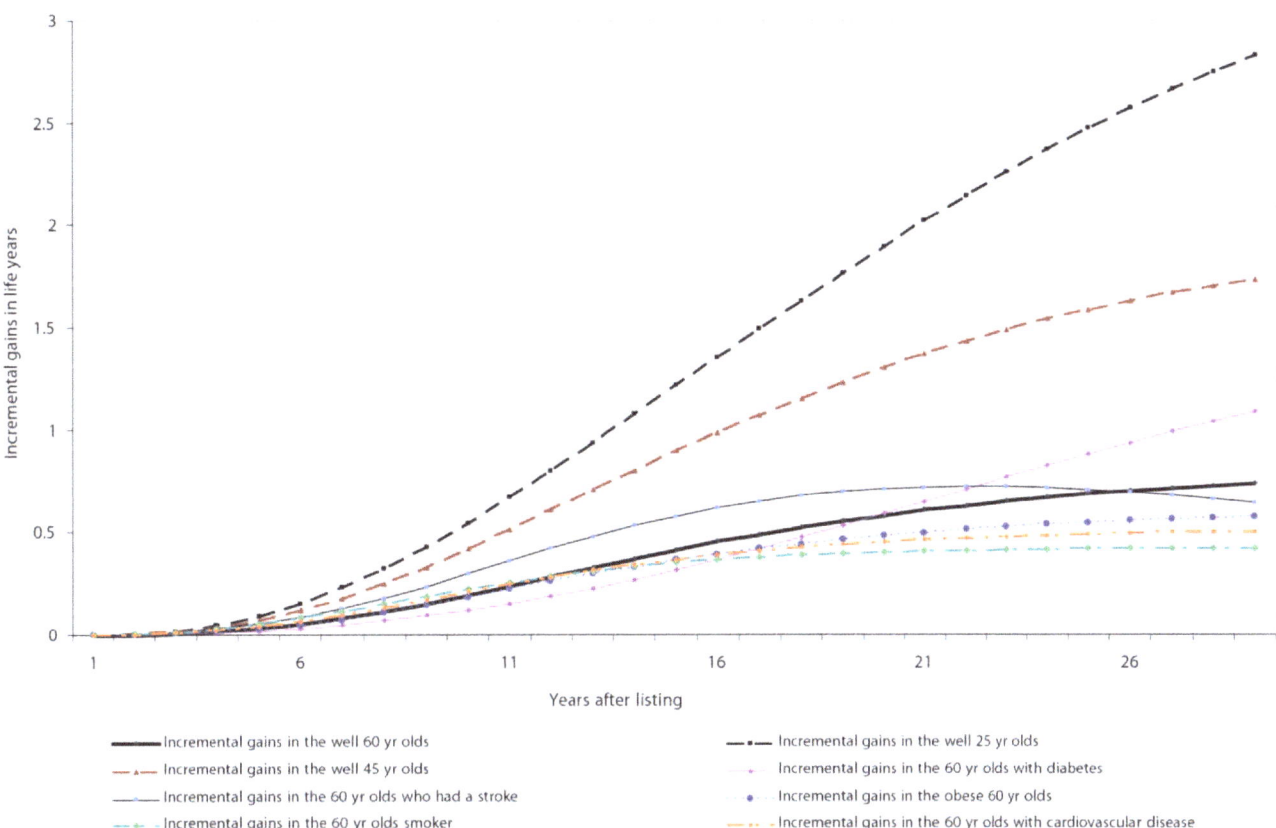

Figure 2. The cumulative incremental benefits of listing compared with non-waitlisting among individuals with ESKD and varying age and co-morbidities.

incremental benefits of transplantation compared to being on dialysis are not apparent until more than 4–5 years after listing. The extent of the survival benefits saved with waitlisting and transplantation is dependent on the underlying characteristics of the potential recipient, with the young and healthy achieving the greatest number of absolute and incremental gains in life years. However, the presence of the co-morbidities does not negate the benefits of waitlisting and transplantation, and indeed among those of older age with known cardiovascular disease and diabetes who are deemed suitable, listing and transplantation achieves comparable survival gains as seen in an older individual with no co-morbidities.

Previous studies have identified factors such as aging, gender, racial and socio-economic issues as being associated with the inequities in access to kidney transplantation. Once accepted on the waiting list, transplantation will achieve a gain in life expectancy of 3–15 years compared with maintenance dialysis [36–39], gains being dependent on donor and recipient characteristics including age at transplantation [36–38,40–43]. Previous studies, however, have not quantified the influence of the underlying co-morbidities on the listing benefits and healthcare expenditure compared to non-waitlisting. Using decision analytic modelling, we have estimated the absolute and incremental gains in survival benefits and costs between listing compared to non-waitlisting among individuals with varying co-morbidities such as cardiovascular disease, obesity, cerebrovascular disease, smoking and aging.

Listing and transplanting the young and healthy individuals will accrue the greatest number of life years over time and achieve the

greatest incremental gains in life expectancy compared to remaining on dialysis. Younger, healthier patients are often considered as "ideal" recipients who will maximally utilise the donated organs in the context of limited resources and will most likely achieve transplant success (i.e. better short and longer-term patient and graft survival compared to the older and sicker population). Whilst the absolute gains in survival among older recipients and those with co-morbidities may never be comparable to those observed for "ideal" candidates, we have shown that even in the face of the prolonged waiting-time under the current allocation algorithm, placing older individuals with co-morbidities such as cardiovascular disease and diabetes mellitus on the waiting list still achieves modest gains in survival.

Listing and transplantation affects the overall organ utilisation and therefore has an impact on all individuals with ESRD regardless of age and co-morbidities. Although the criteria to list are predominantly age and co-morbidity dependent, the allocation process is complex; and is largely dependent upon the notion of fairness and equity, where priority is largely determined by the duration of waiting time. Given the extent of the imbalance between organ demand and supply, only a small proportion of the waitlisted population will live long enough to receive a deceased donor organ before dying on the waiting list. Age and the waiting time on the deceased donor list are not unexpectedly, the most important factors that influence survival benefits from transplantation compared to being on dialysis. Under the optimistic scenario of unlimited organ supplies and no waiting-time for transplantation, transplanting the "middle to older-age" population achieves substantial relative gains in life expectancy by at least

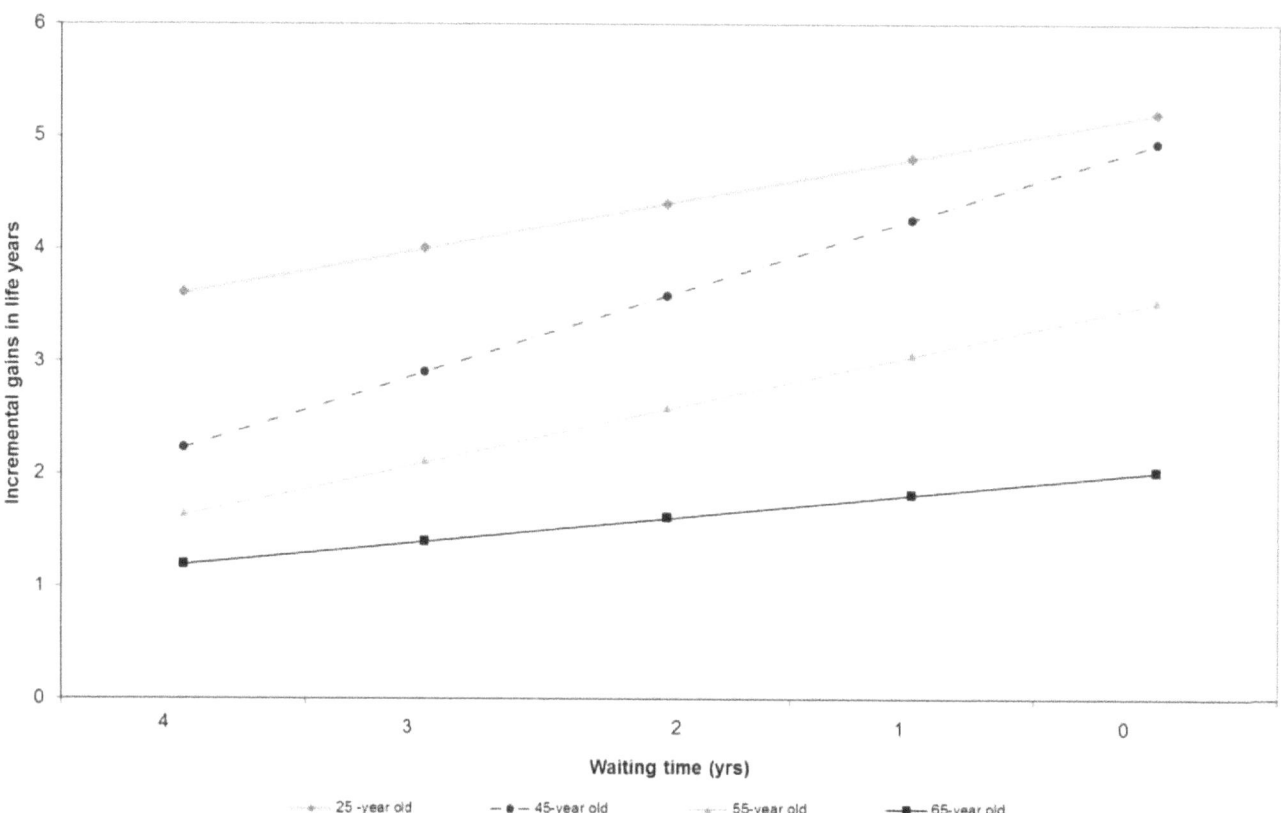

Figure 3. The effects of age and waiting time on the incremental benefits of listing compared with non-waitlisted individuals with ESKD.

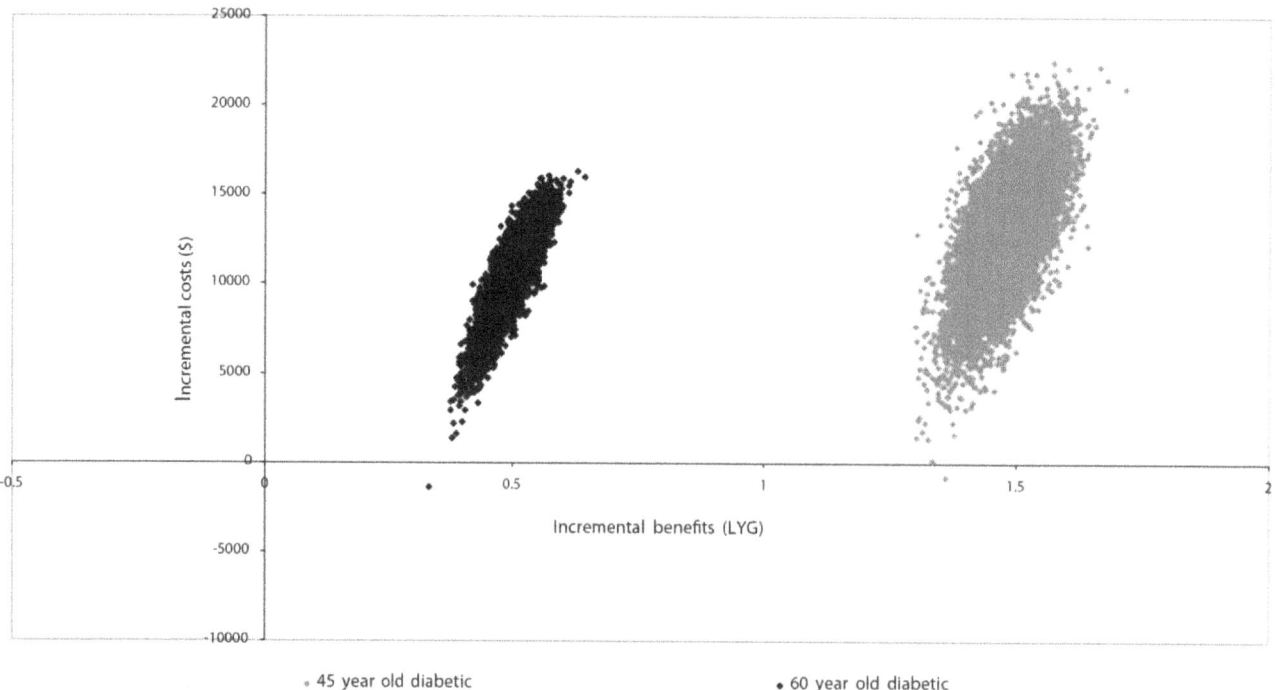

Figure 4. Probabilistic sensitivity analysis showing the uncertainties of the incremental costs and benefits comparing listing and non-waitlisting individuals with ESKD and diabetes.

an extra 3.5 life years, compared to being on dialysis. This somewhat counterintuitive outcome is attributable to the better relative survival on dialysis among the younger population and the synergistically poorer survival outcomes among those who are older and with co-morbidities on dialysis. The annual mortality rates of older people on the waitlisting are phenomenal, varying between 5–10%, with the risk of death increasing exponentially over time, and dependent predominately on age and co-morbidities [2–4]. Our study findings support listing and transplanting this vulnerable group of patients early who are potentially at the greatest risk of death from cardiovascular events on dialysis. It is inevitable and foreseeable that older patients are more likely to die with a functioning graft than their younger counterparts, and many would argue that the opportunity costs (i.e. the extra life years gained from transplanting a younger person with the same deceased organ) do not support the allocation of "better" quality kidneys to older patients. Recent advocates and initiatives have suggested a change in the allocation policy to "age-match" the deceased donor organs to maximise total graft life years on a societal level [44]. Whilst the "age-match" debate is an interesting and relevant issue, this discussion is beyond the scope of our analysis.

Previous studies have shown that transplantation is good value for money, and sometimes cost-saving [45–47]. Conversely, dialysis is expensive, with an annual expenditure of over US$20 billion in the United States and A$ 700 million in Australia annually and the demand for renal replacement therapy worldwide is increasing. Contrary to findings from other economic models, our data have suggested transplanting older individuals with co-morbidities may not necessarily be more costly than transplanting those without co-existent illnesses, driven predominantly by the higher costs of dialysis in elderly with co-morbidities compared to those without co-morbidities [48]. Transplanting individuals with co-morbidities, such as diabetes requires additional resources, for example in management of diabetic-related diseases such as retinopathy and peripheral neuropathy, but the total cumulative costs of transplanting a diabetic are less than a non-diabetic because they die more quickly and thus mitigated the extra costs.

We would hope that the findings of our study will allow greater consistency and equity for patient entry to the waiting list and allocation of scarce transplant resources. Preferential allocation and prioritisation of scarce organs to a specific population, in particular the sicker and older population, would be controversial and would raise ethical concerns by certain groups and authorities, and does not reflect current clinical practice. Kidney transplantation is a valuable medical procedure and should be offered to those who require it equally and fairly. Given the current limited supply of and on-going excess demand for organs, the distribution process should be free from biases such as gender, age, ethnicity, income, co-morbidities and socioeconomic status.

However, historical and registry data have shown that less than 5% of those aged 65 and older are on the deceased donor waiting list and less than 1% of the older population receive a deceased donor kidney annually [2,49,50]. Many would argue against allowing the younger and healthier population to wait for "more years" on the transplant lists because of the cumulative "uraemic" effects on potential vascular and metabolic events, and that the greatest benefits for these younger individuals, the community, the transplant authorities, and the policy-makers are to transplant them early, to ensure maximal absolute gains in graft and patient survival. The prestige and the perceived medical excellence commonly associated with most transplant programs have prompted

transplant authorities/clinicians to achieve optimal transplant outcomes by "cherry-picking" the best candidates for transplantation and not considering the overall benefits for the entire ESKD population. Increasing the numbers of patients wait-listed for transplantation through expanding the criteria to include the sicker and older individuals would likely prolong waiting times, which may adversely effect average outcomes, shorten the overall graft and patient survival, but will potentially extend the survival benefits to the disadvantaged, the sickest and the most needy ESKD population.

There are a number of limitations in our study. First, our estimates of survival gains and cost-savings are limited to patients for whom transplant clinicians had chosen to list and then transplant. For example, of all patients on renal replacement therapy who are listed as having coronary artery disease on the ANZDATA registry, it is probable that those who were transplanted on average have lesser degrees of vascular disease than those who were not listed for transplantation. Therefore, the outcome probabilities used in our models, which are based on actual outcomes, may over-estimate benefits for those with more severe disease. Second, we have not taken into consideration the benefits of living donor transplantation among those who had been listed and waiting for deceased donor transplants, and the harms, benefits and costs of multiple transplantations. Third, we have not valued outcomes in quality-adjusted life years, which may provide a more accurate assessment of both survival and quality of life outcomes in transplant recipients. There is, uniformly, a lack of utility-based quality of life data among recipients with co-morbidities. The extent of the quality of life improvement and the relative gains in quality adjusted life years post transplant in the elderly and those with co-morbid illnesses may be greater than those without co-existent diseases, rendering transplantation a more attractive option for those with co-morbidities than those without. There is therefore a need for future research to assess the utility-based quality of life of having co-morbidities such as diabetes and cardiovascular disease, in the dialysis and transplant populations to ensure a more realistic evaluation of the true impact of the survival and quality of life of having two or more chronic illnesses. Fourth, we have not considered donor factors, which may have a significant impact on the graft survival and potential survival benefits from receiving a transplant. In addition, data about the smoking status, body weight, and stroke history within the ANZDATA registry are incomplete, only collected at the start of the renal replacement therapy (and therefore may not be representative of co-morbidity status at the time of transplantation), and may be subjected to reporting bias. We have also not allowed co-morbidities to co-exist in the modelling and have not modelled re-transplantation which may potentially affect the overall survival benefits through transplantation in the ESKD population. Finally, patients' preferences and perspectives were not considered in this analysis. Previous studies have reported inconsistencies in the preferences concerning the allocation policy of transplant organs between the community, patients and healthcare professionals [50]. A recent systematic review of community preferences for organ allocation found that in addition to maximising efficiency, community preferences were also underpinned by principles relating to social valuation, moral deservingness, fair innings, and medical urgency [51].

While it is important to recognise and understand an individual's need and interests, it is also imperative to consider the interests of the wider community, particularly in the context of the limited organ supply and on-going demand. A better understanding of the absolute and incremental gains in survival and costs will help inform clinicians, decision and policy-makers about the optimal allocation of scarce organs to achieve maximal health gains, both from a societal and an individual's perspective. Excluding older and sicker patients from transplantation may disadvantage the group who actually have the greatest incremental gains in life years. The process of organ allocation is complex and requires careful distillation and consideration of all factors and available evidence, with the ultimate objective to balance the two competing interests of maximising efficiency and maintaining social justice in the distribution of limited resources.

Author Contributions

Conceived and designed the experiments: GW KH JRC JCC. Performed the experiments: GW KH JRC JCC. Analyzed the data: GW KH JRC JCC ACW AT SC NC. Wrote the paper: GW. Revised and advised on the presentation of the manuscript: ACW AT SC NC.

References

1. Lysaght MJ (2002) Maintenance dialysis population dynamics: current trends and long-term implications. Journal of the American Society of Nephrology 13: Suppl-40.
2. Australia and New Zealand Organ Donation Registry (2008) ANZOD Registry Report. Available: http://www.anzdata.org.au/anzod/anzodreport/anzodreport.htm#2008. Accessed 2009 Dec 18.
3. NHS Blood and Transplant (2009) Transplant activity in the UK. Available: http://www.uktransplant.org.uk/ukt/statistics/statistics.jsp. Accessed 2010 Jun 22.
4. Tuttle-Newhall JE, Krishnan SM, Levy MF, McBride V, Orlowski JP, et al. (2009) Organ donation and utilization in the United States: 1998–2007. American Journal of Transplantation 9: 1–93.
5. Takahashi K, Saito K, Takahara S, Okuyama A, Tanabe K, et al. (2004) Excellent long-term outcome of ABO-incompatible living donor kidney transplantation in Japan. American Journal of Transplantation 4: 1089–1096.
6. Tyden G, Kumlien G, Fehrman I (2003) Successful ABO-incompatible kidney transplantations without splenectomy using antigen-specific immunoadsorption and rituximab. Transplantation 76: 730–731.
7. de Klerk M, Witvliet MD, Haase-Kromwijk BJ, Weimar W, Claas FH (2008) A flexible national living donor kidney exchange program taking advantage of a central histocompatibility laboratory: the Dutch model. Clinical Transplants. pp 69–73.
8. Ferrari P, de Klerk M (2009) Paired kidney donations to expand the living donor pool. Journal of Nephrology 22: 699–707.
9. de Klerk M, Zuidema WC, Ijzermans JN, Weimar W (2008) Strategies to expand the living donor pool for kidney transplantation. Frontiers in Bioscience 13: 3373–3380.
10. Ravanan R, Udayaraj U, Ansell D, Collett D, Johnson R, et al. (2010) Variation between centres in access to renal transplantation in UK: longitudinal cohort study. BMJ 341: c3451.
11. Villar E, Rabilloud M, Berthoux F, Vialtel P, Labeeuw M, et al. (2004) A multicentre study of registration on renal transplantation waiting list of the elderly and patients with type 2 diabetes. Nephrology Dialysis Transplantation 19: 207–214.
12. Organ Donation Taskforce (2008) Organs for transplants: a report from the Organ Donation Taskforce. London: Department of Health, Available: http://www.dh.gov.uk/en/Publicationsandstatistics. Accessed 2008 Jan 16.
13. Cass A, Cunningham J, Snelling P, Wang Z, Hoy W (2003) Renal transplantation for Indigenous Australians: identifying the barriers to equitable access. Ethnicity & Health 8: 111–119.
14. Weber CL, Rush DN, Jeffery JR, Cheang M, Karpinski ME (2006) Kidney transplantation outcomes in Canadian aboriginals. American Journal of Transplantation 6: 1875–1881.
15. Garg PP, Furth SL, Fivush BA, Powe NR (2000) Impact of gender on access to the renal transplant waiting list for pediatric and adult patients. Journal of the American Society of Nephrology 11: 958–964.
16. Ojo A, Port FK (1993) Influence of race and gender on related donor renal transplantation rates. American Journal of Kidney Diseases 22: 835–841.
17. Bloembergen WE, Port FK, Mauger EA, Briggs JP, Leichtman AB (1996) Gender discrepancies in living related renal transplant donors and recipients. Journal of the American Society of Nephrology 7: 1139–1144.
18. Klassen AC, Hall AG, Saksvig B, Curbow B, Klassen DK (2002) Relationship between patients' perceptions of disadvantage and discrimination and listing for kidney transplantation. American Journal of Public Health 92: 811–817.
19. Tait BD, Russ GR (2004) Allocation of cadaver donor kidneys in Australia. Transplantation 77: 627–629.
20. Pilmore H, Dent H, Chang S, McDonald SP, Chadban SJ (2010) Reduction in cardiovascular death after kidney transplantation. Transplantation 89: 851–857.
21. Persijn GG (2002) Organ allocation: balancing utility and justice. Transplantation 73: 1536–1537.
22. Gill JS, Johnston O (2007) Access to kidney transplantation: the limitations of our current understanding. Journal of Nephrology 20: 501–506.
23. The Transplantation Society of Australia and New Zealand (2011) Consensus statement on eligibility criteria and allocation protocols. Available: http://www.tsanz.com.au/organallocationprotocols/index. Accessed 2011 Jun 11.
24. Gaylin DS, Held PJ, Port FK, Hunsicker LG, Wolfe RA, et al. (1993) The impact of comorbid and sociodemographic factors on access to renal transplantation. JAMA 269: 603–608.
25. Briggs AH (2000) Handling uncertainty in cost-effectiveness models. Pharmacoeconomics 17: 479–500.
26. Doubilet P, Begg CB, Weinstein MC, Braun P, McNeil BJ (1985) Probabilistic sensitivity analysis using Monte Carlo simulation. A practical approach. Medical Decision Making 5: 157–177.
27. Australia and New Zealand Dialysis and Transplant Registry (ANZDATA) (2009) Special data request. .
28. Australian Government Australia Institute of Health and Welfare (2007) AR-DRG data cube. Available: http://www.aihw.gov.au/data/. Accessed 2008 Jan 23.
29. Australian and New Zealand Dialysis and Transplant Registry (2007) The 30th Annual Report. Available: http://www.anzdata.org.au/v1/report_2007.html. Accessed 2008 Jan 11.
30. Australian Government Department of Health and Ageing (2010) Schedule of Pharmaceutical Benefits. Available: http://www.pbs.gov.au/pbs/home. Accessed 2010 Feb 4.
31. Australian Government Department of Health and Ageing (2010) Medicare Benefits Schedule Book. Available: http://www.mbsonline.gov.au/. Accessed 2010 Feb 2.
32. Australian Institute of Health and Welfare (2001) Australian Hospital Statistics. Available: http://www.aihw.gov.au/data/. Accessed 2001 Feb 18.
33. Raftery J (2000) Costing in economic evaluation. BMJ 320: 1597.
34. TreeAge Software, Inc (2009) Available: http://treeage.com/products/index.html. Accessed 2009 Jul 15.
35. Quinn RR, Naimark DM, Oliver MJ, Bayoumi AM (2007) Should hemodialysis patients with atrial fibrillation undergo systemic anticoagulation? A cost-utility analysis. American Journal of Kidney Diseases 50: 421–432.
36. Schnitzler MA, Whiting JF, Brennan DC, Lentine KL, Desai NM, et al. (2005) The life-years saved by a deceased organ donor. American Journal of Transplantation 5: 2289–2296.
37. Jassal SV, Krahn MD, Naglie G, Zaltzman JS, Roscoe JM, et al. (2003) Kidney transplantation in the elderly: a decision analysis. Journal of the American Society of Nephrology 14: 187–196.
38. Wolfe RA, Ashby VB, Milford EL, Ojo AO, Ettenger RE, et al. (1999) Comparison of mortality in all patients on dialysis, patients on dialysis awaiting transplantation,and recipients of a first cadaveric transplant. New England Journal of Medicine 341: 1725–1730.
39. Ojo AO, Hanson JA, Meier-Kriesche H, Okechukwu CN, Wolfe RA, et al. (2001) Survival in recipients of marginal cadaveric donor kidneys compared with other recipients and wait-listed transplant candidates. Journal of the American Society of Nephrology 12: 589–597.
40. Rao PS, Merion RM, Ashby VB, Port FK, Wolfe RA, et al. (2007) Renal transplantation in elderly patients older than 70 years of age: results from the Scientific Registry of Transplant Recipients. Transplantation 83: 1069–1074.
41. Wolfe RA, McCullough KP, Schaubel DE, Kalbfleisch JD, Murray S, et al. (2008) Calculating life years from transplant (LYFT): methods for kidney and kidney-pancreas candidates. American Journal of Transplantation 8: 1000–1011.
42. Wolfe RA, McCullough KP, Leichtman AB (2009) Predictability of survival models for waiting list and transplant patients: calculating LYFT. American Journal of Transplantation 9: 1523–1527.
43. Oniscu GC, Brown H, Forsythe JL (2004) How great is the survival advantage of transplantation over dialysis in elderly patients? Nephrology Dialysis Transplantation 19: 945–951.
44. Lim WH, Chang S, Chadban S, Campbell S, Dent H, et al. (2010) Donor-recipient age matching improves years of graft function in deceased-donor kidney transplantation. Nephrology Dialysis Transplantation 25: 3082–3089.
45. Laupacis A, Keown P, Pus N, Krueger H, Ferguson B, et al. (1996) A study of the quality of life and cost-utility of renal transplantation. Kidney International 50: 235–242.
46. Eggers P (1992) Comparison of treatment costs between dialysis and transplantation. Seminars in Nephrology 12: 284–289.

47. Karlberg I, Nyberg G (1995) Cost-effectiveness studies of renal transplantation. International Journal of Technology Assessment in Health Care 11: 611–622.

48. Grun RP, Constantinovici N, Normand C, Lamping DL, North Thames Dialysis Study Group (2003) Costs of dialysis for elderly people in the UK. Nephrology Dialysis Transplantation 18: 2122–2127.

49. Danovitch GM, Cohen DJ, Weir MR, Stock PG, Bennett WM, et al. (2005) Current status of kidney and pancreas transplantation in the United States, 1994–2003. American Journal of Transplantation 5: 1–15.

50. Satayathum S, Pisoni RL, McCullough KP, Merion RM, Wikstrom B, et al. (2005) Kidney transplantation and wait-listing rates from the international Dialysis Outcomes and Practice Patterns Study (DOPPS). Kidney International 68: 330–337.

51. Tong A, Howard K, Jan S, Cass A, Rose J, et al. (2010) Community preferences for the allocation of solid organs for transplantation: a systematic review. Transplantation 89: 796–805.

15

Measuring Parathyroid Hormone (PTH) in Patients with Oxidative Stress – Do We Need a Fourth Generation Parathyroid Hormone Assay?

Berthold Hocher[1*9], Franz Paul Armbruster[29], Stanka Stoeva[2], Christoph Reichetzeder[1], Hans Jürgen Grön[2], Ina Lieker[3], Dmytro Khadzhynov[3], Torsten Slowinski[39], Heinz Jürgen Roth[49]

1 Institute of Nutritional Science, University of Potsdam, Potsdam-Rehbrücke, Germany, 2 Immundiagnostik AG, Bensheim, Germany, 3 Department of Nephrology, Charité-Mitte, Berlin, Germany, 4 Department of Endocrinology/Oncology, Limbach Laboratory, Heidelberg, Germany

Abstract

Oxidation of PTH at methionine residues results in loss of biological activity. PTH may be oxidized in patients with renal disease. The aim of this study was to develop an assay considering oxidation of PTH. Oxidized hPTH was analyzed by high resolution nano-liquid chromatography coupled to ESI-FTT tandem mass spectrometry (nanoLC-ESI-FT-MS/MS) directly and after proteolytic cleavage. The oxidized hPTH(1–84) sample shows TIC-peaks at 18–20 min and several mass peaks due to mass shifts caused by oxidations. No significant signal for oxidized hPTH(1–84) species after removal of oxidized PTH molecules by a specific column with monoclonal antibodies (MAB) raised against the oxidized hPTH was detectable. By using this column in samples from 18 patients on dialysis we could demonstrate that measured PTH concentrations were substantially lower when considering oxidized forms of PTH. The relationship between PTH concentrations determined directly and those concentrations measured after removal of the oxidized PTH forms varies substantially. In some patients only 7% of traditionally measured PTH was free of oxidation, whereas in other patients 34% of the traditionally measured PTH was real intact PTH. In conclusion, a huge but not constant proportion of PTH molecules are oxidized in patients requiring dialysis. Since oxidized PTH is biologically inactive, the currently used methods to detect PTH in daily clinical practice may not adequately reflect PTH-related bone and cardiovascular abnormalities in patients on dialysis.

Editor: Rajesh Mohanraj, UAE University, Faculty of Medicine & Health Sciences, United Arab Emirates

Funding: The authors have no support or funding to report.

Competing Interests: Dr. Hocher, Dr. Armbruster and Dr. Roth submitted a patent application. The title is "MEANS AND METHODS OF MEASURING PARATHYROID HORMONE IN PATIENTS SUFFERING FROM OXIDATIVE STRESS." The application number is 12156441.3. This application does not alter the authors' adherence to all the PLoS ONE policies on sharing data and materials. Dr. Armbruster is the CEO of Immundiagnostik AG, Bensheim, Germany. Dr. Stoeva and Dr. Grön are research employees of Immundiagnostik AG, Bensheim, Germany. Dr. Roth is a research employee of the Department of Endocrinology/Oncology, Limbach Laboratory, Heidelberg, Germany. This does not alter the authors' adherence to all the PLoS ONE polices on sharing data and materials.

* E-mail: hocher@uni-potsdam.de

9 These authors contributed equally to this work.

¶ These authors also contributed equally to this work.

Introduction

Secondary hyperparathyroidism occurs frequently in chronic kidney disease as an adaptive response to deteriorating renal function. A combination of factors contribute to the increase of PTH that are additive [1]. Circulating 1,25-dihydroxy vitamin D starts to decrease very early in stage 2 of chronic kidney disease and continues to fall as the glomerular filtration rate (GFR) decreases further, and the renal 1α-hydroxylase is inhibited by hyperphosphataemia, hyperuricaemia, metabolic acidosis as well as 25-hydroxyvitamin D deficiency [1]. As GFR decreases below 60 mL/min/$1 \cdot 73$ m^2, phosphate is retained and stimulates synthesis and secretion of PTH. Hypocalcaemia develops as the GFR decreases below 50 mL/min/$1 \cdot 73$ m^2, further stimulating release of PTH. With disease progression, intact PTH (1–84) half-life increases and C-terminal fragments of the hormone accumulate. A relative state of end-organ resistance to the hormone exists, but chronic elevation of it has major consequences resulting in bone loss (particularly cortical bone), fractures, vascular calcification, cardiovascular disease, and hence an increased cardiovascular mortality [1].

A reliable method to measure PTH is a key for detecting patients with hyperparathyroidism as well as subsequent monitoring of therapeutic interventions. Therefore big efforts have been made in the past decades to develop PTH assays that are suitable for clinical use. So far three generations of PTH assays were developed as outlined below.

The first radioimmunoassay (RIA) for PTH was developed in the early 1960's [2]. This assay used polyclonal sera from guinea pigs and rabbits directed against extracted bovine PTH. Cross-reactivity with human PTH was relatively low, allowing only for measurement of elevated PTH levels (e.g., patients with primary hyperparathyroidism), but not normal to low levels of PTH. About 10 years later, Arnaud and colleagues at the Mayo Clinic published their results measuring PTH with an improved RIA using an antiserum raised against porcine PTH [3]. This assay allowed measurement within the normal range because of the

a

Methionine Oxidation

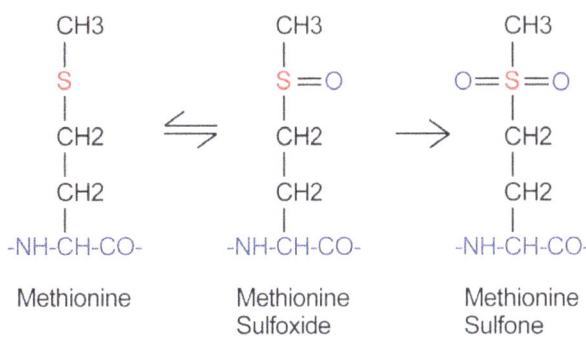

b

hPTH (1-84)

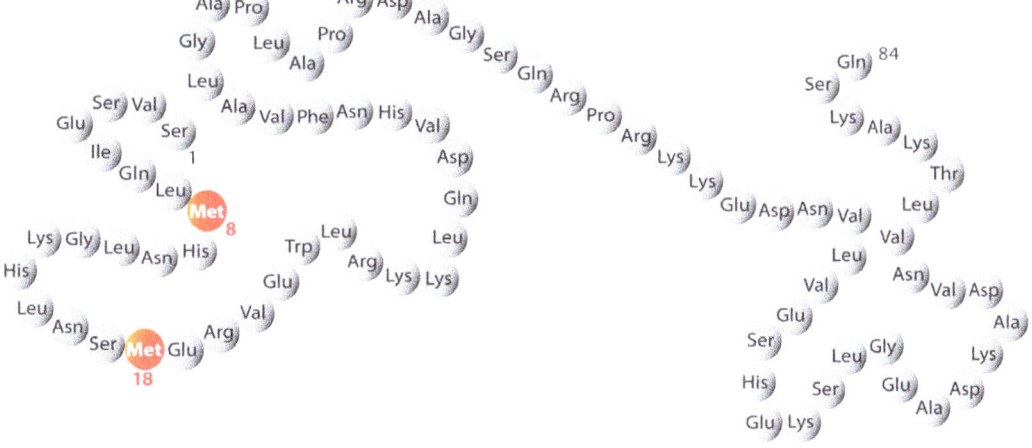

Figure 1. A: Under conditions of oxidative stress the methionine residues at position 8 and 18 may be oxidized to methionine sulfoxide and methionine sulfone. Oxidation to methionine sulfoxide is reversible, whereas the second oxidation step to methionine sulfone is irreversible. Oxidized PTH changes its 3-dimesional structure. This blocks the interaction of PTH with its receptor. B: Schematic diagram of the full length PTH(1–84) molecule ("bioactive" intact PTH). Oxidation at position Met 8 and/or Met 18 (red) alters the receptor binding site of PTH. Oxidized PTH does not bind the PTH receptor anymore and is thus biologically inactive. (see: E. Blind, Clin. Lab. 2008;54:439-446, reference 3).

better cross-reactivity of the antibodies against porcine and human PTH.

When the full structure of the 84–amino acid PTH molecule was determined [4], it became obvious that most of the anti-PTH antibodies used at this time were directed against the carboxyl-terminus of the peptide. The biologic activity of the hormone, however, is located in the amino-terminal residues of the molecule and a major cleavage site in the PTH molecule was identified at residues 33–34 Thus, these PTH assays detected the biologically active 84–amino acid PTH molecule, but also biologically inactive carboxy-terminal breakdown products of PTH. This is especially a problem in patients with renal failure, since inactive carboxyl-terminal PTH fragments accumulate in these patients, leading to falsely elevated results in the assay.

A second-generation assay was described in 1987 [5]. This PTH assay claimed to measure "intact PTH", since it used a pair of affinity purified antibodies, specific for two different regions of the PTH molecule. The capture antibody was directed against the carboxyl-terminal part of the hormone (amino acids 39–84), whereas the detection antibody was specific for the amino-terminal one (amino acids 1–34). PTH was sandwiched between the two antibodies. Only "intact" hormone molecules were detected. In addition to the increased specificity, such "two-site" assays were recognized as providing increased analytical sensitivity.

Third generation PTH assay was developed when it became apparent that patients with renal failure sometimes have intact PTH levels out of proportion to the level of bone disease even when 2nd generation assays were used [6]. At the time, it was suggested that the discrepancy was caused by the presence of a large PTH fragment lacking residues 1–6 [7]. Such a fragment would be expected to bind to PTH receptors but would lack biological activity. It was suggested but never proven that these species represent up to 50% of PTH detected in uremic patients [7]. This has led to the development of 3rd generation assays. They use the same carboxyl-terminal capture antibodies as the 2nd generation assays but the detection antibodies are specific for amino acids 1 to 4. However, even these 3rd generation tests have not improved the diagnosis of bone disease or other clinical manifestations of secondary hyperparathyroidism in uremic patients. Furthermore, there appears to be no difference in the diagnostic sensitivities between 2nd and 3rd generation assays in the diagnosis of primary hyperparathyroidism in patients with normal renal function [8]. Thus, it is so far not clear whether the initial hypothesis that led to the development of the 3rd generation PTH assays is valid or not. It remains still unknown why in particular in uremic patients there is often a discrepancy between bone disease and measured PTH levels.

Patients with more advanced stages of renal disease are subject to oxidative stress; accordingly hormones like PTH are oxidized. The oxidized hormones may lose their biological activity by losing their ability to interact properly with their receptors. PTH has two methionine residues at position 8 and 18 (see figure 1), and indeed studies by independent groups have repeatedly shown that oxidation of PTH diminishes its interaction with its receptor. Oxidized PTH (Figure 1) does not stimulate the PTH receptor to generate cAMP, and is thus most likely biological inactive [9–12]. These studies showed clearly on a cellular level measuring the second messenger and on whole animal approaches measuring calcium, phosphorus and vitamin D that oxidized PTH loses its biological properties. In the current study we describe the development of an assay that is able to distinguish between oxidized PTH and biologically active PTH. We furthermore used this assay in a patient population known to be exposed to oxidative stress: end-stage renal disease patients on intermittent hemodialysis [13].

Methods

Oxidation of hPTH(1–84)

Human PTH(1–84) was purchased from Bachem (Bubendorf, Switzerland). 200 µg hPTH(1–84) were dissolved in 400 µl of 0.1 M acetic acid (final concentration of 0.5 µg/µl), mixed 1:1 with 30% hydrogen peroxide and incubated for 45 min at 37°C. Afterwards, the mixture was cooled on ice, divided into aliquots and lyophilized.

Specificity test of anti-human oxidized PTH monoclonal antibody. The antibody was developed by Immundiagnostik AG, Bensheim, Germany. Based on the previously published methods [14], we now selected hybridoma cell lines from previously generated cell lines (14) producing antibodies against all forms of oxidized parathyroid hormone.

In order to characterize the specificity of the monoclonal antibody (MAB) raised against oxidized human PTH fragments, the antibody was immobilized on CNBr-activated Sepharose 4B (GE Healthcare Bio-Sciences, Uppsala, Sweden). Hundred µl aliquot of the slurry was filled in a column (MobiSpinColumn, MoBiTec, Göttingen, Germany) and equilibrated with PBS buffer, pH 7.4. Then 2.5 µg of lyophilized oxidized hPTH(1–84) were

dissolved in 300 µl of equilibrating buffer and applied on the column. The column was incubated end-over-end for 1 h at room temperature, washed with 300 µl of equilibrating buffer, followed by 3 washes with 300 µl of distilled water, and then eluted 2 times with 200 µl of elution buffer (0.1% TFA). Flow-through, wash fractions (equilibrating buffer and water) as well as eluate of the column were collected separately, lyophilized and analyzed by nanoLC-ESI-FT-MS.

nanoLC-ESI-FT-MS/MS

In order to investigate the amino acid oxidation of human PTH(1–84), the sample was analyzed directly by high resolution nanoLC-ESI-FT-MS/MS to determine the masses of the whole molecule species and after proteolytic cleavage by three endoproteases (ArgC, LysC and chymotrypsin) to characterize the methionine oxidation at positions 8 and/or 18.

The non-digested samples were directly applied to nanoLC-ESI-FT-MS after acidification with 2% formic acid.

Before enzymatic digestion, the oxidized human PTH(1–84) sample (1 nmol) was denatured by 8 M urea containing 20 mM TCEP (tris[2-carboxyl]phosphine) reducing agent for 30 min. Iodoacetamide was added to 50 mM final concentration and the mixture incubated for another 20 min in the dark. After dilution to 0.8 M urea, the sample was digested separately by endoproteases (ArgC, LysC and chymotrypsin; enzyme to protein ratio (w/w): 1:50) according to Proteome Factory's protein digestion SOPs. The acidified peptide sample digests (ArgC, LysC and chymotrypsin) were pooled and applied to nano-LC-ESI-MS (LTQ-FT, Thermo Scientific) analysis using a 35 min nanoLC gradient (Agilent 1100 nanoLC system) with solvent A (0.1% formic acid/5% acetonitrile/94.9% ddH2O) and solvent B (0.1% formic acid/99.9% acetonitrile).

The mass accuracy was better than 5 ppm for MS data. The MS data were analyzed by MASCOT (Matrixscience) and Qualbrowser (Thermo Scientific) according to the predicted peptide masses.

Blood Sample Preparation

For sample preparation, 100 µl aliquots of the slurry with the immobilized monoclonal antibody (MAB) were filled in MobiSpin-columns equilibrated with PBS buffer, pH 7.4. Then 500 µl of each sample were applied on the column, respectively. The columns were incubated mixing end-over-end for 2 h at room temperature, washed with 250 µl of 0.1 M ammonium acetate buffer pH 7.0, followed by a wash with 250 µl of 0.1 M ammonium acetate buffer pH 7.0, containing 20% acetonitrile, and then eluted 2 times with 200 µl of elution buffer (0.05 M formic acid, pH 3.5). Flow-through, wash fractions as well as eluate of the column were collected separately and lyophilized. Then the samples were reconstituted in 500 µl of PBS buffer, pH 7.4 and aliquots analyzed by the Roche Elecsys® PTH, Intact (Roche, Penzberg, Germany) assay, see below.

Sample Spiking with PTHox

To prove the recovery of oxidized PTH, 500 µl of a sample were spiked with 1 ng oxidized PTH. The spiked samples were treated as described in the sample preparation part.

Studying Clinical Specimens

We studied specimens from 18 patients on intermittent haemodialysis treated in our dialysis unit. Specimen (EDTA-whole blood) was taken just before the dialysis session started, centrifuged and stored immediately after plasma was obtained at

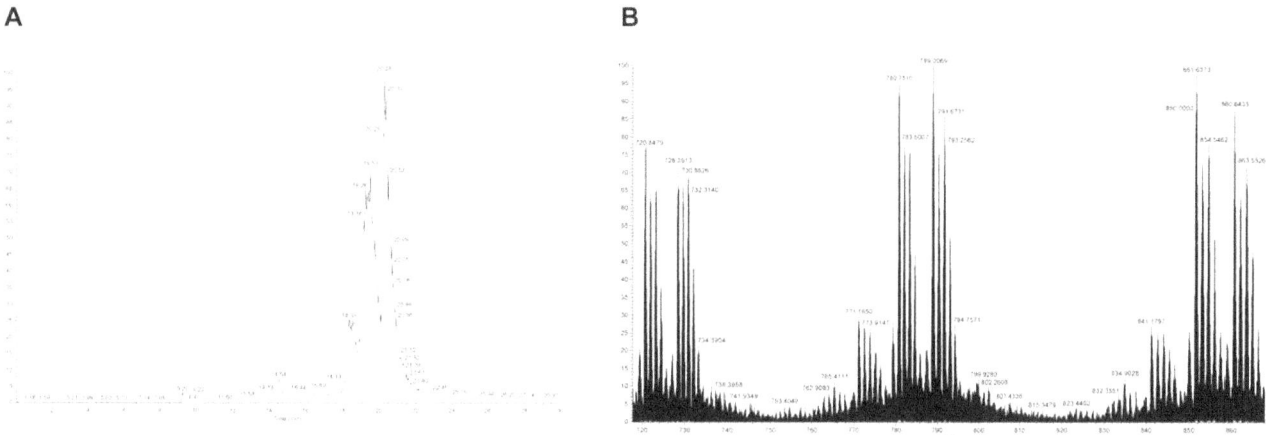

Figure 2. Non-digested oxidized synthetic hPTH(1–84)ox. A: NanoLC-ESI-FTMS total ion chromatogram. B: Magnified summed FTMS spectrum for retention time interval 18.30–20.50 minutes. Several different charged analyte ions were detected.

−80°C until further analysis. The study was approved by the ethical committee of the university hospital Charité, Berlin, Germany. Written informed consent was obtained in each case. Patients' characteristics were obtained from their clinical records. Serum phosphorus, calcium and C-reactive protein (CrP) were analyzed on an automatic analyzer of the clinical laboratory of the university hospital Charité.

Removal of Oxidized PTH from Human Specimens

500 µl of plasma samples were applied on the column with the immobilized monoclonal rat/mouse parathyroid hormone antibody (MAB). The column was exactly prepared as described above for the high resolution nanoLC-ESI-FT-MS/MS experiments.

The columns were incubated mixing end-over-end for 2 h at room temperature, washed with 250 µl of 0.1 M ammonium acetate buffer pH 7.0, followed by a wash with 250 µl of 0.1 M ammonium acetate buffer pH 7.0, containing 20% acetonitrile, and then eluted 2 times with 200 µl of elution buffer (0.05 M formic acid, pH 3.5). Flow-through, wash fractions as well as eluate of the column were collected separately and lyophilized. Then the samples were reconstituted in 500 µl of PBS buffer, pH 7.4 and aliquots analyzed by Roche Intact PTH assay, see below.

PTH Assay

The intact-PTH electrochemiluminescence immunoassay (ECLIA; Roche PTH, Intact [iPTH]) uses a biotinylated monoclonal antibody, which reacts with amino acids 26–32, and a capture ruthenium-complexed monoclonal antibody, which reacts with amino acids 55–64. The determinations were performed on Roche Modular E 170®. The intraassay CV was 4.1% and the interassay CV was 5.8% at concentrations of 35.0 and 180.0 ng/L, respectively. Human samples were either measured directly (named iPTH) or after removal of oxidized PTH by a column with removing oxidized PTH using anti-hPTHox monoclonal antibodies.

Control Tests

In order to be sure that the oxPTH columns remove specifically only oxidized parathyroid-hormone, we also analyzed some samples after purification with a column able to detect 1,25 dihydroxyvitamin D3 using vitamin D specific antibodies (Vit D-AssayK1107–737).

A second control experiment was designed to test the possibility that the monoclonal antibody (MAB) raised against the human oxidized PTH fragments may be released from the column and possibly interfere with the final PTH quantification: the conven-

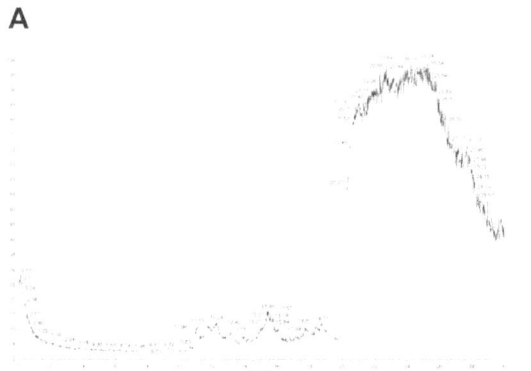

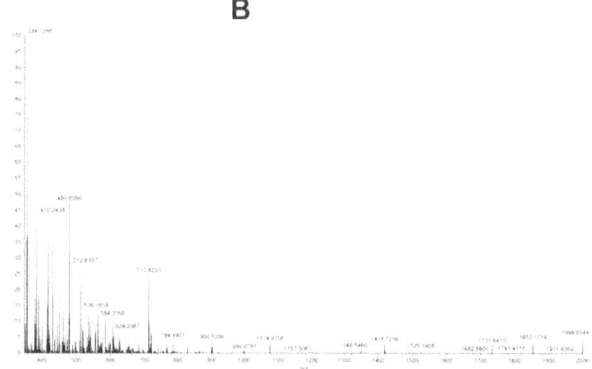

Figure 3. Flow through fraction of non-digested oxidized synthetic hPTH(1–84)ox from the affinity column. A: NanoLC-ESI-FTMS total ion chromatogram. **B**: Magnified summed FTMS spectrum for retention time interval of 16.50–18.50 minutes. The spectrum does not show any analyte masses which belong to PTH or oxidized PTH.

Table 1. Deduced molecular weights from the differently charged peaks in the spectra of the starting material, non-digested oxidized synthetic hPTH(1–84)ox (Fig. 1B), and the eluate from the affinity column (Fig. 3B).

Mass [m/z]	Charge z	MW [Da]	MW increase
728.16	13	9453.08	+32
729.39	13	9469.07	+48
730.62	13	9485.06	+64
731.85	13	9501.05	+80
780.50	12	9354.00	+32
781.83	12	9369.96	+48
783.17	12	9386.04	+64
788.76	12	9453.12	+32
790.09	12	9469.08	+48
791.42	12	9485.04	+64
792.75	12	9501.00	+80
851.36	11	9353.96	+32
852.82	11	9370.02	+48
854.27	11	9385.97	+64
860.28	11	9452.08	+32
861.73	11	9468.03	+48
863.19	11	9484.09	+64
864.64	11	9500.04	+80

The molecular masses correspond to values shifted by +16, +32, +48, +64 Da caused by methionine oxidation (sulfoxide, +16 Da and sulfone, +32 Da for each residue, and combinations thereof, maximal+64 Da) and by +80 Da for the additional oxidation of tryptophan 23.

tional 2-site "sandwich" immunoassay system. We took samples from 2 patients and added high amounts of free monoclonal antibody (MAB) raised against the oxidized PTH fragments or solvent to the probes (the final concentration of the antibodies in the samples was 1.8 µg/ml). The samples were then analyzed by means of the iPTH immunoassay.

Results

nanoLC-ESI-FT-MS and nanoLC-ESI-FT-MS/MS Data

The intact hPTH(1–84)ox sample shows TIC-peaks at 18–20 min and several mass peaks due to +16, +32, +48, +64 and +80 Da mass shifts caused by the oxidations (methionine sulfoxide, +16 Da and sulfone, +32 Da for each methionine residue, and combinations thereof) (Fig. 2A,B).

The digested hPTH(1–84)ox sample shows oxidation of methionines 8 and 18 (methionine sulfoxide, +16 Da and sulfone, +32 Da for each methionine residue) in the analysis of the proteolytic peptides. Oxidation of tryptophan 23 (+16 Da) was observed additionally (data not shown).

No significant mass peaks were observed that can be assigned to any of the hPTH(1–84)ox species by nanoLC-ESI-FT-MS analysis of the flow-through and wash fractions (equilibrating buffer and water) of the column (Fig. 3A,B), whereas several mass peaks corresponding to the different oxidized states of hPTH(1–84)ox were detected in the eluate (Fig. 4A,B; Table 1).

Comparison of the spectra of the starting material, non-digested oxidized synthetic hPTH(1–84)ox (Fig. 2B), and the eluate from the affinity column of non-digested oxidized synthetic hPTH(1–84)ox (Fig. 4B) as illustrated in Fig. 5 reveals the same profile despite the difference in peak intensity.

The results demonstrate that the synthetic hPTH(1–84) was completely oxidized resulting in the formation of a variety of products corresponding to the different oxidized methionine status. In addition, the column with the monoclonal antibody (MAB) raised against the oxidized human PTH is specific for all oxidized forms of hPTH(1–84) and removed them all from the sample.

Clinical Data

The clinical characteristics are shown in table 2. The method to detect oxidized and non-oxidized PTH is illustrated in figure 6. We included 17 patients on chronic hemodialysis as well as one patient requiring dialysis due to acute renal failure. We analyzed the clinical specimens with the iPTH immunoassay. In all patients the measured PTH concentrations were substantially lower when considering oxidized forms of parathyroid-hormone (see table 2 and figure 7). It is of note, however, that the relationship between PTH concentrations determined directly with the iPTH immu-

A

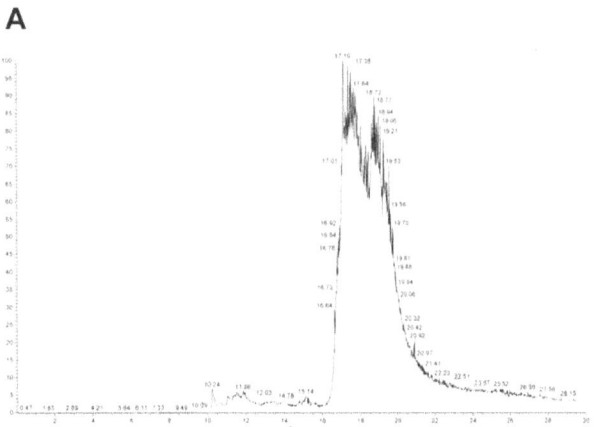

B

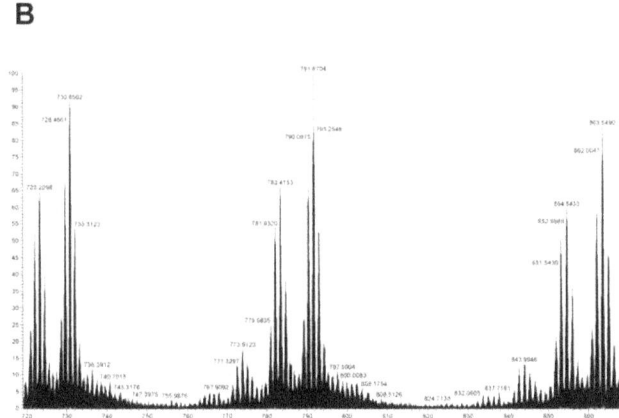

Figure 4. Eluate from the affinity column of non-digested oxidized synthetic hPTH(1–84)ox. A: NanoLC-ESI-FTMS total ion chromatogram. **B:** Magnified summed FTMS spectrum for retention time interval of 16.50–18.50 minutes. Several different charged analyte ions of PTH eluate were detected.

A

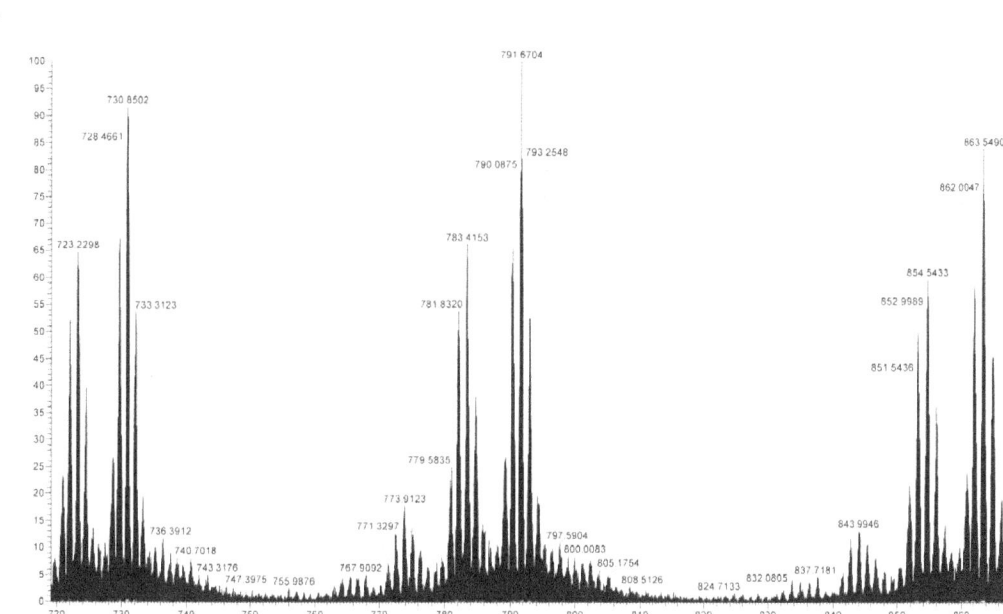

B

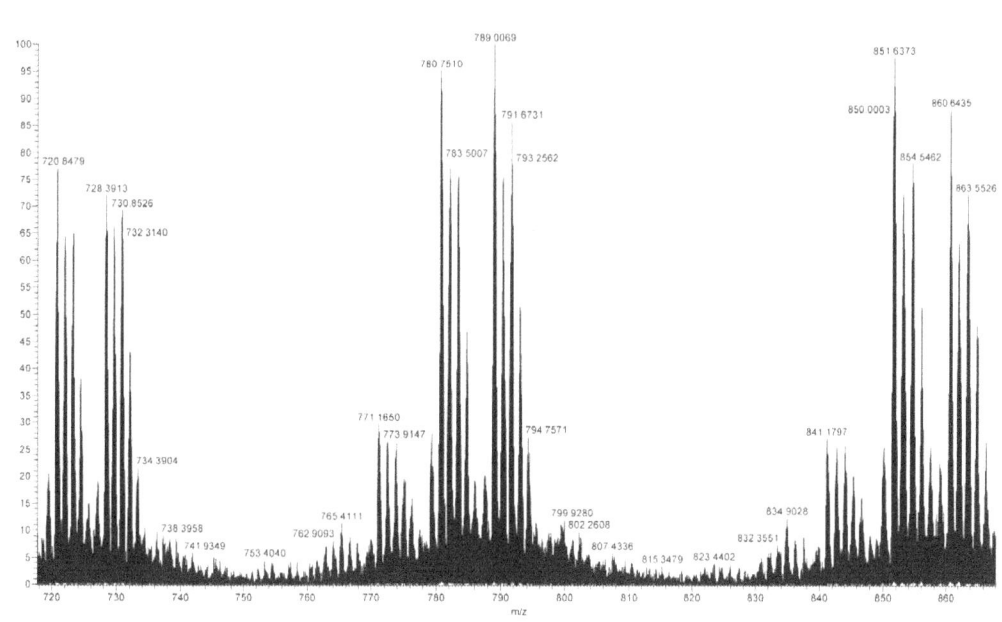

Figure 5. Comparison of the enlarged spectra of the starting material, non-digested oxidized synthetic hPTH(1–84)ox (Fig.1B), and the eluate from the affinity column of non-digested oxidized synthetic hPTH(1–84)ox (Fig. 3B).

noassay and those concentrations measured after removal of the oxidized PTH forms is not constant, by contrast the relationship varies substantially probably due to the different degree of oxidative stress among the studied patients. In some patients only 7% of traditionally measured PTH were free of oxidation, whereas in another patient 34% of the traditionally measured PTH were real intact PTH. Taken together without considering oxidation status of PTH, the traditionally measured PTH concentrations using a modern sandwich detection system are severalfold higher as the concentrations when considering oxidation of PTH. The effect of oxidation of PTH is highly variable among these patients

requiring dialysis. There is only a very weak correlation between traditionally measured PTH and oxidized PTH.

In some patients besides the iPTH immunoassay from Roche we also used the PTH(1–84) assay system from Roche. We basically got similar results as described above with the iPTH assay system. Without considering oxidation status of PTH, the traditionally measured PTH concentrations are detected severalfold higher as compared to the concentrations when considering oxidation of PTH (data not shown). This may indicate that all third generation PTH test systems (see introduction) used nowadays do not consider oxidation status of PTH.

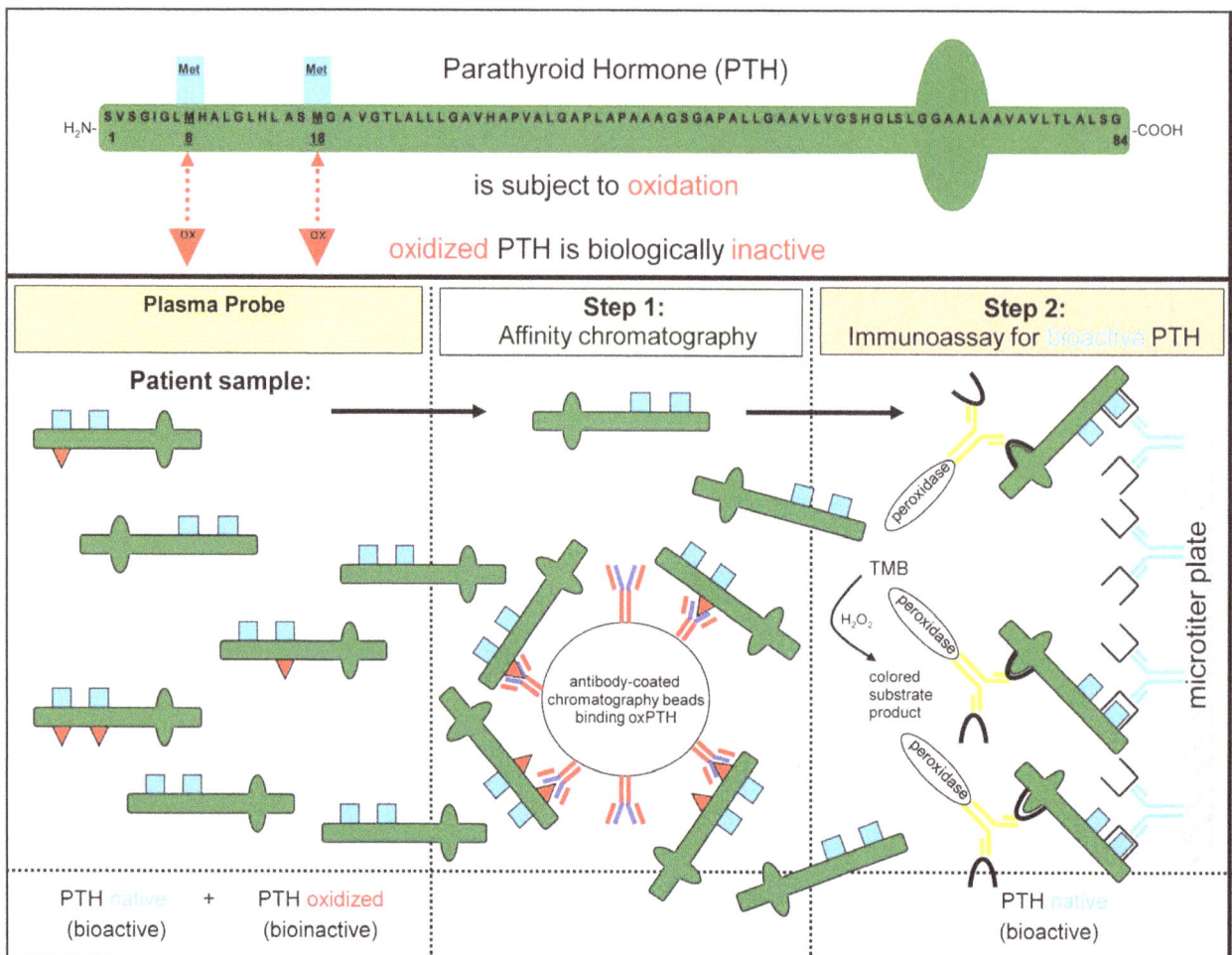

Figure 6. Basic principles of the new assay system for detection of intact and real intact PTH in human samples. The new detection process for real intact bioactive PTH consists of 2 steps: Firstly, any oxidized forms of oxidized PTH at position Met8 and/or position Met18 will be removed from the probe by a specific affinity chromatography column. The column contains monoclonal rat/mouse antibody (MAB) raised against the hPTH(1–34)oxidized fragments. These antibodies are able to remove any oxidized forms of PTH. In the second step the remaining non-oxidized PTH will be analyzed in conventional 2-site "sandwich" immunoassay systems. The antibody on the left (*capture antibody*) is bound to solid phase. The antibody on the right (*label antibody*) relays the signal. These antibodies must bind different sites on the PTH analyte to produce a positive result in the assay.

In order to be sure that the oxPTH columns remove specifically only oxidized PTH, we also analyzed some samples after purification with a column able to bind 1,25 dihydroxyvitamin D3. These data indicate that only approximately 14% of the PTH is non-specifically bound by a "nonsense" (vitamin D) column. In other words, the column on its own when containing no antibodies raised against oxidized forms of PTH but antibodies detecting other epitopes does not significantly influence the test results (table 3).

A second control experiment was designed to test the possibility that the monoclonal rat/mouse antibody (MAB) raised against the hPTH(1–34)oxidized fragments may be released from the column and possibly interfere with final PTH quantification: the conventional 2-site "sandwich" immunoassay system (see figure 6). We took samples from 2 patients and added high amounts of free monoclonal antibodies (MAB) raised against oxidized human PTH fragments or solvent (the final concentration of the antibodies in the samples was 1.8 µg/ml). The samples were then analyzed using the iPTH immunoassay. Those samples where only solvent was added had measured iPTH concentrations of 43.63 [ng/L]

(patient a), and 796,20 [ng/L] (patient b), respectively. Adding the monoclonal antibodies to the samples did not alter the results significantly. In the samples with antibodies we measured 35,70 [ng/L] (patient a) and 753,20 [ng/L] (patient b). This indicates that even in the case that the column may lose monoclonal antibodies (MAB) raised against the oxidized human PTH molecules, these antibodies do not interfere significantly with the final iPTH quantification (see figure 6).

Discussion

Using very sensitive mass spectroscopy approaches, the current study clearly demonstrated that oxidation of human PTH(1–84) resulted in the formation of a variety of products corresponding to the different oxidized methionine resides at position 8 and/or 18 within the parathyroid hormone. A column with the monoclonal antibody raised against the hPTH(1–34)ox fragment is specific for all oxidized forms of hPTH(1–84) and removed them all from the sample. The clinical part of our study demonstrated that without considering oxidation status of PTH, the traditionally measured

Table 2. Clinical Characteristic of the patients on dialysis.

No.	renal disease	Age (years)	Time on dialysis (years)	sex	iPTH (ng/L)	real-iPTH (ng/L)	ox-iPTH (ng/L)	Ratio iPTH/ real-iPTH	Total Ca (mmol/l)	P (mmol/l)	CrP (mg/dl)
1	Hypertensive Nephropathy	62	0,3	m	43,63	8,9	34,73	0.204	2,58	1,24	0,43
2	Diabetic Nephropathy	73	4	m	796,2	70,62	725,6	0.089	2,2	2,15	–
3	unknown	37	0,1	m	52,84	10,35	42,49	0.196	2,53	0,81	0,03
4	Diabetic Nephropathy	68	2,1	f	70,8	11,18	59,62	0.158	2,23	0,91	4,08
5	Acute Kidney Injury	64	0	m	46,49	9,45	37,04	0.203	2,17	1,32	3,26
6	Diabetic Nephropathy	63	1,6	f	42,13	5,37	36,76	0.127	2,08	1,43	12,2
7	ADPKD	70	3,3	f	1029	74,76	954,2	0.073	2,1	1,37	0,53
8	Cardio-Renal-Syndrom	70	3,4	m	240,4	41,89	198,5	0.174	2,38	1,57	0,32
9	unknown	70	9	m	105	18,48	86,52	0.176	2,26	1,5	3,12
10	Diabetic Nephropathy	65	7	m	1301	445,3	855,7	0.342	2,53	2,23	1,74
11	Membranous GN	45	5,4	f	311,8	24,44	287,4	0.078	1,57	2,06	0,52
12	Membranoproliferative GN (Typ1)	52	1,5	m	144,1	19,24	124,9	0.134	1,87	0,73	0,17
13	Hypertensive Nephropathy	61	4,1	m	73,45	15,92	57,53	0.217	2,15	2,35	0,67
14	ADPKD	57	1,2	m	281,9	44,02	237,9	0.156	2,18	1,35	13,4
15	Diabetic Nephropathy	73	4	m	116,9	19,73	97,17	0.169	2,38	1,66	4
16	Mesangioproliferative GN	69	8,1	m	70,81	18,51	52,3	0.261	2,62	2,28	6,7
17	interstitial Nephritis	61	2,6	f	76,28	11,21	65,07	0.147	2,21	1,61	2,9
18	unknown	56	10,6	m	487,1	76,12	411	0.156	2,35	2,41	0,17

PTH concentrations based on current gold standard methods resulted in much higher PTH concentrations in the clinical samples as compared to the concentrations when considering oxidation of PTH. The effect of PTH oxidation is highly variable among patients requiring dialysis. There is only a weak correlation between traditionally measured PTH and PTH data considering the oxidation of this hormone. Given the fact that oxidized PTH (Figure 1) does not stimulate the PTH receptor anymore to generate cAMP, and is thus most likely biologically inactive [9–12], clinical strategies for the treatment of hyperparathyroidism in dialysis patients based on measurements of PTH using classical third generation sandwich ELISA techniques are most likely prone to incorrect decision making.

It is known for example that in uremic patients highly specific assays have measured a 2.5-fold increase in the non-suppressible fraction of PTH compared with healthy subjects [15–20]. Moreover, PTH concentrations measured in uremic serum apparently overestimated PTH-related bone abnormalities also by a factor of 2–2.5 [6]. It was suggested that in patients with chronic renal failure, the presence of high circulating levels of non-1–84 PTH fragments (most likely 7–84 PTH) detected by the second generation assay and the antagonistic effects of 7–84 PTH on the biological activity of 1–84 PTH may explain this [21]. However, this hypothesis was never proven in adequately designed clinical studies using for example HPLC coupled to mass spectrometry to really distinguish between different PTH fragments. Our data on the other hand using modern liquid chromatography linked to tandem mass spectroscopy to detect PTH suggest that this well-known overestimation of PTH in patients on dialysis might be most likely due to the presence of oxidized, biologically inactive forms of PTH in patients on dialysis.

Reactive oxygen species (ROS) such as hydrogen peroxide (H_2O_2) or hypochlorous acid (HOCl), and free radicals such as hydroxyl radical (OH) or others are continuously formed *in vivo*. Additional imbalance between formation of ROS and potent antioxidative defense mechanisms creates oxidative stress. Uraemia in general is associated with enhanced oxidative stress, and haemodialysis or peritoneal dialysis may in particular contribute to oxidative stress and reduced antioxidant levels in such patients [6–10].

One of the preferred highly sensitive targets for oxidation is methionine. The oxidation product methionine sulfoxide can be reversed by reduction with chemicals or biologically, whereas oxidation to the methionine sulfone is biologically irreversible (figure 1). Oxidation of methionine residues can lead to an activation or inactivation of a functional protein, respectively, and the resulting methionine sulfoxide can be reversed enzymatically by a specific reductase. Methionyl sulfoxide reductase has been found in *E. coli* and in mammalian tissues. Oxidation of methionine and its reversal may serve as a regulator for protein activities [12]. The parathyroid hormone contains two methionine residues in the amino-terminal region (position 8 and 18), responsible for the biological activity of the peptide, accessible to alterations by oxidation. Galceran et al. concluded in 1984 that oxidation of bPTH-(1–34) results in loss of both the renal and skeletal effects of PTH *in vivo* in rats and dogs [10]. Horiuchi postulated in 1988 that intact methionine residues at position 8 and 18 of hPTH-(1–34) are necessary for all its major biological actions, including its effect on the renal metabolism of 25-hydroxyvitamin D_3 [11]. The secondary structure of the parathyroid hormone seems to be essential for its receptor binding. The methionine residue 8 is important for the folding of the hormone and proves the key role for this residue in the structure of the

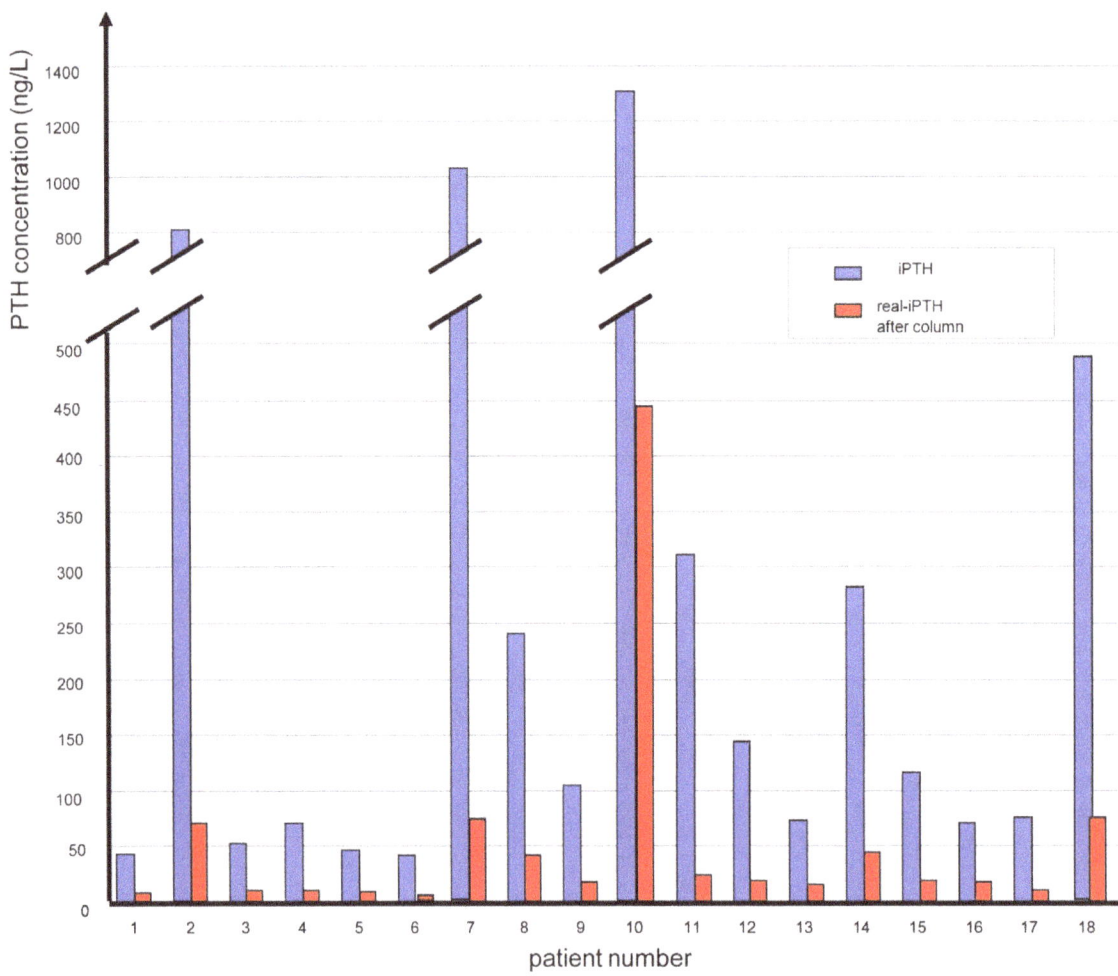

Figure 7. We measured intact PTH using the intact PTH assay as described in the method section in 18 patients on dialysis (blue bars), for further detail see also table 2. When removing the oxidized forms of PTH from the sample as illustrated in figure 6, the results were completely different (red bars). The effect of oxidation of PTH is highly variable among these patients requiring dialysis. There is only a very weak correlation between traditionally measured PTH and PTH data considering the oxidation of this hormone.

amino-terminal domain and its biological activity [12]. Thus oxidation of methionine residue 8, producing fundamental chances in secondary structure of PTH, is implicated both in binding and in activation of adenylyl cyclase. As early as 1974 O'Riordan and his group showed the effect of oxidation and back-reduction on the potency of porcine PTH, measured by its activation of rat renal cortical adenyl-cyclase [22].

Based on published data and our results, we suggest that methionine residues in different peptide hormones, like human growth hormone, somatomammotropin, luteotropin as well as PTH may be subject to oxidation resulting in loss of biological activity or receptor affinity. Methionine oxidation may be a general principle in regulation of hormone activity. However, this hypothesis needs to be proved in detail.

Our new assay system is - for the first time - able to differentiate between oxidized and non-oxidized forms of PTH by removing oxidized PTH fragments with a highly specific antibody able to detect and bind all forms of oxidized PTH. The removal of oxidized forms of PTH can be done either – as it was done in the present study – prior to analysis by a coated column followed by a third generation PTH assays (for assay principle see figure 6) or even as an integrative part of a third generation sandwich immunoassay system. It should also be feasible to combine our approach [14] with modern techniques like liquid chromatography coupled to tandem mass spectrometry [23,24] in clinical practice in the near future by immunocapture oxidized PTH fragments prior to LC-MS/MS. This will improve the diagnostic performance of LC-MS/MS PTH approaches.

Table 3. Control experiment: PTH was measured directly and after washing of the samples from a vitamin D column.

iPTH	iPTH after vitamin D column (ng/L)	Ratio
43,63	32,43	0,743295897
796,2	684,83	0,860123085
52,84	47,45	0,897993944
46,49	41,86	0,90040869
70,6	61,99	0,878045326

In conclusion, by means of nanoLC-ESI-FT-MS/MS, we were able to demonstrate that oxidation of human PTH(1–84) resulted in the formation of a variety of products corresponding to the different oxidized methionine residues at position 8 and/or 18 within the parathyroid hormone. A column with a monoclonal antibody (MAB) raised against the oxidized human PTH fragment is specific for all oxidized forms of hPTH(1–84) and removed them all from the sample. Without considering oxidation status of PTH, the traditionally measured PTH concentrations based on current gold standard methods resulted in much higher PTH concentrations in clinical samples specimens as compared to the concentrations when considering oxidation of PTH. The effect of PTH oxidation is highly variable among patients requiring dialysis. Given the impact of vascular calcification in end-stage renal disease patients on morbidity and mortality [25] further adequately powered studies are needed to demonstrate that measuring whole PTH without "contamination" of oxidized PTH forms improves clinical decision making and better reflects PTH-related bone and cardiovascular abnormalities. Reliable measurements of biologically active PTH are clinically important. Treatment guidelines for patients on dialysis as well as in- and exclusion criteria into clinical trials are based on PTH concentrations. Given the poor clinical performance of currently available assay systems for PTH measurement [26], a recent review even suggested that reliance on PTH concentrations (measured by the classical test systems) alone is a dangerous substitute for the search for, and use of, more precise and reliable biomarkers [27]. We suggest that this is at least partially attributed to the neglection of the oxidation status of the hormone. However, as stated above, this clearly needs to be investigated in detail in suitable clinical studies.

Author Contributions

Conceived and designed the experiments: BH FPA SS TS HR. Performed the experiments: SS HG IL DK. Analyzed the data: BH TS FPA SS CR. Contributed reagents/materials/analysis tools: BH FPA SS TS HR. Wrote the paper: BH.

References

1. Fraser WD (2009) Hyperparathyroidism. Lancet 374: 145–158. doi:10.1016/S0140-6736(09)60507-9.

2. Berson SA, Yalow RS, Aurbach GD, Potts JT (1963) IMMUNOASSAY OF BOVINE AND HUMAN PARATHYROID HORMONE. Proc Natl Acad Sci USA 49: 613–617.

3. Blind E (2008) Twenty years of progress with parathyroid hormone (PTH): from specialized and "difficult" measurement to common laboratory parameter and treatment option in osteoporosis. Clin Lab 54: 439–449.

4. Keutmann HT, Sauer MM, Hendy GN, O'Riordan LH, Potts JT Jr (1978) Complete amino acid sequence of human parathyroid hormone. Biochemistry 17: 5723–5729.

5. Blind E, Schmidt-Gayk H, Armbruster FP, Stadler A (1987) Measurement of intact human parathyrin by an extracting two-site immunoradiometric assay. Clin Chem 33: 1376–1381.

6. Quarles LD, Lobaugh B, Murphy G (1992) Intact parathyroid hormone overestimates the presence and severity of parathyroid-mediated osseous abnormalities in uremia. J Clin Endocrinol Metab 75: 145–150.

7. Lepage R, Roy L, Brossard JH, Rousseau L, Dorais C, et al. (1998) A non-(1–84) circulating parathyroid hormone (PTH) fragment interferes significantly with intact PTH commercial assay measurements in uremic samples. Clin Chem 44: 805–809.

8. Brossard JH, Lepage R, Cardinal H, Roy L, Rousseau L, et al. (2000) Influence of glomerular filtration rate on non-(1–84) parathyroid hormone (PTH) detected by intact PTH assays. Clin Chem 46: 697–703.

9. Vogt W (1995) Oxidation of methionyl residues in proteins: tools, targets, and reversal. Free Radic Biol Med 18: 93–105.

10. Galceran T, Lewis-Finch J, Martin KJ, Slatopolsky E (1984) Absence of biological effects of oxidized parathyroid hormone-(1–34) in dogs and rats. Endocrinology 115: 2375–2378.

11. Horiuchi N (1988) Effects of oxidation of human parathyroid hormone on its biological activity in continuously infused, thyroparathyroidectomized rats. J Bone Miner Res 3: 353–358. doi:10.1002/jbmr.5650030316.

12. Zull JE, Smith SK, Wiltshire R (1990) Effect of methionine oxidation and deletion of amino-terminal residues on the conformation of parathyroid hormone. Circular dichroism studies. J Biol Chem 265: 5671–5676.

13. Witko-Sarsat V, Friedlander M, Capeillère-Blandin C, Nguyen-Khoa T, Nguyen AT, et al. (1996) Advanced oxidation protein products as a novel marker of oxidative stress in uremia. Kidney Int 49: 1304–1313.

14. Tampe J, Broszio P, Manneck HE, Missbichler A, Blind E, et al. (1992) Characterization of antibodies against human N-terminal parathyroid hormone by epitope mapping. J Immunoassay 13: 1–13.

15. Rodriguez M, Felsenfeld AJ, Williams C, Pederson JA, Llach F (1991) The effect of long-term intravenous calcitriol administration on parathyroid function in hemodialysis patients. J Am Soc Nephrol 2: 1014–1020.

16. Felsenfeld AJ, Rodriguez M, Dunlay R, Llach F (1991) A comparison of parathyroid-gland function in haemodialysis patients with different forms of renal osteodystrophy. Nephrol Dial Transplant 6: 244–251.

17. Ramirez JA, Goodman WG, Gornbein J, Menezes C, Moulton L, et al. (1993) Direct in vivo comparison of calcium-regulated parathyroid hormone secretion in normal volunteers and patients with secondary hyperparathyroidism. J Clin Endocrinol Metab 76: 1489–1494.

18. Malberti F, Surian M, Cosci P (1992) Effect of chronic intravenous calcitriol on parathyroid function and set point of calcium in dialysis patients with refractory secondary hyperparathyroidism. Nephrol Dial Transplant 7: 822–828.

19. Messa P, Vallone C, Mioni G, Geatti O, Turrin D, et al. (1994) Direct in vivo assessment of parathyroid hormone-calcium relationship curve in renal patients. Kidney Int 46: 1713–1720.

20. Sanchez CP, Goodman WG, Ramirez JA, Gales B, Belin TR, et al. (1995) Calcium-regulated parathyroid hormone secretion in adynamic renal osteodystrophy. Kidney Int 48: 838–843.

21. Slatopolsky E, Finch J, Clay P, Martin D, Sicard G, et al. (2000) A novel mechanism for skeletal resistance in uremia. Kidney Int 58: 753–761. doi:10.1046/j.1523-1755.2000.00222.x.

22. O'Riordan JL, Woodhead JS, Hendy GN, Parsons JA, Robinson CJ, et al. (1974) Effect of oxidation on biological and immunological activity of porcine parathyroid hormone. J Endocrinol 63: 117–124.

23. Lopez MF, Rezai T, Sarracino DA, Prakash A, Krastins B, et al. (2010) Selected reaction monitoring-mass spectrometric immunoassay responsive to parathyroid hormone and related variants. Clin Chem 56: 281–290. doi:10.1373/clinchem.2009.137323.

24. Kumar V, Barnidge DR, Chen L-S, Twentyman JM, Cradic KW, et al. (2010) Quantification of serum 1–84 parathyroid hormone in patients with hyperparathyroidism by immunocapture in situ digestion liquid chromatography-tandem mass spectrometry. Clin Chem 56: 306–313. doi:10.1373/clinchem.2009.134643.

25. Chaykovska L, Tsuprykov O, Hocher B (2011) Biomarkers for the prediction of mortality and morbidity in patients with renal replacement therapy. Clin Lab 57: 455–467.

26. Garrett G, Goldsmith DJA (2012) Parathyroid hormone measurements, guidelines statements and clinical treatments: a real-world cautionary tale. Ann Clin Biochem 49: 4–6. doi:10.1258/acb.2011.011254.

27. Garrett G, Sardiwal S, Lamb EJ, Goldsmith DJ (2012) PTH–A Particularly Tricky Hormone: Why Measure It at All in Kidney Patients? Clin J Am Soc Nephrol. 2012 Mar 8. [Epub ahead of print].

16

Good Glycemic Control is Associated with Better Survival in Diabetic Patients on Peritoneal Dialysis

Dong Eun Yoo, Jung Tak Park, Hyung Jung Oh, Seung Jun Kim, Mi Jung Lee, Dong Ho Shin, Seung Hyeok Han, Tae-Hyun Yoo, Kyu Hun Choi, Shin-Wook Kang*

Department of Internal Medicine, College of Medicine, Brain Korea 21 for Medical Science, Severance Biomedical Science Institute, Yonsei University, Seoul, Korea

Abstract

Background: The effect of glycemic control after starting peritoneal dialysis (PD) on the survival of diabetic PD patients has largely been unexplored, especially in Asian population.

Methods: We conducted a prospective observational study, in which 140 incident PD patients with diabetes were recruited. Patients were divided into tertiles according to the means of quarterly HbA1C levels measured during the first year after starting PD. We examined the association between HbA1C and all-cause mortality using Cox proportional hazards models.

Results: The mean age was 58.7 years, 59.3% were male, and the mean follow-up duration was 3.5 years (range 0.4–9.5 years). The mean HbA1C levels were 6.3%, 7.1%, and 8.5% in the 1st, 2nd, and 3rd tertiles, respectively. Compared to the 1st tertile, the all-cause mortality rates were higher in the 2nd [hazard ratio (HR), 4.16; 95% confidence interval (CI), 0.91–18.94; p = 0.065] and significantly higher in the 3rd (HR, 13.16; 95% CI, 2.67–64.92; p = 0.002) tertiles (p for trend = 0.005), after adjusting for confounding factors. Cardiovascular mortality, however, did not differ significantly among the tertiles (p for trend = 0.682). In contrast, non-cardiovascular deaths, most of which were caused by infection, were more frequent in the 2nd (HR, 7.67; 95% CI, 0.68–86.37; p = 0.099) and the 3rd (HR, 51.24; 95% CI, 3.85–681.35; p = 0.003) tertiles than the 1st tertile (p for trend = 0.007).

Conclusions: Poor glycemic control is associated with high mortality rates in diabetic PD patients, suggesting that better glycemic control may improve the outcomes of these patients.

Editor: Shree Ram Singh, National Cancer Institute, United States of America

Funding: This work was supported by the Brain Korea 21 Project for Medical Science, Yonsei University, by the National Research Foundation of Korea grant funded by the Korea government (MEST) (No. 2011-0030711), and by a grant of the Korea Healthcare Technology Research & Development Project, Ministry of Health and Welfare, Republic of Korea (A102065). The funders had no role in study design, data collection and analysis, decision to publish, or preparation of the manuscript.

Competing Interests: The authors have declared that no competing interests exist.

* E-mail: kswkidney@yuhs.ac

Introduction

Diabetes mellitus (DM) is the leading cause of end-stage renal disease (ESRD) worldwide, accounting for more than 40% of incident dialysis patients in the United States [1]. To delay diabetic nephropathy from progressing and to improve outcomes for DM patients, a multidisciplinary approach is currently recommended, including glycemic control [2].

Accumulating evidences have shown that tight glycemic control prevents the development and progression of diabetic complications in both type 1 and type 2 DM patients [3–5]. In addition, high blood glucose concentrations were found to be associated with increased incidence of cardiovascular disease in diabetic patients [6]. Moreover, HbA1C levels were revealed as an independent risk factor for coronary heart disease in diabetic patients [7]. Since cardiovascular diseases are the most common cause of death in DM patients, it has been surmised that strict glucose control may be favorable to the outcome in these patients.

However, recent several randomized controlled trials have failed to demonstrate any beneficial effects of strict glycemic control on the cardiovascular morbidity and mortality in type 2 DM patients without advanced renal failure [8–10].

While many previous studies have excluded diabetic patients with advanced renal failure, only a few investigations have explored the impact of glycemic control on the prognosis of DM patients on dialysis, with inconsistent results [11–14]. An American report using a database from a large dialysis organization showed a significant correlation between the levels of HbA1C and prognosis in diabetic patients on hemodialysis (HD) [13], while another recent Canadian study found that higher blood glucose and HbA1C levels were not associated with mortality in maintenance HD patients with DM [14]. Different from HD, peritoneal dialysis (PD) results in a large amount of glucose load that is continuously absorbed from the dialysate. Therefore, glycemic control may be more difficult, and the impact of strict glycemic control on the clinical outcomes may be more obvious in diabetic PD patients, but definite evidence is furthermore lacking in these patients. To date, only one study has investigated the relationship between glycemic control after starting PD and the clinical outcomes in type 2 diabetic PD patients, in which only a few Asians were included [15]. Although there has been a study conducted in Asian population to show the association between glycemic control and patient outcomes, glycemic control before starting dialysis was used as an indicator of glycemic control [16]. In this study, we tried to determine whether glycemic control after starting PD was associated with all-cause and cardiovascular mortality in Asian diabetic PD patients.

Methods

Ethics statement

This study was approved by the Institutional Review Board for human research at Yonsei University College of Medicine, and all participants provided their written informed consent prior to study entry.

Study setting and participants

For this prospective observational study, we recruited 145 incident continuous ambulatory PD patients with DM from a single Korean dialysis center, and followed them at Yonsei University Health System in Seoul, Korea. Enrollment of patients was conducted from Jan 2001 until December 2008. The diagnosis of DM at the initiation of PD was based on the diagnostic criteria of the American Diabetes Association [17]. We excluded patients who were younger than 20 years old (n = 1), had a history of malignancy (n = 1), a history of receiving a kidney transplant (n = 1), or a history of HD for more than three months (n = 1). Patients who failed to maintain PD for more than three months were also excluded (n = 1).

Data Collection

To assess glycemic control, monthly preprandial blood glucose and quarterly HbA1C levels were collected during the first year after starting PD. However, to exclude the possibility of undue hyperglycemia, the HbA1C levels were omitted from mean HbA1C levels when measured during acute illness or when taking medications such as glucocorticoid that can affect blood glucose concentrations. Blood glucose concentrations were determined by the hexokinase-UV method and HbA1C levels were measured by high-performance liquid chromatography. The mean preprandial blood glucose and HbA1C values were used for this analysis.

The following demographic and clinical data were collected for each patient at the beginning of PD: age, gender, height, weight, body mass index (BMI), primary renal disease, duration of DM, smoking status, and comorbid conditions including hypertension, chronic lung disease, chronic liver disease, cardiovascular disease (CVD), and other serious medical illnesses. CVD included coronary artery disease, peripheral vascular disease, and cerebrovascular disease. The Charlson comorbidity index (CCI) score was used to quantify comorbid conditions [18]. Information on blood pressure and antihypertensive medications was collected at 3 months after beginning PD, when the patients' volume status had stabilized. The management of hyperglycemia was categorized into 4 groups; no medication, oral hypoglycemic agents alone, insulin alone, and combined treatment (oral hypoglycemic agents and insulin). The following laboratory data were also measured from blood samples taken 3 months after beginning PD: hemoglobin, white blood cell count, blood urea nitrogen, creatinine, albumin, calcium, phosphorus, intact parathyroid hormone (iPTH), total cholesterol, uric acid, bicarbonate, and high sensitivity c-reactive protein (hsCRP). Residual GFR was calculated as the average of urea and creatinine clearance from a 24-hour urine collection. Kt/V_{urea} was determined from the total urea nitrogen loss in the spent dialysate using the Watson equation [19], and normalized protein catabolic rate (nPCR) [20] was assessed for nutritional status.

Outcomes

Patients were classified into tertile groups, based on their average HbA1Cs during the first year after beginning PD, and prospectively followed from enrollment until death, transfer to an alternative dialysis method, or Dec 2010. Patients who transferred to HD or transplantation were censored for the patient survival analysis. The primary and secondary outcomes for all analyses were all-cause and cardiovascular mortality, respectively.

Statistical analysis

Statistical analysis was performed using SPSS version 13.0 (SPSS, Inc., Chicago, Illinois, USA). Data were basically expressed as mean ± standard deviation (SD) or percentages. Due to the log-normal distributions of hsCRP and iPTH, natural log values were used for analyses. Geometric means for all log-normally distributed continuous variables were calculated and reported with geometric SD. Results were analyzed using ANOVA or chi-square tests for comparisons. Significant differences detected by ANOVA were further confirmed by the Student's t-tests with the Bonferroni corrections. The relationships between HbA1C and preprandial blood glucose or log-transformed hsCRP (log hsCRP) levels were determined by Pearson's correlation analysis. Cox proportional hazards analysis was performed on variables revealed to be significant by univariate analysis to define the effect of HbA1C levels on mortality. A case-mix model was performed after adjusting for age, gender, year of PD start, CCI score. In the fully-adjusted model, mean arterial pressure (MAP), serum creatinine, albumin, and log hsCRP levels were further adjusted in addition to all variables used in the case-mix model. P-values less than 0.05 were considered statistically significant.

Results

Baseline characteristics and laboratory findings of patients

Of the 810 patients who began PD between January 2001 and December 2008, 145 patients had DM. After excluding 5 patients, a total of 140 patients were finally recruited in this study. The baseline characteristics of the study patients are shown in Table 1. The mean age was 58.7 years, 59.3% were male, and the mean follow-up duration was 3.5 years (range 0.4–9.5 years). The primary renal diseases were diabetic nephropathy (85.0%), chronic glomerulonephritis (7.1%), and hypertensive nephrosclerosis (4.3%) in order. Hypertension and CVD were accompanied in 139 (99.3%) and 44 (31.4%) patients, respectively. The mean systolic and diastolic blood pressures were 133.9±19.4 and 77.5±11.5 mmHg, respectively, and 75.7% of patients were taking RAS blockades. The frequency distribution of HbA1C values for all study patients is shown in Figure 1, and 47.1% of patients were within the recommended target HbA1C (less than 7%). Hypoglycemia occurred at the frequency of 1.1 events per 100 patient-year.

During the follow-up, 23 (16.4%) patients died, 28 (20.0%) were transferred to HD, and 7 (5.0%) received a kidney transplant. Cardiovascular disease (39.1%) and infection (39.1%) were the most common causes of death. Among death due to infection, PD-related infection such as PD peritonitis accounted for only 22.2% of all infection-related death, while non-PD-related causes, including pneumonia, wound infection, and necrotizing colitis, contributed to the majority of infection-related death (77.8%).

Table 1. Comparision of demographic, clinical, and laboratory characteristics in each tertile.

	n = 140	I (5.15–6.7) n = 46	II (6.8–7.5) n = 47	III (7.6–13.25) n = 47	P
Age, years (SD)	58.7±10.6	57.2±11.5	59.2±9.2	59.6±11.0	0.493
Male gender	83 (59.3%)	33 (71.7%)	30 (63.8%)	20 (42.6%)	0.012
Follow-up duration, years	3.5±2.0	3.6±1.9	3.9±2.0	3.0±1.9	0.095
Diabetes as the cause of ESRD	119 (85.0%)	37 (80.4%)	40 (85.1%)	42 (89.4%)	0.105
CVD	44 (31.4%)	18 (39.1%)	10 (21.3%)	16 (34.0%)	0.160
CCI score	5.8±1.4	5.6±1.4	5.8±1.2	6.0±1.7	0.352
Year of starting PD					0.306
2001~2004	45 (32.1%)	12 (26.1%)	14 (29.8%)	19 (40.4%)	
2005~2008	95 (67.9%)	34 (73.9%)	33 (70.2%)	28 (59.6%)	
BMI (kg/m^2)	23.2±2.7	23.4±3.0	23.4±2.4	22.8±2.8	0.489
Systolic BP (mmHg)	133.9±19.4	134.1±19.2	135.2±21.2	132.4±17.9	0.796
Diastolic BP (mmHg)	77.5±11.5	77.8±11.0	78.2±11.0	76.6±12.6	0.778
Methods of glycemic control					0.135
Insulin	55 (39.3%)	17 (37.0%)	18 (38.3%)	20 (42.6%)	
Oral hypoglycemic agent	59 (42.1%)	24 (52.2%)	20 (42.6%)	15 (31.9%)	
Combined	19 (13.6%)	3 (6.5%)	5 (10.6%)	11 (23.4%)	
No control	7 (5.0%)	2 (4.3%)	4 (8.5%)	1 (2.1%)	
Hypoglycemic event*	1.1	0.9	1.1	1.2	0.250
Hemoglobin (g/dL)	11.0±1.7	11.0±1.8	11.1±1.8	10.9±1.5	0.842
HbA1C (%)	7.3±1.1	6.3±0.3	7.1±0.3	8.5±1.1	<0.001
Preprandial glucose (mg/dL)	145.3±50.3	104.9±22.6	136.2±16.6	194.0±52.2	<0.001
Creatinine (mg/dL)	6.6±2.4	6.9±2.6	6.9±2.7	6.0±1.9	0.100
Albumin (g/dL)	3.3±0.5	3.4±0.4	3.4±0.4	3.1±0.5$^{(I,II)}$	0.003
Total cholesterol (mg/dL)	184.1±44.6	178.7±45.6	180.2±38.1	193.3±49.0	0.220
Bicarbonate (mmol/L)	27.7±3.1	27.7±3.0	27.6±3.2	28.0±3.3	0.821
Calcium (mg/dL)	8.9±0.9	8.9±1.0	9.1±0.8	8.9±0.9	0.411
Phosphorus (mg/dL)	4.2±1.0	4.4±1.0	4.2±0.9	4.0±0.9	0.125
iPTH (pg/mL)$^\#$	74.9±3.5	98.2±4.1	70.0±3.5	59.3±2.9	0.245
hsCRP (mg/L)$^\#$	1.57±5.38	1.60±5.37	1.31±5.02	1.83±5.85	0.654
Total Kt/V$_{urea}$	2.48±0.62	2.37±0.61	2.54±0.68	2.55±0.58	0.450
RRF (ml/min/1.73 m^2)	4.62±3.20	4.59±2.49	4.50±3.88	4.76±3.38	0.953
nPCR (g/kg/day)	0.97±0.21	0.95±0.21	1.04±0.21	0.94±0.20	0.120

Data are presented as mean ± SD or n (%).
$^\#$expressed as geometric mean ± geometric SD. ESRD, end-stage renal disease; CVD, cardiovascular disease; CCI, Charlson comorbidity index; PD, peritoneal dialysis; BMI, body mass index; BP, blood pressure; iPTH, intact parathyroid hormone; hsCRP, high-sensitivity C-reacitve protein; RRF, residual renal function; nPCR, normalized protein catabolic rate.
*per 100-patient year.

Correlation between preprandial blood glucose and HbA1C

Pearson's correlation analysis revealed a significant correlation between preprandial blood glucose and HbA1C concentrations, as shown in Figure 2 (r = 0.622, p<0.001). Using a linear regression model, the following formula was extracted:

$$HbA1C(\%) = preprandial\ serum\ glucose(mg/dL) \times 0.016 + 5.377$$

On the other hand, there was no significant association between HbA1C and log hsCRP levels (r = 0.029, p = 0.744).

Comparisons of clinical and biochemical parameters among patients according to HbA1C levels

To explore whether patients with good and poor glycemic control had different clinical and biochemical parameters, the study subjects were divided into tertile groups according to their mean of HbA1C levels. The mean HbA1C levels in the 1st, 2nd, and 3rd tertiles were 6.3% (range, 5.2–6.7), 7.1% (6.8–7.5), and 8.5% (7.6–13.3), respectively. The percentage of patients in each tertile with HbA1C levels within the levels recommended by the American Diabetes Association [2] were 100%, 42.6%, and 0% in the 1st, 2nd, and 3rd tertiles, respectively. The proportion of male patients was significantly higher in the 1st and 2nd tertiles than in the 3rd tertile (p<0.05). Serum albumin was significantly lower in

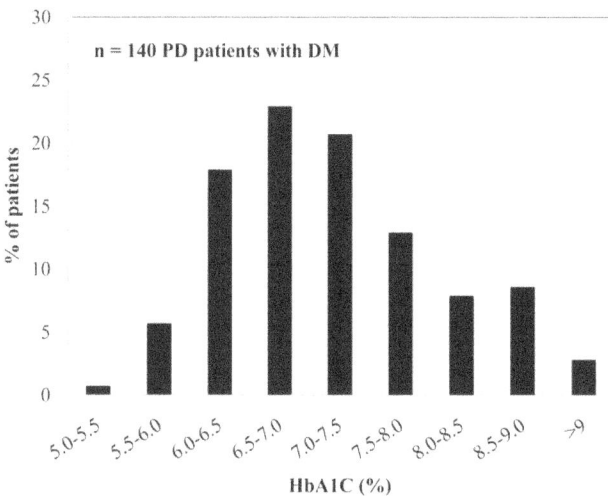

Figure 1. The frequency distribution of HbA1C values for all study patients.

Table 2. Differences in the cause of death among tertiles.

Cause of death	I	II	III	Total
Cardiovascular disease	12.2	22.0	21.3	18.5
Infection	0	16.5	42.6	18.5
Other (Malignancy, Bleeding)	6.1	11.0	7.1	8.2
All-cause	18.3	49.5	71.0	45.2

per 1000-patient-year.

more increased in the 3rd tertile. While cardiovascular disease was the most common cause of death in the 1st (12.2 per 1000-patient year) and 2nd (22.0 per 1000-patient-year) tertiles, infection was the leading cause of death in the 3rd tertile (42.6 per 1000-patient-year).

Factors influencing all-cause mortality

In univariate Cox proportional hazards analysis, age [hazard ratio (HR), 1.07 per 1 year; 95% confidence interval (CI), 1.02–1.13; p = 0.01], CCI score (HR, 1.82 per 1 point; 95% CI, 1.24–2.67; p<0.01), and log hsCRP (HR, 1.43 per 1 unit; 95% CI, 1.10–1.87; p<0.01) were significantly associated with all-cause mortality in diabetic PD patients, whereas there were significant inverse correlations between all-cause mortality and variables such as MAP (HR, 0.95 per 1 mmHg; 95% CI, 0.92–0.99; p = 0.013) and serum creatinine [HR, 0.83 per 1 mg/dL; 95% CI, 0.68–0.99; p = 0.045].

Impact of HbA1C levels on all-cause mortality

Although all-cause mortality in the 3rd tertile group was significantly higher than in the 1st tertile (HR, 4.18; 95% CI, 1.15–15.21; p = 0.030), higher HbA1C levels were not associated with all-cause mortality in the unadjusted Cox proportional hazards analysis (p for trend = 0.089) (Table 3 and Figure 3). Using case-mix and fully-adjusted models, however, there was a significant association between the mean HbA1C levels and all-cause mortality (p for trend, 0.020 and 0.005, respectively). In the case-mix model, there were 2.22- and 6.08-fold increases in the risk of all-cause mortality in the 2nd (95% CI, 0.58–8.41; p = 0.243) and the 3rd tertiles (95% CI, 1.58–23.49; p = 0.009), respectively, compared to the 1st tertile. The risk of all-cause mortality increased further in the 2nd (HR, 4.16; 95% CI, 0.91–18.94; p = 0.065) and 3rd tertiles (HR, 13.16; 95% CI, 2.67–64.92; p = 0.002) using the fully-adjusted model.

Impact of HbA1C levels on cardiovascular mortality

The risk of cardiovascular mortality was comparable among the three tertiles in the unadjusted, case-mix, and fully-adjusted models (p for trend, 0.731, 0.532, and 0.682, respectively) (Table 3 and Figure 3).

Impact of HbA1C on non-cardiovascular mortality

The risk of non-cardiovascular mortality increased in the 2nd (HR, 4.16; 95% CI, 0.49–35.65; p = 0.194) and 3rd tertiles (HR, 8.31; 95% CI, 1.02–51.57; p = 0.048) compared to the 1st tertile, but this trend failed to reach statistical significance (p for trend, 0.107). In the case-mix model, there were 3.01- and 13.03-fold increases in the risk of non-cardiovascular mortality in the 2nd (95% CI, 0.34–26.78; p = 0.323) and the 3rd tertiles (95% CI, 1.47–85.34; p = 0.021), respectively, compared to the 1st tertile (p for trend = 0.029). The risk of non-cardiovascular mortality

the 3rd tertile than the 1st tertile (p<0.05). In contrast, there were no significant differences among the three tertiles in age, proportion of diabetes as the cause of ESRD, CCI score, BMI, systolic and diastolic blood pressure, hemoglobin, creatinine, calcium, phosphorus, total cholesterol, log-transformed iPTH, and log hsCRP levels. Residual renal function, Kt/V$_{urea}$, and nPCR were also comparable among the three groups. In addition, there was no difference in the frequencies of hypoglycemic events among tertiles (Table 1).

Causes of death among patients according to HbA1C levels

The causes of death for each tertile are shown in Table 2. Overall, cardiovascular disease and infection were the most common causes of death (18.5 per 1000-patient-year for each). However, while deaths from cardiovascular diseases occurred at similar frequencies across tertiles, deaths from infection increased according to increasing HbA1C tertiles. Therefore, compare to the 1st tertile, all-cause mortality increased in the 2nd tertile and even

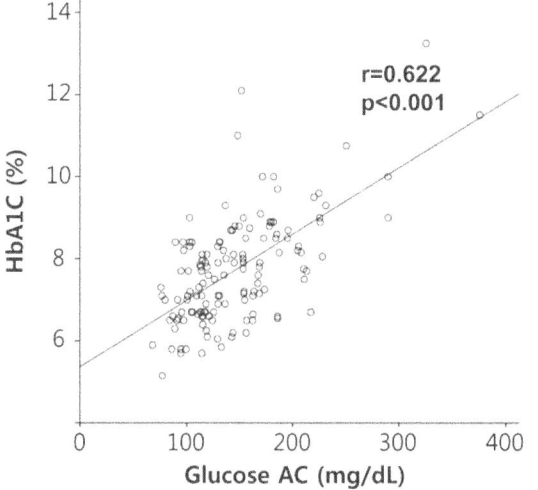

Figure 2. Bivariate correlation analysis between HbA1C and preprandial glucose (Glucose AC).

Table 3. Risk of all-cause, cardiovascular, and non-cardiovascular mortality among tertiles (n = 140).

Model	All-cause HR (95% CI)	Cardiovascular HR (95% CI)	Non-cardiovascular HR (95% CI)
Unadjusted	P for trends 0.089	P for trends 0.731	P for trends 0.107
Tertile I	1.00	1.00	1.00
Tertile II	2.55 (0.69–9.41)	1.74 (0.32–9.54)	4.16 (0.49–35.65)
Tertile III	4.18 (1.15–15.21)	2.02 (0.33–12.17)	8.31 (1.02–51.57)
Case-mix	P for trends 0.020	P for trends 0.532	P for trends 0.029
Tertile I	1.00	1.00	1.00
Tertile II	2.22 (0.58–8.41)	1.76 (0.30–10.21)	3.01 (0.34–26.78)
Tertile III	6.08 (1.58–23.49)	3.09 (0.43–22.28)	13.03 (1.47–85.34)
Fully-adjusted	P for trends 0.005	P for trends 0.682	P for trends 0.007
Tertile I	1.00	1.00	1.00
Tertile II	4.16 (0.91–18.94)	2.80 (0.28–28.40)	7.67 (0.68–86.37)
Tertile III	13.16 (2.67–64.92)	2.46 (0.15–39.67)	51.24 (3.85–340.35)

Case-mix model is adjusted for age, gender, year of PD start, Charlson comorbidity index score. Fully-adjusted model is adjusted for mean arterial pressure, albumin, serum creatinine, and log-transformed hsCRP, in addition to all variables which were used in case-mix model.

significantly increased further in the 2nd (HR, 7.67; 95% CI, 0.68–86.37; p = 0.099) and 3rd tertiles (HR, 51.24; 95% CI, 3.85–340.35; p = 0.003) using the fully-adjusted model (p for trend = 0.007), as shown in Table 3 and Figure 3.

Impact of HbA1C on clinical outcomes in diabetic PD patients, whose etiology of ESRD was diabetic nephropathy

To elucidate whether the impact of glycemic control on clinical outcomes was comparable in diabetic PD patients whose etiology of ESRD was diabetic nephropathy, we performed additional analysis with the data of these patients (n = 119). The risk of all-cause mortality was not significantly increased in the 2nd (HR, 1.40; 95% CI, 0.35–5.60; p = 0.638) and 3rd tertiles (HR, 3.69; 95% CI, 0.99–13.70; p = 0.051) compared to the 1st tertile in the unadjusted model (p for trend = 0.065). In the case-mix model, however, there were 1.2- and 4.68-fold increases in the risk of all-cause mortality in the 2nd (95% CI, 0.29–5.05; p = 0.328) and 3rd tertiles (95% CI, 1.19–18.44; p = 0.028), respectively, compared to the 1st tertile (p for trend = 0.023). The risk of all-cause mortality increased further in the 2nd (HR, 3.30; 95% CI, 0.57–19.28; p = 0.185) and 3rd tertiles (HR, 12.71; 95% CI, 2.23–42.39; p = 0.004) using the fully-adjusted model (p for trend = 0.010). Meanwhile, there was a significant increase in the risk of non-cardiovascular mortality in the 2nd (HR, 4.62; 95% CI, 0.33–44.42; p = 0.255) and 3rd tertiles (HR, 33.92; 95% CI, 2.80–120.22; p = 0.003) relative to the 1st tertile using the fully-adjusted model (p for trend = 0.006), while the risk of cardiovascular mortality was comparable among the three tertiles in the unadjusted, case-mix, and fully-adjusted models (p for trend, 0.898, 0.920, and 0.498, respectively) (Table 4).

Discussion

In this prospective observational study on 140 incident diabetic PD patients from a single center, we found that poor glycemic control was associated with increased risk of mortality in diabetic PD patients, after adjusting for confounding factors. However, there were no differences in cardiovascular mortality rates among patients with different levels of glycemic control. These findings suggest that diabetic patients on PD could benefit from strict glycemic control, even if such control may not decrease cardiovascular mortality.

Tight glycemic control has been demonstrated to prevent the development and progression of microvascular complications and to be associated with reduced risk of coronary heart disease in diabetic patients [3–5]. In addition, previous studies have shown that high blood glucose concentrations are associated with increased incidence of cardiovascular diseases in patients with DM [6,7]. Based on these findings, it has been supposed that strict glucose control could exert a beneficial impact on the survival and cardiovascular outcome in diabetic patients, drawing up current guidelines of a target HbA1C level of 7.0% or less for most DM patients. Against these expectations, however, several recent studies showed that there was no beneficial effect of tight glycemic control on the cardiovascular morbidity and mortality in type 2 DM patients without advanced renal failure [8–10].

Findings regarding the impact of glycemic control on the outcomes of DM patients on dialysis have also been inconsistent. An analysis of 23,618 American diabetic HD patients showed that the adjusted risk for all-cause mortality in patients with HbA1C ≥10.0% was 1.41-higher than patients with HbA1C in the 5–6% range [13]. Most previous studies including East Asian diabetic patients on HD also found that poor glycemic control was associated with reduced survival, which agrees with the results of our study [11,21]. In contrast, a recent study by Shurraw et al [14] showed that higher blood glucose and HbA1C levels were not associated with mortality in 1,484 incident HD patients in Canada. These conflicitng results may be attributed to the differences in ethnicity, body size, the duration of dialysis, and the definition of good glycemic control.

Meanwhile, there has been only one study conducted among PD patients, and it has revealed that poor glycemic control was associated with poor survival in diabetic PD patients [15]. However, few Asian patients were included in that study, and the impact of glycemic control on patient outcomes among Asian diabetic PD patients is still unclear. Although another report by Wu et al [16], which was conducted among Asian PD patients, revealed that glycemic control before starting dialysis was a predictor of survival for type 2 diabetic patients on PD, the importance of glycemic control after starting dialysis was not evaluated. Since PD fluid contains extremely high concentrations of glucose, we hypothesized that the glycemic control in PD patients would be different from the predialysis state. Therefore, we determined glycemic control by using average HbA1C levels during the 1st year after beginning PD, which were supposed to better reflect overall serum glucose concentrations. To exclude the possibility of improper hyperglycemia, moreover, the HbA1C levels around the time of acute illness or when taking medications that could affect serum glucose concentrations were omitted from the mean HbA1C levels.

In this study, poor glycemic control was associated with deleterious outcomes but not cardiovascular mortality which is the most common cause of death in ESRD patients undergoing dialysis. Consistent with these results, most previous studies have failed to demonstrate that good glycemic control improves cardiovascular survival in patients with long duration of DM [8–10]. Since most diabetic ESRD patients already have advanced microvascular and macrovascular complications, there might be a "point of no return", after which patient outcomes are not affected

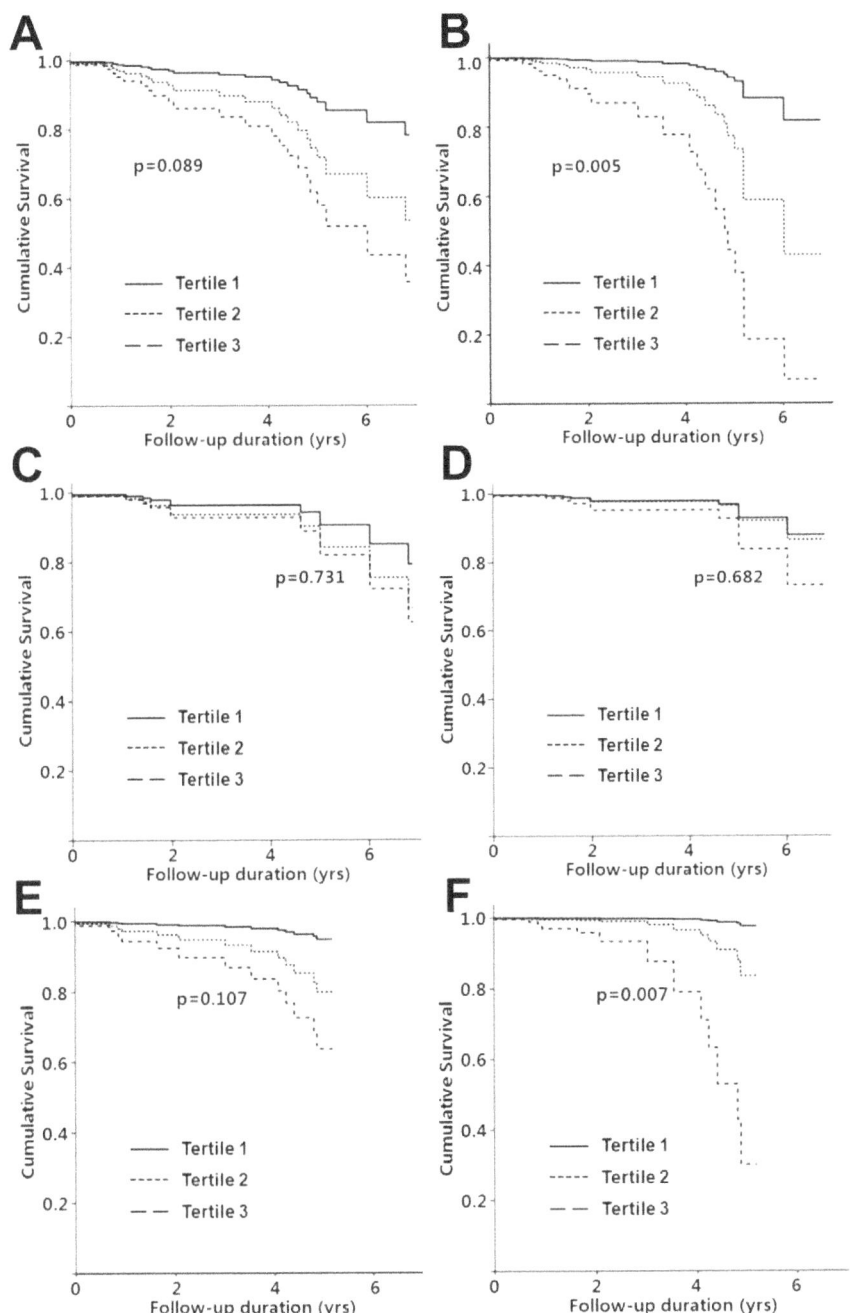

Figure 3. Comparison of cumulative survival among tertiles, plotted by Cox proportional hazards analysis. (A–B) Comparison of all-cause mortality among tertiles in unadjusted (A) and fully-adjusted model (B). (C–D) Comparison of cardiovascular mortality among tertiles in unadjusted (C) and fully-adjusted model (D). (E–F) Comparison of non-cardiovascular mortality among tertiles in unadjusted (E) and fully-adjusted model (F).

by strict glycemic control. Is it also relevant for diabetic ESRD patients whose primary renal diagnosis is not diabetic nephropathy? To answer this issue, we performed an additional subgroup analysis in patients whose primary renal disease was diabetic nephropathy. In result, the all-cause and non-cardiovascular mortality was also significantly higher in the 3rd tertile group compared to the 1st tertile group, whereas the risk of cardiovascular mortality was not different among groups, which were similar to the results with all diabetic PD patients. Therefore, it is surmised that "point of no return" theory can be applied at least to

PD patients in whom the etiology of ESRD was diabetic nephropathy. Meanwhile, a previous American report [13] observed a significantly higher cardiovascular mortality in patients with HbA1C ≥10.0%, while the rates were comparable among patients with HbA1C levels between 5.0% and 10.0%, suggesting that only extremely uncontrolled hyperglycemia may affect cardiovascular outcomes. Only 4 patients (2.8%) in our study sample had mean HbA1C levels greater than 10.0%, and therefore this effect might not be reflected in our study. There is also another possibility that "survival bias" could be involved in

Table 4. Risk of all-cause, cardiovascular, and non-cardiovascular mortality among tertiles in patients whose etiology of ESRD was diabetic nephropathy (n = 119).

Model	All-cause HR (95% CI)	Cardiovascular HR (95% CI)	Non-cardiovascular HR (95% CI)
Unadjusted	P for trends 0.065	P for trends 0.898	P for trends 0.107
Tertile I	1.00	1.00	1.00
Tertile II	1.40 (0.35–5.60)	1.13 (0.19–6.80)	4.16 (0.49–35.65)
Tertile III	3.69 (0.99–13.70)	0.65 (0.06–7.57)	8.31 (1.02–67.57)
Case-mix	P for trends 0.023	P for trends 0.920	P for trends 0.013
Tertile I	1.00	1.00	1.00
Tertile II	1.21 (0.29–5.05)	1.47 (0.23–9.56)	1.43 (0.14–14.47)
Tertile III	4.68 (1.19–18.44)	1.40 (0.10–19.97)	9.22 (1.10–77.37)
Fully-adjusted	P for trends 0.010	P for trends 0.498	P for trends 0.005
Tertile I	1.00	1.00	1.00
Tertile II	3.30 (0.57–19.28)	1.29 (0.28–14.54)	4.62 (0.33–44.42)
Tertile III	12.71 (2.23–42.39)	0.60 (0.10–28.57)	33.92 (2.80–120.22)

Case-mix model is adjusted for age, gender, year of PD start, Charlson comorbidity index score. Fully-adjusted model is adjusted for mean arterial pressure, albumin, serum creatinine, and log-transformed hsCRP, in addition to all variables which were used in case-mix model.

the results of cardiovascular mortality. In our study subjects, CVD was less in tertile II (21.3%), as compared with tertile I (39.1%) and tertile III (34.0%). One explanation to this observation is that patients with moderate glycemic control died of cardiovascular events even before starting PD and reaching at poorer glycemic states, and those who have reached to the 3rd tertile survived from any cardiovascular events.

This study revealed that patients with poor glycemic control had significantly higher non-cardiovascular mortality, mainly due to infection. Similarly, a Taiwanese study [16] and another Korean study on diabetic PD patients [22] also found that the proportion of mortality from infection was high and comparable to that from cardiovascular diseases in their subjects, which raises several questions. Why is there a difference in the proportion of mortality from infection between diabetic HD and PD patients? Why infection-related mortality is influenced by the degree of glycemic control? While the answers are not clear, mounting evidence has shown that diabetic PD patients may be more vulnerable to infections. Frequently exchanging PD fluid could eliminate or dilute phagocytes and immunoglobulins normally present in the peritoneal cavity. In fact, the amount of removed immunoglobulin G and C3 through PD is reported to be significantly greater in DM than non-diabetic patients [23]. Moreover, hypertonic glucose solution used for PD could make patients susceptible to infection, especially in diabetic patients. It is well known that 60 to 80% of glucose in dialysate is systemically absorbed by diffusion and lymphatic absorption during a 6-hour dwell, which makes

strict glycemic control more difficult in PD patients. These local and systemic hyperglycemic conditions have been suggested to be able to modify cytokine production and phagocytotic activity of immune cells by several mechansims, including hyperosmotic stress [24]. Furthermore, the production of advanced glycation endproducts can increase under hyperglycemic conditions, resulting in increased interaction between advanced glycation endproducts and their receptors, which can in turn increase inflammatory response [25].

Several shortcomings of this study should be discussed. First, as a single center study, it is subject to the biases inherent to this study design. In addition, 145 patients out of the total incident PD patients (n = 810) had diabetes, which corresponds to only 18% of incident PD patients. Considering the fact that 35 to 40% of incident ESRD patients in Korea from 2001 to 2009 had diabetes [26], we could not completely affirm that there was no selection bias even though it was not intentional. We surmise that the discrepancy in the proportion of DM patients between incident HD and PD patients in our institute may be partially attributed to our physician's tendency to hesitate to perform PD in DM patients, especially in whom predialysis blood glucose control was not appropriate. In fact, only 2.8% of this study subjects had mean HbA1C greater than 10.0%, which was much lower than 6.6% of enrolled patients in an American report [15]. Second, besides serum glucose and HbA1C levels, laboratory values at 3 months after starting PD were used for analyses in most cases. Therefore, the changes of confounding factors during the follow-up were not reflected. Third, diabetic ESRD patients, whose cause of ESRD was not diabetic nephropathy, could have different response to poor glycemic control. However, due to a small number of these patients (n = 21), subgroup analysis was not able to be performed for this issue. Lastly, there are some limitations for using HbA1C levels as a surrogate marker of glycemic control in dialysis patients. However, tests for better surrogate markers such as glycoalbumin are not widely performed and have been available in our institute only after 2009.

In conclusion, this study demonstrated that poor glycemic control was associated with higher all-cause mortality, mainly non-cardiovascular mortality represented by infection-related deaths, in diabetic PD patients. These findings suggest that better glycemic control may improve the outcome of these patients. Clinical trials are needed to better examine the impact of strict glycemic control on survival in diabetic PD patients.

Acknowledgments

The authors acknowledge our gratitude to the patients who participated in this study. The abstract of this study was presented as a poster at the American Society of Nephrology Annual Meeting 2011, Philadelphia, PA, U.S.A.

Author Contributions

Conceived and designed the experiments: DEY JTP. Analyzed the data: SHH T-HY KHC. Contributed reagents/materials/analysis tools: HJO SJK MJL DHS. Wrote the paper: DEY S-WK.

References

1. United States Renal Data System (2010) Atlas of End-Stage Renal Disease in the United States - Introduction. Am J Kidney Dis 52: S212.
2. American Diabetes Association (2011) Standards of medical care in diabetes-2011. Diabetes Care 34 Suppl 1: S11–61.
3. The Diabetes Control and Complications Trial Research Group (1993) The effect of intensive treatment of diabetes on the development and progression of long-term complications in insulin-dependent diabetes mellitus. N Engl J Med 329: 977–986.
4. UK Prospective Diabetes Study Group (1998) Intensive blood-glucose control with sulphonylureas or insulin compared with conventional treatment and risk of complications in patients with type 2 diabetes (UKPDS 33). UK Prospective Diabetes Study (UKPDS) Group. Lancet 352: 837–853.

5. Ohkubo Y, Kishikawa H, Araki E, Miyata T, Isami S, et al. (1995) Intensive insulin therapy prevents the progression of diabetic microvascular complications in Japanese patients with non-insulin-dependent diabetes mellitus: a randomized prospective 6-year study. Diabetes Res Clin Pract 28: 103–117.

6. Wei M, Gaskill SP, Haffner SM, Stern MP (1998) Effects of diabetes and level of glycemia on all-cause and cardiovascular mortality. The San Antonio Heart Study. Diabetes Care 21: 1167–1172.

7. Selvin E, Marinopoulos S, Berkenblit G, Rami T, Brancati FL, et al. (2004) Meta-analysis: glycosylated hemoglobin and cardiovascular disease in diabetes mellitus. Ann Intern Med 141: 421–431.

8. Gerstein HC, Miller ME, Byington RP, Goff DC, Jr., Bigger JT, et al. (2008) Effects of intensive glucose lowering in type 2 diabetes. N Engl J Med 358: 2545–2559.

9. Duckworth W, Abraira C, Moritz T, Reda D, Emanuele N, et al. (2009) Glucose control and vascular complications in veterans with type 2 diabetes. N Engl J Med 360: 129–139.

10. Patel A, MacMahon S, Chalmers J, Neal B, Billot L, et al. (2008) Intensive blood glucose control and vascular outcomes in patients with type 2 diabetes. N Engl J Med 358: 2560–2572.

11. Oomichi T, Emoto M, Tabata T, Morioka T, Tsujimoto Y, et al. (2006) Impact of glycemic control on survival of diabetic patients on chronic regular hemodialysis: a 7-year observational study. Diabetes Care 29: 1496–1500.

12. Williams ME, Lacson E, Jr., Teng M, Ofsthun N, Lazarus JM (2006) Hemodialyzed type I and type II diabetic patients in the US: Characteristics, glycemic control, and survival. Kidney Int 70: 1503–1509.

13. Kalantar-Zadeh K, Kopple JD, Regidor DL, Jing J, Shinaberger CS, et al. (2007) A1C and survival in maintenance hemodialysis patients. Diabetes Care 30: 1049–1055.

14. Shurraw S, Majumdar SR, Thadhani R, Wiebe N, Tonelli M (2010) Glycemic control and the risk of death in 1,484 patients receiving maintenance hemodialysis. Am J Kidney Dis 55: 875–884.

15. Duong U, Mehrotra R, Molnar MZ, Noori N, Kovesdy CP, et al. (2011) Glycemic control and survival in peritoneal dialysis patients with diabetes mellitus. Clin J Am Soc Nephrol 6: 1041–1048.

16. Wu MS, Yu CC, Wu CH, Haung JY, Leu ML, et al. (1999) Pre-dialysis glycemic control is an independent predictor of mortality in type II diabetic patients on continuous ambulatory peritoneal dialysis. Perit Dial Int 19 Suppl 2: S179–183.

17. Genuth S, Alberti KG, Bennett P, Buse J, Defronzo R, et al. (2003) Follow-up report on the diagnosis of diabetes mellitus. Diabetes Care 26: 3160–3167.

18. Charlson ME, Pompei P, Ales KL, MacKenzie CR (1987) A new method of classifying prognostic comorbidity in longitudinal studies: development and validation. J Chronic Dis 40: 373–383.

19. Watson PE, Watson ID, Batt RD (1980) Total body water volumes for adult males and females estimated from simple anthropometric measurements. Am J Clin Nutr 33: 27–39.

20. Blagg CR (1991) Importance of nutrition in dialysis patients. Am J Kidney Dis 17: 458–461.

21. Morioka T, Emoto M, Tabata T, Shoji T, Tahara H, et al. (2001) Glycemic control is a predictor of survival for diabetic patients on hemodialysis. Diabetes Care 24: 909–913.

22. Chung SH, Han DC, Noh H, Jeon JS, Kwon SH, et al. (2010) Risk factors for mortality in diabetic peritoneal dialysis patients. Nephrol Dial Transplant 25: 3742–3748.

23. Krediet RT, Zuyderhoudt FM, Boeschoten EW, Arisz L (1986) Peritoneal permeability to proteins in diabetic and non-diabetic continuous ambulatory peritoneal dialysis patients. Nephron 42: 133–140.

24. Wade CE (2008) Hyperglycemia may alter cytokine production and phagocytosis by means other than hyperosmotic stress. Crit Care 12: 182.

25. Bopp C, Bierhaus A, Hofer S, Bouchon A, Nawroth PP, et al. (2008) Bench-to-bedside review: The inflammation-perpetuating pattern-recognition receptor RAGE as a therapeutic target in sepsis. Crit Care 12: 201.

26. Jin DC (2011) Current status of dialysis therapy in Korea. Korean J Intern Med 26: 123–131.

17

Sensitive Troponins – Which Suits Better for Hemodialysis Patients? Associated Factors and Prediction of Mortality

Ferruh Artunc[1]*, Christian Mueller[2], Tobias Breidthardt[2], Raphael Twerenbold[2], Andreas Peter[1], Claus Thamer[1], Peter Weyrich[1], Hans-Ulrich Haering[1], Bjoern Friedrich[1,3]

1 Department of Internal Medicine, Division of Endocrinology, Diabetology, Vascular Disease, Nephrology and Clinical Chemistry, University of Tuebingen, Germany, 2 Department of Internal Medicine, Division of Cardiology, University of Basel, Basel, Switzerland, 3 Dialysis Center, Leonberg, Germany

Abstract

Background: In hemodialysis patients, elevated plasma troponin concentrations are a common finding that has even increased with the advent of newly developed sensitive assays. However, the interpretation and relevance of this is still under debate.

Methods: In this cross-sectional study, we analyzed plasma concentrations of sensitive troponin I (TnI) and troponin T (TnT) in stable ambulatory hemodialysis patients (n = 239) and investigated their associations with clinical factors and mortality.

Results: In all of the enrolled patients, plasma TnI or TnT was detectable at a median concentration of 14 pg/ml (interquartile range: 7–29) using the Siemens TnI ultra assay and 49 pg/ml (31–74) using the Roche Elecsys high sensitive TnT assay. Markedly more patients exceeded the 99th percentile for TnT than for TnI (95% vs. 14%, p<0.0001). In a multivariate linear regression model, TnT was independently associated with age, gender, systolic dysfunction, time on dialysis, residual diuresis and systolic blood pressure, whereas TnI was independently associated with age, systolic dysfunction, pulse pressure, time on dialysis and duration of a HD session. During a follow-up period of nearly two years, TnT concentration above 38 pg/mL was associated with a 5-fold risk of death, whereas elevation of TnI had a gradual association to mortality.

Conclusion: In hemodialysis patients, elevations of plasma troponin concentrations are explained by cardiac function and dialysis-related parameters, which contribute to cardiac strain. Both are highly predictive of increased risk of death.

Editor: Wolf-Hagen Schunck, Max Delbrueck Center for Molecular Medicine, Germany

Funding: These authors have no support or funding to report.

Competing Interests: The authors have declared that no competing interests exist.

* E-mail: ferruh.artunc@med.uni-tuebingen.de

Introduction

Elevations of cardiac troponins in the plasma define are indicative of myocardial injury and necrosis [1]. According to the universal definition of myocardial infarction (MI) published in 2007, MI can be diagnosed based on a rise and fall in the plasma troponin concentrations above the 99th percentile when there is evidence of myocardial ischemia [2]. However, in patients with end-stage renal failure (ESRD), chronic elevations at the subclinical level have been shown to occur without signs of myocardial ischemia [3–5]. Several longitudinal studies have consistently shown that elevated troponin concentrations in ESRD patients add prognostic information and are associated with increased mortality [6–10]. A meta-analysis concluded that increases in plasma troponin T or troponin I concentrations conferred a 2.64 or 1.74-fold increase, respectively, in mortality risk in ESRD patients [11]. The current view is that an elevated troponin concentration reflects chronic myocardial strain and damage during the course of renal failure and ESRD [12] rather

than reduced clearance [13] or cross-reactivity with troponins from skeletal muscle [14,15]. The cardiac work load of ESRD patients is greatly increased by several conditions, such as hypertension, shunt flow, chronic extracellular volume expansion, anemia or increased pulse pressure. These factors induce profound alterations in cardiac structure [16] and may lead to subsequent troponin release. In addition to a chronically increased cardiac work load, acute hemodialysis sessions induce cardiac stress due to circulatory alterations and may trigger myocardial stunning [17].

Typically, plasma troponin concentrations in ESRD patients are slightly elevated above the 99th percentile touching the lower detection limit of many troponin assays employed in routine diagnostics. At this point, the analytical precision of conventional troponin measurements is reduced, and the coefficient of variation (CV) can reach 10–20% [18]. To overcome this problem, sensitive assays with a CV of <10% at the 99th percentile have been developed and have shown improved accuracy in the diagnosis of MI [19]. Some of these tests can be designated as highly sensitive based on a high proportion (>50%) of subjects with measurable

Table 1. Patient characteristics of the cohort (n = 239).

median age		70 (61; 77) years (n = 239)
gender distribution		64% male (n = 153)/36% female (n = 86)
renal disease	diabetic nephropathy	26% (n = 63)
	hypertension	8% (n = 19)
	glomerulonephritis	30% (n = 71)
	polycystic disease	5% (n = 11)
	other/unknown	31% (n = 75)
cardiac comorbidities	coronary heart disease	31% (n = 74)
	revascularized	19% (n = 31)
	valvular heart disease	26% (n = 61)
	atrial fibrillation	23% (n = 55)
	pulmonary hypertension	7% (n = 16)
	AICD carrier	2% (n = 4)
other comorbidities	diabetes mellitus	38% (n = 90)
	peripheral vascular disease	33% (n = 80)
	stroke	16% (n = 38)
	vasculitis	3% (n = 8)
	malignoma	14% (n = 34)
	COPD	8% (n = 19)
length of time on dialysis		46 (19; 85) months (n = 239)
duration of dialysis session		4.0 (4.0; 4.5) hours (n = 239)
dialysis access	arteriovenous fistula	71% (n = 169)
	PTFE graft	13% (n = 31)
	tunneled catheter	16% (n = 38)
dialysis membrane	high-flux	92% (n = 219)
	low-flux	8% (n = 20)
residual diuresis		250 (0; 1000) mL/day (n = 239)
anuric patients		39% (n = 93)
interdialytic weight gain		1.85 (1.29; 2.47) kg (n = 239)
blood pump speed		300 (280; 340) mL/min (n = 239)
shunt flow		1080 (733; 1475) mL/min (n = 187)
blood pressure		134 (122; 144)/69 (63; 74) mm Hg (n = 239)
pulse pressure		65 (54; 74) mm Hg (n = 239)
singe pool Kt/V		1.55 (1.40; 1.73) (n = 239)
laboratory data	hemoglobin	11.5 (11.1; 12.0) g/dL (n = 239)
	C-reactive protein	8.6 (4.6; 15.0) mg/L (n = 239)
	albumin	37.1 (35.4; 39.3) g/L (n = 239)
	parathormone	204 (130; 348) pg/mL (n = 239)
	β2-microglobulin	23.4 (19.4; 25.4) mg/L (n = 239)
LV systolic function	normal	59% (n = 140)
	mildly reduced	13% (n = 32)
	moderately or severely reduced	12% (n = 29)
	unknown	16% (n = 38)

Values shown are the median and interquartile range. N indicates number of patients from which data were available.
abbreviations:
PTFE = polytetrafluorethylene, LV = left ventricle, AICD = automated implantable cardioverter-defibrillator.

values that fall below the 99th percentile [18,20]. Currently, only few clinically available assays, such as the Roche Elecsys high sensitive (hs) TnT, fulfill this criterion [18]. There are only a few studies that have applied sensitive troponin assays in ESRD patients [21–23]. In one study, sensitive troponin T was found to be the most powerful predictor of mortality in ESRD patients among other established cardiac biomarkers [22].

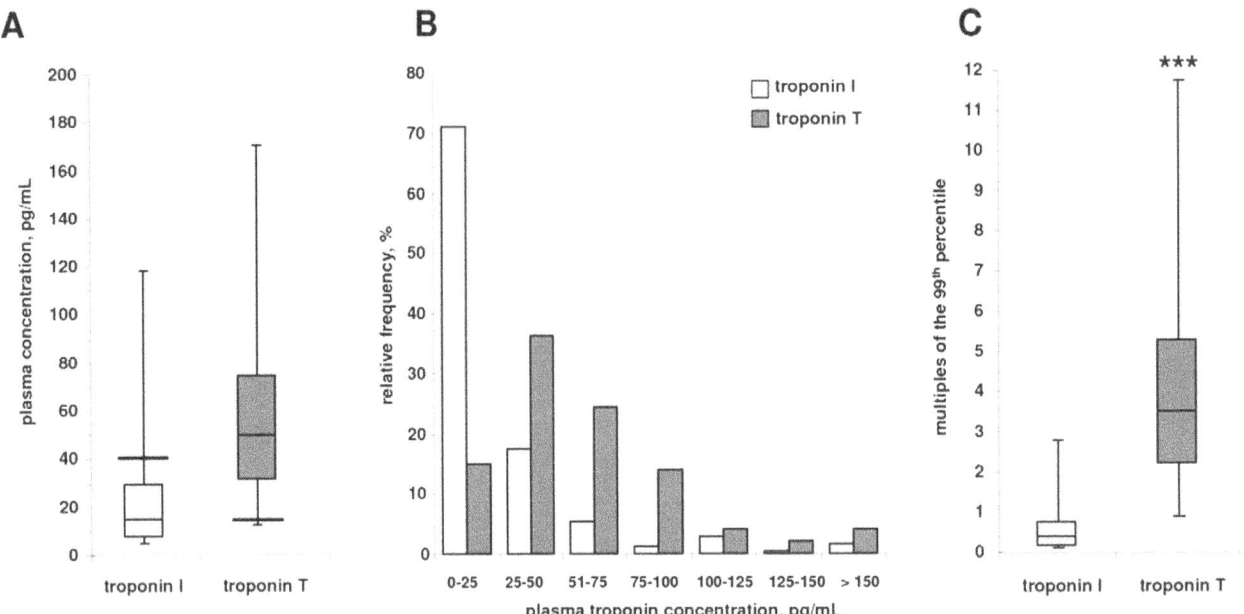

Figure 1. Depiction of the plasma troponin I and T concentrations in the cohort. A Box-and-Whiskers-Plot of the plasma troponin I and T concentrations indicating the median, interquartile range and the range between the 2.5th and 97.5th percentile. Solid lines represent the 99th percentile of the assay [19]. **B** Distribution of the plasma troponin I and T concentrations in the cohort (n = 239). **C** Box-and-Whiskers-Plot of the plasma troponin I and T concentrations expressed as multiples of the 99th percentile [19]. *** indicates a significant difference (p<0.0001) between the troponin T and troponin I concentrations.

With the advent of sensitive assays, cardiac troponins are now detected to a larger extent in hemodialysis patients raising questions about interpretation and relevance to nephrologists and cardiologists alike. The increased sensitivity and resolution of the assays, however, also improve the chance to identify factors that are associated with elevated plasma troponin concentrations, such as loss of residual renal function [24] or volume overload [25], both of which contribute to cardiac strain and are predictive of increased mortality. Since both troponins (I and T) can be measured with sensitive assays, results might also reflect different biochemical properties. Therefore, we measured both troponin I and T with sensitive assays in a comparative approach to investigate associated factors and to analyze the diagnostic performance in predicting death during a follow-up period of two years.

Methods

Patients and cohort

This cross-sectional, prospective multicenter study was conducted in stable, ambulatory hemodialysis patients from four dialysis centers in southwest Germany between September 2009 and April 2010. Patients without evidence of an acute illness and cardiac event or procedure within two months were included in the study after providing written informed consent. Patients with cardiac diseases leading to increased plasma troponin concentrations independent of ESRD, such as amyloidosis, were excluded. The study was approved by the local ethics committee of the University hospital Tuebingen.

Laboratory assays

Plasma concentrations of troponin I and troponin T were measured in three independent samples collected within two weeks. Each sample was collected prior to the start of a dialysis

Table 2. Univariate correlations (Pearson's r) of the plasma troponin concentration with general and dialysis-specific parameters (n = 210–239).

	troponin I, pg/ml	troponin T, pg/ml
age, y	0.32 ***	0.43 ***
systolic LVF, classes	0.44 ***	0.38 ***
time on dialysis, months	0.15 *	0.18 **
residual diuresis, ml/day	−0.13 *	−0.29 ***
interdialytic weight gain, kg	0.13 *	0.25 **
shunt flow, ml/min	−0.16 *	−0.14 #
systolic blood pressure, mm Hg	0.11 #	n.s.
diastolic blood pressure, mm Hg	−0.13 *	−0.19 **
pulse pressure, mm Hg	0.21 *	0.22 **
duration of a HD session	n.s.	n.s.
blood pump speed, ml/min	n.s.	0.15 *
Kt/V	n.s.	n.s.
hemoglobin, g/dL	n.s.	n.s.
plasma albumin, g/L	n.s.	n.s.
C-reactive protein, mg/L	n.s.	0.21 **
parathormone, pg/mL	0.16 *	0.14 *
β2-microglobulin, mg/dL	n.s	n.s.

#p<0.10, * p<0.05, ** p<0.01, *** p<0.001, n.s. = not significant (p>0.10).

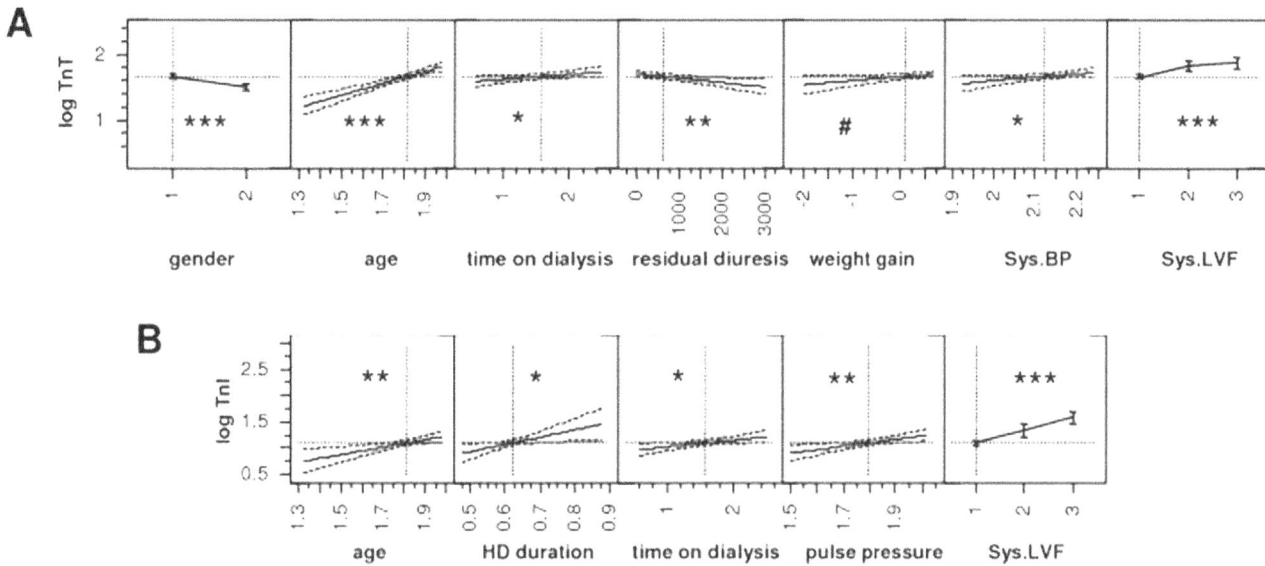

Figure 2. Plot showing the influence of single predictors in the multivariate model for troponin T (A) and troponin I (B). # p<0.10, * p<0.05, ** p<0.01, *** p<0.001.

session. Blood was collected in lithium-heparinized tubes (Sarstedt, Nuembrecht, Germany), cooled at 4°C, and centrifuged within 4 hours. The sera were stored at −80°C until further analysis. Plasma concentrations of troponin I were measured using the Troponin I Ultra assay on a Siemens ADVIA Centaur system (Siemens Healthcare Diagnostics, Eschborn, Germany) with a detection limit of 6 pg/ml, a 99th percentile at 40 pg/ml, and a CV of less than 10% at 30 pg/ml, as specified by the manufacturer. Plasma concentrations of troponin T were measured using an automated Roche assay on an Elecsys 2010 system with a detection limit of 2 pg/ml, a 99th percentile at 14 pg/ml, and a coefficient of variation of less than 10% at 13 pg/ml [19]. Plasma beta-2-microglobulin concentrations were measured using a turbidimetric assay (Randox Laboratories, Antrim,

United Kingdom) on a Siemens ADVIA 1800 system with a measurable range between 0.56–20.9 mg/l and an upper reference concentration of 3 mg/l [26]. All other laboratory values (parathormone, hemoglobin, albumin and C-reactive protein) were extracted from the patients' medical records and represent an average of the available values from the previous year (4–12 values).

Clinical data

The following data were extracted from each patient: residual diuresis, as measured by 24 h urine collection: single pool Kt/V (mean of the most recent 4 values collected), interdialytic weight gain, predialytic systolic and diastolic blood pressure (mean of the most recent 12 values), dialysis access and membrane, length of

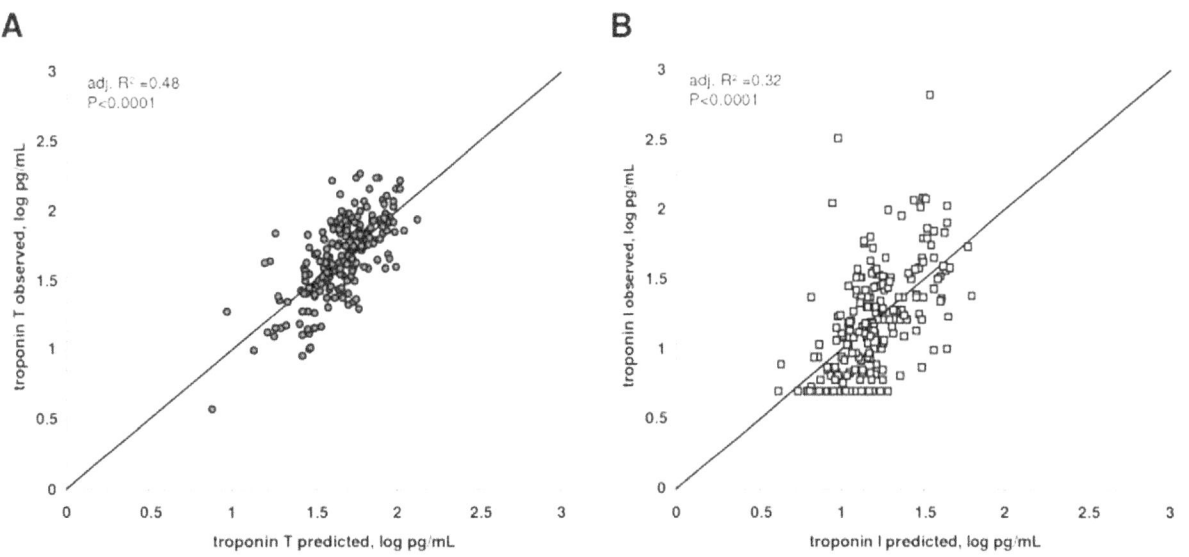

Figure 3. Agreement between predicted and observed log troponin I and T concentrations. Plot of the predicted and observed troponin values for troponin T (**A**) and troponin I (**B**) as a result of the models shown in table 4. The diagonal line represents the line of identity.

Table 3. Independent factors determining plasma troponin concentrations by multivariate linear modeling (n = 201).

	covariate	estimate ± SD	standardized estimate ± SD	p-value
troponin T, pg/ml	y-intercept	−1.25±0.61	1.59±0.02	0.0410
	age, y	0.84±0.14	0.27±0.05	<.0001
	systolic LVF, classes [2 vs. 1]	0.14±0.04	0.14±0.04	0.0016
	systolic blood pressure, mmHg	0.55±0.27	0.09±0.04	0.0432
	residual diuresis, ml/24 h	$-6\ 10^{-5}\pm2\ 10^{-5}$	-0.09±0.03	0.0050
	gender [1 = male]	0.08±0.02	0.08±0.02	<.0001
	interdialytic weight gain, kg	0.06±0.03	0.07±0.04	0.0688
	time on dialysis. months	0.08±0.04	0.07±0.04	0.0395
	systolic LVF, classes [3 vs. 2]	0.04±0.27	0.06±0.06	0.4715
	atrial fibrillatiom [1 = yes]	0.08±0.04	0.04±0.02	0.0324
troponin I, pg/ml	y-intercept	−2.32±0.69	1.10±0.03	0.0009
	duration of a HD session, h	1.30±0.58	0.26±0.12	0.0274
	systolic LVF, classes [3 vs. 2]	0.22±0.07	0.25±0.08	0.0042
	systolic LVF, classes [2 vs. 1]	0.25±0.08	0.22±0.07	0.0013
	age, y	0.62±0.24	0.20±0.08	0.0104
	pulse pressure, mm Hg	0.71±0.24	0.18±0.06	0.0032
	time on dialysis, months	0.11±0.06	0.11±0.05	0.0410
	valvular disease [1 = yes]	0.10±0.06	0.05±0.03	0.0767

time on dialysis, blood pump flow and shunt flow measured using a Transonic system (Ithaca, NY, USA). The left ventricular (LV) systolic function was classified from available echocardiography examinations in which class 1 indicated normal function, 2 was mildly reduced, and 3 was moderately or severely reduced. Determination of the LV systolic function was done at the discretion of the cardiologist and not standardized. Echocardiography was available in 84% of all patients within one year (plus-minus) relative to study enrollment.

Statistical analysis

Three samples were available in 87% of the patients and were averaged to calculate the arithmetic mean without excluding possible outliers. For further analysis, plasma troponin concentrations and continuous clinical data were log transformed to approximate normal distribution. The association of the plasma troponin concentrations with clinical or dialysis-related factors was analyzed by univariate parametric correlation. Multivariate linear regression analyses were performed to identify independent determinants of the plasma troponin concentrations. Selection of the variables entering the model were derived from forward, stepwise multiple linear regression, and all variables with a p-value <0.05 were included in the multivariate linear regression models. The residuals of each model were tested for normality. Averaged values of the deceased patients were compared to those from the surviving patients using t-Test or Wilcoxon's test. Kaplan-Meier curves were generated after stratification into tertiles of the variable according to its distribution. The follow-up period started on the first day of blood draw and was censored as of 31 December 2011. The diagnostic performance was analyzed using receiver-operator curves (ROC or c-index) and the best cut-off value was considered as the maximal difference of sensitivity and 1-specificity (Youden index). C-Index was calculated using Wessa, P. (2012), Free Statistics Software, Office for Research Develop-

ment and Education, version 1.1.23-r7, http://www.wessa.net/. Univariate and multivariate proportional hazards were calculated to analyze the risk ratios of each predictor and the independence of the predictors. Data analysis was performed using the statistical software package JMP 10.0.1 (SAS Institute, Cary, NC).

Results

Patients

Of the n = 250 available patients that were treated in the participating centers, n = 239 were included in the study. The reasons for exclusion of the n = 11 patients were the following: patients declined to participate (n = 6), deaths occurred following the initial plasma collection (n = 2), cardiac amyloidosis (n = 2) and a recent enrollment in dialysis (n = 1). The characteristics of the study cohort are provided in table 1. Participants were primarily geriatric, with a median age of 70. They had been in a dialysis-dependent state for a median of 45 months and were dialyzed mainly using an arteriovenous (AV) fistula (71%) or a high flux membrane (95%). The dialysis sessions, which lasted 4 hours, had a Kt/V value above the recommended K/DOQI target value of 1.3. Median shunt flow was approximately 1 L/min. Residual diuresis was low (median of 250 ml/day), and 39% of the patients were anuric. The median plasma albumin concentration was slightly below the recommended KDOQI target of 40 g/L, although hemoglobin and parathormone levels were within the target range. Plasma β2-microglobulin concentrations were highly elevated (median concentration of 23.5 mg/L), indicating an accumulation due to reduced renal and low dialysis-driven clearance.

Cardiac comorbidities were present in a large proportion of the patients. Ischemic heart disease was the most frequent condition (31%). Systolic LV dysfunction was found in 26% of all of the patients (table 1).

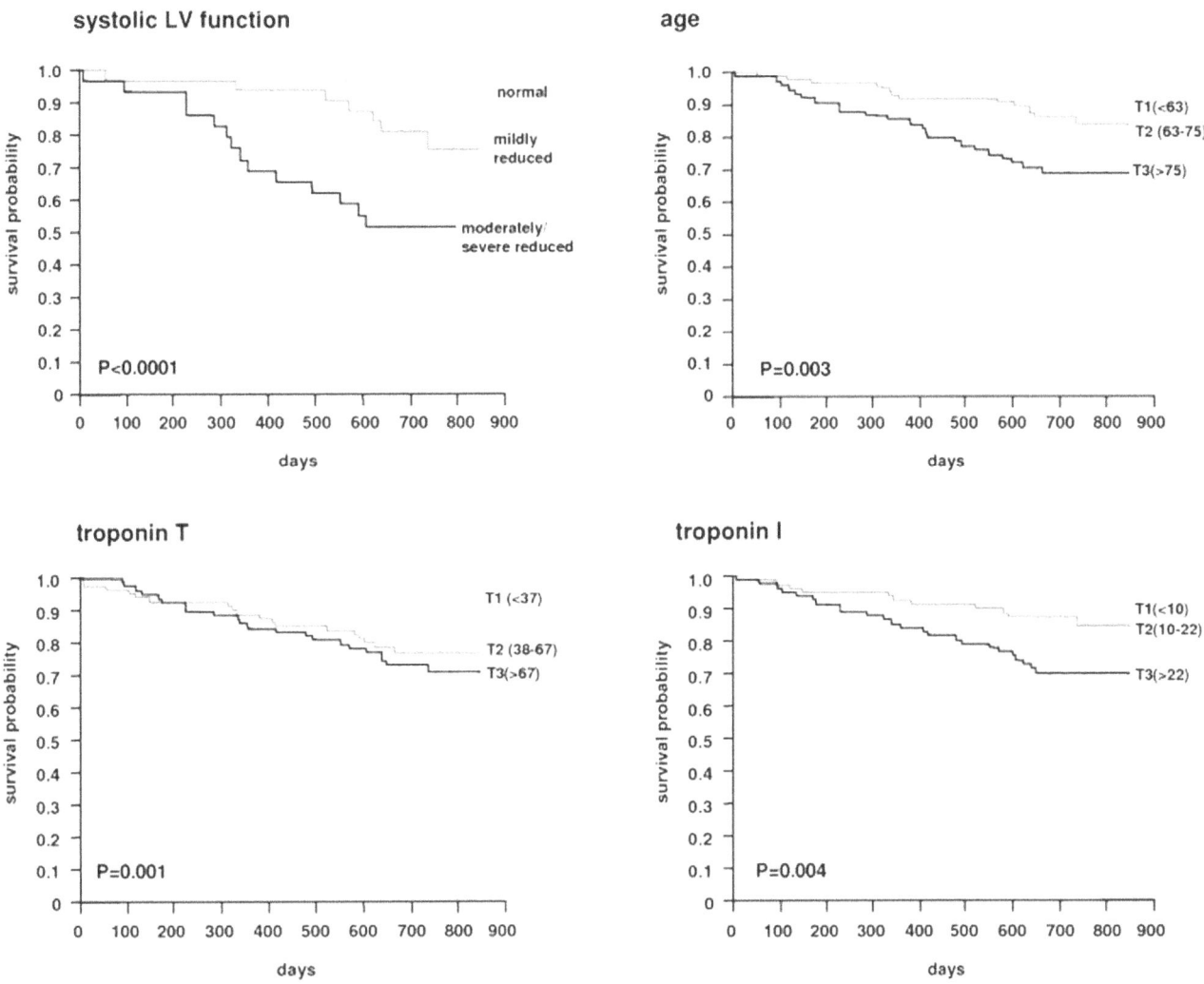

Figure 4. Survival curves of the cohort stratified according to classes of systolic LV function and tertiles of age, troponin T and troponin I.

Plasma troponin concentrations in the cohort

Plasma troponin I or T was detectable with the applied sensitive assays in all of the enrolled patients. The median TnT and TnI concentrations were 49 pg/ml and 14 pg/ml, with an interquartile range of 31 to 73 pg/ml and 7 to 28 pg/ml, respectively (Fig. 1A). The distributions of the plasma troponin concentrations are shown in Figure 1B. A large proportion of patients (95%) had a plasma TnT concentration above the 99th percentile at 14 pg/ml, while only 14% of the patients had a plasma TnI concentration above the 99th percentile at 40 pg/ml. Expressed as multiples of the 99th percentile, the TnT concentration was elevated 3.5 fold (interquartile range: 2.2 to 5.2) compared to 0.4 fold for TnI (interquartile range: 0.2 to 0.7; Figure 1C), which represented a highly significant difference (p<0.0001). Plasma troponin concentrations were moderately correlated with each other (r = 0.63, p<0.0001). TnI had a greater variability within the three samples with a variation of 26±24% compared to 8±8% for TnT.

Univariate analyses

Table 2 lists the results of univariate correlation analyses of the plasma TnI and TnT concentrations with the collected parameters. Both troponins showed a significant positive correlation with age, degree of systolic dysfunction, interdialytic weight gain, pulse pressure and parathormone concentration. The troponins were negatively correlated with residual diuresis, diastolic blood pressure and shunt flow. TnT was positively correlated with blood pump speed and C-reactive protein concentrations. There was no correlation with the plasma β2-microglobulin concentration. Variations in TnT and TnI, expressed as the standard deviation of the three samples obtained from each patient, were not correlated to any of the parameters studied.

Multivariate analyses

To analyze independent determinants of the plasma TnI and TnT concentrations, multivariate linear regression modeling was performed. The parameters that entered the final model were selected using a stepwise forward approach with a p-value of <0.05. Table 3 and Figure 2 show the results of the multivariate linear regression models that were applied. Besides age and gender, the independent determinants of the plasma TnT concentration were systolic LV function, systolic blood pressure, time on dialysis and residual diuresis. The influence of interdialytic weight gain was close to reaching statistical significance (p = 0.0688). Overall, the adjusted r^2 of the model was 0.48,

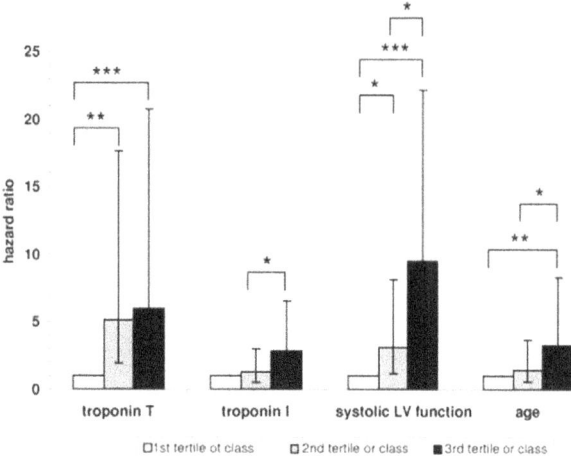

Figure 5. Hazard ratio of mortality according to tertiles of troponin T (<37; 38–67; >67 pg/ml), troponin I (<10; 10–22; >22 pg/ml), age (<63; 63–75; >75 years) and classes of systolic LV function (1 = normal, 2 = mildly reduced; 3 = moderately and severe reduced). Error bars represent lower and upper 95% confidence interval. The hazard ratio of the first tertile or class, respectively, was set to 1. ** p<0.01, *** p<0.001.

indicating that 48% of the variability in plasma TnT concentrations could be explained by these factors (Figure 3A). In contrast, the best model for TnI had an adjusted r^2 of 0.32, and age, systolic LV function, pulse pressure, length of time on dialysis and duration of a HD session were independent predictors (Figure 3B).

Prognostic value

After the initial blood draw, the cohort was followed for survival to analyze the prognostic value of elevated plasma troponin concentrations. During a median follow-up time of 710 days (679; 761), 44 patients died corresponding to an annual mortality rate of 9.2%. Compared to surviving patients, deceased patients were significantly older (77 years [68;82] vs. 69 [59; 76]; p<0.0001), were more likely to have LV dysfunction (68% vs. 24%; p<0.0001) and had lower diastolic blood pressure (65 mm Hg [59;72] vs. 69 [63; 74]; p = 0.0087). They had higher plasma CRP and parathormone concentrations (12.9 mg/L [8.8;20.1] vs. 7.7 [4.2; 13.6]; p<0.0001 and 240 pg/mL [169;431] vs. 203 [124; 326]; p = 0.0011, respectively). Plasma troponin T and I concentrations were also significantly (p<0.0001) higher in deceased patients (67 [46;87] pg/mL and 24 [11;46] pg/mL, respectively) compared to surviving patients (44 [29;70] pg/mL and 13 [7;24] pg/mL, respectively).

The survival curves stratified for tertiles of age, plasma troponin T and I concentrations as well as classes of systolic LV function are shown in Figure 4. The relative risk compared to the first tertile or class is shown in Figure 5. Systolic LV function was the strongest

predictor of death during follow-up, followed by increased plasma troponin T concentration. When analyzing the diagnostic performance of plasma troponin T and I concentrations using contingency tables and receiver-operator curves (Table 4), both troponins showed similar AUC-values, however, plasma troponin T concentration had a higher sensitivity (91%) and negative predictive value (95%) compared to troponin I (61% and 77%, respectively). For each increase of the plasma troponin T or I concentration by 10 pg/ml, the risk ratio was increased by 13.9% and 5.2%, respectively. In a multivariate proportional hazards model with age, systolic function and troponin concentration, only systolic function and age remained independent predictors (data not shown).

Discussion

This study shows that plasma troponin T concentrations measured using a highly sensitive assay were elevated in the vast majority of the hemodialysis cohort studied and that both cardiac and dialysis-related parameters determined its concentrations. Compared to sensitive troponin I, TnT was elevated in more patients, reflected dialysis-related factors to a greater extent and tended to be a stronger predictor of mortality. This study is in agreement with previous studies of patients without ESRD that showed an association between increased plasma troponin concentrations and impaired systolic function [27,28]. In addition, plasma troponin concentrations were independently associated with dialysis-related parameters, such as time on dialysis, residual diuresis, interdialytic weight gain or duration of a HD session. These factors, which can be termed "dialysis heritage", are strongly interrelated to each other in that residual function was lost with an increasing time on dialysis, which favors volume overload. Residual function and interdialytic weight gain are both independent risk factors for increased mortality in ESRD patients [24,25]. The association between residual diuresis and plasma troponin concentration has been reported earlier [29].

Most of the studies evaluating plasma troponin concentrations in ESRD patients have investigated the prognostic value and association with mortality. However, only a few studies have addressed the determinants of plasma troponin concentration in ESRD patients. Several studies found that elevated troponin concentrations were associated with the extent of coronary disease [30,31], calcification [32] or left ventricular hypertrophy or dysfunction [33]. Interestingly, in our study shunt flow was negatively correlated with plasma troponin T or I concentrations and was an independent predictor with a borderline statistical significance in the multivariate analysis (p = 0.07). Despite the possible detrimental effects of a high shunt flow on the heart [16], our results suggest that a high shunt flow can be interpreted as a sign of better cardiac status as judged by a lower plasma troponin concentration. This also highlights the fact that association studies cannot distinguish between cause and consequence and can be influenced by phenomena such as reverse causation (i.e., a failing

Table 4. Prognostic performance of the plasma troponin concentration in predicting death during follow-up.

	AUC (c-index)	cut-off, pg/ml	Youden index	sensitivity, %	specificity, %	positive predictive value, %	negative predictive value, %
troponin T	0.684	38	0.32	91	41	26	95
troponin I	0.665	21	0.32	61	70	16	77

heart that leads to increased plasma troponin concentrations and low shunt flow).

In studies comparing troponin T to troponin I, ESRD patients were 2–3 times more likely to have elevated concentrations of troponin T than troponin I [34,35]. In this study, TnT was elevated in nearly all of the patients (95%) compared to TnI (14%). This is similar to the findings of Jacobs et al., who found elevations of TnT measured with the high sensitive Roche assay in all of the patients studied whereas TnI measured using a conventional assay was elevated in only 28% of the cases [21]. Using a sensitive troponin I assay and a cut-off point of 35 pg/ml, this proportion was increased to 37% [23]. This difference can be partially explained with our data, which showed a slight accumulation of troponin T during the course of ESRD in that residual diuresis and the length of time on dialysis were independent predictors of the plasma concentration of only TnT, but not TnI. The finding that plasma troponin I concentrations were not influenced by residual renal clearance is in agreement with a study in ESRD patients that showed no differences in the clearance of troponin I after an acute MI [36].

However, there should be caution when interpreting high troponin T values as mere accumulation [5,37]. Elevated troponin T and troponin I concentrations are both strong predictors of mortality. Accumulation of troponin T can only occur following release after myocyte damage and should be regarded as a pathologic finding in any ESRD patients. Furthermore, accumulation can only occur when residual renal function declines, which is a strong predictor of survival in hemodialysis patients [38]. Therefore, plasma troponin T concentrations provide information about cardiac release and dialysis heritage, which might explain the improved prognostic value of troponin T compared to troponin I, as seen in our study or in the study of Jacobs et al. [18,20].

A more meaningful cut-off point than the 99th percentile would be levels that are linked to an increased mortality risk. We found that a plasma troponin T concentration above 38 pg/mL which is roughly three-times the 99th percentile was associated with a 5-fold risk of death during 2 years of follow-up. In contrast, we could not find a clear cut-off for troponin I as the association with death was more gradual. So far, only one study reported the association of hs TnT with mortality and found reduced survival rates at levels above 24.15 pg/ml [22]. In our study, both troponins were not independent predictors of death such as age or systolic LV function and did not add prognostic information. However, they

can be used as alternative markers to identify patients at risk when echocardiography or other cardiac workup is not available. Additional studies are needed to clarify the diagnostic value of sensitive TnT and sensitive TnI in terms of mortality and risk stratification in ESRD patients.

On average, patients in this cohort had a TnT value that was 3.5-fold greater than the 99th percentile. Given these elevated baseline values, acute MI can only be diagnosed or ruled out when one or more subsequent samples show a significant rise or fall. Sensitive troponin I offers advantages in this respect, as the plasma concentration of a minority of the patients (14%) was above the 99th percentile.

The study is limited by the paucity of cardiac parameters that were collected, which might have contributed to an unexplained variability of roughly 70% and 50% in plasma troponin I and troponin T concentrations during multivariate modeling. Survival analyses might be limited by the low mortality during the follow-up period. This study focused on nephrological parameters that are commonly available and accessible during hemodialysis treatment, such as residual diuresis or shunt flow. Systolic left ventricular function served as a surrogate for cardiac status and showed a high correlation to the plasma troponin concentration. Other cardiac morbidities, such as valvular disease or atrial fibrillation were also contributors of the plasma troponin concentration. Again it should be emphasized that association studies cannot prove causality between the studied parameters and elevated troponin concentrations and cannot distinguish between cause and consequence.

In summary, elevations of plasma troponin concentrations in hemodialysis patients measured with sensitive assays are influenced by cardiac function and dialysis-related parameters. Both are strong predictors of mortality in the short-term and are useful markers to identify patients at risk, however, troponin T is more retained during ESRD compared to troponin I.

Acknowledgments

We thank Andrea Janessa, Claudia Stelzig, Boris Huegle, MD & M.Sc. and Aline Naumann for their valuable assistance during the study.

Author Contributions

Conceived and designed the experiments: FA BF. Analyzed the data: HUH TB RT CT PW. Contributed reagents/materials/analysis tools: AP. Wrote the paper: FA BF CM.

References

1. Wu AH, Ford L (1999) Release of cardiac troponin in acute coronary syndromes: ischemia or necrosis? Clin Chim Acta 284: 161–174.

2. Thygesen K, Alpert JS, White HD (2007) Universal definition of myocardial infarction. Eur Heart J 28: 2525–2538.

3. Freda BJ, Tang WH, Van Lente F, Peacock WF, Francis GS (2002) Cardiac troponins in renal insufficiency: review and clinical implications. J Am Coll Cardiol 40: 2065–2071.

4. Artunc F, Haap M, Heyne N, Weyrich P, Wolf S (2010) [Interpretation of elevated serum troponin levels in end stage renal disease – case 2/2010]. Dtsch Med Wochenschr 135: 240.

5. Katus HA, Haller C, Muller-Bardorff M, Scheffold T, Remppis A (1995) Cardiac troponin T in end-stage renal disease patients undergoing chronic maintenance hemodialysis. Clin Chem 41: 1201–1203.

6. Porter GA, Norton T, Bennett WB (1998) Troponin T, a predictor of death in chronic haemodialysis patients. Eur Heart J 19 Suppl N: N34–N37.

7. Stolear JC, Georges B, Shita A, Verbeelen D (1999) The predictive value of cardiac troponin T measurements in subjects on regular haemodialysis. Nephrol Dial Transplant 14: 1961–1967.

8. Dierkes J, Domrose U, Westphal S, Ambrosch A, Bosselmann HP, et al. (2000) Cardiac troponin T predicts mortality in patients with end-stage renal disease. Circulation 102: 1964–1969.

9. Apple FS, Murakami MM, Pearce LA, Herzog CA (2002) Predictive value of cardiac troponin I and T for subsequent death in end-stage renal disease. Circulation 106: 2941–2945.

10. Mallamaci F, Zoccali C, Parlongo S, Tripepi G, Benedetto FA, et al. (2002) Troponin is related to left ventricular mass and predicts all-cause and cardiovascular mortality in hemodialysis patients. Am J Kidney Dis 40: 68–75.

11. Khan NA, Hemmelgarn BR, Tonelli M, Thompson CR, Levin A (2005) Prognostic value of troponin T and I among asymptomatic patients with end-stage renal disease: a meta-analysis. Circulation 112: 3088–3096.

12. Wang AY, Lai KN (2008) Use of cardiac biomarkers in end-stage renal disease. J Am Soc Nephrol 19: 1643–1652.

13. Diris JH, Hackeng CM, Kooman JP, Pinto YM, Hermens WT, et al. (2004) Impaired renal clearance explains elevated troponin T fragments in hemodialysis patients. Circulation 109: 23–25.

14. Bodor GS, Survant L, Voss EM, Smith S, Porterfield D, et al. (1997) Cardiac troponin T composition in normal and regenerating human skeletal muscle. Clin Chem 43: 476–484.

15. Zumrutdal A, Bakinen O, Ucan H, Atalay HV, Bodur H (2000) Relationship between uremic myopathy and false-positive cardiac troponin T test. Nephron 86: 522–523.

16. London GM (2002) Left ventricular alterations and end-stage renal disease. Nephrol Dial Transplant 17 Suppl 1: 29–36.

17. Breidthardt T, McIntyre CW (2011) Dialysis-induced myocardial stunning: the other side of the cardiorenal syndrome. Rev Cardiovasc Med 12: 13–20.

18. Apple FS (2009) A new season for cardiac troponin assays: it's time to keep a scorecard. Clin Chem 55: 1303–1306.

19. Reichlin T, Hochholzer W, Bassetti S, Steuer S, Stelzig C, et al. (2009) Early diagnosis of myocardial infarction with sensitive cardiac troponin assays. N Engl J Med 361: 858–867.

20. Keller T, Munzel T, Blankenberg S (2011) Making it more sensitive: the new era of troponin use. Circulation 123: 1361–1363.

21. Jacobs LH, van de KJ, Mingels AM, Kleijnen VW, van der Sande FM, et al. (2009) Haemodialysis patients longitudinally assessed by highly sensitive cardiac troponin T and commercial cardiac troponin T and cardiac troponin I assays. Ann Clin Biochem 46: 283–290.

22. McGill D, Talaulikar G, Potter JM, Koerbin G, Hickman PE (2010) Over time, high-sensitivity TnT replaces NT-proBNP as the most powerful predictor of death in patients with dialysis-dependent chronic renal failure. Clin Chim Acta 411: 936–939.

23. Kumar N, Michelis MF, DeVita MV, Panagopoulos G, Rosenstock JL (2011) Troponin I levels in asymptomatic patients on haemodialysis using a high-sensitivity assay. Nephrol Dial Transplant 26: 665–670.

24. van der Wal WM, Noordzij M, Dekker FW, Boeschoten EW, Krediet RT, et al. (2011) Full loss of residual renal function causes higher mortality in dialysis patients; findings from a marginal structural model. Nephrol Dial Transplant.

25. Kalantar-Zadeh K, Regidor DL, Kovesdy CP, Van Wyck D, Bunnapradist S, et al. (2009) Fluid retention is associated with cardiovascular mortality in patients undergoing long-term hemodialysis. Circulation 119: 671–679.

26. Evrin PE, Wibell L (1972) The serum levels and urinary excretion of 2 - microglobulin in apparently healthy subjects. Scand J Clin Lab Invest 29: 69–74.

27. Peacock WF, De Marco T, Fonarow GC, Diercks D, Wynne J, et al. (2008) Cardiac troponin and outcome in acute heart failure. N Engl J Med 358: 2117–2126.

28. Horwich TB, Patel J, MacLellan WR, Fonarow GC (2003) Cardiac troponin I is associated with impaired hemodynamics, progressive left ventricular dysfunc-tion, and increased mortality rates in advanced heart failure. Circulation 108: 833–838.

29. Fernandez-Reyes MJ, Mon C, Heras M, Guevara P, Garcia MC, et al. (2004) Predictive value of troponin T levels for ischemic heart disease and mortality in patients on hemodialysis. J Nephrol 17: 721–727.

30. deFilippi C, Wasserman S, Rosanio S, Tiblier E, Sperger H, et al. (2003) Cardiac troponin T and C-reactive protein for predicting prognosis, coronary atherosclerosis, and cardiomyopathy in patients undergoing long-term hemodi-alysis. JAMA 290: 353–359.

31. Hayashi T, Obi Y, Kimura T, Iio K, Sumitsuji S, et al. (2008) Cardiac troponin T predicts occult coronary artery stenosis in patients with chronic kidney disease at the start of renal replacement therapy. Nephrol Dial Transplant 23: 2936–2942.

32. Jung HH, Ma KR, Han H (2004) Elevated concentrations of cardiac troponins are associated with severe coronary artery calcification in asymptomatic haemodialysis patients. Nephrol Dial Transplant 19: 3117–3123.

33. Mallamaci F, Zoccali C, Parlongo S, Tripepi G, Benedetto FA, et al. (2002) Diagnostic value of troponin T for alterations in left ventricular mass and function in dialysis patients. Kidney Int 62: 1884–1890.

34. Kanderian AS, Francis GS (2006) Cardiac troponins and chronic kidney disease. Kidney Int 69: 1112–1114.

35. Hickman PE, Koerbin G, Southcott E, Tate J, Dimeski G, et al. (2007) Newer cardiac troponin I assays have similar performance to troponin T in patients with end-stage renal disease. Ann Clin Biochem 44: 285–289.

36. Ellis K, Dreisbach AW, Lertora JL (2001) Plasma elimination of cardiac troponin I in end-stage renal disease. South Med J 94: 993–996.

37. Giannitsis E, Katus HA (2004) Troponin T release in hemodialysis patients. Circulation 110: e25–e26.

38. Termorshuizen F, Dekker FW, van Manen JG, Korevaar JC, Boeschoten EW, et al. (2004) Relative contribution of residual renal function and different measures of adequacy to survival in hemodialysis patients: an analysis of the Netherlands Cooperative Study on the Adequacy of Dialysis (NECOSAD)-2. J Am Soc Nephrol 15: 1061–1070.

18

Pre-Dialysis Systolic Blood Pressure-Variability is Independently Associated with All-Cause Mortality in Incident Haemodialysis Patients

Viknesh Selvarajah[1,2]*, Laura Pasea[3], Sanjay Ojha[2], Ian B. Wilkinson[4], Laurie A. Tomlinson[4]

1 Clinical Pharmacology Unit, Department of Medicine, University of Cambridge, Cambridge, United Kingdom, 2 Department of Nephrology, Cambridge University Hospitals NHS Foundation Trust, Cambridge, United Kingdom, 3 Centre for Applied Medical Statistics, Department of Public Health and Primary Care, Institute of Public Health, University of Cambridge, Cambridge, United Kingdom, 4 Cambridge Clinical Trials Unit, University of Cambridge, Cambridge, United Kingdom

Abstract

Systolic blood pressure variability is an independent risk factor for mortality and cardiovascular events. Standard measures of blood pressure predict outcome poorly in haemodialysis patients. We investigated whether systolic blood pressure variability was associated with mortality in incident haemodialysis patients. We performed a longitudinal observational study of patients commencing haemodialysis between 2005 and 2011 in East Anglia, UK, excluding patients with cardiovascular events within 6 months of starting haemodialysis. The main exposure was variability independent of the mean (VIM) of systolic blood pressure from short-gap, pre-dialysis blood pressure readings between 3 and 6 months after commencing haemodialysis, and the outcome was all-cause mortality. Of 203 patients, 37 (18.2%) patients died during a mean follow-up of 2.0 (SD 1.3) years. The age and sex-adjusted hazard ratio (HR) for mortality was 1.09 (95% confidence interval (CI) 1.02–1.17) for a one-unit increase of VIM. This was not altered by adjustment for diabetes, prior cardiovascular disease and mean systolic blood pressure (HR 1.09, 95% CI 1.02–1.16). Patients with VIM of systolic blood pressure above the median were 2.4 (95% CI 1.17–4.74) times more likely to die during follow-up than those below the median. Results were similar for all measures of blood pressure variability and further adjustment for type of dialysis access, use of antihypertensives and absolute or variability of fluid intake did not alter these findings. Diastolic blood pressure variability showed no association with all cause mortality. Our study shows that variability of systolic blood pressure is a strong and independent predictor of all-cause mortality in incident haemodialysis patients. Further research is needed to understand the mechanism as this may form a therapeutic target or focus for management.

Editor: Rudolf Kirchmair, Medical University Innsbruck, Austria

Funding: IBW and VS are supported by the British Heart Foundation and the Cambridge Biomedical Research Centre. The funders had no role in study design, data collection and analysis, decision to publish, or preparation of the manuscript.

Competing Interests: The authors have declared that no competing interests exist.

* E-mail: vs321@cam.ac.uk

Introduction

Mortality is high among patients undergoing haemodialysis treatment for end-stage renal disease (ESRD), and cardiovascular disease is the main cause of death [1]. Hypertension is common in ESRD but, unlike in the general population, is not linearly associated with adverse outcomes [2].

Blood pressure (BP) variability is more closely associated with adverse outcomes in patients with or at risk of vascular disease than 'usual' BP [3] and may play a causal role in the progression of organ damage and in triggering vascular events [4]. BP variability is known to be increased in patients with ESRD [5,6]. Among patients undergoing haemodialysis potential causes of high BP variability such as baroreceptor dysfunction, aortic stiffness and variations in intravascular volume, as well as plausible outcomes such as cerebral small-vessel disease, cerebral haemorrhage and cardiac sudden death are increased compared to the general population [7,8]. Therefore increased BP variability could provide a strong potential explanation for the increased cardiovascular morbidity and mortality among patients undergoing haemodialysis.

BP variability can be quantified over both the short term, using 24-hour ambulatory BP measurements, and long-term using visit-to-visit BP readings [9]. The optimum method for evaluating BP variability for patients with ESRD is unclear. Previous studies have suggested that visit-to-visit pre-dialysis BP variability is associated with mortality among haemodialysis patients [6,10,11]. However, these studies are limited by lack of power and short duration of follow-up, [10,11] inclusion of prevalent haemodialysis patients [6,10] and use of measures of blood pressure variability that are associated with average blood pressure levels [10]. Therefore, we planned to investigate whether visit-to-visit pre-dialysis blood pressure variability was associated with mortality among a cohort of patients commencing incident haemodialysis, independently of confounders including average blood pressure.

Subjects and Methods

Study Design

We performed a longitudinal cohort study of patients who commenced maintenance haemodialysis between January 1st 2005 and December 12th 2010. Patients were from Addenbrookes

Hospital and four satellite units in East Anglia, England. Each underwent haemodialysis three times a week and each dialysis session was at the same time of day and lasted for 3–4 hours.

Inclusion & Exclusion Criteria

We included all patients who were aged over 18 years at the start of dialysis, had no history of prior renal replacement therapy including transplantation, and remained on dialysis for more than 180 days with no recovery of kidney function. To avoid reverse causality (where underlying cardiovascular disease causes variable blood pressure), we excluded patients who died or suffered cardiovascular events (stroke, transient ischaemic attack (TIA), myocardial infarction, angina or heart failure) in the first 180 days after starting haemodialysis.

Exposure: Blood Pressure Measurements

BP was measured was measured at the beginning and end of each dialysis session in a seated position by trained dialysis nurses in accordance with routine unit practice and entered immediately into an electronic database. BP was measured using validated oscillometric BP monitor equipped haemodialysis machines (Fresenius 4008S or Nikisso DBB-05), which were maintained as per dialysis unit protocols. For each patient we analysed pre-dialysis BP readings obtained over a consecutive 3-month period, from the 4th to 6th months after commencing haemodialysis. BP readings from the first 3 months after commencing dialysis were not used because this period is associated with acute illness and frequent adjustments to fluid weight and medications, which may have led to overestimation of BP variability in more unwell patients. We used pre-dialysis BP readings to minimise the effect of change in BP due to fluid removal during haemodialysis. We excluded BP readings taken on the first dialysis session of each week to avoid the possible confounding effects of fluid gains over the extended three-day weekend break. Therefore over the 3-month observation period all patients included in the analysis had almost identical numbers of BP readings included in the measurement of the exposure and these were 2 BP readings per week taken 2 days apart on the same day and same time of day for each individual.

Exposure: Blood Pressure Variability

We measured intra-individual BP variability for both pre-dialysis systolic and diastolic BP using standard deviation, coefficient of variation (standard deviation/mean) and variation independent of the mean (VIM) as previously described [3]. VIM is a transformation of the standard deviation that is uncorrelated with mean BP and is calculated as follows:

$$VIM = \frac{k \times \text{Standard Deviation (SBP)}}{\text{Mean (SBP)}^x}$$

Where x is calculated from fitting a power model:

$$SD(SBP) = \text{constant} \times \text{Mean(SBP)}^x$$

And $k = \text{Mean(Mean(SBP))}^x$.
(i.e. the mean of all SBP readings across all patients to the power of x).
For this study, $x = 0.789$ and $k = 50.552$.

Outcome: All-cause Mortality

The outcome was all-cause mortality during the study period, i.e. from 6 months after the commencement of haemodialysis (at the end of the 3–6 month measurement of the exposure) until the end of follow-up (May 12th 2011). Follow-up was censored if patients received a kidney transplant, switched to peritoneal dialysis or transferred to a different renal unit.

Demographic data, comorbidities and details and dates of censoring events were obtained from the regional renal electronic database and verified using local medical records. Data on medications, interdialytic weight changes, intradialytic weight changes and type of dialysis access were also available. Previous cardiovascular disease (including clinically evident: stroke, transient ischaemic attack (TIA), myocardial infarction, angina, heart failure or peripheral vascular disease) and diabetes were defined as present if recorded in the medical notes. Data on cause of death was not available so it was not possible to analyse cardiovascular mortality separately.

Statistical Analysis

The definitions of the exposure (including all BP measurements that contributed to the measurement of the exposure and outcome) were defined a priori. The demographic characteristics of groups above and below the median of VIM were compared using Mann-Whitney U tests for continuous variables and chi-squared tests for categorical variables.

We used Cox proportional hazards models to obtain hazard ratios (HR) and 95% confidence intervals (95% CI) for mortality for people with intraindividual visit-to-visit BP variability as a continuous covariate, and also as a categorical covariate, with BP variability dichotomized at the median. We examined whether the proportional hazards assumption was met using partial residual plots for continuous covariates and log (-log) plots for categorical covariates. Kaplan-Meier plots and log-rank tests were also used to compare survival between the two BP variability groups. We carried out univariate analyses of the effect of intraindividual visit-to-visit blood pressure variability on all-cause mortality. We present results adjusted for age and sex as these were considered important a priori confounders. Further covariates examined in multivariate analysis were based on potential evidence of association with mortality among haemodialysis patients; mean systolic BP (SBP), previous cardiovascular events and diabetes. This dataset was complete for all patients. Data on ethnicity was not available but in this region more than 90% of patients are of Caucasian ethnicity. In further separate analyses we adjusted for type of dialysis access (arteriovenous fistula vs indwelling venous catheter), the use of antihypertensive medication (yes vs no) and the number of antihypertensives taken at three months after start of haemodialysis (start of BP variability measurement), the mean intradialytic weight change and the standard deviation of weight change between dialysis sessions as a marker of variability of fluid intake. For this analysis the standard deviation of interdialytic weight change was log transformed due to skewness. We performed the analysis using SPSS version 21.0 (IBM Corp., Armonk, NY).

Ethics Statement

The study received approval from the Hertfordshire Research Ethics Committee (REC 11/H0311/3). Data was anonymised at source so individual patient consent was not required.

Data Availability

We are able to provide anonymized data to researchers upon request.

Results

Patient Demographics

During the study period 219 patients who were eligible for inclusion commenced maintenance haemodialysis in this region with a total follow up time of 409.4 person years. Of these, we did not include in the analysis 7 patients who died or recovered kidney function and 9 who had cardiovascular events within the first 180 days of haemodialysis. Therefore 203 patients were included in the analysis. From a mean of 25 dialysis sessions, the mean number of BP readings used for the analyses was 25 (SD 1.63). Over a mean follow-up period of 2.0 (SD 1.3) years, 37 patients (18.2%) died. Follow-up was censored for 24 (11.8%) patients who underwent kidney transplantation and 5 (2.5%) who switched to peritoneal dialysis. No patients changed renal units during the follow-up period.

Baseline characteristics of the study population and patients above and below the median VIM of intraindividual visit-to-visit BP variability are shown in Table 1. Patients with VIM of BP variability above the median were more likely to have diabetes but otherwise there were no significant difference between the groups.

Intraindividual Visit-to-visit Systolic Blood Pressure Variability

Standard deviation.   At an individual level, the mean SD of SBP was 17.4 mmHg (SD 5.1 mmHg). After adjusting for age and sex, the HR for total mortality was 1.07 (95% CI 1.01, 1.13) for every mmHg increase in SD of SBP. This was not attenuated after further adjustment for mean SBP, previous cardiovascular events and diabetes (HR 1.08, 95% CI 1.01, 1.16) (Table 2). After adjusting for age, gender, mean SBP, previous cardiovascular events and diabetes, patients with SD of SBP above the median had a 48% increased risk of death during follow-up but this was not statistically significant (HR 1.48, 95% CI 0.75, 2.91).

Coefficient of variation.   For the purpose of regression modelling the coefficient of variation (COV) was multiplied by 100 for each patient to allow sensible interpretation of the hazard ratio. The HR for total mortality, adjusted for age and gender, was 1.13 (95% CI 1.02, 1.24) for every 0.01 increase in COV. After adjusting for age, sex, previous cardiovascular disease, diabetes and mean SBP the HR for total mortality was 1.13 (95% CI 1.02, 1.24) for every 0.01 increase in COV (table 2). After full adjustment, patients with COV of SBP above the median had more than double the risk of death during follow-up (HR 2.08, 95%CI 1.04, 4.16).

Variation independent of the mean.   After adjusting for age and sex, the HR for total mortality was 1.09 (95% CI 1.02, 1.16) for a one-unit increase of VIM. Again, this was not attenuated in the fully adjusted model (HR 1.09, 95% CI 1.02, 1.16). Patients with VIM of SBP above the median were 2.4 (95% CI 1.17, 4.74) times more likely to die during follow-up than those below or equal to the median after adjustment for diabetes, prior cardiovascular disease, gender, age and mean SBP (figure 1).

Further Analyses

The relationship between VIM of systolic BP and all-cause mortality was not affected by adjustment for the type of dialysis

Table 1. Demographic characteristics of whole study population and groups above and below the median of blood pressure variability.

	Whole group	VIM below or equal to median	VIM above median	P-value*
	n = 203	n = 100	n = 103	
Age (yrs)	66±15	65±17	68±13	0.55
Male	133 (66)	68 (68)	65 (63)	0.46
Diabetes	61 (30)	20 (20)	41 (40)	0.002
Cardiovascular disease	68 (33)	28 (28)	39 (38)	0.14
Number of SBP readings	23.9±2.6	24.0±2.9	23.8±2.3	0.59
Mean SBP (mmHg)	144±16	145±16	144±17	0.78
Mean DBP (mmHg)	75±10	75±11	74±9	0.31
Blood pressure medications at 3 months:				
ACE-I or ARB	69 (34)	31 (31)	38 (37)	0.61
CCB	92 (45)	44 (44)	48(47)	0.90
β-blocker	71 (35)	31 (31)	40 (39)	0.43
Other	109 (54)	46 (46)	63 (61)	0.03
Mean number of agents	2.0±1.3	1.9±1.3	2.2±1.3	0.17
Dialysis access at 3 months:				
Arteriovenous fistula	88 (43)	44 (44)	44 (43)	0.85
Venous catheter	115 (57)	56 (56)	59 (57)	
Interdialytic weight gain (kg)	1.10±0.97	1.04±1.06	1.17±0.87	0.05

Values are expressed as mean ± SD or n (%). ACE-I - Angiotensin Converting Enzyme Inhibitor; ARB - Angiotensin receptor blocker; CCB –Calcium channel blocker, Other – Alpha-blocker, Nitrate, Diuretic, Aldosterone antagonist.
*Mann-Whitney U tests and chi-squared tests were used to compute p-values for continuous and categorical variables respectively.

Table 2. Hazard ratios for one unit increase in measures of systolic BP variability and other covariates from fully adjusted model.

	SD	COV	VIM
	Hazard Ratio	**Hazard Ratio**	**Hazard Ratio**
	(95% CI)	**(95% CI)**	**(95% CI)**
BP Variability	1.08	1.13	1.09
	(1.01, 1.16)	(1.02, 1.24)	(1.02, 1.16)
Age	1.03	1.03	1.03
	(0.99, 1.06)	(0.99, 1.06)	(0.99, 1.06)
Sex	1.36	1.35	1.35
	(0.65,2.83)	(0.65,2.81)	(0.65,2.82)
Cardiovascular disease	0.91	0.92	0.92
	(0.44,1.90)	(0.44, 1.93)	(0.44, 1.92)
Diabetes	1.33	1.33	1.33
	(0.63,2.81)	(0.63,2.82)	(0.63,2.82)
Mean SBP	0.99	0.99	0.99
	(0.97,1.01)	(0.98, 1.02)	(0.98, 1.02)

SD – standard deviation; COV – coefficient of variation; VIM – Variation independent of the mean; SBP – Systolic blood pressure.

access, the use of antihypertensives, number of antihypertensives used or mean weight change during dialysis sessions (tables S1–S4). In an analysis including the variability of weight change between dialysis sessions (likely to reflect variability of fluid intake) this parameter is also associated with all-cause mortality but does not attenuate the relationship between BP variability and mortality (table S5).

Inclusion of mean diastolic BP in the fully adjusted models made no important difference to the association between any measure of intraindividual visit-to-visit SBP variability and mortality (data not shown).

Intraindividual visit-to-visit diastolic blood pressure variability. Measures of intraindividual visit-to-visit diastolic BP variability were not associated with mortality in univariate or multivariate analyses. The age and sex adjusted HR for a one-unit increase in VIM of DBP is 1.02 [95% CI 0.91, 1.14].

Discussion

Our study shows that intraindividual visit-to-visit variability of systolic BP is associated with all-cause mortality in incident haemodialysis patients, independently of confounders such as age, cardiovascular disease and diabetes. This is seen across measures of BP variability including VIM, which importantly is not correlated with systolic BP. The association between mortality and intraindividual visit-to-visit BP variability is not explained by the type of dialysis access, the use of antihypertensives, absolute fluid intake or variability in fluid intake.

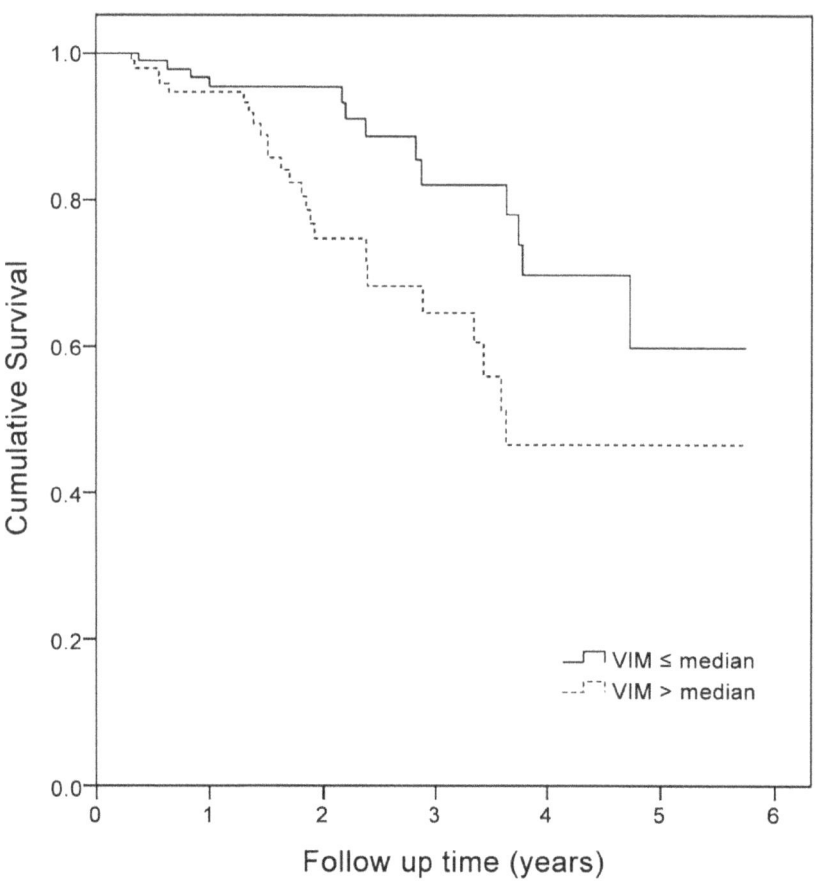

Figure 1. Mortality for patients with high versus low variability of systolic blood pressure.

This study has a number of strengths. Duration of haemodialysis is associated with aortic stiffening and autonomic neuropathy, and thus previous renal replacement therapy may be associated with increased BP variability in prevalent cohorts [12,13]. Therefore, demonstrating these results in a cohort of only incident haemodialysis patients provides greater evidence that this association may be important. We measured intraindividual visit-to-visit BP variability only after 90 days of dialysis, avoiding the early period which may be complicated by acute illness, changes in medications and unstable fluid balance. We only included measurement of pre-dialysis systolic BP taken after the two-day gap to minimize the potential confounding effect of poor compliance with fluid restriction. In addition, we included readings of BP over a prolonged period with very complete data and analyzed the results using three different measures of BP variability. Reverse causality was minimized by excluding patients who had cardiovascular events during measurement of BP variability. This cohort is reasonably large with over two years of follow-up on average and includes all eligible patients in standard clinical care.

However, there are also important limitations. We were not able to adjust for a number of potential cardiovascular risk factors such as smoking, body mass index and cholesterol, as these data were not available. However, among patients with ESRD, the relationship between classic risk factors and risk of adverse events is often weak or reversed and these data may not have affected our findings [14]. We retrospectively analysed routine clinical measurements of blood pressure where technique was as per routine unit practice and not standardized as part of a clinical study protocol. However, it is not clear that use of clinical blood pressure measurements would have led to systematic misclassification of blood pressure variability. Since random measurement error is likely to bias findings to the null, we may have underestimated the strength of the association between BP variability and mortality. Use of routine measurements in an unselected population also means that these results are likely to be generalizable across the United Kingdom and in other countries with similar dialysis schedules and patient populations. In addition, there is potential for selection bias in our findings as follow up was censored when patients received a kidney transplant or transferred to peritoneal dialysis. These people are likely to be healthier, and may have lower BP variability. However, this represents less than 15% of the initial cohort and there was no other loss-to follow-up. Finally, we were not able to examine cause-specific mortality which might have provided greater etiological insight.

Mortality in haemodialysis patients is markedly higher than in the general population and cardiovascular disease is the main cause of death [1]. Conventional measures of BP are linearly associated with cardiovascular risk in the general population [15]. However, among patients undergoing haemodialysis, many studies demonstrate a non-linear relationship between mean BP and mortality [2]. In this group there is increasing evidence that BP variability may be more closely associated with adverse outcomes than conventional measures of BP. Patients with ESRD have greater visit to visit BP variability compared to the general population [5]. Tozawa et al showed that systolic BP variability, quantified by coefficient of variation, predicted all-cause but not cardiovascular mortality in a cohort of 144 Japanese dialysis patients [10]. However, this study was limited by a small number of deaths during the study period (n = 13). A further study by Rossignol and colleagues examined the role of BP variability in a cohort of 397 haemodialysis patients with left ventricular hypertrophy enrolled in an interventional study [16]. They showed that visit-to-visit systolic and diastolic BP variability was

associated with a composite end-point of cardiovascular events during follow-up while baseline SBP and DBP were not. A recent study by Chang et al in a cohort of 1844 haemodialysis patients from the HEMO study showed that visit-to-visit SBP variability, quantified by coefficient of variation and average real variability, predicted all-cause and cardiovascular mortality [6]. All three of these studies were limited by inclusion of prevalent haemodialysis patients. Only one study has demonstrated an association between pre-dialysis systolic and diastolic BP variability and all-cause mortality in an incident dialysis cohort [11]. However this study was limited by an extremely short-follow-up (6 months) meaning that reverse causality was a strong potential explanation of their findings. BP variability during haemodialysis has also been associated with all-cause and cardiovascular mortality, as has changing pre-dialysis systolic and diastolic BP over time [17–19]. While examining slightly different hypotheses, it is likely that they reflect similar underlying pathophysiology to studies of pre-dialysis systolic BP variability.

The mechanisms that contribute to increased BP variability in patients with ESRD are complex and poorly understood. They include changes in intravascular volume and vasoactive factors (angiotensin 2, endothelin, nitric oxide), reduced arterial compliance, increased sympathetic innervation and alterations of arterial and cardiopulmonary reflexes [20]. Poor or variable compliance with fluid restriction and antihypertensive therapy could also contribute to BP fluctuations. Whether increased BP variability is causal in cardiovascular events and mortality, or whether it is a marker of vascular disease and autonomic dysfunction, is still subject to debate. Strong arguments have been made for changes in BP as a direct mechanism of event causation in cohorts without CKD [4]. The increased BP variability seen in patients with ESRD as well as the high incidence of outcomes plausibly linked to changes in BP such as dementia due to cerebral small vessel disease, hemorrhagic stroke and sudden cardiac death suggest that changes in BP may directly trigger events among dialysis patients. This is important as the use of antihypertensive drugs associated with reduced BP variability are also associated with reduced incidence of stroke [21]. Evidence for improved outcomes with therapeutic regimes targeted to reduce BP variability and prospective data on the effects of different classes of antihypertensives on BP variability in ESRD are still lacking. However, the growing evidence of a link between BP variability and adverse outcomes among haemodialysis patients raises the hope that future strategies to reduce BP fluctuations may be able to improve outcomes for this vulnerable group of patients.

Conclusions

In summary, this study shows that in standard care, variability of systolic BP from clinical measurements is a strong and independent predictor of all-cause mortality in incident HD patients, even after adjustments for factors such as age, cardiovascular disease and diabetes. This effect is consistent across different measures of BP variability, including VIM, which avoids the confounding effect of average BP. Further research is needed to understand the mechanism as this may form an important therapeutic target or focus for management in this group.

Supporting Information

Table S1 Results of fully adjusted model for analysis examining the effect of type of dialysis access on relationship between VIM and mortality.

Table S2 Results of fully adjusted model for analysis examining the effect of antihypertensive use on relationship between VIM and mortality.

Table S3 Results of fully adjusted model for analysis examining the effect of number of antihypertensives on relationship between VIM and mortality.

Table S4 Results of fully adjusted model for analysis examining the effect of mean intradialytic weight change (kg) on relationship between VIM and mortality.

Table S5 Results of fully adjusted model for analysis examining the effect of interdialytic weight variability on relationship between VIM and mortality.

Acknowledgments

Disclaimer: The results presented in this paper have not been published previously in whole or part, except in abstract format.

Author Contributions

Conceived and designed the experiments: VS LT IBW SO. Analyzed the data: VS LP LT. Wrote the paper: VS LP SO IBW LT.

References

1. Parfrey PS, Foley RN (1999) The Clinical Epidemiology of Cardiac Disease in Chronic Renal Failure. Journal of the American Society of Nephrology 10: 1606–1615.
2. Chang TI (2011) Systolic blood pressure and mortality in patients on hemodialysis. Curr Hypertens Rep 13: 362–369.
3. Rothwell PM, Howard SC, Dolan E, O'Brien E, Dobson JE, et al. (2010) Prognostic significance of visit-to-visit variability, maximum systolic blood pressure, and episodic hypertension. The Lancet 375: 895–905.
4. Rothwell PM (2010) Limitations of the usual blood-pressure hypothesis and importance of variability, instability, and episodic hypertension. The Lancet 375: 938–948.
5. Rohrscheib RM, Myers OB, Servilla KS, Adams CD, DD M, et al. (2008) Age-related Blood Pressure Patterns and Blood Pressure Variability among Hemodialysis Patients. Clinical Journal of the American Society of Nephrology 3: 1407–1414.
6. Chang TI, Flythe JE, Brunelli SM, Muntner P, Greene T, et al. (2013) Visit-to-visit systolic blood pressure variability and outcomes in hemodialysis. J Hum Hypertens: 1–7. doi:10.1038/jhh.2013.49.
7. Lacy P, Carr SJ, O'Brien D, Fentum B, Williams B, et al. (2006) Reduced glomerular filtration rate in pre-dialysis non-diabetic chronic kidney disease patients is associated with impaired baroreceptor sensitivity and reduced vascular compliance. Clinical Science 110: 101–108.
8. Wang AYM, Lam CWK, Chan IHS, Wang M, Lui SF, et al. (2010) Sudden Cardiac Death in End-Stage Renal Disease Patients: A 5-Year Prospective Analysis. Hypertension 56: 210–216.
9. Mallamaci F, Tripepi G (2013) Blood pressure variability in chronic kidney disease patients. Blood Purif 36: 58–62.
10. Tozawa M, Iseki K, Yoshi S, Fukiyama K (1999) Blood pressure variability as an adverse prognostic risk factor in end-stage renal disease. Nephrology Dialysis Transplantation 14: 1976–1981.
11. Brunelli SM, Thadhani RI, Lynch KE, Ankers ED, Joffe MM, et al. (2008) Association between long-term blood pressure variability and mortality among incident hemodialysis patients. Am J Kidney Dis 52: 716–726.

12. Vita G, Bellinghieri G, Trusso A, Costantino G, Santoro D, et al. (1999) Uremic autonomic neuropathy studied by spectral analysis of heart rate. Kidney International 56: 232–237.
13. Blacher J, Guerin AP, Pannier B, Marchais SJ, London GM (2001) Arterial Calcifications, Arterial Stiffness, and Cardiovascular Risk in End-Stage Renal Disease. Hypertension 38: 938–942.
14. Baigent C, Landray MJ, Wheeler DC (2007) Misleading associations between cholesterol and vascular outcomes in dialysis patients: the need for randomized trials. Seminars in Dialysis 20: 498–503.
15. Lewington S, Clarke R, Qizilbash N, Peto R, Collins R, et al. (2002) Age-specific relevance of usual blood pressure to vascular mortality: a meta-analysis of individual data for one million adults in 61 prospective studies. Lancet 360: 1903–1913.
16. Rossignol P, Cridlig J, Lehert P, Kessler M, Zannad F (2012) Visit-to-visit blood pressure variability is a strong predictor of cardiovascular events in hemodialysis: insights from FOSIDIAL. Hypertension 60: 339–346.
17. Flythe JE, Inrig JK, Shafi T, Chang TI, Cape K, et al. (2013) Association of Intradialytic Blood Pressure Variability With Increased All-Cause and Cardiovascular Mortality in Patients Treated With Long-term Hemodialysis. AJKD: 1–9.
18. Di Iorio B, Di Micco L, Torraca S, Sirico ML, Guastaferro P, et al. (2013) Variability of blood pressure in dialysis patients: a new marker of cardiovascular risk. J Nephrol 26: 173–182.
19. Raimann JG, Usvyat LA, Thijssen S, Kotanko P, Rogus J, et al. (2012) Blood pressure stability in hemodialysis patients confers a survival advantage: results from a large retrospective cohort study. Kidney International 81: 548–558.
20. Parati G, Ochoa JE, Bilo G (2012) Blood pressure variability, cardiovascular risk, and risk for renal disease progression. Curr Hypertens Rep 14: 421–431.
21. Webb AJS, Fischer U, Mehta Z, Rothwell PM (2010) Effects of antihypertensive-drug class on interindividual variation in blood pressure and risk of stroke: a systematic review and meta-analysis. Lancet 375: 906–915.

19

Aldosterone and Mortality in Hemodialysis Patients: Role of Volume Overload

Szu-Chun Hung[1]⁹, Yao-Ping Lin[2]⁹, Hsin-Lei Huang[3], Hsiao-Fung Pu[3], Der-Cherng Tarng[2,3]*

1 Division of Nephrology, Buddhist Tzu Chi General Hospital, Taipei Branch, Taipei, Taiwan, **2** Division of Nephrology, Department of Medicine, and Immunology Research Center, Taipei Veterans General Hospital, Taipei, Taiwan, **3** Department and Institute of Physiology, School of Medicine, National Yang-Ming University, Taipei, Taiwan

Abstract

Background: Elevated aldosterone is associated with increased mortality in the general population. In patients on dialysis, however, the association is reversed. This paradox may be explained by volume overload, which is associated with lower aldosterone and higher mortality.

Methods: We evaluated the relationship between aldosterone and outcomes in a prospective cohort of 328 hemodialysis patients stratified by the presence or absence of volume overload (defined as extracellular water/total body water >48%, as measured with bioimpedance). Baseline plasma aldosterone was measured before dialysis and categorized as low (<140 pg/mL), middle (140 to 280 pg/mL) and high (>280 pg/mL).

Results: Overall, 36% (n = 119) of the hemodialysis patients had evidence of volume overload. Baseline aldosterone was significantly lower in the presence of volume overload than its absence. During a median follow-up of 54 months, 83 deaths and 70 cardiovascular events occurred. Cox multivariate analysis showed that by using the low aldosterone as the reference, high aldosterone was inversely associated with decreased hazard ratios for mortality (0.49; 95% confidence interval, 0.25–0.76) and first cardiovascular event (0.70; 95% confidence interval, 0.33–0.78) in the presence of volume overload. In contrast, high aldosterone was associated with an increased risk for mortality (1.97; 95% confidence interval, 1.69–3.75) and first cardiovascular event (2.01; 95% confidence interval, 1.28–4.15) in the absence of volume overload.

Conclusions: The inverse association of aldosterone with adverse outcomes in hemodialysis patients is due to the confounding effect of volume overload. These findings support treatment of hyperaldosteronemia in hemodialysis patients who have achieved strict volume control.

Editor: Leighton R James, University of Florida, United States of America

Funding: This study was supported by grants from the National Science Council (NSC 96-2628-B-010-001-MY3 and 99-2314-B-010-004-MY3), Taipei City Hospital (97001-62-002), National Yang-Ming University Hospital (RD2011-025), and Ministry of Education's aim for the Top University Plan. The funders had no role in study design, data collection and analysis, decision to publish, or preparation of the manuscript.

Competing Interests: The authors have declared that no competing interests exist.

* E-mail: dctarng@vghtpe.gov.tw

⁹ These authors contributed equally to this work.

Introduction

Cardiovascular disease (CVD) in patients with end-stage renal disease (ESRD) [1]. There is accumulating evidence that aldosterone, in addition to its classical role in regulating fluid and electrolyte balance, plays a significant role in the pathogenesis of CVD [2]. Patients with chronic kidney disease (CKD) have higher aldosterone concentrations than the general population [3], suggesting that aldosterone might modulate the development of CVD in CKD. However, higher aldosterone levels are associated with lower mortality in CKD patients on hemodialysis [4,5], which is in marked contrast to findings from prospective studies in the general population and in early CKD [6,7]. A similar inverse association of serum cholesterol levels with mortality has been previously documented in dialysis patients [8–10]. It has been suggested that this paradoxical association results from a confounding effect of inflammation and/or malnutrition, which leads to lower cholesterol levels and higher mortality (the so called reverse epidemiology).

Volume overload is a common finding in dialysis patients and has been recognized as an important contributor to an adverse prognosis [11,12]. This factor may explain the inverse association between aldosterone level and mortality because volume overload is strongly associated with lower aldosterone levels and higher mortality [13]. In view of the particularly high incidence of CVD in dialysis patients, a better understanding of the diagnostic implications of aldosterone levels in these patients is needed. Therefore, we investigated whether the association between aldosterone levels and mortality would be modified by the presence of volume overload.

Materials and Methods

Ethics Statement

The study complied with the Declaration of Helsinki and was approved by the institutional review board of National Yang-Ming University Hospital. All participants gave their written informed consent before inclusion.

Patient Population

This prospective cohort study was conducted at the dialysis centers of affiliated hospitals of National Yang-Ming University, Taipei. The study subjects were recruited from November 1 to December 31, 2004. Initially, all patients (n = 418) undergoing hemodialysis were screened, and 366 clinically stable patients aged older than 20 years, who had been on hemodialysis for more than 6 months, were included. Exclusion criteria were dialysis for less than 12 h per week; inadequacy of dialysis, defined as Kt/V urea <1.2; conditions of malignancy, infectious disease, sepsis, or hepatobiliary disease; and unwillingness to participate in this study. Finally, the study population of 328 patients (188 men and 140 women; mean age of 59 years) was followed up until June 30, 2009. All the patients were subjected to a standard bicarbonate dialysis session with use of 137 mEq/L sodium and 2.0 mEq/L potassium dialysate. Hemodialysis was performed three times weekly using single-use dialyzers with a membrane surface area of 1.6–1.7 m^2.

Laboratory Investigations

Blood samples were drawn from patients who had fasted overnight before the start of a mid-week dialysis session, and heparin was then administered. Plasma and serum were separated and kept frozen at –70°C when not analyzed immediately. Plasma aldosterone levels were measured according to the manufacturer's instructions using a commercially available radioimmunoassay kit (Diagnostic Systems Laboratories, Webster, TX). The intra- and inter-assay coefficients of variation were 3.4% and 8.9%, respectively, at an aldosterone level of 60 pg/mL, 4.7% and 7.6%, respectively, at a level of 250 pg/mL, and 4.0% and 5.2%, respectively, at a level of 500 pg/mL. Albumin, urea, creatinine, calcium, phosphate, iron, and total iron-binding capacity (TIBC) in serum were determined with a Hitachi 7600 autoanalyzer (Roche Modular; Hitachi Ltd, Tokyo, Japan) using commercial kits. Serum high-sensitivity C-reactive protein (hs-CRP) levels were measured using an immunoturbidimetric assay and rate nephelometry (IMMAGE; Beckman Coulter, Galway, Ireland). The adequacy of dialysis was estimated by measuring mid-week urea clearance (Kt/V urea) using the standard method [14]. Blood pressure (BP) was measured and recorded by an automated sphygmomanometer. Pre-dialysis BP (before placement of a dialysis needle) was measured in the nonaccess arm after a 5-minute rest while the patient was seated with both feet on the floor.

Bioimpedance Study

Multifrequency bioimpedance method (Model 310 Bioimpedance Analyzer; Biodynamics, Seattle, WA) was performed within 30 minutes after a dialysis session at presumed dry weight. The ratio of extracellular water to total body water (ECW/TBW) was then taken as a measure of volume status. To avoid inter-observer variation, a single well-trained dietitian was involved in the measurement of bioimpedance.

Outcomes

In all patients, a thorough medical history was taken at the time of study enrollment. Presence of CVD was defined as a medical history and clinical findings of congestive heart failure, coronary artery disease, cerebrovascular disease, and/or peripheral vascular disease. No major modifications were made in dialysis treatments during the follow-up period. The primary outcome measures were death from any cause and CV events from the time of inclusion in the study. CV events included fatal and nonfatal myocardial infarction, stroke and congestive heart failure, as well as complicated peripheral vascular disease and sudden death. A trained physician who had no knowledge of the results of plasma aldosterone measurements independently reviewed all suspected CV events by examining each medical chart.

Statistical Analysis

All variables were expressed as percentages for categorical data and as means ± SDs or medians and interquartile ranges (IQRs) for continuous data with or without a normal distribution, respectively. The baseline characteristics of the 2 study subgroups with ECW/TBW ≤48% and >48% were compared using a t-test, x^2 statistics, and Mann-Whitney U test as appropriate. Potential differences among the 3 patient groups for each baseline plasma aldosterone tertile were assessed by an analysis of variance (ANOVA), x^2 statistics, or the Kruskal-Wallis test, as appropriate. Receiver operating characteristic (ROC) curves were constructed for prediction of mortality using ECW/TBW at baseline. The optimal cutoff point for volume overload (ECW/TBW >48%) is listed in Figure 1, along with the sensitivity, specificity and accuracy for predicting mortality at the end of the follow-up period. Confidence intervals (CI) for the area under the ROC curves were calculated using nonparametric assumptions. Univariate correlations between ECW/TBW or plasma aldosterone and potentially explanatory variables were assessed by Pearson correlation analyses.

The Kaplan-Meier method was used to describe survival curves. Individuals were censored at the time of kidney transplantation, peritoneal dialysis, and withdrawal from the study, or at the end of the follow-up period on June 30, 2009. Cox proportional hazards models were used to investigate the role of volume overload as a potential effect modifier for relationships between diverse independent variables and either all-cause mortality or first CV event. For all multivariate survival analyses, clinically relevant variables with a P value ≤0.1 in the univariate analysis were fitted and the backward selection procedure was used for model selection [15]. The aldosterone variables were modeled as categorical variables (<140, 140–280, and >280 pg/mL) or continuous variables (per 100 pg/mL). Adjusted hazard ratios with 95% CI were reported. P values less than 0.05 were considered statistically significant. P values for interactions between the volume indicators and the aldosterone levels were computed using likelihood ratio tests. All statistical analyses were performed using the computer software Statistical Package for the Social Science, version 16.0 (SPSS Inc., Chicago, IL).

Results

Clinical Characteristics

The mean baseline age of the 328 patients was 59±13 years, 57.3% were male, and 29.3% had diabetes. The baseline characteristics for the patient groups divided by the absence or presence of volume overload [defined as ECW/TBW >48%] are presented in Table 1. Overall, 36% (n = 119) of the dialysis patients had evidence of volume overload. The presence of volume overload was associated with older age, diabetes, prior CVD, hypertension, higher inflammatory markers, and lower aldosterone, albumin, calcium, phosphate, and hemoglobin levels. There

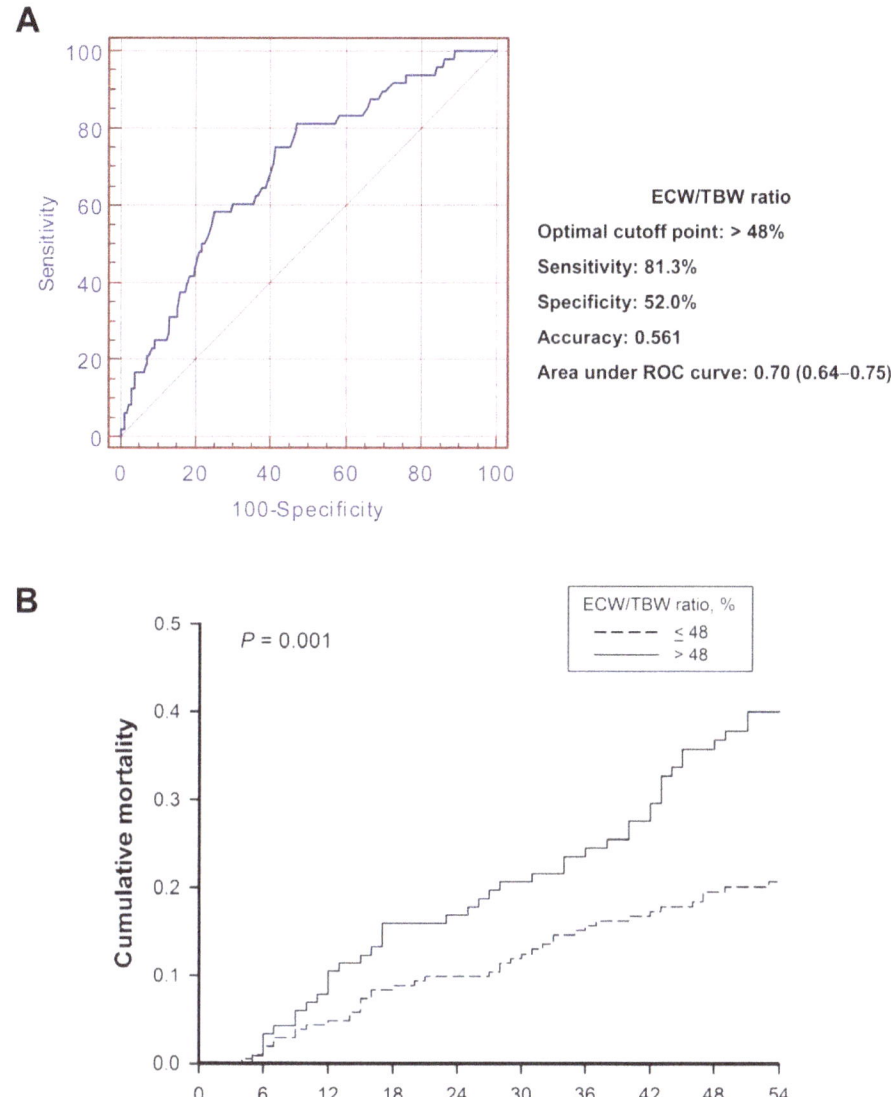

ECW/TBW ratio

Optimal cutoff point: > 48%

Sensitivity: 81.3%

Specificity: 52.0%

Accuracy: 0.561

Area under ROC curve: 0.70 (0.64–0.75)

Figure 1. Volume status for predicting mortality. The receiver operating characteristic (ROC) curve for prediction of all-cause mortality constructed using the ratio of extracellular water to total body water (ECW/TBW) at baseline (A). The optimal cutoff point for ECW/TBW is listed in the attached table, along with the sensitivity, specificity and accuracy for predicting mortality at the end of the follow-up period. The area under ROC curve is significantly larger than 0.5. Kaplan-Meier analysis curve for all-cause mortality in relation to the ECW/TBW at baseline, stratified by the cutoff point among hemodialysis patients (B).

were no significant differences between groups regarding the type of antihypertensive medications, dialysis prescription, and serum potassium levels. The median plasma aldosterone concentration was 184 pg/mL (IQR: 97–484 pg/mL), which is above the 75th percentile for aldosterone in a large cohort of non-CKD patients referred for coronary angiography [3]. Table 2 shows the baseline characteristics stratified by both volume status and plasma aldosterone categories. In patients without volume overload, hs-CRP and interleukin-6 (IL-6) levels were significantly higher in patients in the >280 pg/mL aldosterone category than in patients in the <140 pg/mL aldosterone category (P<0.05). This relationship was inversed in patients with volume overload. The number

of antihypertensive medication was positively and significantly associated with the aldosterone categories for patients without volume overload, but the trend was reversed for patients with volume overload.

Table 3 shows univariate correlations between ECW/TBW or plasma aldosterone levels and potentially explanatory variables. The ECW/TBW was negatively correlated with plasma aldosterone, hemoglobin, albumin, calcium, and phosphate levels and was positively correlated with age, hs-CRP, IL-6, ferritin levels, and systolic BP. In contrast, plasma aldosterone was positively associated with albumin and phosphate levels and was negatively associated with age, ECW/TBW, ferritin and systolic BP.

Table 1. Baseline characteristics of the study participants by categories of ECW/TBW.

Baseline values	Total patients (n = 328)	ECW/TBW ≤48% (n = 209)	ECW/TBW >48% (n = 119)	P-value[a]
Age (years)	59±13	55±12	65±11	<0.001[b]
Male (%)	57.3	59.8	52.9	0.23[c]
Smoking history (%)	31.7	32.1	31.1	0.86[c]
Diabetes mellitus (%)	29.3	19.1	47.1	<0.001[c]
Prior CVD (%)	23.4	18.2	32.8	0.002[c]
Hypertension (%)	48.2	40.6	61.3	<0.001[c]
Systolic BP (mmHg)	136±24	134±22	140±26	0.04[b]
Diastolic BP (mmHg)	76±12	76±11	76±14	0.99[b]
RAAS blockade (%)	27.1	24.9	31.1	0.22[c]
Calcium channel blocker (%)	62.2	59.8	66.4	0.31[c]
β-blocker (%)	32.6	32.0	33.6	0.53[c]
No. of antihypertensives	2.0±1.3	2.0±1.1	2.1±1.5	0.72[b]
Statin use (%)	15.9	16.3	15.1	0.79[c]
HD duration (months)	66±54	67±53	65±56	0.84[b]
Kt/V urea	2.0±0.6	2.0±0.5	2.1±0.7	0.11[b]
Intradialytic UF (L)	2.9±0.6	2.9±0.7	2.8±0.5	0.87[b]
BMI (kg/m^2)	22.6±3.5	22.0±3.1	23.3±4.1	0.02[b]
ECW (L)	13.0±2.1	12.5±2.1	13.7±2.0	<0.001[b]
TBW (L)	28.4±4.6	29.3±4.8	26.9±3.9	<0.001[b]
ECW/TBW (%)	45.8±5.0	42.9±3.4	50.9±2.8	<0.001[b]
Aldosterone (pg/mL)	184 (97–484)	215 (99–768)	166 (95–263)	0.02[d]
hs-CRP (mg/L)	3.94 (1.29–7.86)	3.74 (1.55–6.74)	4.10 (1.24–8.09)	0.04[d]
IL-6 (pg/mL)	2.92 (2.21–7.87)	2.80 (1.78–5.53)	4.59 (2.66–9.67)	<0.001[d]
Albumin (g/L)	39.3±3.5	39.9±3.2	38.2±3.7	<0.001[b]
Total cholesterol (mg/dL)	186±33	188±32	180±35	0.16[b]
Triglyceride (mg/dL)	127±61	130±64	121±57	0.18[b]
Potassium (mmol/L)	4.01±0.36	4.02±0.37	3.98±0.37	0.28[b]
Calcium (mg/dL)	9.7±0.7	9.8±0.7	9.6±0.8	0.03[b]
Phosphate (mg/dL)	5.0±1.4	5.2±1.4	4.8±1.3	0.002[b]
Hemoglobin (g/dL)	10.5±1.5	10.8±1.5	9.8±1.4	<0.001[b]
EPO dose (u/kg/wk)	66±46	55±47	87±36	<0.001[b]
Ferritin (µg/L)	344 (201–538)	291 (129–439)	361 (255–606)	0.001[d]
Transferrin saturation (%)	27±13	27±13	27±14	0.77[b]

Abbreviations: BMI denotes body mass index; BP, blood pressure; CVD, cardiovascular disease; ECW, extracellular water; ECW/TBW, ratio of extracellular water to total body water; EPO, erythropoietin; HD, hemodialysis; hs-CRP, high-sensitivity C-reactive protein; IL-6, inerleukin-6; RAAS, renin-angiotensin-aldosterone system; TBW, total body water; UF, ultrafiltration.
[a]Comparison between two groups of patients with ECW/TBW ≤48% and >48%.
Statistical analysis by [b]Student t-test, [c]Pearson x^2 test, and [d]Mann-Whitney U test.
Prior CVD category consisted of congestive heart failure, coronary artery disease, cerebrovascular disease, and peripheral arterial disease.

Follow-up Data

During the follow-up period, 16 patients received kidney transplants, and 4 patients transitioned to peritoneal dialysis. Thirty-three patients who were transferred to other dialysis units were followed up using questionnaire forms completed by the attending physicians at the units. At the end of the follow-up period, 225 patients were confirmed to be alive on hemodialysis treatment, and 83 patients died while being treated; 37 (44.6%) of these deaths were due to CVD-related causes. There were 70 CV events in the median follow-up period of 54 months (IQR: 27–107 months). In unadjusted analysis, lower aldosterone levels were

associated with higher mortality in the overall cohort (P for trend = 0.006) (Fig. 2) and in the presence of volume overload (P for trend = 0.001) (Fig. 3A), respectively. However, in the absence of volume overload, the association was reversed, with higher aldosterone levels associated with higher mortality (P for trend = 0.042) (Fig. 3B).

Multivariate analysis with plasma aldosterone, age, gender, prior CVD, presence of diabetes mellitus, smoking status, body mass index, systolic blood pressure, dialysis vintage, baseline levels of serum albumin, total cholesterol, hemoglobin, ferritin, calcium×phosphate, Kt/V urea, and IL-6 as the independent

Table 2. Baseline characteristics of the study participants by categories of ECW/TBW and plasma aldosterone.

	ECW/TBW ≤48%			ECW/TBW >48%		
	Plasma aldoterone, pg/mL			Plasma aldoterone, pg/mL		
	<140	140–280	>280	<140	140–280	>280
Baseline values	(n = 69)	(n = 53)	(n = 87)	(n = 39)	(n = 56)	(n = 24)
Age (years)	55±12	57±11	54±11	67±9	66±13	64±9
Male (%)	63.8	54.7	59.8	51.3	53.6	54.2
Smoking history (%)	34.8	32.1	29.9	30.8	28.6	37.5
Diabetes mellitus (%)	23.2	24.5	12.6	38.5	51.8	50.0
Prior CVD (%)	20.3	22.6	13.8	38.5	30.4	29.2
Hypertension (%)	39.4	41.8	41.3	67.9	66.7	41.6[b,c]
Systolic BP (mmHg)	132±19	134±24	135±24	143±27	140±25	135±26[b,c]
Diastolic BP (mmHg)	76±9	76±11	75±11	74±12	77±18	76±7
RAAS blockade (%)	15.9	28.3	29.9	28.2	30.4	37.5
No. of antihypertensives	1.5±1.0	2.0±1.0	2.4±1.5[b]	2.5±1.5	2.4±1.5	1.4±1.0[b,c]
Statin use (%)	11.6	17.0	19.5	17.9	14.3	12.5
HD duration (months)	67±49	65±53	68±56	59±47	67±52	74±74
Kt/V urea	2.0±0.6	2.0±0.3	2.0±0.4	2.0±0.4	2.3±0.9	2.0±0.3
BMI (kg/m^2)	21.8±3.1	21.7±2.8	22.6±3.1	23.1±5.2	23.5±3.4	22.5±4.8
ECW (L)	12.4±1.5	12.3±2.2	12.8±2.2	13.9±2.2	13.0±1.9	13.6±2.1
TBW (L)	28.2±3.7	28.±9 4.8	30.1±5.1	27.1±4.6	26.7±3.4	27.3±4.4
ECW/TBW (%)	44.2±2.9	42.7±4.1[b]	42.7±3.1[b]	51.4±2.9	50.9±2.8	49.9±2.0[b,c]
hs-CRP (mg/L)	2.53 (1.09–4.99)	3.85 (1.26–5.79)	4.76 (1.62–7.55)[b]	6.12 (2.28–8.63)	4.70 (0.94–8.06)	1.53 (0.59–5.82)[b]
IL-6 (pg/mL)	2.42 (1.62–4.44)	3.10 (1.87–5.84)	3.85 (2.19–6.04)[b]	5.42 (2.52–11.57)	4.86 (3.04–12.36)	3.62 (2.55–6.43)[b]
Albumin (g/L)	39.5±3.1	39.9±3.4	40.0±3.2	36.8±1.3	38.9±3.5	39.3±4.0[b]
Total cholesterol (mg/dL)	193±45	189±40	183±30	177±32	180±34	185±38
Triglyceride (mg/dL)	133±68	130±60	128±48	122±53	120±47	121±49
Potassium (mmol/L)	4.03±0.37	4.02±0.37	4.01±0.37	4.00±0.36	3.99±0.37	3.98±0.37
Calcium (mg/dL)	9.8±0.7	9.6±0.7	9.8±0.7	9.4±0.9	9.7±0.8	9.4±0.6
Phosphate (mg/dL)	4.8±1.2	5.1±1.4	5.5±1.5	4.5±1.2	4.8±1.3	4.8±1.2
Hemoglobin (g/dL)	10.8±1.2	10.6±1.6	10.8±1.6	9.7±1.3	9.8±1.4	10.0±1.2
EPO dose (u/kg/wk)	51±44	72±50[b]	52±45[c]	89±31	87±41	77±36
Ferritin (µg/L)	323 (157–407)	277 (142–541)	271 (101–466)	370 (272–675)	393 (264–593)	278 (239–514)
Transferrin saturation (%)	29±12	24±10	28±14	27±14	27±14	26±15

For abbreviations see Table 1.
[a]Comparisons among three groups in patients with ECW/TBW ≤48% and >48%, respectively. Statistical analysis by one-way ANOVA test, Pearson x^2 test, and Kruskal-Wallis test as appropriate.
[b]P<0.05 versus patients with plasma aldosterone of <140 pg/mL.
[c]P<0.05 versus patients with plasma aldosterone of 140–280 pg/mL.
Prior CVD category consisted of congestive heart failure, coronary artery disease, cerebrovascular disease, and peripheral arterial disease.

variables demonstrated that plasma aldosterone, age, prior CVD, serum albumin, and IL-6 were independently related to mortality and first CV event. The inverse association of aldosterone level with mortality, both in the entire patient population and in the presence of volume overload (ECW/TBW >48%), was also seen in adjusted analysis (Table 4). Furthermore, volume overload was found to modify the risk relationship between aldosterone and first CV event in the Cox regressions with plasma aldosterone level as a categorical (interaction, P = 0.02) or a continuous measure (interaction, P = 0.03). In the absence of volume overload (ECW/TBW ≤48%), the aldosterone category was positively associated with all-cause mortality and first CV event. Analyzing aldosterone

as a continuous variable also showed the similar association of aldosterone with all-cause mortality and first CV event.

Discussion

This study demonstrates an inverse association of aldosterone levels with all-cause mortality and CV event rates in the presence of volume overload. This represents a paradoxical effect of volume status on mortality. In contrast, there was a significant, graded, and positive association of aldosterone levels with all-cause mortality and CV event rates in the 64% of participants without volume overload. Accordingly, some ESRD patients with low aldosterone levels have a low risk of adverse outcomes, as in the general population, whereas others have a high risk because they

Table 3. Univariate correlations between ECW/TBW or plasma aldosterone and potentially explanatory variables.

Variables	ECW/TBW		Aldosterone	
	r	P-value	r	P-value
Age (years)	−0.555	<0.001	−0.286	<0.001
Body mass index (kg/m²)	−0.136	0.02	−0.038	0.54
ECW/TBW (%)	–	–	−0.200	0.001
Aldosterone (pg/mL)	−0.200	0.001	–	–
hs-CRP (mg/L)	−0.180	0.002	−0.013	0.81
IL-6 (pg/mL)	−0.310	<0.001	−0.069	0.22
Hemoglobin (g/dL)	−0.368	<0.001	−0.067	0.24
Serum ferritin (μg/L)	−0.208	<0.001	−0.169	0.003
Transferrin saturation (%)	−0.092	0.10	−0.029	0.61
Albumin (g/L)	−0.337	<0.001	−0.189	0.001
Calcium (mg/dL)	−0.123	0.03	−0.082	0.15
Phosphate (mg/dL)	−0.177	0.001	−0.222	<0.001
Potassium (mmol/L)	−0.080	0.19	−0.024	0.69
Systolic BP (mmHg)	−0.123	0.03	−0.135	0.02
Diastolic BP (mmHg)	−0.032	0.57	−0.081	0.16
Kt/V urea	−0.089	0.06	−0.028	0.63

For abbreviations see Table 1.

are in a state of volume overload, which lowers aldosterone levels and increases the risk of mortality and CV events. These findings underline the importance of hyperaldosteronemia as a risk factor for adverse long-term outcomes among patients with ESRD, and of the masking of this association among individuals with volume overload.

A growing body of evidence has linked aldosterone excess to the development and progression of different CVD processes, including hypertension, congestive heart failure, and coronary artery disease [16,17]. Plasma aldosterone levels are markedly elevated among patients with CKD [3–5] which is similar to the remnant kidney model in the rat [18]. In a study of 28 selected patients with varying degrees of CKD and normal serum potassium levels and plasma renin activity, Hene et al. showed that aldosterone levels were elevated when creatinine clearance was less than 50% of normal, increasing three- to four-fold above normal levels as clearance values decreased [3]. Therefore, aldosterone-mediated CV damage might be amplified by decreased kidney function, which by itself is a potent CV risk factor [7].

Plasma aldosterone levels are influenced by a number of factors, including potassium and volume status. Our results showed that a relatively lower aldosterone level was in fact a surrogate marker of volume overload in hemodialysis patients. In healthy volunteers with salt loading and in hemodialysis patients with increased inter-dialytic weight gain, expansions of ECW led to reciprocal declines in plasma aldosterone concentrations. The relationship was more profound in healthy volunteers than in hemodialysis patients. As a result, the shift of the volume-aldosterone curve in hemodialysis patients suggests that ESRD is a state of high volume and

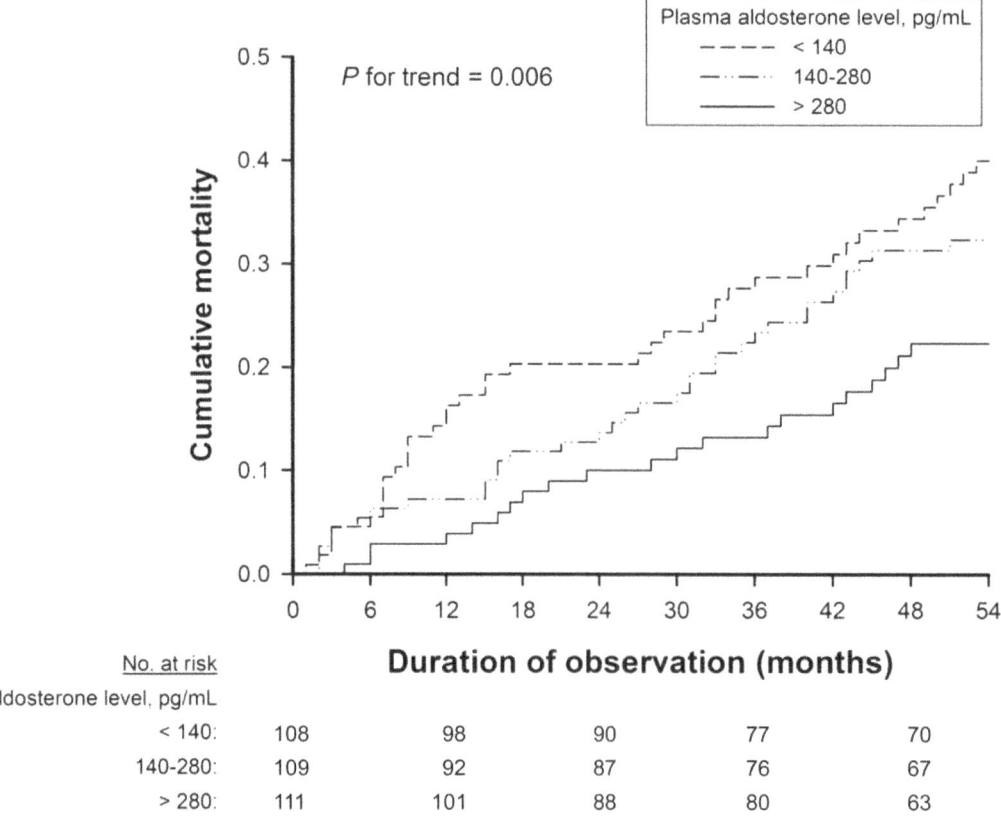

Figure 2. Kaplan-Meier mortality curves according to aldosterone tertile. All-cause mortality in relation to plasma aldosterone levels at baseline among hemodialysis patients.

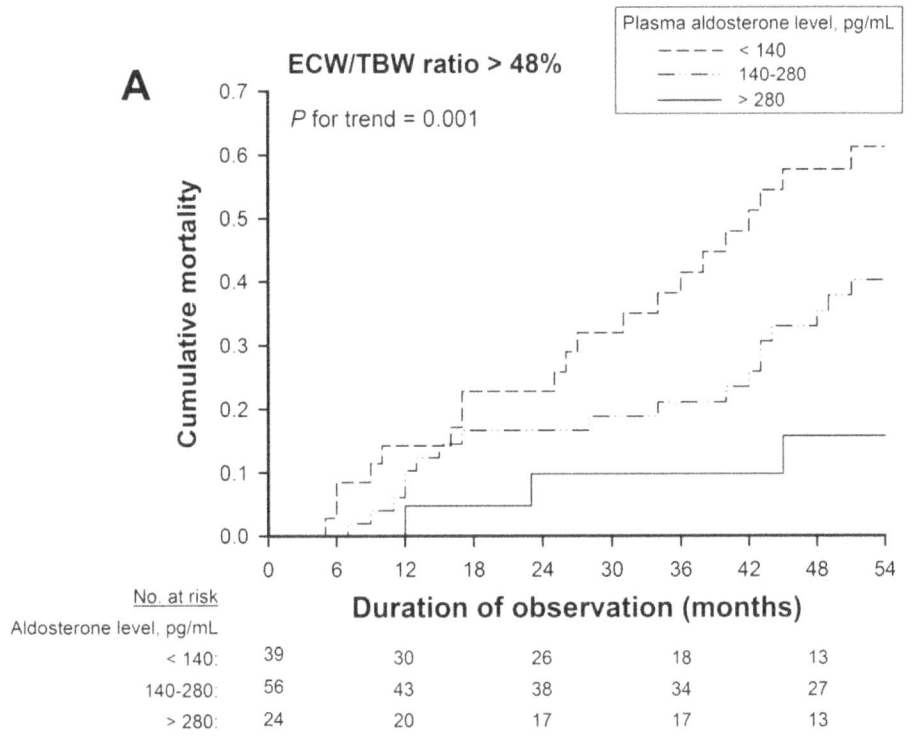

No. at risk

Aldosterone level, pg/mL					
< 140:	39	30	26	18	13
140-280:	56	43	38	34	27
> 280:	24	20	17	17	13

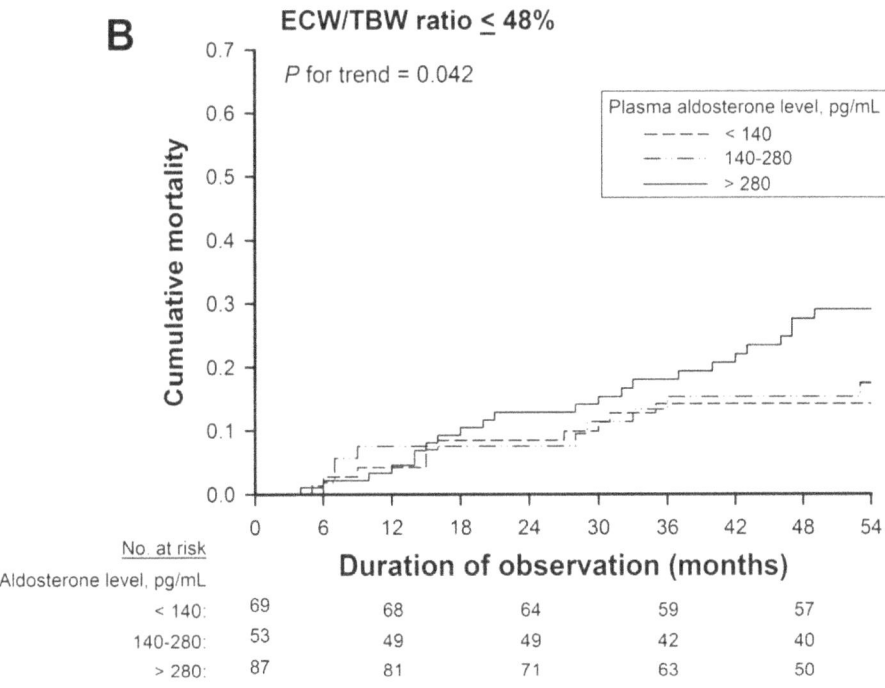

No. at risk

Aldosterone level, pg/mL					
< 140:	69	68	64	59	57
140-280:	53	49	49	42	40
> 280:	87	81	71	63	50

Figure 3. Kaplan-Meier mortality curves according to aldosterone tertile, modified by volume status. All-cause mortality in relation to plasma aldosterone levels at baseline modified by the ratio of extracellular water to total body water (ECW/TBW) >48% (A) and ≤48% (B) among hemodialysis patients.

inappropriately high aldosterone levels [19]. ESRD patients are particularly vulnerable to sudden cardiac death resulting from left ventricular hypertrophy (LVH) and fibrosis [20]. Cumulative evidence has indicated that aldosterone, beyond its classical actions on epithelial cells with BP-dependent organ damage, exerts non-classical effects on interstitial tissues, which are involved in

cardiac and renal fibrosis [21–24]. These non-epithelial effects of aldosterone are exaggerated in conditions of elevated aldosterone levels and expanded ECW, such as ESRD [25].

In a large cohort of non-CKD patients scheduled for coronary angiography, variations in aldosterone concentrations within the normal range were associated with increased all-cause and CV

Table 4. Hazard ratios for mortality and first cardiovascular event by categorical or continuous measure of plasma aldosterone modified by ECW/TBW.

	Overall (n = 328)	ECW/TBW >48% (n = 119)	ECW/TBW ≤48% (n = 209)	P-value[a]
All-cause Mortality, Adjusted HR (95% Confidence Interval)				
Categorical measure				
Aldosterone <140 pg/mL	1.00	1.00	1.00	0.01
Aldosterone 140–280 pg/mL	0.87 (0.58−1.31)	0.82 (0.43−1.45)	1.15 (0.91−2.23)	
Aldosterone >280 pg/mL	0.65 (0.48−0.91)	0.49 (0.25−0.76)	1.97 (1.69−3.75)	
Age, per 1 year	1.05 (1.03−1.07)	1.03 (1.00−1.08)	1.07 (1.02−1.12)	
Prior CVD	2.54 (1.54−4.17)	5.29 (2.44−11.49)	2.35 (1.87−6.36)	
Albumin, per 1 g/L	0.92 (0.85−0.98)	0.87 (0.75−0.91)	0.91 (0.79−0.92)	
IL-6, per 1 pg/mL	1.07 (1.01−1.14)	1.11 (1.01−1.23)	1.08 (1.04−1.12)	
Continuous measure				
Aldosterone, per 100 pg/mL	0.75 (0.60−0.91)	0.84 (0.67−0.96)	1.61 (1.20−2.73)	0.03
Age, per 1 year	1.05 (1.03−1.08)	1.03 (0.99−1.07)	1.07 (1.02−1.12)	
Prior CVD	2.58 (1.40−4.76)	5.52 (2.53−12.07)	2.14 (1.80−5.67)	
Albumin, per 1 g/L	0.92 (0.85−0.99)	0.85 (0.77−0.94)	0.93 (0.89−0.97)	
IL-6, per 1 pg/mL	1.05 (1.02−1.13)	1.11 (1.02−1.27)	1.07 (1.03−1.11)	
First CV Event, Adjusted HR (95% Confidence Interval)				
Categorical measure				
Aldosterone <140 pg/mL	1.00	1.00	1.00	0.02
Aldosterone 140–280 pg/mL	0.89 (0.65−1.41)	0.81 (0.51−1.89)	1.21 (0.92−2.43)	
Aldosterone >280 pg/mL	0.79 (0.41−0.81)	0.70 (0.33−0.78)	2.01 (1.28−4.15)	
Age, per 1 year	1.03 (1.02−1.06)	1.02 (0.97−1.08)	1.04 (0.99−1.10)	
Prior CVD	5.08 (2.57−10.09)	6.45 (2.52−16.52)	3.41 (1.24−9.39)	
Albumin, per 1 g/L	0.89 (0.80−0.99)	0.80 (0.65−0.98)	0.82 (0.68−0.98)	
IL-6, per 1 pg/mL	1.14 (1.04−1.25)	1.14 (1.02−1.29)	1.21 (1.01−1.45)	
Continuous measure				
Aldosterone, per 100 pg/mL	0.80 (0.69−0.95)	0.69 (0.57−0.90)	1.67 (1.12−2.89)	0.03
Age, per 1 year	1.04 (1.01−1.08)	1.03 (0.97−1.09)	1.05 (0.99−1.12)	
Prior CVD	5.10 (2.26−11.56)	6.45 (2.52−16.52)	3.42 (1.24−9.39)	
Albumin, per 1 g/L	0.89 (0.79−0.96)	0.81 (0.65−0.99)	0.82 (0.68−0.98)	
IL-6, per 1 pg/mL	1.13 (1.02−1.25)	1.15 (1.02−1.29)	1.21 (1.01−1.45)	

Abbreviations: CI denotes confidence interval; CV, cardiovascular; CVD, cardiovascular disease; ECW/TBW, ratio of extracellular water to total body water; HR, hazard ratio; IL-6, inerleukin-6.
[a]The interaction P values assessed the modifying effect of volume overload (ECW/TBW >48%) on the risk relationship between plasma aldosterone and overall mortality and CV events.

mortality independent of major established CV risk factors [6]. In the same cohort, the association of higher plasma aldosterone concentrations with overall CV mortality and sudden cardiac death was stronger for patients with decreased kidney function [7]. Furthermore, a recent study by Edwards et al. also showed that the use of spironolactone reduced left ventricular (LV) mass and improved arterial stiffness in early-stage CKD [26]. Unfortunately, the largest trials to date that used mineralocorticoid receptor antagonists and demonstrated a mortality benefit in patients with severe heart failure due to systolic LV dysfunction or acute myocardial infarction [27,28], excluded patients with moderate to advanced CKD. Once CKD patients have progressed to ESRD, aldosterone levels may remain elevated [29–31]. The markedly elevated levels of aldosterone levels seen in ESRD suggest that mineralocorticoid receptor blockade could emerge as a crucial

strategy against CVD in this population [32]. Randomized controlled trials are required to confirm our preliminary findings and define the risk of potential hazards, particularly those involving hyperkalemia [33].

The present study has a number of limitations. First, the modifying effect of volume overload on the risk relationship between aldosterone and mortality may still be subject to residual confounding. Furthermore, as with any cohort study, this study cannot establish causality between volume overload or aldosterone levels and mortality, and we caution against translating the results of observational studies into therapeutic practice. Finally, the impact of volume overload on the association between aldosterone and mortality might be different at different stages of CKD. It is unclear whether findings from our study of patients on dialysis can be extrapolated to patients who have moderate to advanced CKD and are not yet on dialysis.

Our study has biological plausibility and important therapeutic implications. In CKD patients, a progressive decline in glomerular filtration rate, activation of the renin-angiotensin-aldosterone system (RAAS), and superimposed CV comorbidities contribute to salt and water retention. Volume overload and inappropriately high aldosterone levels in CKD patients resulted in more severe LVH and increased arterial stiffness [34,35], both of which are independent predictors of CV mortality in dialysis patients [36,37]. Achieving strict volume control appears to be an imperative therapeutic strategy for inducing regression of LVH and arterial compliance, and lowering the CVD risk in dialysis patients. However, our study provides strong evidence that favorable effects of volume correction might be negated by the simultaneous stimulation of RAAS and thus may become apparent only if this response is inhibited [38,39].

In summary, aldosterone level is inversely associated with adverse outcomes in hemodialysis patients. Volume overload underlies this paradox. In the absence of volume overload, aldosterone is an independent risk factor for all-cause mortality and CV events in this population. These data provide evidence for the confounding and effect modification of the association of aldosterone with adverse outcomes by volume overload. Hence, further research is warranted to clarify the pathophysiological mechanisms that link volume overload and hyperaldosteronemia to increased mortality and CV events and whether therapeutic interventions to mitigate volume overload and lower aldosterone concentrations may lead to improved outcomes in dialysis patients.

Acknowledgments

We are deeply indebted to Miss P.C. Lee for her expert secretarial assistance and graphic design.

Author Contributions

Conceived and designed the experiments: DCT. Performed the experiments: HLH HFP. Analyzed the data: SCH YPL. Wrote the paper: SCH.

References

1. Foley RN, Parfrey PS, Sarnak MJ (1998) Clinical epidemiology of cardiovascular disease in chronic kidney disease. Am J Kidney Dis 32: 112–119.
2. Rossignol P, Ménard J, Fay R, Gustafsson F, Pitt B, et al. (2011) Eplerenone survival benefits in heart failure patients post-myocardial infarction are independent from its diuretic and potassium-sparing effects: Insights from an EPHESUS (Eplerenone Post-Acute Myocardial Infarction Heart Failure Efficacy and Survival Study) Substudy. J Am Coll Cardiol 58: 1958–1966.
3. Hene R, Boer P, Koomans H, Mees E (1982) Plasma aldosterone concentrations in chronic renal disease. Kidney Int 21: 98–101.
4. Diskin CJ, Stokes TJ, Dansby LM, Carter TB, Radcliff L (2004) The clinical significance of aldosterone in ESRD: Part II. Nephrol Dial Transplant 19: 1331–1332.
5. Kohagura K, Higashiuesato Y, Ishiki T, Yoshi S, Ohya Y, et al. (2006) Plasma aldosterone in hypertensive patients on chronic hemodialysis: distribution, determinants and impact on survival. Hypertens Res 29: 597–604.
6. Tomaschitz A, Pilz S, Ritz E, Meinitzer A, Boehm BO, et al. (2010) Plasma aldosterone levels are associated with increased cardiovascular mortality: the Ludwigshafen Risk and Cardiovascular Health (LURIC) Study. Eur Heart J 31: 1237–1247.
7. Tomaschitz A, Pilz S, Ritz E, Grammer T, Drechsler C, et al. (2011) Association of plasma aldosterone with cardiovascular mortality in patients with low estimated GFR: the Ludwigshafen Risk and Cardiovascular Health (LURIC) Study. Am J Kidney Dis 57: 403–414.
8. Lowrie EG, Lew NL (1990) Death risk in hemodialysis patients: the predictive value of commonly measured variables and an evaluation of death rate differences between facilities. Am J Kidney Dis 15: 458–482.
9. Liu Y, Coresh J, Eustace JA, Longenecker JC, Jaar B, et al. (2004) Association between cholesterol level and mortality in dialysis patients: Role of inflammation and malnutrition. JAMA 291: 451–459.
10. Contreras G, Hu B, Astor BC, Greene T, Erlinger T, et al. (2010) Malnutrition-Inflammation modifies the relationship of cholesterol with cardiovascular disease. J Am Soc Nephrol 21: 2131–2142.
11. Kalantar-Zadeh K, Regidor DL, Kovesdy CP, Van Wyck D, Bunnapradist S, et al. (2009) Fluid retention is associated with cardiovascular mortality in patients undergoing long-term hemodialysis. Circulation 119: 671–679.
12. Agarwal R (2010) Hypervolemia is associated with increased mortality among hemodialysis patients. Hypertension 56: 512–517.
13. Klemmer PJ, Bomback AS (2009) Extracellular volume and aldosterone interaction in chronic kidney disease. Blood Purif 27: 92–98.
14. Daugirdas JT (1993) Second generation logarithmic estimates of single-pool variable volume Kt/V: an analysis of errors. J Am Soc Nephrol 4: 1205–1213.
15. Parmar MKB, Machin D (1995) Survival Analysis. A Practical Approach. New York, John Wiley & Sons.
16. Guder G, Bauersachs J, Frantz S, Weismann D, Allolio B, et al. (2007) Complementary and incremental mortality risk prediction by cortisol and aldosterone in chronic heart failure. Circulation 115: 1754–1761.
17. Beygui F, Collet JP, Benoliel JJ, Vignolles N, Dumaine R, et al. (2006) High plasma aldosterone levels on admission are associated with death in patients presenting with acute ST-elevation myocardial infarction. Circulation 114: 2604–2610.
18. Ibrahim HN, Hostetter TH (1998) The renin-aldosterone axis in two models of reduced renal mass in the rat. J Am Soc Nephrol 9: 72–76.
19. Bomback AS, Kshirsagar AV, Ferris ME, Klemmer PJ (2009) Disordered aldosterone-volume relationship in end-stage kidney disease. J Renin Angiotensin Aldosterone Syst 10: 230–236.
20. Green D, Roberts PR, New DI, Kalra PA (2011) Sudden cardiac death in hemodialysis patients: an in-depth review. Am J Kidney Dis 57: 921–929.
21. Hostetter TH, Ibrahim HN (2003) Aldosterone in chronic kidney and cardiac disease. J Am Soc Nephrol 14: 2395–2401.
22. Weber KT, Brilla CG (1991) Pathological hypertrophy and cardiac interstitium. Fibrosis and renin-angiotensin-aldosterone system. Circulation 83: 1849–1865.
23. Young M, Funder JW (2004) Eplerenone, but not steroid withdrawal, reverses cardiac fibrosis in deoxycorticosterone/salt-treated rats. Endocrinology 145: 3153–3157.
24. Juknevicius I, Segal Y, Kren S, Lee R, Hostetter TH (2004) Effect of aldosterone on renal transforming growth factor-beta. Am J Physiol Renal Physiol 286: F1059–F1062.
25. Sato A, Saruta T (2004) Aldosterone-induced organ damage: plasma aldosterone level and inappropriate salt status. Hypertens Res 27: 303–310.
26. Edwards NC, Steeds RP, Stewart PM, Ferro CJ, Townend JN (2009) Effect of spironolactone on left ventricular mass and aortic stiffness in early-stage chronic kidney disease: a randomized controlled trial. J Am Coll Cardiol 54: 505–512.
27. Pitt B, Zannad F, Remme WJ, Cody R, Castaigne A, et al. (1999) The effect of spironolactone on morbidity and mortality in patients with severe heart failure. Randomized Aldactone Evaluation Study Investigators. N Engl J Med 341: 709–717.
28. Pitt B, Remme W, Zannad F, Neaton J, Martinez F, et al. (2003) Eplerenone, a selective aldosterone blocker, in patients with left ventricular dysfunction after myocardial infarction. N Engl J Med 348: 1309–1321.
29. Berl T, Katz FH, Henrich WL, de Torrente A, Schrier RW (1978) Role of aldosterone in the control of sodium excretion in patients with advanced chronic renal failure. Kidney Int 14: 228–235.
30. Ratge D, Augustin R, Wisser H (1983) Catecholamines, renin, aldosterone and arterial pressure in patients on chronic hemodialysis treatment. Int J Artif Organs 6: 255–260.
31. McLaughlin N, Gehr TW, Sica DA (2004) Aldosterone-receptor antagonism and end-stage renal disease. Curr Hypertens Rep 6: 327–330.
32. Covic A, Gusbeth-Tatomir P, Goldsmith DJ (2006) Is it time for spironolactone therapy in dialysis patients? Nephrol Dial Transplant 21: 854–858.
33. Ritz E, Koleganova N (2010) Aldosterone in uremia–beyond blood pressure. Blood Purif 29: 111–113.
34. Barenbrock M, Spieker C, Laske V, Heidenreich S, Hohage H, et al. (1994) Studies of the vessel wall properties in hemodialysis patients. Kidney Int 45: 1397–1400.
35. London GM, Pannier B, Vicaut E, Guerin A, Marchais SJ, et al. (1996) Antihypertensive effects and arterial haemodynamic alterations during angiotensin converting enzyme inhibition. J Hypertens 14: 1139–1146.
36. London GM, Pannier B, Guerin AP, Blacher J, Marchais SJ, et al. (2001) Alterations of left ventricular hypertrophy in and survival of patients receiving hemodialysis: follow-up of an interventional study. J Am Soc Nephrol 12: 2759–2767.
37. Blacher J, Guerin AP, Pannier B, Marchais SJ, Safar ME, et al. (1999) Impact of aortic stiffness on survival in end-stage renal disease. Circulation 99: 2434–2439.
38. Tycho Vuurmans JL, Boer WH, Bos WJ, Blankestijn PJ, Koomans HA (2002) Contribution of volume overload and angiotensin II to the increased pulse wave velocity of hemodialysis patients. J Am Soc Nephrol 13: 177–183.
39. Cice G, Di Benedetto A, D'Isa S, D'Andrea A, Marcelli D, et al. (2010) Effects of telmisartan added to angiotensin-converting enzyme inhibitors on mortality and morbidity in hemodialysis patients with chronic heart failure: A double-blind, placebo-controlled trial. J Am Coll Cardiol 56: 1701–1708.

20

Predicting Mortality of Incident Dialysis Patients in Taiwan

Ping-Hsun Wu[1,4], **Yi-Ting Lin**[2,3], **Tzu-Chi Lee**[2], **Ming-Yen Lin**[1], **Mei-Chuan Kuo**[1,5]*, **Yi-Wen Chiu**[1,5], **Shang-Jyh Hwang**[1,5], **Hung-Chun Chen**[1,5]

1 Division of Nephrology, Department of Internal Medicine, Kaohsiung Medical University Hospital, Kaohsiung, Taiwan, **2** Department of Family Medicine, Kaohsiung Medical University Hospital, Kaohsiung, Taiwan, **3** Department of Public Health, College of Medicine, Kaohsiung Medical University, Kaohsiung, Taiwan, **4** Department of Internal Medicine, College of Medicine, Kaohsiung Medical University, Kaohsiung, Taiwan, **5** Faculty of Renal Care, College of Medicine, Kaohsiung Medical University, Kaohsiung, Taiwan

Abstract

Background: Comorbid conditions are highly prevalent among patients with end-stage renal disease (ESRD) and index score is a predictor of mortality in dialysis patients. The aim of this study is to perform a population-based cohort study to investigate the survival rate by age and Charlson comorbidity index (CCI) in incident dialysis patients.

Methods: Using the catastrophic illness registration of the Taiwan National Health Insurance Research Database for all patients from 1 January 1998 to 31 December 2008, individuals newly diagnosed with ESRD and receiving dialysis for more than 90 days were eligible for our study. Individuals younger than 18 years or renal transplantation patients either before or after dialysis were excluded. We calculated the CCI, age-weighted CCI by Deyo-Charlson method according to ICD-9 code and categorized CCI into six groups as index scores <3, 4–6, 7–9, 10–12, 13–15, >15. Cox regression models were used to analyze the association between age, CCI and survival, and the risk markers of survival.

Results: There were 79,645 incident dialysis patients, whose mean age (± SD) was 60.96 (±13.92) years; 51.43% of patients were women and 51.2% were diabetic. In cox proportional hazard models and stratifying by age, older patients had significantly higher mortality than younger patients. The mortality risk was higher in persons with higher CCI as compared with low CCI. Mortality increased steadily with higher age or comorbidity both for unadjusted and for adjusted models. For all age groups, mortality rates increased in different CCI groups with the highest rates occurring in the oldest age groups.

Conclusions: Age and CCI are both strong predictors of survival in Taiwan. The older age or higher comorbidity index in incident dialysis patient is associated with lower long-term survival rates. These population-based estimates may assist clinicians who make decisions when patients need long-term dialysis.

Editor: Utpal Sen, University of Louisville, United States of America

Funding: No current external funding sources for this study.

Competing Interests: The authors have declared that no competing interests exist.

* E-mail: mechku@kmu.edu.tw

Introduction

End-stage renal disease (ESRD) patients have a high prevalence of comorbid conditions [1,2], high mortality rate [3–5], and poor prognosis. Although the prognosis for patients with ESRD treated by dialysis has improved in recent years, mortality rates remain high. The ESRD population is high in Taiwan and patients start dialysis with very low residual renal function and in poor clinical conditions [6]. Compared with populations in western countries, cardiovascular disease occurs less frequently among Asians [7] and late dialysis in Taiwan with low mortality [6] is quite different from other countries. Besides, there is no difference in survival rates between hemodialysis and peritoneal dialysis patients in Taiwan [8,9]. The median serum creatinine and glomerular filtration rate (GFR) are 10.1 mg/dL and 4.7 mL/min/1.73m^2 in Taiwan and lower GFR at dialysis initiation is associated with lower

mortality [10]. This finding is similar to the result in an IDEAL (Initiating Dialysis Early and Late) study that mentioned early initiation of dialysis principle was not associated with an improvement in survival or clinical outcomes [11]. Although late dialysis strategy is applied in Taiwan, comorbidity is still a major confounder but also a predictor of the patient's natural course and outcomes. Therefore, comorbidity should be assessed in dialysis patients and simplified comorbidity indexes are more applicable. Comorbidity scales have been evaluated in dialysis patients, such as Charlson comorbidity index (CCI) [12], index of co-existent diseases (ICED) [13], Davies [14], and Wright-Khan indices [3]. Of the comorbidity scales developed for general medical patients, CCI is the most popular [12] and easiest to apply. CCI was originally developed to create a single-value summary for several comorbid conditions for breast cancer patients in 1984 and is suitable for general medical inpatient populations. It is also applied to the dialysis population and also validated in ESRD patients [5,15]. ICED works better than CCI in analyses of ESRD patients but ICED is difficult to apply [13]. CCI is also a better predictor for mortality compared with the Davies comorbidity index for peritoneal dialysis patients [16]. However, previous studies examining on incident dialysis populations were performed in single centers, involved small numbers of patients, and had short-term duration. Few reports predict long-term mortality in dialysis patients [17,18] and publications on this subject in Asian populations are rare [19]. Age with CCI as a good predictor of long term prognosis in dialysis patients in Taiwan is still unknown. The objective of the present study is to predict long term survival in large sample incident dialysis patients using CCI and age-weight CCI in a 10-year nationwide cohort study. We used claims data from the National Health Insurance program in Taiwan to evaluate the comorbidities during pre-dialysis care and to investigate the relationship between CCI and survival in incident patients. Population-based data often contains all patients with a given disease, and administrative data offer a picture of the "real world" effectiveness of interventions as they are being practiced.

Methods

Data Source

This study is based on a longitudinal health insurance database, the National Health Insurance Research Database (NHIRD), provided by the Taiwan National Health Research Institute. Taiwan launched its compulsory social insurance program, National Health Insurance (NHI), to provide health care for all the island's residents since 1995. The annual coverage rate of the NHI program ranged from 96.16% to 99.6% and includes contracts with 97% of hospitals and clinics, with more than 23 million Taiwanese residents enrolled since 1997. It covers all medical benefit claims of ambulant and inpatient care and is extensively applied to many epidemiological studies. The NHIRD established a registry system for "Catastrophic Illnesses", including cancer, chronic mental illness, end-stage renal disease, congenital illness, and several autoimmune diseases. Insured persons with major diseases can

apply for catastrophic illness registration cards from the Bureau of National Health Insurance (BNHI) and do not need to make co-payments when seeking health care for catastrophic illness. Both outpatient and inpatient claims of beneficiaries with a catastrophic illness certificate are collected in the catastrophic illness profile and are distributed as a package. The BNHI performs routine validations of the diagnoses by reviewing the original medical charts of all of the patients who apply for catastrophic illness registration. In this study, all cases of dialysis patients are obtained from the Registry of Catastrophic Illness Database, a subpart of the NHIRD. The issuance of catastrophic illness certificates is validated by at least 2 specialists, based on careful examination of the medical records, laboratory studies, imaging studies, and dialysis treatment. Only individuals who meet the diagnostic criteria for major diseases are issued a catastrophic illness certificate. The database included all relevant information about the "catastrophic illness certificate" status, such as diagnostic codes in the format of the *International Classification of Disease, Ninth Revision, Clinical Modification* (ICD-9-CM), date of diagnosis, date of death, date of receiving dialysis, date of every clinic visits, details of prescriptions, expenditure amounts, and outpatient/inpatient claimed data for the beneficiaries with catastrophic illnesses during the period 1998–2008. During the study period, International Classification of Diseases, Ninth Revision (ICD-9) codes are used to define diseases. Personal information including family history, lifestyle, and habits such as smoking and alcohol use are not available from the NHIRD.

Study Cohorts

From the Registry for Catastrophic Illness Patient Database, we selected all patients diagnosed ESRD defined as those who had catastrophic illness registration cards for ESRD (ICD-9-CM code 585) and started hemodialysis or peritoneal dialysis of more than 90 days of renal replacement therapy between Jan,1, 1998, and Dec, 31, 2008. The NHIRD are enrolled since 1997, so the study cohort started from 1998, as a wash-out period for one year, and we also extended the observation time until 2009 in this cohort study. We excluded individuals younger than 18 years (n = 377) or those who had renal transplantation either

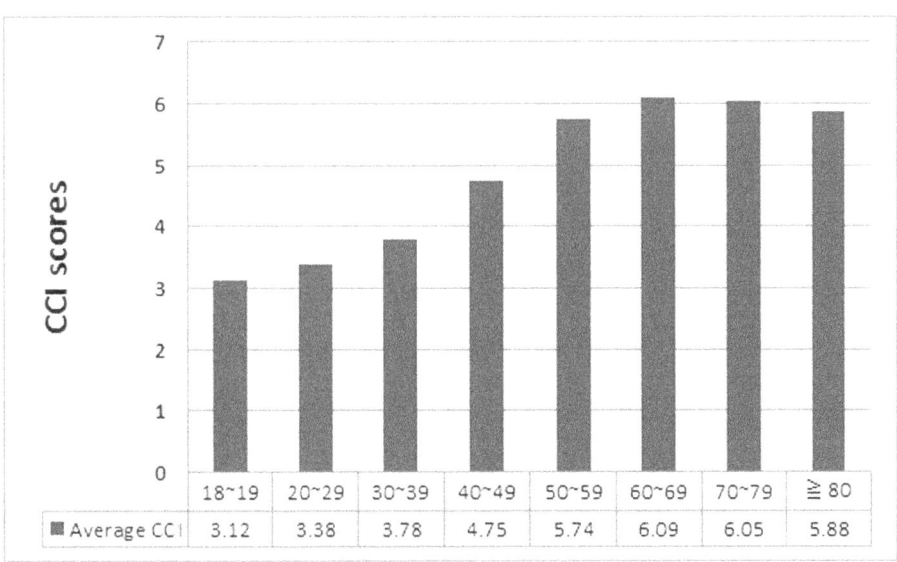

	18~19	20~29	30~39	40~49	50~59	60~69	70~79	≧ 80
■ Average CCI	3.12	3.38	3.78	4.75	5.74	6.09	6.05	5.88

Figure 1. Average comorbidity scores by age group.

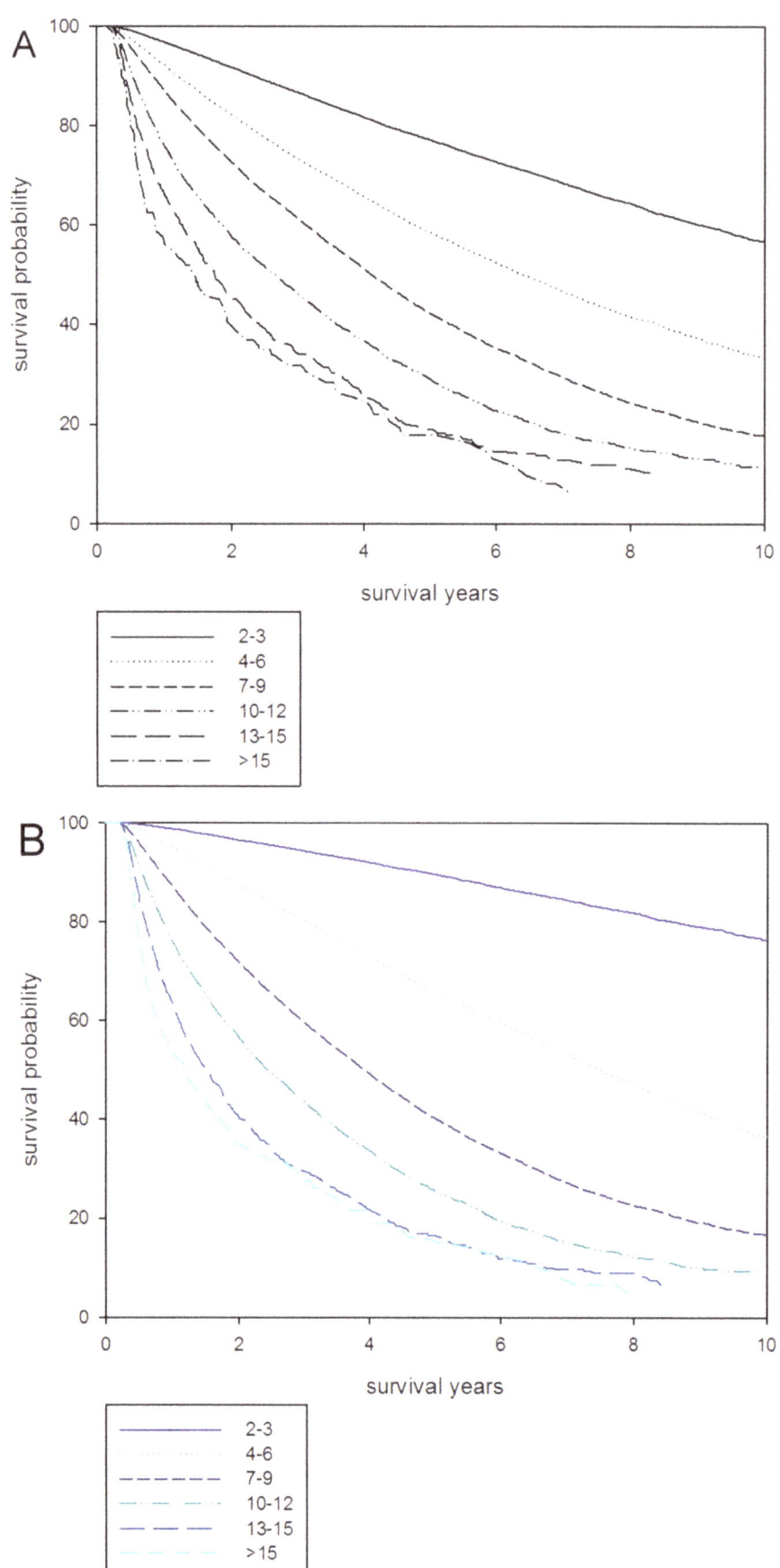

Figure 2. Survival curve stratified by Charlson comorbidity index (CCI) and age-weighted CCI. (A) Kaplan-Meier curves for 10 year survival by CCI score in incident patients. (B) Kaplan-Meier curves for 10 year survival by age-weighted CCI score. Survival is calculated beginning 90 days after starting dialysis. The survival rate of incident patients declined as CCI increased. A similar phenomenon is observed in incident patients in age-weighted CCI.

before or after dialysis (n = 1585). Patients receiving regular dialysis without catastrophic illness certificate were not included in this study.

Under the reimbursement system, hospitals have to claim medical expenses from the NHI based on the diagnosis or treatment codes for the disease presented by their patients. We used all diagnosis codes for a full year to define the existing comorbidities, including outpatient and inpatient diagnosis codes before the date of starting dialysis, which is defined as the index date. CCI and age-weighted CCI are calculated according to all diagnosis codes for a full year before the index date on every inpatient or outpatient to define the existing comorbidities [20]. Follow-up began on the index date until death or remaining alive at the end of the study period (Dec, 31, 2009). The CCI is defined by Charlson et al [12] and the Deyo-Charlson comorbidity index (table S1), based on ICD-9 codes in claims data, has been widely used in the analyses of the impact of comorbidities on mortality [21]. The CCI contains the following components: 1 point is assigned for history of myocardial infarction, congestive heart failure, peripheral vascular disease, cerebrovascular disease, dementia, chronic pulmonary disease, connective tissue disorder, peptic ulcer disease, mild liver disease and diabetes without end organ damage; 2 points for hemiplegia, moderate to severe renal disease (excluded in our scale because all patients had diagnosis of ESRD) diabetes with end organ damage, tumor without metastases, leukemia, lymphoma and myeloma; 3 points for moderate or

severe liver disease; and 6 points for metastatic solid tumor or full-blown acquired immunodeficiency syndrome (still included in this study's scale because of small numbers of dialysis patients) (table S2). As for Age-weighted-CCI, 1 point is added to the score for every decade more than 40 years of age (0 points for 18–49 years, 1 point for 50–59 years, 2 points for 60–69 years, 3 points for 70–79 years, 4 points for 80–89 years, 5 points for 90–99 years) (table S3). Because all patients are on dialysis, the minimum Charlson score is 2. All dialysis patients with diabetes are defined as diabetes with end organ damage. We categorized CCI into six groups as index scores ≦3, 4–6, 7–9, 10–12, 13–15, >15. Hazard ratio of mortality in dialysis patients by six comorbidity index groups and different age groups were analyzed.

Statistical Analysis

Data is summarized using proportions, and means (±standard deviation) as appropriate. The association between CCI and mortality was assessed using Cox proportional hazards model and Kaplan–Meier estimate with log rank tests declaring survival in the follow-up period for dialysis patients for each CCI level. In the mortality analyses, the patients were followed until event (death) or censoring (lost to follow-up or end of follow-up period); which ever happened first. The variables were analyzed initially by univariate analysis, and statistically significant variables were chosen for multivariate analysis. Analyses were performed using the SAS statistical package (version 9.2; SAS Institute Inc, www.sas.com).

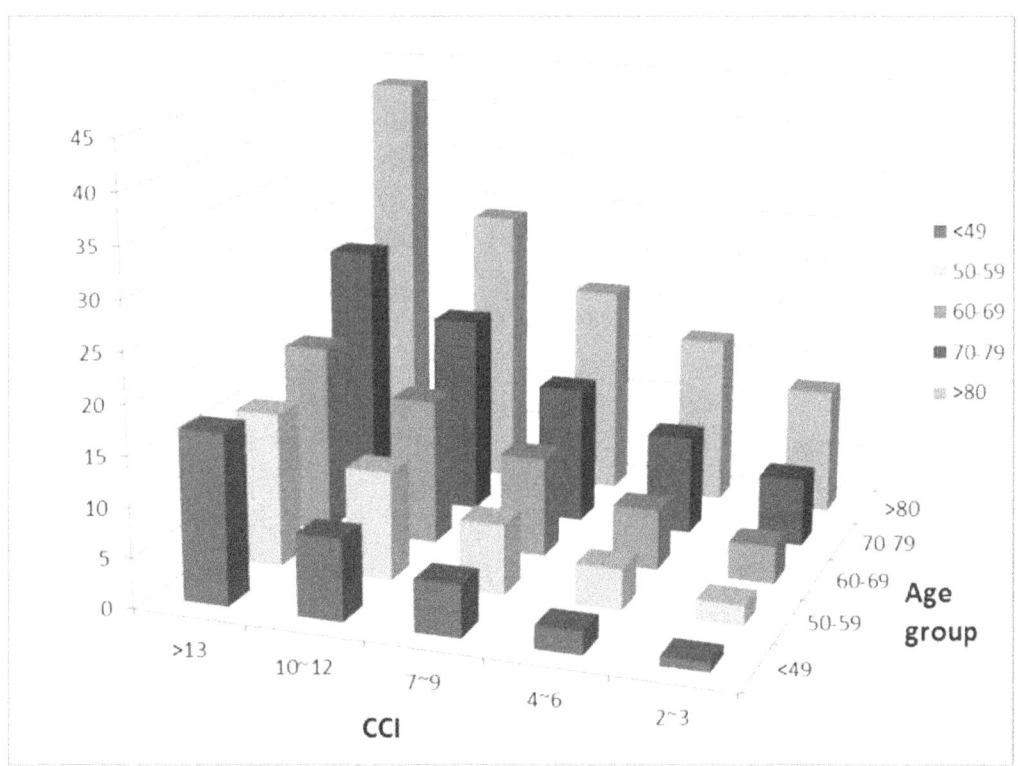

Figure 3. Increase of mortality with old age and high CCI in incident dialysis cohort. All the bars represent hazard ratio by age group and CCI.

Table 1. Basic demographics and characteristics of incident dialysis patients.

N = 79645	N	%
Age group		
18–19	136	0.2
20–29	1670	2.1
30–39	4386	5.5
40–49	11417	14.3
50–59	17697	22.2
60–69	21128	26.5
70–79	17751	22.3
≥80	5460	6.9
Gender		
Male	38683	48.6
Female	40962	51.4
Specific comorbidity		
Myocardial infarction	7873	9.9
Congestive heart failure	37168	46.7
Peripheral vascular disease	10,996	13.8
Cerebral vascular disease	29564	37.1
Dementia	5819	7.3
Chronic lung disease	31443	39.5
Rheumatological disorder	3614	4.5
Peptic ulcer disease	43637	54.8
Mild liver disease	21542	27.1
Diabetes with complications	40780	51.2
Paraplegia	3135	4.0
Neoplasia	15212	19.1
Moderate/severe liver disease	16559	20.8
Metastatic disease	2666	3.4
Human immunodeficiency virus	47	0.1
Conventional CCI		
≤3(n %)	10604	13.3
4–6	30930	38.8
7–9	24993	31.4
10–12	9637	12.1
13–15	2630	3.3
>15	851	1.1
Age-weighted-CCI		
≤3(n %)	5521	7.0
4–6	18330	23.1
7–9	27755	35.0
10–12	18921	23.8
13–15	6695	8.4
>15	2178	2.8

Footnotes: CCI, Charlson comorbidity index.

All statistical tests were 2 sided. p-value <0.05 was considered statistically significant.

Table 2. The effect of age and CCI on the survival of dialysis patients by cox regression (univariate and multivariable).

Variable	Crude HR	95% CI	p-value	Adjust HR	95% CI	p-value
Age group, years						
18–29	1(Ref.)	–		1(Ref.)	–	–
30–39	1.26	1.08–1.48	0.004	1.20	1.02–1.40	0.025
40–49	2.15	1.87–2.49	<0.001	1.74	1.51–2.01	<0.001
50–59	3.89	3.38–4.47	<0.001	2.71	2.36–3.12	<0.001
60–69	6.05	5.26–6.95	<0.001	4.11	3.57–4.72	<0.001
70–79	9.04	7.87–10.39	<0.001	6.27	5.45–7.21	<0.001
≥80	14.57	12.64–16.80	<0.001	10.40	9.02–12.00	<0.001
Sex						
Men	1.13	1.11–1.16	<0.001	1.16	1.13–1.182	<0.001
Women	1(Ref.)	–		1(Ref.)	–	
CCI						
≤3	1(Ref.)	–		1(Ref.)	–	
4–6	2.49	2.35–2.63	<0.001	1.91	1.81–2.02	<0.001
7–9	3.53	3.34–3.73	<0.001	2.39	2.26–2.53	<0.001
10–12	3.66	3.45–3.88	<0.001	2.42	2.28–2.57	<0.001
13–15	4.12	3.84–4.42	<0.001	2.62	2.44–2.81	<0.001
>15	4.42	4.02–4.86	<0.001	2.78	2.53–3.05	<0.001

Footnotes: CCI, Charlson comorbidity index; HR, Hazard ratio.

Results

The study population in the analyses was representative of the Taiwan dialysis population and enrolled 79645 incident patients with ESRD. Patient's clinical characteristics and comorbid conditions are listed in Table 1. The patient's mean age (±SD) was 60.96 (±13.92) years, 51.4% of patients were women, 51.2% were diabetic. After ranking subjects according to CCI scores, we categorized them into score quartiles with 10604, 30930, 24993, 9637, 2630, 851 numbers of patients in the six groups respectively. The distribution of CCI into six groups were 13.3% in index scores ≤ 3, 38.8% in index scores 4–6, 31.4% in index scores 7–9, 12.1% in index scores 10–12, 3.3% in index scores 13–15, and 1.1% in index scores >15. We made the same categorization in age-weighted CCI into six groups as listed in Table 1. Older patients were more likely to be in the higher comorbidity index (Figure 1). In cox proportional hazard models and stratifying by age, older patients had significantly higher mortality than younger patients: at age 30 to 39 years, the adjusted hazard ratio [aHR] was 1.20 (95% confidence interval [CI], 1.02–1.40), at age 40 to 49 years, the aHR was 1.74 (95% CI, 1.51–2.01), at age 50 to 59 years, the aHR was 2.71 (95% CI, 2.36–3.12), at age 60 to 69 years, the aHR was 4.11 (95% CI, 3.57–4.72), at age 70 to 79 years, the aHR was 6.27 (95% CI, 5.45–7.21), at age older than 80 years, the aHR was 10.40 (95% CI, 9.02–12.00), respectively. For every increased age of one year, the relative risk of death was 1.050 (95% CI 1.049–1.050, p-value <0.001) (data not shown). Males had higher risk of all-cause mortality compared to females significantly (aHR was 1.16, p-value <0.001). For CCI scores, mortality increased steadily with higher comorbidity both for unadjusted and for adjusted models. Compared to the lowest comorbidity group (reference group), fully adjusted models of CCI 4–6, CCI 7–9, CCI 10–12, CCI 13–15, CCI >15 showed hazard ratios for mortality of 1.91 (95% CI 1.81–2,02), 2.39 (95% CI 2.26–2.53), 2.42 (95% CI 2.28–2.57), 2.62 (95% CI 2.44–2.81), 2.78 (95% CI 2.53–3.05), respectively. For every increase of one point in the CCI score, the relative risk of death was 1.085 (95% CI 1.085–1.092, *p*-value <0.001) (data not shown). Mortality increased steadily with higher age or comorbidity both for unadjusted and for adjusted models. Figure 2A shows the survival curve for CCI stratified according to six comorbidity index groups. The same survival curve is illustrated in Figure 2B as age-weighted CCI. Death rates increased both with increasing age and increasing CCI score (Figure 3). Baseline mortality rates among elderly patients with CCI scores 2 to 3 points were higher than for younger patients. Among elderly patients with age more than 80 years and CCI more than 13 points, mortality rates were extremely higher than the CCI 10- to 12- point group (Figure 3). For all age groups, mortality rates increased in different CCI groups with the highest rates occurring in the oldest age groups.

Discussion

The present study used a nationally representative dialysis dataset to evaluate the ability of the Charlson comorbidity index to predict long-term survival in a large population of incident dialysis patients. Results suggest that the CCI is a good tool to assess comorbidity and predict survival in general dialysis population as previous studies validated [16,22–24]. When CCI is compared directly to the Wright-Khan Index, Davies Index, and ICED, the areas under the Receiver Operator Characteristic (ROC) curve are 0.67, 0.68, 0.68, and 0.72 respectively. Furthermore, the CCI requires only 15 minutes (often less) to complete [25], and a useful comorbidity index should be a simplified utilitarian substitute for individual comorbid conditions.

Our study population demographics and clinical characteristics are not obviously different from a previously reported 1995–2002 Taiwan Renal Registry study [26] and other NHI published population based study [20]. The comorbid conditions are the same in other Taiwan dialysis cohort studies, as myocardial infarction [20], peripheral vascular disease [27], and diabetes mellitus [28]. In Taiwan, the national health insurance covers all expenses in the health-care system including hemodialysis and peritoneal dialysis. We calculated all the inpatient and outpatient diagnosis codes one year before dialysis to define the CCI, and expect missing comorbidity information to be rare and unlikely to influence the result. We demonstrated that old age, higher CCI, or higher age-weighted CCI posit lower survival rates (Table 2 and Figure 2). Age is still the strongest predictor of mortality in dialysis patients but is a better predictor when combined with CCI. The *p* for trend hazard ratio is higher in age-weighted CCI than age or CCI only. In the elderly patient, dramatically increased hazard ratio by CCI groups are found (Figure 3). Thus, we should pay more attention to incident elderly dialysis patients with higher comorbidity conditions, which cause higher mortality and lower survival rates. Though it is controversial to judge patients with ESRD as for dialysis no matter how many comorbid conditions exist -or with short survival expectation, and this involves ethical and medical problems, and quality of life and life expectancies should be considered in this elderly and high comorbidity group.

Our study has several limitations. First, laboratory data and measures of physical functioning are not available in the National Health Insurance Research Database. Though clinical parame-

ters, such as predialysis systolic blood pressure [29,30], calcium × phosphate product [31], hematocrit [32], novel inflammatory markers such as C-reactive protein or Il-6 [33], BMI [34], or nutritional status related to survival cannot be obtained from this data set, this study still showed an index of comorbidity is the strongest statistical predictor of mortality previously [24]. CCI was a better predictor than models containing age, diabetes, cardiovascular disease, or albumin [16]. Second, certain parameters that may have improved the performance of our study population, such as information for dialysis access, dialysis dose, modality, residual renal function, or other treatment factors during follow up were not included because of unavailability in the database. However, this was consonant with the study objective, to assess baseline risk factors for survival in an incident dialysis population. Third, we were unable to link some nonhospital deaths, thus we had to define the date of cancellation of health insurance as the date of death. Previous study had link data with the real death registration showings that, on average, most cancellation dates were within 1 week of the real death registration for dialysis patients [9]. Fourth, patients who received dialysis <90 days were excluded from this study because of the possibility of including patients with acute renal failure or terminal illness with renal failure patients. Our study also had several strengths. Firstly, claims data from universal medical coverage in Taiwan allow for identification of population samples free from selection bias and of sufficient size to document outcomes. Secondly, by using insurance records that consist of comorbidity information, we could unambiguously analyze comorbid conditions and survival rates in the incident dialysis patients.

Conclusion

In conclusion, age and CCI, an index of overall comorbidity, assessed at the onset of dialysis, was the strong predictor of survival. Long-term survival rate was low in incident dialysis patients in the elderly and with higher comorbidity indexes. The simply CCI score should be emphasized in every incident dialysis patient to predict long term mortality and also evaluate his/her quality of life.

Acknowledgments

This study is based in part on data from the NHIRD provided by the Bureau of National Health Insurance, Department of Health, and managed by the National Health Research Institutes (Registered number 99324). The interpretation and conclusions contained herein do not represent the views of the Bureau of National Health Insurance, Department of Health or National Health Research Institutes. The authors thank the help from the Statistical Analysis Laboratory, Department of Internal Medicine, Kaohsiung Medical University Hospital.

Author Contributions

Conceived and designed the experiments: PHW YTL MCK YWC SJH HCC. Analyzed the data: YTL TCL MYL. Wrote the paper: PHW YTL MCK.

References

1. Bradbury BD, Fissell RB, Albert JM, Anthony MS, Critchlow CW, et al. (2007) Predictors of early mortality among incident US hemodialysis patients in the Dialysis Outcomes and Practice Patterns Study (DOPPS). Clin J Am Soc Nephrol 2: 89–99.
2. Collins AJ, Foley RN, Herzog C, Chavers B, Gilbertson D, et al. (2009) United States Renal Data System 2008 Annual Data Report. Am J Kidney Dis 53: S1–374.
3. Khan IH, Catto GR, Edward N, Fleming LW, Henderson IS, et al. (1993) Influence of coexisting disease on survival on renal-replacement therapy. Lancet 341: 415–418.
4. Nicolucci A, Cubasso D, Labbrozzi D, Mari E, Impicciatore P, et al. (1992) Effect of coexistent diseases on survival of patients undergoing dialysis. ASAIO J 38: M291–295.
5. van Manen JG, Korevaar JC, Dekker FW, Boeschoten EW, Bossuyt PM, et al. (2002) How to adjust for comorbidity in survival studies in ESRD patients: a comparison of different indices. Am J Kidney Dis 40: 82–89.
6. Yang WC, Hwang SJ (2008) Incidence, prevalence and mortality trends of dialysis end-stage renal disease in Taiwan from 1990 to 2001: the impact of national health insurance. Nephrol Dial Transplant 23: 3977–3982.
7. Ueshima H, Okayama A, Saitoh S, Nakagawa H, Rodriguez B, et al. (2003) Differences in cardiovascular disease risk factors between Japanese in Japan and Japanese-Americans in Hawaii: the INTERLIPID study. J Hum Hypertens 17: 631–639.
8. Lee CC, Sun CY, Wu MS (2009) Long-term modality-related mortality analysis in incident dialysis patients. Perit Dial Int 29: 182–190.
9. Chang YK, Hsu CC, Hwang SJ, Chen PC, Huang CC, et al. (2012) A comparative assessment of survival between propensity score-matched patients with peritoneal dialysis and hemodialysis in taiwan. Medicine (Baltimore) 91: 144–151.
10. Hwang SJ, Yang WC, Lin MY, Mau LW, Chen HC (2010) Impact of the clinical conditions at dialysis initiation on mortality in incident haemodialysis patients: a national cohort study in Taiwan. Nephrol Dial Transplant 25: 2616–2624.
11. Cooper BA, Branley P, Bulfone L, Collins JF, Craig JC, et al. (2010) A randomized, controlled trial of early versus late initiation of dialysis. N Engl J Med 363: 609–619.
12. Charlson ME, Pompei P, Ales KL, MacKenzie CR (1987) A new method of classifying prognostic comorbidity in longitudinal studies: development and validation. J Chronic Dis 40: 373–383.
13. Athienites NV, Miskulin DC, Fernandez G, Bunnapradist S, Simon G, et al. (2000) Comorbidity assessment in hemodialysis and peritoneal dialysis using the index of coexistent disease. Semin Dial 13: 320–326.
14. Davies SJ, Russell L, Bryan J, Phillips L, Russell GI (1995) Comorbidity, urea kinetics, and appetite in continuous ambulatory peritoneal dialysis patients: their interrelationship and prediction of survival. Am J Kidney Dis 26: 353–361.
15. Hall SF (2006) A user's guide to selecting a comorbidity index for clinical research. J Clin Epidemiol 59: 849–855.
16. Fried L, Bernardini J, Piraino B (2001) Charlson comorbidity index as a predictor of outcomes in incident peritoneal dialysis patients. Am J Kidney Dis 37: 337–342.
17. Geddes CC, van Dijk PC, McArthur S, Metcalfe W, Jager KJ, et al. (2006) The ERA-EDTA cohort study–comparison of methods to predict survival on renal replacement therapy. Nephrol Dial Transplant 21: 945–956.
18. Miskulin D, Bragg-Gresham J, Gillespie BW, Tentori F, Pisoni RL, et al. (2009) Key comorbid conditions that are predictive of survival among hemodialysis patients. Clin J Am Soc Nephrol 4: 1818–1826.
19. Chae JW, Song CS, Kim H, Lee KB, Seo BS, et al. (2011) Prediction of mortality in patients undergoing maintenance hemodialysis by Charlson Comorbidity Index using ICD-10 database. Nephron Clin Pract 117: c379–384.
20. Ng YY, Hung YN, Wu SC, Ko PJ, Hwang SM (2012) Progression in comorbidity before hemodialysis initiation is a valuable predictor of survival in incident patients. Nephrol Dial Transplant.
21. Deyo RA, Cherkin DC, Ciol MA (1992) Adapting a clinical comorbidity index for use with ICD-9-CM administrative databases. J Clin Epidemiol 45: 613–619.
22. Miskulin DC, Martin AA, Brown R, Fink NE, Coresh J, et al. (2004) Predicting 1 year mortality in an outpatient haemodialysis population: a comparison of comorbidity instruments. Nephrol Dial Transplant 19: 413–420.
23. Hemmelgarn BR, Manns BJ, Quan H, Ghali WA (2003) Adapting the Charlson Comorbidity Index for use in patients with ESRD. Am J Kidney Dis 42: 125–132.
24. Miskulin DC, Meyer KB, Martin AA, Fink NE, Coresh J, et al. (2003) Comorbidity and its change predict survival in incident dialysis patients. Am J Kidney Dis 41: 149–161.
25. Beddhu S, Bruns FJ, Saul M, Seddon P, Zeidel ML (2000) A simple comorbidity scale predicts clinical outcomes and costs in dialysis patients. Am J Med 108: 609–613.
26. Huang CC, Cheng KF, Wu HD (2008) Survival analysis: comparing peritoneal dialysis and hemodialysis in Taiwan. Perit Dial Int 28 Suppl 3: S15–20.
27. Lee CC, Wu CJ, Chou LH, Shen SM, Chiang SF, et al. (2012) Peripheral artery disease in peritoneal dialysis and hemodialysis patients: single-center retrospective study in Taiwan. BMC Nephrol 13: 100.
28. Luo JC, Leu HB, Huang KW, Huang CC, Hou MC, et al. (2011) Incidence of bleeding from gastroduodenal ulcers in patients with end-stage renal disease receiving hemodialysis. CMAJ 183: E1345–1351.
29. Port FK, Hulbert-Shearon TE, Wolfe RA, Bloembergen WE, Golper TA, et al. (1999) Predialysis blood pressure and mortality risk in a national sample of maintenance hemodialysis patients. Am J Kidney Dis 33: 507–517.
30. Mazzuchi N, Carbonell E, Fernandez-Cean J (2000) Importance of blood pressure control in hemodialysis patient survival. Kidney Int 58: 2147–2154.
31. Kopple JD (1994) Effect of nutrition on morbidity and mortality in maintenance dialysis patients. Am J Kidney Dis 24: 1002–1009.
32. Ma JZ, Ebben J, Xia H, Collins AJ (1999) Hematocrit level and associated mortality in hemodialysis patients. J Am Soc Nephrol 10: 610–619.
33. Honda H, Qureshi AR, Heimburger O, Barany P, Wang K, et al. (2006) Serum albumin, C-reactive protein, interleukin 6, and fetuin a as predictors of malnutrition, cardiovascular disease, and mortality in patients with ESRD. Am J Kidney Dis 47: 139–148.
34. Kopple JD, Zhu X, Lew NL, Lowrie EG (1999) Body weight-for-height relationships predict mortality in maintenance hemodialysis patients. Kidney Int 56: 1136–1148.

21

Left Ventricular Mass in Dialysis Patients, Determinants and Relation with Outcome: Results from the COnvective TRansport STudy (CONTRAST)

Ira M. Mostovaya[1]*, Michiel L. Bots[2], Marinus A. van den Dorpel[3], Roel Goldschmeding[4], Claire H. den Hoedt[1,3], Otto Kamp[5], Renée Levesque[6], Albert H. A. Mazairac[1], E. Lars Penne[1,7], Dorine W. Swinkels[8], Neelke C. van der Weerd[1,7], Piet M. ter Wee[7,9], Menso J. Nubé[7,9], Peter J. Blankestijn[1], Muriel P. C. Grooteman[7,9]

1 Department of Nephrology, University Medical Center Utrecht, Utrecht, the Netherlands, 2 Julius Center for Health Sciences and Primary Care, University Medical Center Utrecht, Utrecht, the Netherlands, 3 Department of Internal Medicine, Maasstad Hospital, Rotterdam, the Netherlands, 4 Department of Pathology, University Medical Center Utrecht, Utrecht, the Netherlands, 5 Department of Cardiology, Vrije Universiteit Medical Center, Amsterdam, the Netherlands, 6 Department of Nephrology, Centre Hospitalier de l'Université de Montréal St. Luc Hospital, Montréal, Canada, 7 Department of Nephrology, Vrije Universiteit Medical Center, Amsterdam, the Netherlands, 8 Department of Laboratory Medicine, Laboratory of Genetic, Endocrine and Metabolic diseases, Radboud University Medical Centre Nijmegen, the Netherlands, 9 Institute for Cardiovascular Research Vrije Universiteit Medical Center, Vrije Universiteit Medical Center, Amsterdam, the Netherlands

Abstract

Background and Objectives: Left ventricular mass (LVM) is known to be related to overall and cardiovascular mortality in end stage kidney disease (ESKD) patients. The aims of the present study are 1) to determine whether LVM is associated with mortality and various cardiovascular events and 2) to identify determinants of LVM including biomarkers of inflammation and fibrosis.

Design, Setting, Participants, & Measurements: Analysis was performed with data of 327 ESKD patients, a subset from the CONvective TRansport STudy (CONTRAST). Echocardiography was performed at baseline. Cox regression analysis was used to assess the relation of LVM tertiles with clinical events. Multivariable linear regression models were used to identify factors associated with LVM.

Results: Median age was 65 (IQR: 54–73) years, 203 (61%) were male and median LVM was 227 (IQR: 183–279) grams. The risk of all-cause mortality (hazard ratio (HR) = 1.73, 95% CI: 1.11–2.99), cardiovascular death (HR = 3.66, 95% CI: 1.35–10.05) and sudden death (HR = 13.06; 95% CI: 6.60–107) was increased in the highest tertile (>260grams) of LVM. In the multivariable analysis positive relations with LVM were found for male gender (B = 38.8±10.3), residual renal function (B = 17.9±8.0), phosphate binder therapy (B = 16.9±8.5), and an inverse relation for a previous kidney transplantation (B = −41.1±7.6) and albumin (B = −2.9±1.1). Interleukin-6 (Il-6), high-sensitivity C-reactive protein (hsCRP), hepcidin-25 and connective tissue growth factor (CTGF) were not related to LVM.

Conclusion: We confirm the relation between a high LVM and outcome and expand the evidence for increased risk of sudden death. No relationship was found between LVM and markers of inflammation and fibrosis.

Editor: Leighton R. James, University of Florida, United States of America

Funding: CONTRAST is partly supported by unrestricted grants from Fresenius Medical Care (The Netherlands) and Gambro Lundia AB (Sweden). Additional support for CONTRAST was also received from Roche, the Netherlands. There are no patents, products in development or marketed products to declare. IM Mostovaya, CH den Hoedt, O Kamp, ML Bots, NC van der Weerd, EL Penne and AHA Mazairac report receiving no lecture fees, no consulting support, or grant support. MPC Grooteman reports research funded by Fresenius, Gambro, and Baxter. PJ Blankestijn reports research funded by Fresenius, Gambro, Roche, Amgen and Novartis, consultant fee and honoraria for lectures from Fresenius, Gambro, Solvay, Medtronic, and Novartis. R Lévesque reports research funded by Amgen Canada. PM ter Wee reports research funded by Abbott, Baxter, Gambro, Fresenius, and Roche; honoraria for lectures received from Amgen, Roche, Genzyme, Fresenius. MJ Nubé reports research funded by Baxter and Fresenius; honoraria for lectures received from Fresenius and Baxter. MA van den Dorpel reports research funded by Amgen. This does not alter the authors' adherence to all the PLOS ONE policies on sharing data and materials. The funders had no role in study design, data collection and analysis, decision to publish, or preparation of the manuscript.

Competing Interests: The authors have the following interests: CONTRAST is partly supported by unrestricted grants from Fresenius Medical Care (The Netherlands) and Gambro Lundia AB (Sweden). Additional support for CONTRAST was also received from Roche, the Netherlands. There are no patents, products in development or marketed products to declare. IM Mostovaya, CH den Hoedt, O Kamp, ML Bots, NC van der Weerd, EL Penne, and AHA Mazairac report receiving no lecture fees, no consulting support, or grant support. MPC Grooteman reports research funded by Fresenius, Gambro, and Baxter. PJ Blankestijn reports research funded by Fresenius, Gambro, Roche, Amgen, and Novartis; consultant fee and honoraria for lectures from Fresenius, Gambro, Solvay, Medtronic, and Novartis. R Lévesque reports research funded by Amgen Canada. PM ter Wee reports research funded by Abbott, Baxter, Gambro, Fresenius, and Roche; honoraria for lectures received from Amgen, Roche, Genzyme, Fresenius. MJ Nubé reports research funded by Baxter and Fresenius; honoraria for lectures received from Fresenius and Baxter. MA van den Dorpel reports research funded by Amgen. This does not alter the authors' adherence to all the PLOS ONE policies on sharing data and materials.

* E-mail: I.M.Mostovaya@umcutrecht.nl

Introduction

Increased left ventricular mass (LVM) has been well described as a frequent component of end stage kidney disease (ESKD) [1]. In fact, more than seventy percent of patients starting dialysis show left ventricular hypertrophy (LVH) on echocardiography [2]. An increase in left ventricular mass (LVM) is associated with cardiovascular morbidity and mortality [3,4]. Although the relation between LVM and overall mortality and cardiovascular events has been well established in ESKD patients, the association between LVM and certain types of cardiovascular morbidity (such as coronary heart disease: CHD) and mortality (such as sudden death) has not yet been thoroughly investigated.

Several inflammatory biomarkers associated with cardiovascular pathology and morbidity have been described for patients with chronic kidney disease (CKD). High sensitivity C-reactive protein (hsCRP and interleukin-6 (Il-6) are both well accepted markers of inflammation, related to increased risk of death and cardiovascular disease [5]. HsCRP is an acute phase reactant, which has been associated with an increased risk of major cardiovascular disease [6]. HsCRP levels are higher in HD patients than in healthy individuals [7] and have been shown to be independent predictors of LVM indexed for body surface area (LVMi) in CKD patients [8]. Il-6 is a short acting protein secreted by cells of the immune system in response to inflammatory stimuli, and is suspected to be a central regulator in the inflammatory process that leads to atherosclerosis [9]. Several studies have reported the relation between a high Il-6 and increased risk of developing CVD [10–12]. In patient deceased from acute myocardial infarction, Il-6 has been associated with mechanisms of cardiac hypertrophy [13]. Furthermore, Il-6 levels are increased in dialysis patients [7,14].

Connective tissue growth factor (CTGF) is a signalling protein involved in the pathogenesis of renal and cardiac fibrosis [15]. In animal studies CTGF has been described to contribute to development of cardiac hypertrophy [16,17]. CKD patients have a higher plasma CTGF level then healthy individuals, since CTGF is eliminated predominantly by the kidney [18].

Hepcidin-25 is a peptide produced by the liver, which regulates intestinal absorption of iron and its distribution through the body [19]. The gene encoding for hepcidin-25 is regulated in response to anemia, hypoxia and inflammation [20]. Furthermore, hepcidin-25 is related to increased risk of cardiovascular events in chronic hemodialysis patients [21].

Although several studies have described a relationship between hsCRP and left ventricle geometry and function [8,22,23], the relationship between LVM and the four described biomarkers has not been examined in a large population of HD patients.

We hypothesize that a high LVM will be related to a higher risk of mortality and cardiovascular events in our study, as is the case in previously studied dialysis populations. Furthermore we expect to find a positive relation between specific cardiovascular events such as risk of CHD or sudden death and LVM. Regarding hsCRP, Il-6, CTGF and hepcidin-25, since these markers are related to pathophysiological mechanisms that could theoretically promote increase of LVM, we assume to find a positive relation between the magnitude of LVM and hsCRP, Il-6, CTGF and hepcidin-25. Hence, the aims of this study are 1) to determine whether LVM is associated with mortality and various cardiovascular events in our population of ESKD patients and 2) to identify determinants of LVM including biomarkers of inflammation, systemic iron homeostasis and fibrosis in HD patients.

Materials and Methods

Patients

The present study included a subset of patients participating in the CONvective TRAnsport STudy (CONTRAST): 327 hemodialysis patients from 15 dialysis centres (14 Dutch centers and 1 Canadian center). CONTRAST has been designed to investigate the effects of increased convective transport by online HDF as compared with low-flux HD on all-cause mortality and cardiovascular morbidity and mortality (ISRCTN38365125) and included a total of 714 patients [24].

The study was conducted in accordance with the Declaration of Helsinki and approved by the medical ethics review boards of all participating dialysis centres. Written informed consent was obtained from all patients prior to enrolment. The names of the medical ethics committees/review boards that have approved this study are listed in the appendix S1 in File S1.

Data collection

Baseline patient and dialysis characteristics were used for this analysis: information on demography, anthropometrics, medical history, medication and standard laboratory values. A history of cardiovascular disease was defined as a previous acute myocardial infarction, coronary artery bypass graft, percutaneous transluminal coronary angioplasty, angina pectoris, stroke, transient ischemic attack, intermittent claudication, amputation, percutaneous transluminal angioplasty, peripheral bypass surgery and renal percutaneous transluminal angioplasty.

Systolic and diastolic blood pressure was measured before and after three consecutive dialysis sessions at baseline using a standard electronic sphygmomanometer. The average of these measurements was computed and used for analysis.

The primary outcome of CONTRAST was all cause mortality. Cause of death was recorded and subdivided into cardiovascular mortality (fatal myocardial infraction, fatal cerebrovascular accident, fatal decompensatio cordis, a rupture of the abdominal aorta or sudden death) and non-cardiovascular mortality. Sudden death was defined as death within 1 hour of the onset of symptoms as verified by a witness.

The main secondary endpoint was a composite of fatal and non-fatal cardiovascular events. Cardiovascular events were defined as death from cardiovascular causes, non-fatal myocardial infarction, non-fatal stroke, therapeutic coronary procedure (percutaneous transluminal coronary angioplasty and/or stenting), therapeutic carotid procedure (endartrectomy and/or stenting), and vascular intervention not related to vascular access (revascularisation, percutaneous transluminal angioplasty and/or stenting) or amputation. Congestive heart failure was excluded as a cardiovascular event, since the distinction with fluid overload is often difficult to make in patients with end stage renal disease.

Follow-up of patients with respect to mortality and non-fatal cardiovascular events was continued even after they stopped with the randomized treatment because of a renal transplant (n = 71), a switch to peritoneal dialysis (n = 5), a move to another non-CONTRAST hospital (n = 11) or a stop of participation for other reasons (n = 58).

An independent Endpoint Adjudication Committee reviewed source documentation for all primary outcome events (deaths), as well as non-fatal cardiovascular events and infections.

Table 1. Demographic, anthropometric, biochemical, hemodynamic and dialysis characteristics of the study population.

	Total Cohort	Echo cor cohort
	n = 714	n = 327
Demographic data		
Male gender	445 (62%)	200 (61%)
Race, Caucasian	304 (85%)	263 (80%)
Age, years	64.1±13.7	63.0±13.3
Smoking	133 (19%)	66 (20%)
Anthropometrics		
Length (cm)	168±10	168±11
Weight (kg)	72.4±14.4	72.1±14.3
BMI (kg/m²)	25.4±14.4	25.5±4.9
Body Surface Area (m²)	1.85 (0.28)*	1.85 (0.30)*
Dialysis Properties		
Dialysis vintage (years)	1.8 (1.0–4.0)*	2.0 (1.0–4.0)*
Duration of dialysis (minutes)	226±23	225±23
Blood flow (mL/minute)	300 (300–348)*	300 (300–350)*
spKt/Vurea	1.40±0.22	1.39±0.20
AV fistula	279 (78%)	260 (80%)
Patients with residual kidney function	186 (52%)	171 (52%)
Comorbidities		
Cardiovascular disease	313 (44%)	146 (45%)
Diabetes	170 (24%)	83 (25%)
Previous kidney transplant	78 (11%)	30 (9%)
Laboratory parameters		
Hemoglobin (g/dL)	11.8±0.40	11.8±1.3
Phosphate (mmol/L)	1.64±0.49	1.67±0.50
Calcium (mmol/L)	2.31±0.18	2.30±0.18
Albumin (g/L)	40.4±3.8	41.2 (37.9–43.5)*
Creatinine (μmol/L), pre-dialysis	861±255	883±252
hsCRP (mg/L)	-	4.0 (1.6–11.9)*
Il-6 (pg/mL)	-	2.0 (1.2–3.8)*
CTGF (nmol/L)	-	3.6 (2.8–4.3)*
Hepcidin -25 (nM)	-	14.2 (6.3–22.4)*
Ferritin (ng/mL)	-	377 (211–597)*
TSAT (%)	-	22 (15–29)*
Medication		
Erythropietin therapy	314 (88%)	295 (91%)
Diuretic therapy	250 (35%)	129 (39%)
Beta-blocker therapy	184 (51%)	174 (53%)
RAS inhibitor therapy	179 (50%)	162 (50%)
Lipid lowering therapy	196 (55%)	152 (47%)
Vitamin D administration	227 (63%)	222 (68%)
Phosphate binding therapy	445 (62%)	194 (59%)
Platelet aggregation therapy or coumarines	111 (34%)	122 (36%)
Iron supplements	476 (67%)	213 (65%)
Hemodynamic measurements		
Systolic blood pressure (mm Hg)	147±21	142±19

Table 1. Cont.

	Total Cohort	Echo cor cohort
	n = 714	n = 327
Diastolic blood pressure (mm Hg)	75±12	74±10
LVEDD (mm)	-	10 (9–11)*
LVESD (mm)	-	32 (27–38)*
EFLV (%)	-	65 (55–72)*
LVM (g)	-	227 (183–279)*
LVH	-	230 (71%)

*:median and IQR (P25–P75).
AV: arterio-venous;BMI: mody mass index; CTGF: connective tissue growth factor; EFLV: ejection fraction of left ventricle; hsCRP: high sensitivity C-reactive protein; Il-6: interleukin 6; LVEDD: left ventricular end diastolic diameter; LVESD: left ventricular end systolic diameter; LVH: left ventricular hypertrophy; LVM: left ventricular mass; RAS: renin-angiotensin system; TSAT: transferrin saturation.

Laboratory measurements

Standard laboratory samples were analysed in the local laboratories of the participating hospitals by standard laboratory techniques.

Furthermore, in centres where storage of blood samples was logistically feasible, additional blood samples were drawn for the analysis of hsCRP, Il-6, CTGF and hepcidin prior to dialysis. Samples were placed on ice, and centrifuged within 30 min, at 1500 g for 10 minutes, and were stored at −80°C until assayed. A total of 248 patients, out of the 327 who underwent echocardiography, were treated in such centers and therefore had additional measurements of hsCRP, Il-6, CTGF and hepcidin.

High sensitivity CRP, hepcidin-25, CTGF and IL-6 levels were measured centrally. Measurements of the bioactive hepcidin-25 were performed with time of flight mass spectrometry which has been described previously [25]. High sensitivity CRP (mg/L) was measured with a particle-enhanced immunoturbidimetric assay on a Roche-Hitachi analyzer as described elsewhere [21]. IL-6 (pg/mL) was measured with an ELISA (Sanquin, Amsterdam, The Netherlands), details have been described earlier [26]. CTGF levels in plasma were determined by sandwich ELISA, using two specific antibodies (FibroGen Inc., San Francisco, CA, USA) directed against two distinct isotopes in the amino-terminal fragment of CTGF, detecting both full length CTGF and the N-fragment, as shown earlier [18].

Echocardiographic measurements

In 15 centres, patients were requested to undergo 2-dimensional echocardiography next to the standard CONTRAST baseline data collection.

Transthoracic echocardiography studies were performed on a mid-week non-dialysis day by an echocardiographer at the participating local hospital. From the parasternal long axis position the left ventricular end-diastolic diameter (LVEDD), end-systolic diameter (LVESD) as well as the posterior and septal wall thickness were determined. The ultrasound investigations were then assessed by an independent experienced echocardiographer at the core laboratory (VU medical Center, Amsterdam, the Netherlands), who was blinded for other patient data. LVM was calculated using the formula of Devereux and Reickek [27], modified in accordance with the recommendations of the American Society of Echocardiography [28]. LVH was defined as an LVM/height$^{2.7}$ >44g/m$^{2.7}$ for women and >48 g/m$^{2.7}$ for men [3].

Table 2. Hazard ratio of clinical events by LVM in grams divided into tertiles.

	T1: <201	T2: 201<LVM<260	95% CI	T3: >260	95% CI
Crude					
Mortality	1	1.61*	1.01–2.55	2.17*	1.39–3.38
Cardiovascular death	1	2.24	0.90–5.55	3.76*	1.61–8.82
Sudden death	1	8.93*	1.12–71.4	17.8*	2.35–135.0
Cardiovascular events	1	1.47	0.92–2.44	1.66*	1.06–2.67
CHD events	1	1.04	0.51–2.13	1.13	0.56–2.31
Adjusted[a]					
Mortality	1	1.50	0.92–2.10	1.73*	1.11–2.99
Cardiovascular death	1	1.80	0.64–5.07	3.69*	1.35–10.05
Sudden death	1	6.29	0.72–52.70	13.06*	6.60–107.16
Cardiovascular events	1	1.27	0.74–2.18	1.49	0.85–2.60
CHD events	1	1.22	0.71–2.09	1.51	0.87–2.64

*$p < 0.05$.
[a]Adjusted with a propensity score containing determinants of LVM (male gender, residual renal function, history of kidney transplantation, albumin, use of RAS-inhibitors, use of phosphate binders, systolic blood pressure) and history of cardiovascular disease, diabetes, height, post-dialysis weight and dialysis modality (intervention).

Data analysis

Data were reported as proportions or as means with standard deviation (SD) or medians with inter-quartile ranges (IQR) when appropriate.

The average percentage of missing values per variable was 7.7%. No data were missing regarding clinical events. Multiple imputation was performed on all variables, where <40% of data were missing. One variable was not imputed due to a higher percentage of missing values, namely blood flow. Imputation was performed to prevent bias in reported estimates and to improve statistical power [29].

To study the independent relation of each variable with LVM, linear regression analysis was used. Patient and dialysis related variables that showed a univariable relation with LVM using a cut-off p-value <0,20 were entered in a multivariate model in consequent groups: demographic data, patient history, dialysis properties, therapeutic parameters and haemodynamic measurements. In addition, height and weight were added into the model upfront.

In a separate analysis, the variables hsCRP, Il-6, hepcidin-25 and CTGF were added to the constructed multivariate model one at a time. The old and new models were compared based on direction of the estimate and the significance of the regression coefficient of the added marker.

The relations between LVM and all-cause mortality, as well as cardiovascular events, cardiovascular death, sudden death and CHD were evaluated by Cox proportional hazards models, involving the time to the first relevant endpoint in any individual patient. For this analysis LVM was both analysed as a linear variable and divided into categories (tertiles). The number of events (in particular sudden death and CHD events) was small, and thus adjusting for all relevant possible confounders would lead to an overfitted model. Propensity scores as opposed to individual variables were used to adjust the models thus omitting the problem of an overfitted model. The propensity score [30] model estimated each individuals probability of having an LVM above the median of the studied population. Propensity score was built using a logistic model including all variables associated with LVM with p<0.20. Moreover, height, post-dialysis baseline weight and

dialysis modality (intervention) were added into the propensity score model upfront.

Results were considered statistically significant when p<0.05 (two-sided). All calculations were made by use of a standard statistical package (SPSS for Windows Version 18.0.1; SPSS Inc. Headquarters, Chicago, Illinois, US).

Results

327 patients participating in CONTRAST underwent echocardiography. Out of this group, in 248 patients blood was collected for a measurement of markers of inflammation and fibrosis. Median age was 65 (IQR: 54–73) years, 203 were male (61%) and the median dialysis vintage was 2.0 (IQR: 1.0–4.0) years. Median LVM was 227 (IQR: 183–279) grams. A total of 230 patients (71%) had LVH. The baseline characteristics of the whole CONTRAST cohort and of the echocardiography population are shown in table 1. The mean follow-up time was 2.0 (minimum 0.1, maximum 6.5) years. Within the group of patients with an LVM measurement 130 (39.8%) patients died from any cause and 116 (35.5%) had a cardiovascular event, out of which 43 (13.1%) were fatal. CHD (angina pectoris or acute myocardial infarction) occurred in 53 (16.2%) patients, of whom 3 (0.9%) died. Sudden death occurred in 24 (7.3%) patients.

Relation to LVM and outcome

Table 2 shows proportional hazard ratios for all-cause mortality, cardiovascular death, sudden death, combined fatal and non-fatal cardiovascular events and CHD events; both crude and adjusted using propensity scores. Risk of all-cause mortality, cardiovascular death and sudden death was increased in the highest tertile (>260grams) of LVM; while no difference in risk was found for overall cardiovascular events and CHD events in the LVM tertiles. Figure 1 shows survival curves for the clinical events described above stratified by LVM tertiles.

As shown in Table S1a and S1b in File S1, when LVM was indexed for BSA or height$^{2.7}$, relations with clinical events were similar.

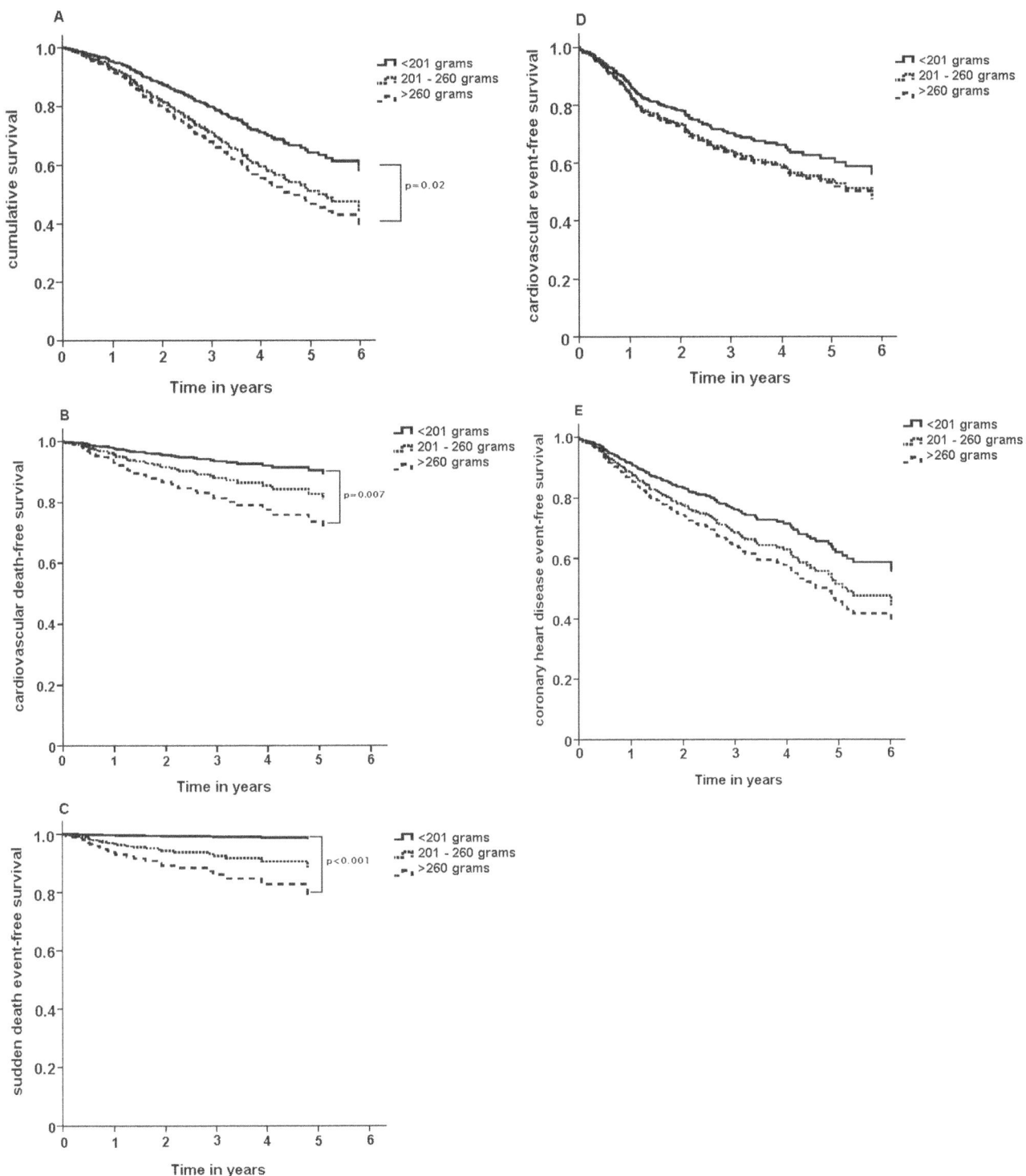

Figure 1. Survival curves for (A) time to death from any cause, (B) cardiovascular death, (C) sudden death, (D) cardiovascular events (both fatal and non-fatal), (E) coronary heart disease events (both fatal and non-fatal, all stratified by LVM tertiles and adjusted using propensity scores.

Determinants of LVM

The univariable and multivariable analysis results of LVM are shown in Table 3. In the multivariate analysis significant positive relations with LVM were found for male gender, presence of residual renal function and phosphate binder therapy. There were

inverse relations for a history of kidney transplantation and albumin. The complete-case multivariate regression analysis showed similar results as demonstrated in Table S2 in File S1.

Table 4 shows that hsCRP, Il-6, hepcidin-25 and CTGF were not related to LVM.

Table 3. Determinants of LVM in dialysis patients: univariable and multivariable regression analysis.

Determinant	Univariable model		Multivariable model	
	B	95% CI	B	95% CI
Demographic data				
Male gender	56.47	39.03 to 73.90	38.80	18.64 to 58.96
Race, Caucasian	12.92	−9.75 to 35.60		
Age (years)	0.75	0.08 to 1.42		
Smoking	22.20	−0.47 to 44.87		
Dialysis Properties				
Duration of dialysis (hours)	35.14	10.95 to 59.33		
spKt/Vurea	−102.7	−145.7 to −59.75		
AV fistula	17.59	−4.66 to 38.83		
Comorbidities				
Cardiovascular disease	16.54	−1.50 to 34.58		
Diabetes	1.94	−18.45 to 22.37		
Previous kidney transplant	−49.76	−80.38 to −19.01	−41.12	−55.94 to −26.31
Dialysis vintage (years)	−5.45	−8.61 to −2.30		
Residual kidney function	29.28	−11.52 to 47.04	17.88	2.16 to 33.61
Laboratory parameters				
Hemoglobin (g/dL)	−1.00	−12.53 to 10.53		
Phosphate (mmol/L)	0.89	−17.17 to 18.94		
Calcium (mmol/L)	13.37	−32.36 to 63.99		
Calcium*Phosphate	1.28	−6.48 to 9.03		
Albumin (g/L)	−1.99	−4.17 to 0.20	−2.94	−5.08 to −0.81
Creatinin (μmol/L)	−0.02	−0.05 to 0.02		
Therapeutic parameters				
Erythropietin	−9.68	−38.78 to 19.38		
Diuretic	0.97	−18.99 to 20.94		
Beta-blocker	16.26	−1.70 to 34.21		
Alpha-blocker	21.44	−13.64 to 56.51		
RAS inhibitor	21.67	3.82 to 39.51	14.08	−2.46 to 30.62
Lipid lowering therapy	0.95	−17.06 to 18.95		
Vitamin D administration	5.15	−14.16 to 22.45		
Phosphate binder	17.82	−0.420 to 36.05	16.87	0.14 to 33.56
Platelet aggregation inhibitor	10.35	−8.44 to 29.13		
Coumarine derivates	22.50	−14.09 to 59.08		
Iron supplements	22.56	3.81 to 41.32		
Hemodynamic measurements				
Systolic blood pressure (mm Hg)	0.54	0.08 to 1.00	0.37	−0.77 to 0.82

The B reflects the change of total LVM (in grams) related with one unit increment of the determinant.
R^2 of the multivariable model = 0.22.

Discussion

The present study confirmed the relation between a high LVM and outcome [2,4,31,32]. Furthermore we expanded the evidence for a strongly increased risk of sudden death in patients with a high LVM. After confirming that LVM was a strong predictor of cardiovascular and overall mortality we wanted to study what factors determine the magnitude of LVM, and in particular if these determinants were potentially modifiable. In our analysis, factors related to LVM were: male gender, history of kidney transplantation, residual kidney function (RKF), albumin and use of phosphate binders. Thus we did not find determinants of LVM that could easily be altered in daily clinical practice. Lastly, we explored whether novel markers of inflammation, fibrosis and iron homeostasis (hsCRP, Il-6, CTGF and hepcidin-25), which in theory could lead to a higher LVM, were related to LVM in a large population of hemodialysis patients. Apparently, although hsCRP, Il-6, CTGF, hepcidin-25 have previously been found to be associated with cardiovascular damage, no relation exists between these biomarkers and the magnitude of LVM in ESKD patients.

Table 4. Hepcidin, hsCRP, Il-6 and CTGF as determinants of LVM.

Determinant	Univariable model		Adding to 'basic' multivariable model		
	B	95% CI	B	95% CI	ΔR^2
Hepcidin-25 (nM)	−0.04	−0.46 to 0.38	0.04	−0.38 to 0.45	−0.003
hsCRP (mg/L)	0.22	−0.46 to 0.90	0.07	−0.43 to 0.57	−0.003
Il-6 (pg/mL)	0.03	−0.17 to 0.22	0.06	−0.13 to 0.23	−0.002
CTGF (nmol/L)	0.05	−3.92 to 4.01	0.67	−3.45 to 4.78	−0.001

The B reflects the change of total LVM (in grams) related with one unit increment of the determinant.

LVM and clinical events

A summary of previous papers in which the relation between left ventricular geometry and clinical events was studied in dialysis patients is shown in Table 5. Foley et al studied the relation between LVM and mortality risks in 433 ESKD patients and found a significant linear association between LVM and overall mortality as well as cardiovascular mortality in particular [2]. Zoccali et al studied the prognostic impact of LVM indexed for body surface are or height$^{2.7}$ in 254 dialysis patients and found that both types of LVMi were related to both overall mortality and cardiovascular mortality [31].

We are among the first to describe the relationship between LVM and sudden death specifically in ESKD patients. In fact, ESKD patients in the highest tertile of LVM had an almost 14-fold higher risk of sudden death when compared to the lowest LVM tertile, while their risk of dying from a cardiac cause in general was 'only' increased by a factor 3.5. The underlying mechanism may be through a decrease in myocardial capillary density, diastolic and systolic dysfunction, disturbances in interventricular conduction, chamber dilatation and eventually more compensatory hypertrophy. These processes lead to an increased risk of triggering a fatal arrhythmia [1,33]. Autopsy studies in ESKD patients point to the presence of diffuse inter-myocardiocyte fibrosis specific for this group, which may indicate an electrical instability predisposing to sudden death [34]. The percentage of sudden deaths (56%) from all cardiac deaths in our population was similar to those of earlier studies [33].

For a combination of fatal- and non-fatal cardiovascular events no relation with LVM size was found. To our knowledge, no such relation has been described in earlier literature; although Zoccali et al found a significant relation between LVM indexed for height$^{2.7}$ and fatal- and non-fatal cardiovascular events combined [31]. Since there were only 3 lethal CHD events in our study, this association could not be explored in our population.

Determinants of LVM

Factors related to LVM were: male gender, history of kidney transplantation, residual kidney function (RKF), albumin and use of phosphate binders.

It was a surprising finding that a history of CVD and blood pressure (BP) were not found to be associated with LVM. Regarding the lack of relation between LVM and CVD this could be attributed to the fact that our definition of CVD encompassed several periphery vasculature diseases/interventions, which do not necessarily lead to an enlargement of LVM. Also, many ESKD patients have a high LVM without a history of CVD [2]. While BP is very variable over time in dialysis patients (mostly due to rigorous changes in extracellular volume during and in-between dialysis treatments), our BP results are an average of three pre- and three post-dialysis BP measurements. Hence our BP

Table 5. Summary of previous studies in which the relation between LV geometry and clinical events was examined in dialysis patients.

Author	patient nr	LV measurement	event	Risk measure	Conclusion
Silverberg et al 1989 (33)	133	LVMi (g/m^2)	mortality	RR: 2.9 (p = 0.013)	LVH is an important determinant of survival
			CV mortality	RR: 2.7 (0.08)	in incident dialysis patients
Foley et al 1995 (2)	433	LVMi (g/m^2)	mortality	RR: 1.003 (p = 0.11)	LVH is highly prevalent in th dialysis
			late (>2 yr) mortality	RR: 1.009 (p<0.001)	population and is a risk factor for mortality
London et al 2001 (4)	153	more than 10% decrease in LVMi (g/height$^{2.7}$)	mortality	RR: 0.78 (p = 0.001)	partial regression of LVM has a favorable
			CV mortality	RR: 0.72 (p = 0.002)	effect on mortlity and CV-mortality
Zoccali et al 2001 (32)	254	LVMi (g/m^2) LVMi (g/height$^{2.7}$)	mortality	HR: 1.01 (p<0.001)/1.03 (p<0.001)	LVM indexed for height$^{2.7}$ provides a more
			CV mortality	HR: 1.01 (p<0.001)/1.03 (p<0.001)	powerful predictor for death and CV events
			CV event	HR: 1.00 (ns)/1.02 (p = 0.004)	compared to LVM indexed for BSA
Zoccali et al 2004 (3)	161	in top 75% progression in LVMi (g/height$^{2.7}$)	mortality	HR: 3.07 (p = 0.008)	Changes in LVMi have an independent
			CV event	HR: 3.02 (p = 0.02)	prognostic value for death and CV events

CV events are defined as a combination of both fatal and non-fatal cardiovascular events.
BSA: body surface area; CV: cardiovascular; HR: hazard ratio; LV: left ventricular; LVH: left ventricular hypertrophy; LVM: left ventricular mass; LVMi: left ventricular mass index; nr: number; RR: relative risk.

measurements could be a poor representative of the total BP burden of a patient (which is truly related to LVM).

The relation between LVM and a history of kidney transplantation [35,36] and albumin [37] is in accordance with earlier literature.

The positive relation between LVM and RKF may be explained by a 'survivor bias': patients that still have RKF have been on dialysis for a shorter period of time. As time passes, the patients with a high LVM are more likely to die, the patient with a lower LVM remain and lose their RKF. In our population, the dialysis vintage differs significantly between patient with RKF (1.92 ± 1.58 years) and without RKF (4.00 ± 3.4 years).

Previous studies on predictors of LVM and LVMi in HD patients identified phosphate and the calcium-phosphate product as patient characteristics associated with LVH [38–40]. In our analysis however, these laboratory values were not significantly related to LVM, while there was a positive association between LVM and use of phosphate binders. The serum calcium and phosphate are well controlled in our dialysis population, and phosphate binders were prescribed to 74% of the patients (mainly sevelamer, a non-calcium containing phosphate binder: 54%). Hyperphosphatemia can lead to vascular calcification and myocardial fibrosis, resulting in increased cardiovascular risk [41]. Thus, it is plausible that in our population the prescription of phosphate binders is a reflection of higher phosphate intake at present and/or hyperphosphatemia in the past, resulting in higher LVM.

Relation between LVM and hsCRP, Il-6, CTGF, hepcidin

We are among the first to investigate the association between LVM and the biomarkers hsCRP, Il-6, CTGF and hepcidin in a population of ESKD patients, which is also large enough to perform appropriate corrections for clinically relevant variables without creating an overfitted model. Although there is a theoretical incentive, as described in the Introduction, to hypothesize that these biomarkers may contribute to LVM, we do not find such a relation in our population. Apparently, although hsCRP, Il-6, CTGF, hepcidin-25 have previously been found to be associated with cardiovascular damage, no relation exists between these biomarkers and the magnitude of LVM in ESKD patients.

In earlier papers concerning LVM and prognosis, LVM was indexed for body surface are, or divided by height$^{2.7}$. It was shown that these indexations, especially LVM/height$^{2.7}$ are better predictors of clinical events than LVM. [3,4]) A downside of ratios is that observed relation may be due to the nominator, the denominator or both. Therefore in the present analyses we chose to use LVM for our analyses only with correction for height and weight in the propensity scores for optimal statistical adjustment. As shown in Tables S1a and S1b in File S1, when LVM was adjusted for height and weight, the relation with clinical events was similar to that of LVM indexed for BSA or height$^{2.7}$.

Strengths and limitations

This study had several limitations. First, 7.7% of data was missing and biomarkers were measured in only 75.5% of the patients. However, since multiple imputation was performed for missing variables included in the multivariable analysis, this prevents the drawing of wrong conclusions due to the fact that data may be missing in specific patients for a reason, and not by chance and by increasing the power of our analyses [29]. Furthermore, our sensitivity analyses of complete cases showed no marked differences with the regression performed on the imputed data. Second, the number of CHD events and sudden deaths was small, thus limiting the precision of our estimates. Third, since cross-sectional data was used to determine variables related to LVM, causality of relations cannot be established. Fourth, measurements of LVM by echocardiography is less precise and reliable than measurement by cardiac magnetic resonance imaging (CMRI) [1]. However, while CMRI is recognized as the "gold standard" for ventricular geometry measurements, it is less often applied in clinical practice since it is more expensive, not widely available and has contra-indications such as claustrophobia and use of cardiac implantable devices [1]. Thus it was not feasible to perform CMRI measurements in our relatively large cohort of dialysis patients. This may have led to misclassification, which generally leads to an underestimation of the magnitude of the relations under study.

The strengths of this study are the large sample size, the concise and prospective data collection, the independent review of source documentation for all primary and secondary outcomes and the double independent analysis of the echocardiography recordings blinded for patient characteristics.

Conclusion

In this study we confirmed the relation between LVM and all-cause mortality. Furthermore we demonstrated a markedly increased risk of sudden death in patients with a high LVM.

No relationship was found for markers of inflammation (except for a negative association with albumin) and fibrosis.

Acknowledgments

The authors are grateful to the patients and nursing staff participating in this project.

Author Contributions

Conceived and designed the experiments: MB MD PW MN PB MG RL. Performed the experiments: MB MD PW MN PB MG CH AM NW LP RL. Analyzed the data: IM MB. Contributed reagents/materials/analysis tools: RG DS OK. Wrote the paper: IM MB PB.

References

1. Glassock RJ, Pecoits-Filho R, Barberato SH (2009) Left ventricular mass in chronic kidney disease and ESRD. Clin J Am Soc Nephrol 4 Suppl 1: S79–S91.

2. Foley RN, Parfrey PS, Harnett JD, Kent GM, Martin CJ, et al (1995) Clinical and echocardiographic disease in patients starting end-stage renal disease therapy. Kidney Int 47: 186–192.

3. Zoccali C, Benedetto FA, Mallamaci F, Tripepi G, Giacone G, et al. (2004) Left ventricular mass monitoring in the follow-up of dialysis patients: prognostic value of left ventricular hypertrophy progression. Kidney Int 65: 1492–1498.

4. London GM, Pannier B, Guerin AP, Blacher J, Marchais SJ, et al. (2001) Alterations of left ventricular hypertrophy in and survival of patients receiving hemodialysis: follow-up of an interventional study. J Am Soc Nephrol 12: 2759–2767.

5. Panichi V, Migliori M, De PS, Taccola D, Bianchi AM, et al. (2000) C-reactive protein as a marker of chronic inflammation in uremic patients. Blood Purif 18: 183–190.

6. Mora S, Musunuru K, Blumenthal RS (2009) The clinical utility of high-sensitivity C-reactive protein in cardiovascular disease and the potential implication of JUPITER on current practice guidelines. Clin Chem 55: 219–228.

7. El-Shehaby AM, El-Khatib MM, Battah AA, Roshdy AR (2010) Apelin: a potential link between inflammation and cardiovascular disease in end stage renal disease patients. Scand J Clin Lab Invest 70: 421–427.

8. Cottone S, Nardi E, Mule G, Vadala A, Lorito MC, et al. (2007) Association between biomarkers of inflammation and left ventricular hypertrophy in moderate chronic kidney disease. Clin Nephrol 67: 209–216.

9. Jones SA, Horiuchi S, Topley N, Yamamoto N, Fuller GM (2001) The soluble interleukin 6 receptor: mechanisms of production and implications in disease. FASEB J 15: 43–58.

10. Ridker PM, Rifai N, Stampfer MJ, Hennekens CH (2000) Plasma concentration of interleukin-6 and the risk of future myocardial infarction among apparently healthy men. Circulation 101: 1767–1772.

11. Biasillo G, Leo M, Della BR, Biasucci LM (2010) Inflammatory biomarkers and coronary heart disease: from bench to bedside and back. Intern Emerg Med 5: 225–233.

12. Vasan RS, Sullivan LM, Roubenoff R, Dinarello CA, Harris T, et al. (2003) Inflammatory markers and risk of heart failure in elderly subjects without prior myocardial infarction: the Framingham Heart Study. Circulation 107: 1486–1491.

13. Kaneko K, Kanda T, Yokoyama T, Nakazato Y, Iwasaki T, et al. (1997) Expression of interleukin-6 in the ventricles and coronary arteries of patients with myocardial infarction. Res Commun Mol Pathol Pharmacol 97: 3–12.

14. Ayerden EF, Ebinc H, Derici U, Aral A, Aybay C, et al. (2009) The relationship between adiponectin levels and proinflammatory cytokines and left ventricular mass in dialysis patients. J Nephrol 22: 216–223.

15. Clarkson MR, Gupta S, Murphy M, Martin F, Godson C, et al. (1999) Connective tissue growth factor: a potential stimulus for glomerulosclerosis and tubulointerstitial fibrosis in progressive renal disease. Curr Opin Nephrol Hypertens 8: 543–548.

16. Zhang J, Chang L, Chen C, Zhang M, Luo Y, et al. (2011) Rad GTPase inhibits cardiac fibrosis through connective tissue growth factor. Cardiovasc Res 91: 90–98.

17. Hayata N, Fujio Y, Yamamoto Y, Iwakura T, Obana M, et al. (2008) Connective tissue growth factor induces cardiac hypertrophy through Akt signaling. Biochem Biophys Res Commun 370: 274–278.

18. Gerritsen KG, Peters HP, Nguyen TQ, Koeners MP, Wetzels JF, et al. (2010) Renal proximal tubular dysfunction is a major determinant of urinary connective tissue growth factor excretion. Am J Physiol Renal Physiol 298: F1457–F1464.

19. Fleming RE, Sly WS (2001) Hepcidin: a putative iron-regulatory hormone relevant to hereditary hemochromatosis and the anemia of chronic disease. Proc Natl Acad Sci U S A 98: 8160–8162.

20. Nicolas G, Chauvet C, Viatte L, Danan JL, Bigard X, et al. (2002) The gene encoding the iron regulatory peptide hepcidin is regulated by anemia, hypoxia, and inflammation. J Clin Invest 110: 1037–1044.

21. van der Weerd NC, Grooteman MP, Bots ML, van den Dorpel MA, den Hoedt CH, et al. (2013) Hepcidin-25 is related to cardiovascular events in chronic haemodialysis patients. Nephrol Dial Transplant 28: 3062–3071.

22. Nozari Y, Geraiely B (2011) Correlation between the serum levels of uric acid and HS-CRP with the occurrence of early systolic failure of left ventricle following acute myocardial infarction. Acta Med Iran 49: 531–535.

23. Tatasciore A, Zimarino M, Renda G, Zurro M, Soccio M, et al. (2008) Awake blood pressure variability, inflammatory markers and target organ damage in newly diagnosed hypertension. Hypertens Res 31: 2137–2146.

24. Penne EL, Blankestijn PJ, Bots ML, van den Dorpel MA, Grooteman MP, et al. (2005) Resolving controversies regarding hemodiafiltration versus hemodialysis: the Dutch Convective Transport Study. Semin Dial 18: 47–51.

25. Kroot JJ, Laarakkers CM, Geurts-Moespot AJ, Grebenchtchikov N, Pickkers P, et al. (2010) Immunochemical and mass-spectrometry-based serum hepcidin assays for iron metabolism disorders. Clin Chem 56: 1570–1579.

26. van der Weerd NC, Grooteman MP, Bots ML, van den Dorpel MA, den Hoedt CH, et al. (2012) Hepcidin-25 in chronic hemodialysis patients is related to residual kidney function and not to treatment with erythropoiesis stimulating agents. PLoS One 7: e39783.

27. Devereux RB, Casale PN, Hammond IW, Savage DD, Alderman MH, et al. (1987) Echocardiographic detection of pressure-overload left ventricular hypertrophy: effect of criteria and patient population. J Clin Hypertens 3: 66–78.

28. Schiller NB, Shah PM, Crawford M, DeMaria A, Devereux R, et al. (1989) Recommendations for quantitation of the left ventricle by two-dimensional echocardiography. American Society of Echocardiography Committee on Standards, Subcommittee on Quantitation of Two-Dimensional Echocardiograms. J Am Soc Echocardiogr 2: 358–367.

29. Greenland S, Finkle WD (1995) A critical look at methods for handling missing covariates in epidemiologic regression analyses. Am J Epidemiol 142: 1255–1264.

30. Sjolander A (2009) Propensity scores and M-structures. Stat Med 28: 1416–1420.

31. Zoccali C, Benedetto FA, Mallamaci F, Tripepi G, Giacone G, et al. (2001) Prognostic impact of the indexation of left ventricular mass in patients undergoing dialysis. J Am Soc Nephrol 12: 2768–2774.

32. Silberberg JS, Barre PE, Prichard SS, Sniderman AD (1989) Impact of left ventricular hypertrophy on survival in end-stage renal disease. Kidney Int 36: 286–290.

33. Ritz E, Wanner C (2008) The challenge of sudden death in dialysis patients. Clin J Am Soc Nephrol 3: 920–929.

34. Aoki J, Ikari Y, Nakajima H, Mori M, Sugimoto T, et al. (2005) Clinical and pathologic characteristics of dilated cardiomyopathy in hemodialysis patients. Kidney Int 67: 333–340.

35. Larsson O, Attman PO, Beckman-Suurkula M, Wallentin I, Wikstrand J (1986) Left ventricular function before and after kidney transplantation. A prospective study in patients with juvenile-onset diabetes mellitus. Eur Heart J 7: 779–791.

36. Guizar-Mendoza JM, mador-Licona N, Lozada EE, Rodriguez L, Gutierrez-Navarro M, et al. (2006) Left ventricular mass and heart sympathetic activity after renal transplantation in children and young adults. Pediatr Nephrol 21: 1413–1418.

37. Zoccali C, Mallamaci F, Tripepi G (2003) Traditional and emerging cardiovascular risk factors in end-stage renal disease. Kidney Int Suppl : S105–S110.

38. Achinger SG, Ayus JC (2006) Left ventricular hypertrophy: is hyperphosphatemia among dialysis patients a risk factor? J Am Soc Nephrol 17: S255–S261.

39. Nitta K, Akiba T, Uchida K, Otsubo S, Otsubo Y, et al. (2004) Left ventricular hypertrophy is associated with arterial stiffness and vascular calcification in hemodialysis patients. Hypertens Res 27: 47–52.

40. Chue CD, Edwards NC, Moody WE, Steeds RP, Townend JN, et al. (2012) Serum phosphate is associated with left ventricular mass in patients with chronic kidney disease: a cardiac magnetic resonance study. Heart 98: 219–224.

41. Tonelli M, Pannu N, Manns B (2010) Oral phosphate binders in patients with kidney failure. N Engl J Med 362: 1312–1324.

22

Circulating Angiopoietin-2 is a Marker for Early Cardiovascular Disease in Children on Chronic Dialysis

Rukshana C. Shroff[1], Karen L. Price[1], Maria Kolatsi-Joannou[1], Alexandra F. Todd[1], David Wells[2], John Deanfield[3], Richard J. Johnson[4], Lesley Rees[1], Adrian S. Woolf[5], David A. Long[1]*

1 Nephro-Urology Unit, UCL Institute of Child Health and Great Ormond Street Hospital for Children NHS Trust, London, United Kingdom, 2 Department of Chemical Pathology, Great Ormond Street Hospital for Children NHS Trust, London, United Kingdom, 3 National Centre for Cardiovascular Disease Prevention and Outcomes, University College London, London, United Kingdom, 4 Division of Renal Diseases and Hypertension, University of Colorado, Denver, Colorado, United States of America, 5 Institute of Human Development, University of Manchester and the Royal Manchester Children's Hospital, Manchester, United Kingdom

Abstract

Cardiovascular disease (CVD) is increasingly recognised as a complication of childhood chronic kidney disease (CKD) even in the absence of diabetes and hypertension. We hypothesized that an alteration in angiopoietin-1 and -2, growth factors which regulate endothelial and vascular function could be involved. We report that the endothelial survival factor, angiopoietin-1 is low in children with pre-dialysis CKD whereas the pro-inflammatory angiopoietin-2 is elevated in children on dialysis. In dialysis patients, angiopoietin-2 positively correlated with time on dialysis, systolic blood pressure, and carotid artery intima media thickness. Elevated angiopoietin-2 levels in dialysis versus pre-dialysis CKD patients were also associated with an anti-angiogenic (high soluble VEGFR-1 and low VEGF-A) and pro-inflammatory (high urate, E-selectin, P-selectin and VCAM-1) milieu. Ang-2 was immunodetected in arterial biopsy samples whilst the expression of VEGF-A was significantly downregulated in dialysis patients. Serum urate correlated with angiopoietin-2 levels in dialysis patients and addition of uric acid was able to induce rapid release of angiopoietin-2 from cultured endothelial cells. Thus, angiopoietin-2 is a marker for cardiovascular disease in children on chronic dialysis and may act as an anti-angiogenic and pro-inflammatory effector in this context. The possibility that the release of angiopoietin-2 from endothelia is mediated by urate should be explored further.

Editor: Samir M. Parikh, Beth Israel Deaconess Medical Center, United States of America

Funding: This work was supported by a project grant from the Great Ormond Street Hospital and UCL Institute of Child Health Biomedical Research Centre (to D.A.L., R.C.S. and L.R.) and a studentship from Kids Kidney Research (to L.R., D.A.L. and R.C.S.). D.A.L. is supported by a Kidney Research UK Senior Non-Clinical Fellowship and a Medical Research Council New Investigator Award. A.S.W. acknowledges grant support from the Manchester Biomedical Research Centre. The funders had no role in study design, data collection and analysis, decision to publish, or preparation of the manuscript.

Competing Interests: The authors have declared that no competing interests exist.

* E-mail: d.long@ucl.ac.uk

Introduction

Children with chronic kidney disease (CKD) develop early onset cardiovascular disease (CVD). [1] Manifestations of CVD in childhood CKD include arterial stiffening [2] and calcification, [3] premature atherosclerosis, [4] and left ventricular hypertrophy. [5] Over time, CKD developing in children is associated with increased cardiovascular mortality that markedly accelerates once dialysis is initiated. [6,7]

One of the earliest signs of CVD in individuals with CKD is endothelial damage and dysfunction, [8] and this has been shown even in children with pre-dialysis CKD. [9] In this context, potential causes of endothelial damage and aberrant repair are disturbances in growth factors involved in the formation of vascular networks. [10] Angiopoietin-1 (Ang-1) binds and activates the Tie-2 receptor on endothelia where it promotes cell survival and decreases vascular permeability. [11] As such, Ang-1 is usually considered beneficial for endothelial cell function. In contrast, Ang-2 is released from Weibel-Palade bodies by various stimuli [12,13] and acts as an antagonist of Ang-1. [14] Ang-2 has pro-inflammatory actions [15,16] and can also promote or retard angiogenesis dependent on the ambient levels of vascular endothelial growth factor-A (VEGF-A). [14] Other evidence exists that, in certain circumstances, Ang-2 may have biological effects, independent of the antagonism of Ang-1. [17,18]

Elevated circulating Ang-2 has been reported in adults with CKD. David and colleagues [19] found an inverse relationship between circulating Ang-2 levels and glomerular filtration rate in adults with CKD. Two other studies reported that Ang-2 levels were elevated in adults on hemodialysis (HD) or peritoneal dialysis (PD) compared with healthy controls. [20,21] In one of these studies Ang-2 correlated with scoring for coronary and peripheral arterial disease. [20] In the other study, Ang-2 correlated with cholesterol, high-sensitive C-reactive protein and osteoprotegerin and was an independent predictor of mortality. [21]

To date, no clinical studies have examined angiopoietins in childhood CKD, despite the latter having similar cardiovascular complications as adults with CKD, but at a proportionately earlier age. [1] These effects are more likely to be directly attributed to the uremic milieu because children seldom have diabetes or dyslipidaemia, uncontrolled hypertension or are smokers which themselves predispose to CVD. We hypothesized that an imbalance of angiopoietin vascular growth factors, which would be detrimental to endothelial structure and function, might be present in children with CKD. Specifically, we predicted that childhood CKD would be associated with elevated Ang-2 and that it would correlate with inflammatory markers.

Materials and Methods

Patient cohort

Informed written consent was obtained from the next of kin, caretakers, or guardians on the behalf of the minors/children participants, and children also gave their assent where appropriate. The study was approved by the Great Ormond Street Hospital and UCL Institute of Child Health research ethics committee. From January to December 2010, 20 children in pre-dialysis CKD stages 4-5 and 30 on dialysis (14 PD, 16 on HD) were recruited from Great Ormond Street Hospital. Primary diagnoses included renal dysplasia (n = 20), posterior urethral valves (n = 9), focal segmental glomerulosclerosis (n = 6), nephronophthisis (n = 4), cortical necrosis (n = 3), and 2 each with autosomal recessive polycystic kidney disease, congenital nephrotic syndrome, bilateral Wilms' tumors and unknown causes. None of the children had diabetes and none were smokers. Children with underlying inflammatory disorders, such as glomerulonephritis and vasculitides were excluded. Patients were compared with healthy age- and gender- matched children who formed part of a contemporaneous study and are previously described. [22]

Clinical, biochemical and vascular parameters

All measures were taken at the same clinical visit; pre a mid-week session of HD or at clinic review for pre-dialysis CKD and PD patients. All children had their weight, height, body mass index (BMI) and Doppler blood pressure measured; these were expressed as standard deviation score (SDS) for age and gender. [23] Routine blood tests (including creatinine, calcium, ionized calcium, phosphate, parathyroid hormone and serum urate) were performed. All children above 5 years of age (n = 24 children on dialysis [11 on PD, 13 on HD]; 14 children in pre-dialysis CKD and 25 healthy controls) underwent vascular scans to assess carotid artery intima media thickness (cIMT) and aortic pulse wave velocity (PWV) using methods previously described [24] and expressed as SDS for age. [25,26] Serum was obtained and ELISA used to assess circulating levels of human Ang-1, Ang-2, VEGF-A, Flt-1, E-selectin, P-selectin, intracellular adhesion molecule 1 (ICAM-1) and vascular cell adhesion molecule 1 (VCAM-1) (R & D Systems). In some cases, serum samples were taken both pre- and post- HD.

Immunolocalisation of Ang-1, Ang-2 and VEGF-A in intact arteries

Medium-sized muscular arteries routinely removed at omentectomy during a peritoneal dialysis catheter insertion or at renal transplantation were obtained from some of the pre-dialysis CKD and dialysis patients (n = 4 in each group). [3] Tissues were fixed in formalin, embedded, then sections cut for immunohistochemistry as described [27] for the following antibodies: rabbit anti-mouse Ang-1 (ADI); rabbit anti-mouse Ang-2 (ADI); rabbit anti-human VEGF-A (Santa Cruz) and rabbit anti-human von Willebrand factor (DAKO). Intensity of staining was quantified by a blinded observed and scored between 0 (no reactivity) to 3 (strong staining); at least four images were obtained from each vessel and a mean value obtained for each specimen.

Uric acid stimulation of human umbilical vein endothelial (HUVEC) and aortic smooth muscle cells (HAoSMC)

HUVEC and HAoSMC (Lonza) were cultured in either EGM-MV or DMEM supplemented with 20% FBS, 25 mM HEPES, 100 U/ml penicillin and 100 mg/ml streptomycin respectively. Cells from passage 2–4 were grown to 70% confluence, placed in low-serum media for 24 hours and challenged with varying concentrations of uric acid (3–12 mg/dl) [28] for 15 minutes, 24 hours and 72 hours. Conditioned media was collected at all time-points to assess Ang-2 levels and cell lysates extracted for protein measurements. In other experiments, RNA was extracted from cells stimulated with uric acid for 6 hours and used for RT-PCR for *Ang1*, *Ang2*, organic anion transporters 1–4 (*Oat1-4*) *Tie1*, *Tie2*, Toll-like receptor 4 *(Tlr4)* and human uric acid transporter 1 (*Urat1*) using previously described methods. [28] Quantitative RT-PCR was also performed for *Ang2* on HUVEC exposed to uric acid (n = 3 for each dose) with hypoxanthine-guanine phosphoribosyltransferase (HPRT) used as a house-keeping gene. Primer details available on request.

Statistics. Results are presented as mean ± SD or median and inter quartile range (IQR), depending on the distribution. Univariate comparisons of continuous variables were performed using unpaired *t*-test for normally distributed data, or non-parametric Mann-Whitney U-test for non-normally distributed variables. For multiple comparisons of several groups, ANOVA or Kruskall-Wallis test were performed. Within group comparisons of continuous variables were performed using paired *t*-test or Wilcoxon test, as appropriate. Spearman tests were used for correlation analyses. Interactions between Ang-2 and biochemical data or vascular scans were tested by two way ANOVA and the difference between each pair of means compared by Tukey's test with appropriate adjustment for the multiple testing. Factors affecting the two outcome variables, Ang-2 and cIMT, were explored using multiple regression analysis, including all variables with $p \leq 0.15$ from univariate analysis in the stepwise multiple regression models. For all analyses, $p < 0.05$ was considered statistically significant.

Results

Circulating Ang levels in pre-dialysis CKD and dialysis patients

Demographic and clinical parameters of the groups studied are summarized in **Table 1**. The pre-dialysis CKD and dialysis patients were similar in all demographic, clinical and biochemical markers except that 25-hydroxyvitamin D was lower and serum cholesterol and urinary albumin/creatinine ratio higher in dialysis patients (**Table 1**). The healthy controls had significantly higher BMI SDS and lower blood pressure SDS and urate levels *versus* the patients.

Ang-1 levels were modestly but significantly (p = 0.02) lower in pre-dialysis CKD patients compared with healthy controls (respective means±SD being 2.9±1.8 and 4.3±1.8 ng/ml). In dialysis patients, Ang-1 levels (mean±SD 5.0±3.5 ng/ml) were similar to values found in healthy controls. Circulating Ang-2 levels were not significantly different between healthy children and those with pre-dialysis CKD, but were markedly and significantly increased in the dialysis group (means±SD in controls 2.7±1.2, pre-dialysis CKD 2.7±0.9, dialysis 10.5±6.9 ng/ml, p<0.0005 in comparisons between dialysis patients and both the other groups). As explained in the *Introduction*, Ang-2 acts an endogenous antagonist to Ang-1, such that comparative levels may be relevant; hence we evaluated the Ang-2/Ang-1 ratio. There was no difference in the Ang-2/Ang-1 ratios (**Figure 1C**) between control

Table 1. Demographic, clinical, anthropometric, and biochemical characteristics of patients and control subjects.

Characteristics	Pre-dialysis CKD (n = 20)	Dialysis (n = 30)	Healthy Controls (n = 25)	p
Age (yr)	10.7±4.1	14.2±3.9	13.1±2.8	0.68
Sex (males/females)	12/8	17/13	14/11	0.82
Race (White/Asian/Black/other)	14/5/1/0	19/7/2/2	16/7/2/0	0.85
eGFR (ml/min per 1.73 m^2)	18.3±6.0	-	113±9.8	-
Time in CKD4-5 pre-dialysis (yr; median [IQR])	4.5 (1.1–9.2)	3.9 (0.2–7.9)	-	0.70
Time on dialysis (yr; median [IQR])	-	1.4 (0.2–3.9)	-	-
Dialysis modality (PD/HD)	-	14/16	-	-
BMI SDS	−0.6±1.1	−0.7±0.3	1.1±0.7	0.42
Systolic BP index*	1.9±0.8	1.5±2.5	0.8±0.2	0.21
Numbers on antihypertensive medications	11	4	0	0.6
Numbers on ACEi or ARB	4	0	0	0.1
Hemoglobin (g/dl)	12.3±1.9	11.4±0.8	12.1±0.9	0.51
Albumin (g/L)	39.0±4.1	41±4.8	40±0.6	0.34
Total cholesterol (mmol/L)	3.5±1.3	4.1±0.9	3.1±0.7	0.07
Triglycerides (mmol/L)	1.1±0.7	1.4±2.1	0.9±0.6	0.11
No. on statins	0	1	0	-
Albumin-adjusted calcium (mmol/L)	2.4±0.2	2.4±0.1	2.4±0.2	0.9
Serum phosphate levels (mmol/L)	1.4±0.6	1.6±0.8	1.2±0.2	0.9
Parathyroid hormone (pmol/L)	5.2±1.1	8.9±3.7	-	0.06
Serum urate level (μmol/L)	260±20.8	278±29.3	184±33.0	0.88
25-hydroxyvitamin D (nmol/L)	40.1±16.2	12.9±9.8	-	0.04
Urinary albumin / creatinine ratio (mg/mmol)	122.8±18.6	260.0±64.3 (n = 21)	-	0.04

All values are presented as mean±SD; p value indicates comparisons between the pre-dialysis CKD and dialysis groups. Parathyroid hormone, 25-hydroxyvitamin D and urinary albumin / creatinine ratio were not measured in healthy controls due to small volumes of serum and lack of urine samples. * Systolic BP index = measured BP/ 95th centile BP for age, gender, and height. ARB, angiotensin II receptor blocker; ACEi, angiotensin-converting enzyme inhibitor; BMI, body mass index; SBP, systolic BP; SDS, SD score.

and pre-dialysis CKD individuals but it was significantly higher in dialysis patients compared with the other groups (means±SD in controls 0.8±0.7, pre-dialysis CKD patients 1.2±0.7 and dialysis patients 2.5±1.4 ng/ml, p<0.0005 in comparisons between dialysis and both the other groups)

Correlation of Ang levels with clinical and vascular measures

Ang-2 levels had no significant relation to age or gender, but increased linearly with time on dialysis (r = 0.37, p = 0.002) whereas there was no association of Ang-2 levels with the time spent in pre-dialysis CKD (p = 0.8, **Figure 2A**). There was no

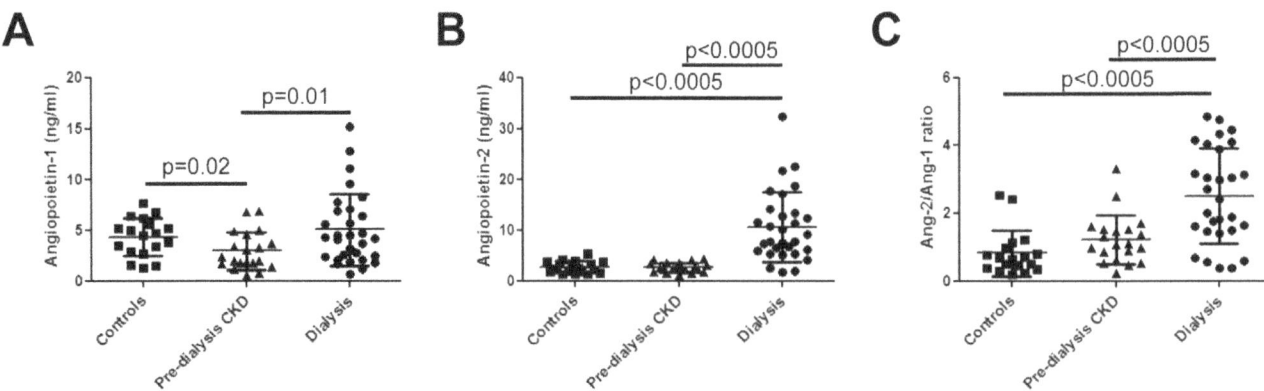

Figure 1. Circulating Ang levels in pre-dialysis CKD and dialysis patients. Serum Ang-1 levels (A) were significantly lower in pre-dialysis CKD patients compared with healthy controls. In dialysis patients Ang-1 levels were similar to values found in healthy controls. Similar levels of both circulating Ang-2 (B) and Ang-2/Ang-1 (C) were found in healthy children and those with pre-dialysis CKD, but these were significantly increased in the dialysis group.

difference in Ang-2 levels between HD and PD patients. Circulating Ang-2 levels was also not significantly related to the presence of residual renal function. To determine whether Ang-2 was cleared by HD, we obtained serum samples pre- and post-HD from 5 individuals. There was no significant differences in Ang-2 levels (means±SD 5.0±1.1 and 4.6±0.9 ng/ml, p = 0.7).

Serum urate levels were significantly increased in both pre-dialysis CKD and dialysis patients compared with controls (**Table 1**) and showed a weak positive correlation with systolic blood pressure SDS in these patients (r = 0.12, p = 0.048). Urate levels positively correlated with Ang-2 levels in the dialysis group (r = 0.52, p = 0.004, **Figure 2B**). There was a strong positive correlation between Ang-2 levels and systolic blood pressure SDS in the dialysis patients (r = 0.64, p = 0.003), but not in the pre-dialysis CKD group, **Figure 2C**. No significant correlations were found between Ang-1 or Ang-2/Ang-1 ratio with any clinical, biochemical or vascular parameters.

Three out of 14 (21%) pre-dialysis CKD patients had increased cIMT compared with age-matched controls (0.37±0.03 versus 0.38±0.02 mm respectively), but there was no significant correlation between Ang-2 and cIMT in this group (p = 0.82, **Figure 2D**). In contrast, cIMT was increased in 16 of 24 (66%) dialysis patients (0.46±0.05 mm) and showed a strong positive correlation with Ang-2 (r = 0.62, p = 0.0005, **Figure 2D**). PWV was increased in two out of 14 children with pre-dialysis CKD

(5.1±0.2 m/sec in pre-dialysis CKD versus 5.0±0.3 m/sec in controls) and 7 out of 24 (5.6±0.5 m/sec) on dialysis but did not show any correlation with Ang-2 in either group. Ang-2 levels were not significantly correlated with blood cholesterol, triglyceride, albumin, calcium, phosphate, parathyroid hormone, 25-hydroxyvitamin D or urinary albumin/creatinine levels in pre-dialysis CKD or dialysis patients. On multiple regression analysis the significant determinants of Ang-2 levels were systolic blood pressure and serum urate levels (**Table 2**). Carotid IMT was significantly and independently influenced by the time on dialysis, calcium x phosphate product and Ang-2 levels (**Table 2**).

Circulating levels of VEGF-A and sFlt-1

The biological actions of Ang-2 on blood vessels are dependent on VEGF-A availability; [14] so we measured circulating levels of this growth factor and the endogenous VEGF-A inhibitor, sFlt-1. Ang-2 levels were similar in healthy controls and pre-dialysis CKD patients and therefore VEGF-A and sFlt-1 levels were only measured in pre-dialysis CKD and dialysis patients. VEGF-A levels were significantly lower in individuals on dialysis compared with pre-dialysis CKD patients (respective medians being 6.9 and 33.5 pg/ml, p = 0.003, **Figure 3A**). In contrast, sFlt-1 levels were significantly higher in dialysis patients compared with pre-dialysis CKD (respective means±SD of 222±78 and 121±54 pg/ml respectively, p<0.0001, **Figure 3B**). There were no significant

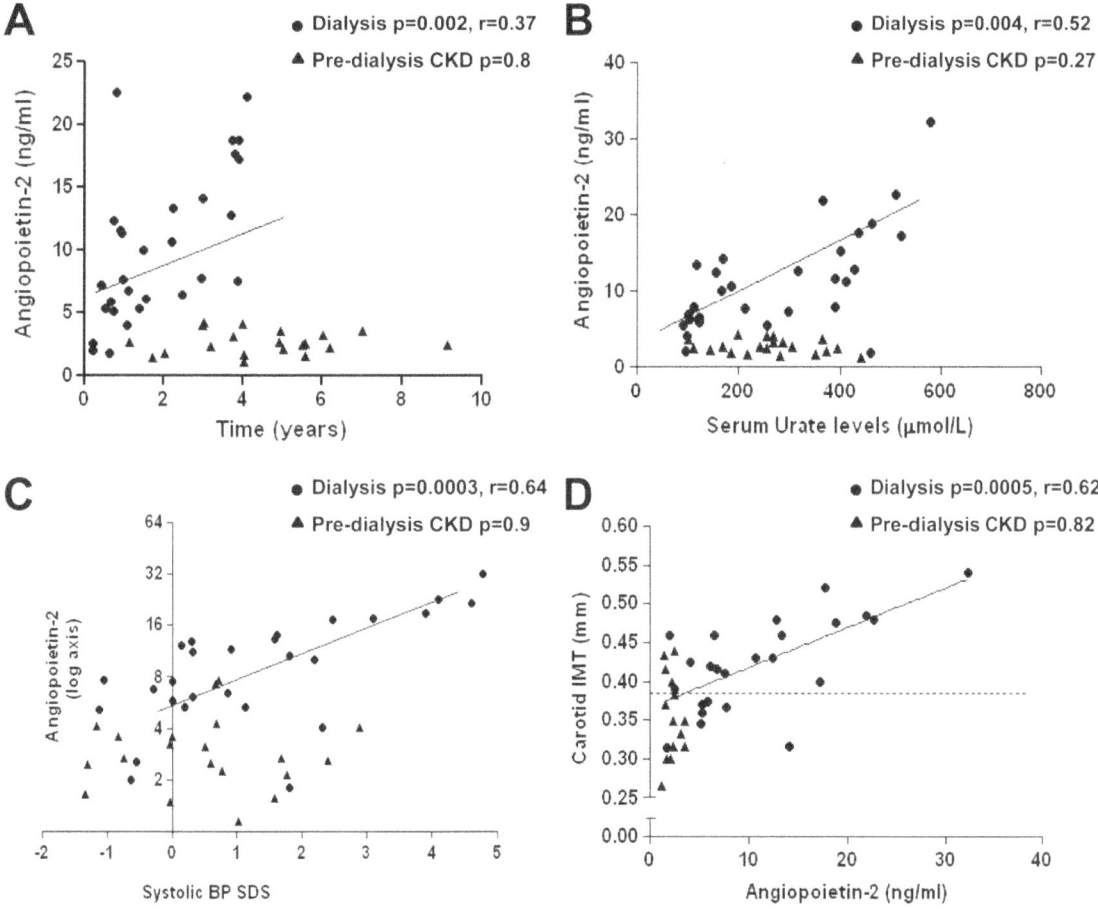

Figure 2. Correlation of Ang-2 levels with clinical and vascular parameters. Ang-2 levels in dialysis individuals correlated positively with time on dialysis (A), serum urate levels (B), systolic blood pressure SDS (C) and cIMT (D). Independent variables are shown on the x-axis. Regression lines account for dialysis patients only. Dotted line in D indicates the value for cIMT in healthy age-matched controls. There was no correlation between Ang-2 and any clinical and vascular measures in pre-dialysis CKD patients.

Table 2. Multiple regression analyses for independent predictors of Angiopoietin-2 (Ang2) and carotid intima media thickness (cIMT).

Variables	β	SE	p	Model R²
Ang2				71%
Systolic BP	2.54	0.21	<0.001	
Serum urate level	0.14	0.006	0.03	
cIMT				68%
Time on dialysis	0.50	0.02	0.008	
Ca x P product	0.37	0.12	0.02	
Ang2	0.26	0.06	0.05	

β - Unstandardized regression coefficient; indicates the difference in the outcome variable (Ang2 or cIMT) per unit change in the independent variables.
SE – standard error
Model R² - The amount of variance in the dependent variable that can be explained by the model.

correlations of either VEGF-A or sFlt-1 with time or mode of dialysis, urate levels, blood pressure SDS or any other vascular measures.

Circulating levels of soluble cell adhesion molecules

Ang-2 has been shown to have pro-inflammatory actions. [16,17] Therefore, circulating levels of cell adhesion molecules which attract inflammatory cells were measured. [29] Compared with pre-dialysis CKD individuals, patients treated with dialysis had significantly elevated levels of soluble E-selectin (respective means±SD being 72±31 and 54±21 ng/ml, p=0.03, **Figure 4A**), soluble P-selectin (75±27 *versus* 52±17 ng/ml, p=0.001, **Figure 4B**) and soluble VCAM-1 (1.9±0.5 *versus* 1.3±0.4 µg/ml, p<0.0001, **Figure 4C**) but there was no difference in ICAM-1 (354±99 versus 341±91 ng/ml, **Figure 4D**). In the dialysis population, circulating levels of Ang-2 positively correlated with soluble VCAM-1 (r=0.41, p=0.02),

but there were no significant correlations with E-selectin, ICAM-1 or P-selectin.

Immunolocalisation of vascular growth factors in arteries

To seek potential source(s) of Ang-1, Ang-2 and VEGF-A immunohistochemistry was undertaken on intact arteries obtained from a subset of the pre-dialysis CKD and dialysis patients. [3] Ang-1 protein was detected in the media of vessels from pre-dialysis CKD (**Figure 5A**) and dialysis patients (**Figure 5B**). As scored by an observer blinded to the source of the samples, there was no difference in staining intensity between the two groups (**Figure 5C**). Ang-2 was also immunodetected in the media of both pre-dialysis CKD (**Figure 5D**) and dialysis (**Figure 5E**) vessels with a similar intensity in each group (**Figure 5F**). Ang-2 expression was also detected in the endothelial layer which was also positive for von Willebrand factor (**Figure 5G, 5H**). VEGF-A immunostaining was prominent in the media of pre-dialysis CKD vessels (**Figure 5I**), but was significantly decreased in dialysis patients (**Figure 5J and K**).

Effect of uric acid exposure on Ang-2 release in-vitro

As demonstrated above, Ang-2 levels strongly and positively correlated with urate levels in dialysis patients. We hypothesized that elevated urate might increase Ang-2 expression by, and/or release from, endothelial and/or vascular smooth muscle cells. There has been a previous report that uric acid can stimulate release of contents from Weibel-Palade bodies including Ang-2. [13] We first examined how urate may enter HUVEC and detected the urate transporter, *Urat1*, but not *Oat1-4*; the mRNA levels of *Urat1* showed a tendency to decrease with increasing doses of uric acid stimulation (**Figure 6A**). HUVEC also expressed *Ang-1, Ang-2, Tie-1* and *Tie-2* (**Figure 6A**).

Exposure of HUVECs to uric acid for 15 minutes led to an increase in Ang-2 release *versus* control media as evaluated by the proportion of Ang-2 protein in the conditioned media. The most prominent response was observed with 12 mg/dl with Ang-2 levels significantly elevated compared with all other groups (**Figure 6B**). This was an acute effect because longer term stimulation with uric acid for 72 hours did not enhance the release of Ang-2 protein in the conditioned media (**Figure 6C**). Within the cells, uric acid

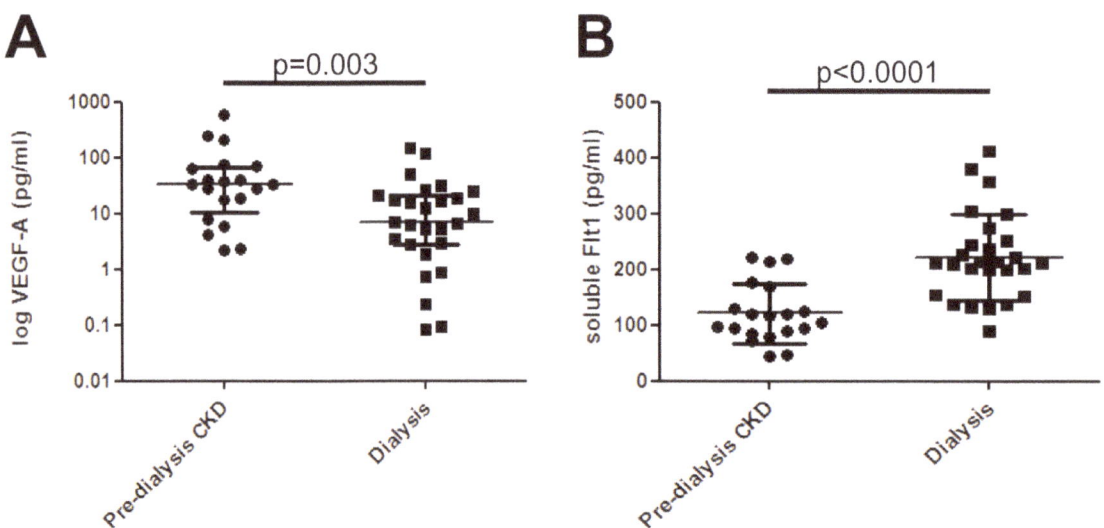

Figure 3. Circulating levels of VEGF-A and sFlt-1 in pre-dialysis CKD and dialysis patients. VEGF-A levels were significantly lower in individuals on dialysis compared with pre-dialysis CKD patients (A). In contrast, sFlt-1 were significantly higher in the dialysis patients (B)

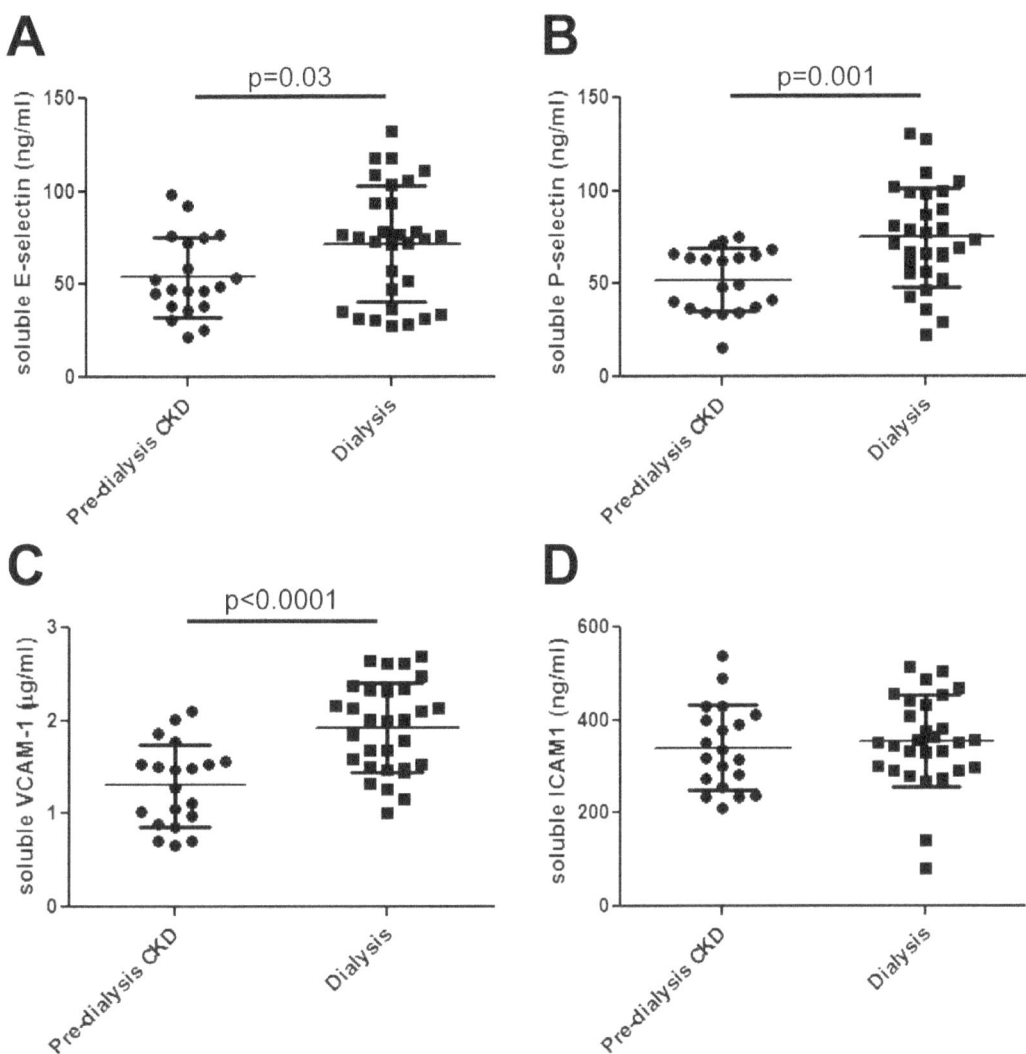

Figure 4. Circulating levels of soluble cell adhesion molecules. Compared with pre-dialysis CKD individuals, patients treated with dialysis had significantly elevated levels of soluble E-selectin (A), P-selectin (B) and VCAM-1 (C); there was no difference in ICAM-1 levels (D).

stimulation led to a decreased abundance of *Ang-2* mRNA after 6 hours of stimulation (**Figure 6D**), compared with controls. It has been suggested that the acute release of Ang-2 from endothelia is mediated by *Tlr4* [13] and we detected mRNA levels of *Tlr4* on HUVECs (**Figure 6A**). Prior studies have shown that HAoSMC express the *Urat1* receptor [28] and in the current study they were also found to express transcripts for *Ang-1*, *Ang-2* and *Tie-2*, but not *Tie-1* (data not shown); however, we did not detect Ang-2 protein in the conditioned media with/without addition of uric acid.

Discussion

Our study demonstrated that circulating Ang-2 levels were markedly elevated in dialysis patients compared with healthy controls and pre-dialysis CKD individuals. Amongst the dialysis patients, Ang-2 positively correlated with time on dialysis, systolic blood pressure and cIMT, but not PWV. These findings may indicate that circulating Ang-2 is a marker for the early cardiovascular changes occurring in children with CKD on dialysis. Previous studies have demonstrated that in the more compliant vessels of children with CKD structural changes precede functional alterations with increases in cIMT observed

before alterations in PWV. [30] Furthermore, our work examining intact vessels from children on dialysis indicated that the vessel calcium load showed a strong linear association with cIMT but not with PWV or the coronary calcification score. [3]

Our findings concur with several studies that have shown a relationship between circulating Ang-2 levels and cardiovascular complications in adults. Elevated circulating Ang-2 is associated with scores for coronary and peripheral arterial disease in adults with CKD on PD or HD [20] and positively correlated with systolic blood pressure and left ventricular hypertrophy in 4000 young to middle-aged individuals. [31]. A further study [21] demonstrated that Ang-2 was an independent predictor of mortality in CKD patients and correlated with markers of vascular disease (cholesterol, hsCRP and osteoprotegerin) but not the degree of vascular calcification or arterial stiffness. The observation that circulating Ang-2 is also elevated in children on dialysis suggests that the uraemic environment may directly influence vascular growth factor expression. This is because children do not have many of the cardiovascular comorbidities that are commonly seen in adults. In addition, the pathophysiology of CVD in children may be different to that found in adults, for example, our

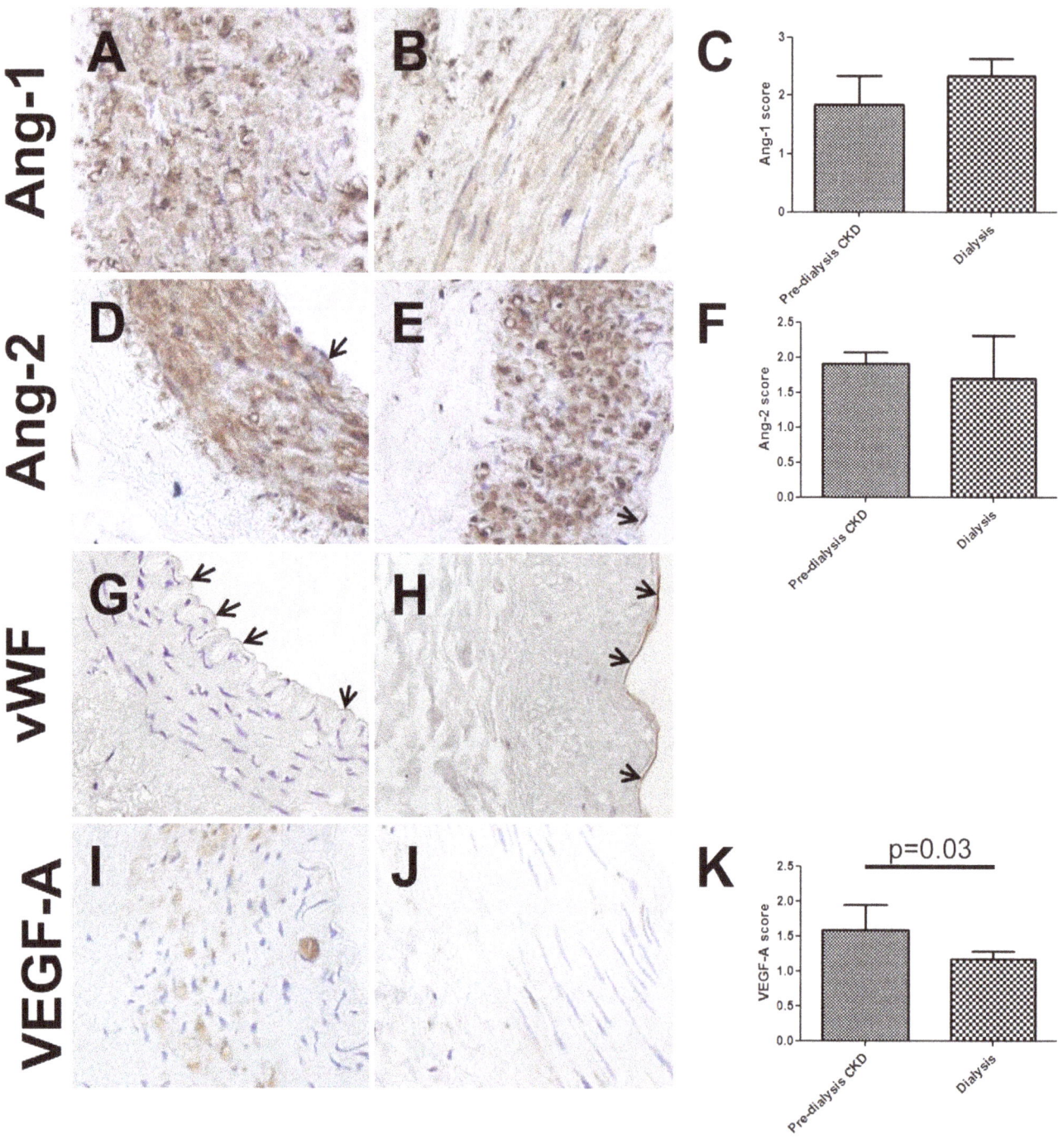

Figure 5. Immunolocalisation of vascular growth factors in arteries. Ang-1 was detected in the media of vessels from both pre-dialysis CKD (A) and dialysis patients (B); no differences in staining intensity were observed between the two groups (C). Ang-2 was immunodetected in both the media and endothelia (arrows) in pre-dialysis CKD (D) and dialysis (E) vessels with similar intensity (F). The endothelial later was also positive for von Willebrand factor (arrows, G and H). VEGF-A immunostaining was prominent in the media of pre-dialysis CKD vessels (I), but was significantly decreased in dialysis patients (J and K). All fields taken with ×40 objective.

previous work has shown that children on dialysis develop arteriosclerosis with exclusively medial involvement [3] whereas adults are much more likely to have both intimal lesions as well as medial damage [32]. Therefore results from adults may not be able to be directly extrapolated to the paediatric population and studies in children with CKD are necessary.

Our studies found that the elevation in circulating Ang-2 levels were similar immediately before and after a HD session. Both Ang-1 and Ang-2 form multimeric structures composed of monomers of 55 kDa [33] and therefore unlikely to be affected by dialytic clearance. In contrast to adults with CKD [19,21] we did not detect different Ang-2 levels in children with pre-dialysis CKD compared with healthy controls. One explanation for this

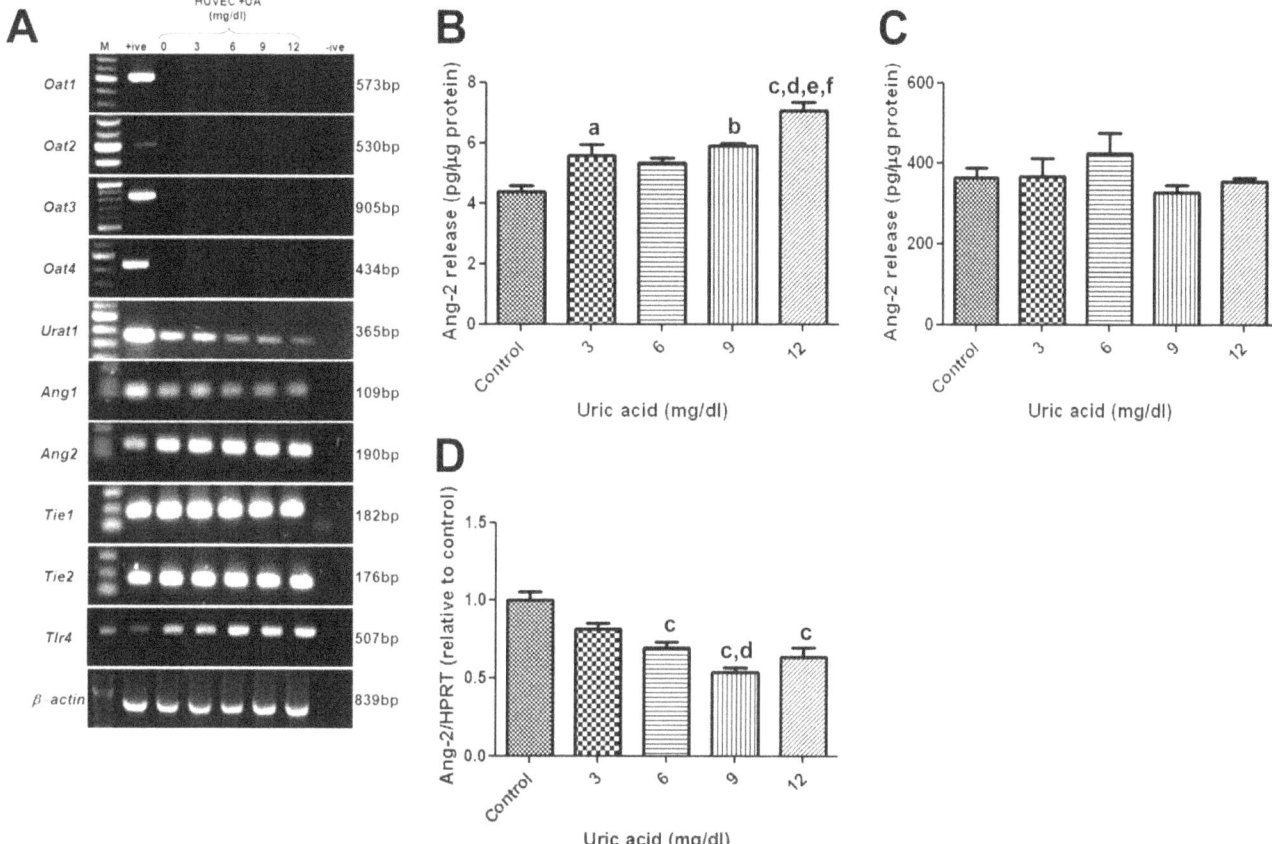

Figure 6. Effect of uric acid on Ang-2 secretion in HUVECs. A) Both non-stimulated and uric acid stimulated HUVECs expressed the mRNA for the transporter *Urat1* but not *Oat1-4*; they were also positive for *Ang-1, Ang-2, Tie-1, Tie-2* and *Tlr4*. Sizes were determined using a 100 bp marker (m), positive (+ive) controls consisted of total kidney cDNA and negative controls were without cDNA addition. (B) Uric acid stimulation for 15 minutes, but not 72 hours (C) led to elevated Ang-2 secretion in the conditioned media of HUVEC cells. Within the cells, uric acid stimulation led to a decreased abundance of Ang-2 mRNA after 6 hours of stimulation (D). a = $p < 0.05$ compared with controls, b = $p < 0.01$ compared with controls, c = $p < 0.001$ compared with controls, d = $p < 0.01$ compared with HUVEC stimulated with 3 mg/dl uric acid, e = $p < 0.01$ compared with HUVEC stimulated with 6 mg/dl uric acid, f = $p < 0.05$ compared with HUVEC stimulated with 9 mg/dl uric acid.

discrepancy could be that the children under study had not been exposed to diabetes mellitus, and that dyslipidaemia and hypertension were less common than in adults with CKD. Indeed, each of these factors have been shown to be associated with elevated Ang-2. [31,34] Instead, children with pre-dialysis CKD had decreased circulating Ang-1 compared with healthy controls. This loss of Ang-1 in pre-dialysis CKD children may decrease blood vessels stability and be an early sign of the endothelial dysfunction which occurs in these patients. [9] Potential sources of Ang-1 not only include the vessel wall, but also platelets [35] and one caveat to consider when measuring circulating Ang-1 in serum samples is that ex-vivo activation may increase Ang-1 levels within serum tubes. [36] In future studies, it would be of interest to quantify both circulating Ang-1 and platelet-derived Ang-1.

Elevated circulating Ang-2 levels in dialysis *versus* non-dialysis CKD children were associated with an anti-angiogenic environment as demonstrated by decreased circulating VEGF-A and elevated soluble sFlt-1 (**Table 3**). Increased sFlt-1 [37] and reduced circulating VEGF-A [38] have been demonstrated in adult populations with CKD. In the presence of low VEGF-A, Ang-2 will destabilise blood vessels leading to vessel regression. [14] This milieu of growth factors may therefore contribute to the impaired endothelial function seen in CKD children on dialysis. [9,39]

Increased circulating Ang-2 in CKD children on dialysis was also associated with pro-inflammatory responses with high urate, E-selectin, P-selectin and VCAM-1 (**Table 3**). Systemic inflammation is seen in children with CKD with dialysis [3,40] and Ang-2 may play a direct role in this process. Ang-2 can sensitise the endothelium to inflammatory responses; [16] and directly affect the biology of inflammatory cells which express the Tie-2 receptor themselves. [41,42] Although, we demonstrated that Ang-2/Ang-1 was also elevated in CKD children on dialysis it did not correlate with any cardiovascular parameters. This suggests that the total Ang-2 levels are important in biological responses in dialysis patients, rather than the relative balance between Ang-2 and Ang-1.

We detected Ang-2 in the endothelium of intact arteries isolated from children with CKD and cultured HUVECs indicating this cell type is a potential source of the increased Ang-2 in dialysis patients. Our studies detected Ang-2 in the walls of intact arteries from both pre-dialysis CKD and dialysis patients and *Ang-2* transcripts were detected in cultured HoASMCs. Using *Ang-2/ LacZ* mice positive expression in renal arterial walls during kidney development has been observed; [43] whilst Ang-2 has been detected in cultured mouse embryonic fibroblasts [44] and smooth muscle cells derived from the heart microvasculature. [45] We could not detect any Ang-2 released from HoASMCs suggesting

Table 3. Changes in circulating angiogenic and inflammatory markers between pre-dialysis CKD and dialysis patients.

Circulating marker	Levels in dialysis compared with pre-dialysis CKD patients
Angiogenic factors	
Ang-1	No change
Ang-2	↑
Ang-2/Ang-1 ratio	↑
VEGF-A	↓
sFlt-1	↑
Inflammatory markers	
E-selectin	↑
P-selectin	↑
VCAM-1	↑
ICAM-1	No change

vascular smooth muscle cells may not contribute to the increase in Ang-2 seen in dialysis patients. We cannot rule this out completely as the cells used in these experiments were not derived from patients, nor did we reproduce the uremic milieu they will be exposed to *in-vivo*. Another potential source of Ang-2 are macrophages. [41,46] Although prior studies [3] have demonstrated that macrophages are not present in the intact arteries of children on dialysis they may be found in the circulation and increase Ang-2.

There are several potential mechanisms for the increase in circulating Ang-2 in patients with CKD. The increase in Ang-2 may be a direct consequence of elevated blood pressure. Korff and colleagues [47] demonstrated that hypertension in mice led to release of stored Ang-2 from Weibel-Palade bodies. There is also evidence that mediators of vascular tone such as angiotensin II can directly alter Ang-2 expression. [48] A lack of endothelial nitric oxide may also predispose to a release of Weibel-Palade bodies that would theoretically increase Ang-2 levels. [49]

One potential factor that could bring these various mechanisms together is uric acid. Urate is retained in CKD and found to correlate with Ang-2 levels in the dialysis patients. We showed that uric acid could directly induce the release of Ang-2 from HUVEC with a corresponding decrease in mRNA abundance within the

cell, consistent with prior reports that uric acid stimulates release of Weibel-Palade bodies. [13] These effects are likely to be mediated by *Urat1* and *Tlr4* [13], both of which were found to be expressed on endothelia. Future studies using inhibitors specific for *Urat1* (probenecid [28] and *Tlr4* (TAK-242 [50] would help to determine the specific role of these molecules in Ang-2 release from endothelia exposed to uric acid. In addition, there is increasing evidence that urate may have a role in hypertension via effects that include inducing endothelial dysfunction, oxidative stress and the production of angiotensin II. [51] These findings might account for why urate can contribute to cardiovascular complications. [52,53]

In conclusion, Ang-2 is a marker for cardiovascular disease in children on chronic dialysis. Furthermore, we suggest that Ang-2 may also be an anti-angiogenic and pro-inflammatory effector in this context.

Author Contributions

Conceived and designed the experiments: RCS LR ASW DAL. Performed the experiments: RCS KLP MKJ AFT DAL. Analyzed the data: RCS KLP DAL. Contributed reagents/materials/analysis tools: DW JD. Wrote the paper: RCS RJJ ASW DAL.

References

1. Goodman WG, Goldin J, Kuizon BD, Yoon C, Gales B, et al. (2000) Coronary-artery calcification in young adults with end-stage renal disease who are undergoing dialysis. N Engl J Med 342: 1478–1483.
2. Covic A, Mardare N, Gusbeth-Tatomir P, Brumaru O, Gavrilovici C, et al. (2006) Increased arterial stiffness in children on haemodialysis. Nephrol Dial Transplant 21: 729–735.
3. Shroff RC, McNair R, Figg N, Skepper JN, Schurgers L, et al. (2008) Dialysis accelerates medial vascular calcification in part by triggering smooth muscle cell apoptosis. Circulation 118: 1748–1757.
4. Dursun I, Poyrazoglu HM, Gunduz Z, Ulger H, Yykylmaz A, et al. (2009) The relationship between endothelial microparticles and arterial stiffness and atherosclerosis in children with chronic kidney disease. Nephrol Dial Transplant 24: 2511–2518.
5. Mitsnefes MM, Barletta GM, Dresner IG, Chand DH, Geary D, et al. (2006) Severe cardiac hypertrophy and long-term dialysis: the Midwest Pediatric Nephrology Consortium study. Pediatr Nephrol 21: 1167–1170.
6. McDonald SP, Craig JC, Australian and New Zealand Paediatric Nephrology Association (2004) Long-term survival of children with end-stage renal disease. N Engl J Med 350: 2654–2662.
7. Oh J, Wunsch R, Turzer M, Bahner M, Raggi P, et al. (2002) Advanced coronary and carotid arteriopathy in young adults with childhood-onset chronic renal failure. Circulation 106: 100–105.
8. Lilien MR, Groothoff JW (2009) Cardiovascular disease in children with CKD or ESRD. Nat Rev Nephrol 5: 229–235.

9. Kari JA, Donald AE, Vallance DT, Bruckdorfer KR, Leone A, et al. (1997) Physiology and biochemistry of endothelial function in children with chronic renal failure. Kidney Int 52: 468–472.
10. Long DA, Norman JT, Fine LG (2012) Restoring the renal microvasculature to treat chronic kidney disease. Nat Rev Nephrol 8: 244–250.
11. Kim KT, Choi HH, Steinmetz MO, Maco B, Kammerer RA, et al. (2005) Oligomerization and multimerization are critical for angiopoietin-1 to bind and phosphorylate Tie2. J Biol Chem 280: 20126–20131.
12. Fiedler U, Scharpfenecker M, Koidl S, Hegen A, Grunow V, et al. (2004) The Tie-2 ligand angiopoietin-2 is stored and rapidly released upon stimulation from endothelial cell Weibel-Palade bodies. Blood 103: 4150–4156.
13. Kuo MC, Patschan D, Patschan S, Cohen-Gould L, Park HC, et al. (2008) Ischemia-induced exocytosis of Weibel-Palade bodies mobilizes stem cells. J Am Soc Nephrol 19: 2321–2330.
14. Maisonpierre PC, Suri C, Jones PF, Bartunkova S, Wiegand SJ, et al. (1997) Angiopoietin-2, a natural antagonist for Tie2 that disrupts in vivo angiogenesis. Science 277: 55–60.
15. Scholz A, Lang V, Henschler R, Czabanka M, Vajkoczy P, et al. (2011) Angiopoietin-2 promotes myeloid cell infiltration in a β2-integrin-dependent manner. Blood 118: 5050–5059.
16. Fiedler U, Reiss Y, Scharpfenecker M, Grunow V, Koidl S, et al. (2006) Angiopoietin-2 sensitizes endothelial cells to TNF-alpha and has a crucial role in the induction of inflammation. Nat Med 12: 235–239.

17. Felcht M, Luck R, Schering A, Seidel P, Srivastava K, et al. (2012) Angiopoietin-2 differentially regulates angiogenesis through TIE2 and integrin signaling. J Clin Invest 122: 1991–2005.

18. Krausz S, Garcia S, Ambarus CA, de Launay D, Foster M, et al. (2012) Angiopoietin-2 promotes inflammatory activation of human macrophages and is essential for murine experimental arthritis. Ann Rheum Dis 71: 1402–1417.

19. David S, Kumpers P, Lukasz A, Fliser D, Martens-Lobenhoffer J, et al. (2010) Circulating angiopoietin-2 levels increase with progress of chronic kidney disease. Nephrol Dial Transplant 25: 2571–2576.

20. David S, Kümpers P, Hellpap J, Horn R, Leitolf H, et al. (2009) Angiopoietin-2 and cardiovascular disease in dialysis and kidney transplantation. *Am J Kidney Dis* 53: 770–778.

21. David S, John SG, Jefferies HJ, Sigrist MK, Kümpers P, et al. (2012) Angiopoietin-2 levels predict mortality in CKD patients. Nephrol Dial Transplant 27: 1867–1872.

22. Kracht D, Shroff R, Baig S, Doyon A, Jacobi C, et al. (2011) Validating a new oscillometric device for aortic pulse wave velocity measurements in children and adolescents. Am J Hypertens 24: 1294–1299.

23. Cole TJ, Green PJ (1992) Smoothing reference centile curves: the LMS method and penalized likelihood. Stat Med 11:1305–1319.

24. Shroff RC, Donald AE, Hiorns MP, Watson A, Feather S, et al. (2007) Mineral metabolism and vascular damage in children on dialysis. J Am Soc Nephrol 18: 2996–3003.

25. Jourdan C, Wühl E, Litwin M, Fahr K, Trelewicz J, et al. (2005) Normative values for intima-media thickness and distensibility of large arteries in healthy adolescents. J Hypertens 23: 1707–1715.

26. Reusz GS, Cseprekal O, Temmar M, Kis E, Cherif AB, et al. (2010) Reference values of pulse wave velocity in healthy children and teenagers. Hypertension 56: 217–224.

27. Long DA, Woolf AS, Suda T, Yuan HT (2001) Increased renal angiopoietin-1 expression in folic acid-induced nephrotoxicity in mice. J Am Soc Nephrol 12: 2721–2731.

28. Price KL, Sautin YY, Long DA, Zhang L, Miyazaki H, et al. (2006) Human vascular smooth muscle cells express a urate transporter. J Am Soc Nephrol 17: 1791–1795.

29. Mestas J, Ley K (2008) Monocyte-endothelial cell interactions in the development of atherosclerosis. Trends Cardiovasc Med 18: 228–232.

30. Litwin M, Wuhl E, Jourdan C, Trelewicz J, Niemirska A, et al. (2005) Altered morphologic properties of large arteries in children with chronic renal failure and after renal transplantation. J Am Soc Nephrol 16: 1494–1500.

31. Lieb W, Zachariah JP, Xanthakis V, Safa R, Chen MH, et al. (2010) Clinical and genetic correlates of circulating angiopoietin-2 and soluble Tie-2 in the community. Circ Cardiovasc Genet 3: 300–306.

32. London GM, Marchais SJ, Guerin AP, Metivier F, Adda H (2002) Arterial structure and function in end-stage renal disease. Nephrol Dial Transplant 17: 1713–1724.

33. Davis S, Papadopoulos N, Aldrich TH, Maisonpierre PC, Huang T, et al. (2003) Angiopoietins have distinct modular domains essential for receptor binding dimerization and superclustering. Nat Struct Biol 10: 38–44.

34. Lim HS, Lip GY, Blann AD (2005) Angiopoietin-1 and angiopoietin-2 in diabetes mellitus: relationship to VEGF, glycaemic control, endothelial damage/dysfunction and atherosclerosis. Atherosclerosis 180: 113–118.

35. Li JJ, Huang YQ, Basch R, Karpatkin S (2001) Thrombin induces the release of angiopoietin-1 from platelets. Thromb Haemost 85: 204–206.

36. Lukasz A, Hellpap J, Horn R, Kielstein JT, David S, et al. (2008) Circulating angiopoietin-1 and angiopoietin-2 in critically ill patients: development and clinical application of two new immunoassays. Crit Care 12: R94.

37. Di Marco GS, Reuter S, Hillebrand U, Amler S, König M, et al. (2009) The soluble VEGF receptor sFlt1 contributes to endothelial dysfunction in CKD. J Am Soc Nephrol 20: 2235–2245.

38. Futrakul N, Butthep P, Laohareungpanya N, Chaisuriya P, Ratanabanangkoon K (2008) A defective angiogenesis in chronic kidney disease. Ren Fail 30: 215–217.

39. Lilien MR, Koomans HA, Schröder CH (2005) Hemodialysis acutely impairs endothelial function in children. Pediatr Nephrol 20: 200–204.

40. Goldstein SL, Leung JC, Silverstein DM (2006) Pro- and anti- inflammatory cytokines in chronic pediatric dialysis patients: effect of aspirin. Clin J Am Soc Nephrol 1: 979–986.

41. Long DA, Price KL, Ioffe E, Gannon CM, Gnudi L, et al. (2008) Angiopoietin-1 therapy enhances fibrosis and inflammation following folic acid-induced acute renal injury. Kidney Int 74: 300–309.

42. Murdoch C, Tazzyman S, Webster S, Lewis CE (2007) Expression of Tie-2 by human monocytes and their responses to angiopoietin-2. J Immunol 178: 7405–7411.

43. Yuan HT, Suri C, Landon DN, Yancopoulos GD, Woolf AS (2000) Angiopoietin-2 is a site-specific factor in differentiation of mouse renal vasculature. J Am Soc Nephrol 11: 1055–1066.

44. Lee SW, Moskowitz MA, Sims JR (2007) Sonic hedgehog inversely regulates the expression of angiopoietin-1 and angiopoietin-2 in fibroblasts. Int J Mol Med 19: 445–451.

45. Phelps ED, Updike DL, Bullen EC, Grammas P, Howard EW (2006) Transcriptional and posttranscriptional regulation of angiopoietin-2 expression mediated by IGF and PDGF in vascular smooth muscle cells. Am J Physiol Cell Physiol 290: C352–C361.

46. Hubbard NE, Lim D, Mukutmoni M, Cai A, Erickson KL (2005) Expression and regulation of murine macrophage angiopoietin-2. Cell Immunol 234: 102–109.

47. Korff T, Ernst E, Nobiling R, Feldner A, Reiss Y, et al. (2012) Angiopoietin-1 mediates inhibition of hypertension-induced release of angiopoietin-2 from endothelial cells. Cardiovasc Res 94: 510–518.

48. Otani A, Takagi H, Oh H, Koyama S, Honda Y (2001) Angiotensin II induces expression of the Tie2 receptor ligand, angiopoietin-2, in bovine retinal endothelial cells. Diabetes 50: 867–875.

49. Nakayama T, Sato W, Yoshimura A, Zhang L, Kosugi T, et al. (2010) Endothelial von Willebrand factor release due to eNOS deficiency predisposes to thrombotic microangiopathy in mouse aging kidney. Am J Pathol 176: 2198–2208.

50. Matsunaga N, Tsuchimori N, Matsumoto T, Ii M (2011) TAK-242 (resatorvid), a small-molecule inhibitor of Toll-like receptor (TLR) 4 signaling, binds selectively to TLR4 and interferes with interactions between TLR4 and its adaptor molecules. Mol Pharmacol 79: 34–41.

51. Yu MA, Sanchez-Lozada LG, Johnson RJ, Kang DH (2010) Oxidative stress with an activation of the renin-angiotensin system in human vascular endothelial cells as a novel mechanism of uric acid-induced endothelial dysfunction. J Hypertens 28: 1234–1242.

52. Feig DI, Kang DH, Johnson RJ (2008) Uric acid and cardiovascular risk. N Engl J Med 359: 1811–1821.

53. Silverstein DM, Srivaths PR, Mattison P, Upadhyay K, Midgley L, et al. (2011) Serum uric acid is associated with high blood pressure in pediatric hemodialysis patients. Pediatr Nephrol 26: 1123–1128.

23

An Assessment of Survival among Korean Elderly Patients Initiating Dialysis

Shina Lee[1]ꝯ, Jung-Hwa Ryu[1]ꝯ, Hyunwook Kim[2], Kyoung Hoon Kim[3], Hyeong Sik Ahn[4], Hoo Jae Hann[5], Yongjae Cho[5], Young Mi Park[5], Seung-Jung Kim[1], Duk-Hee Kang[1], Kyu Bok Choi[1], Dong-Ryeol Ryu[1]*

1 Department of Internal Medicine, School of Medicine, Ewha Womans University, Seoul, Korea, **2** Department of Internal Medicine, Wonkwang University College of Medicine Sanbon Hospital, Gunpo, Korea, **3** Department of Public Health, Graduate School, Korea University, Seoul, Korea, **4** Department of Preventive Medicine, College of Medicine, Korea University, Seoul, Korea, **5** Ewha Medical Research Institute, School of Medicine, Ewha Womans University, Seoul, Korea

Abstract

Background: Although the proportion of the elderly patients with incident end-stage renal disease (ESRD) patients has been increasing in Korea, there has been a lack of information on outcomes of dialysis treatment. This study aimed to assess the survival rate and to elucidate predictors for all-cause mortality among elderly Korean patients initiating dialysis.

Methods: We analyzed 11,301 patients (6,138 men) aged 65 years or older who had initiated dialysis from 2005 to 2008 and had followed up (median, 37.8 months; range, 3–84 months). Baseline demographics, comorbidities and mortality data were obtained using the database from the Health Insurance Review & Assessment Service.

Results: The unadjusted 5-year survival rate was 37.6% for all elderly dialysis patients, and the rate decreased with increasing age categories; 45.9% (65~69), 37.5% (70~74), 28.4% (75~79), 24.1% (80~84), and 13.7% (≥85 years). The multivariate Cox proportional hazard model revealed that age, sex, dialysis modality, the type of insurance, and comorbidities such as diabetes mellitus, myocardial infarction, congestive heart failure, peripheral vascular disease, cerebrovascular disease, dementia, chronic pulmonary disease, hemiparesis, liver disease, and any malignancy were independent predictors for mortality. In addition, survival rate was significantly higher in patients on hemodialysis compared to patients on peritoneal dialysis during the whole follow-up period in the intention-to-treat analysis.

Conclusions: Survival rate was significantly associated with age, sex, and various comorbidities in Korean elderly patients initiating dialysis. The results of our study can help to provide relevant guidance on the individualization strategy in elderly ESRD patients requiring dialysis.

Editor: Ramon Andrade de Mello, Department of Medicine and Biomedical Sciences, University of Algarve, Portugal

Funding: This study was supported by a 2011 grant from the Korean Academy of Medical Sciences; and by the Ewha Global Top5 Grant of Ewha Womans University. The funders had no role in study design, data collection and analysis, decision to publish, or preparation of the manuscript.

Competing Interests: The authors have declared that no competing interest exist.

* E-mail: drryu@ewha.ac.kr

ꝯ These authors contributed equally to this work.

Introduction

The incidence of dialysis in elderly patients with end-stage renal disease (ESRD) has been growing throughout the world [1]. The US Renal Data System revealed that the majority of patients initiating dialysis were 65 years or older at the time of their first treatment and also indicated that the rapid growing portion was the population aged over 75 years [2]. However, elderly patients are thought to represent a different proportion across countries as shown in the results from the Dialysis Outcomes and Practice Patterns Study (DOPPS) [3].

According to the 2010 annual report from the Korean nationwide registry program, the incidence and the prevalence of the patients undergoing renal replacement therapy were 181.5 and 1,144.4 per million population, respectively [4], which are less

than those reported in epidemiology studies form Taiwan, the United States, or Japan [2]. However, the annual increase in the prevalence has been about 12% during the past decade in Korea [5]. Meanwhile, peak age of patients undergoing dialysis therapy was shifted to older populations, with mean age increasing from 55.2 in 2005 to 58.0 in 2010 [4]. In addition, the percentage of dialysis patients over 65 years had increased to more than 35.0% of overall dialysis population in 2010 [4].

Despite the increasing incidence of elderly ESRD patients initiating dialysis in Korea, there has been a lack of reports regarding outcomes for this population. Moreover, there are many controversies regarding the appropriateness of dialysis initiation in elderly ESRD patients, because age is the most important risk factor for death in the general elderly population and because most elderly ESRD patients have many comorbid conditions affecting

Table 1. Baseline characteristics.

Age categories	65~69 (N = 4,491)		70~74 (N = 3,591)		75~79 (N = 2,102)		80~84 (N = 849)		85~ (N = 268)		Total (N = 11,301)		P-value*
Vintage													0.0000
2005	1,101	(24.5)	755	(21.0)	440	(20.9)	176	(20.7)	45	(16.8)	2,517	(22.3)	–
2006	1,055	(23.5)	872	(24.3)	501	(23.8)	200	(23.6)	54	(20.1)	2,682	(23.7)	–
2007	1,115	(24.8)	953	(26.5)	519	(24.7)	209	(24.6)	74	(27.6)	2,870	(25.4)	–
2008	1,220	(27.2)	1,011	(28.2)	642	(30.5)	264	(31.1)	95	(35.4)	3,232	(28.6)	–
Male	2,559	(57.0)	1,977	(55.1)	1,043	(49.6)	419	(49.4)	140	(52.2)	6,138	(54.3)	0.0000
Dialysis modality (ITT)													0.0000
Peritoneal dialysis	976	(21.7)	657	(18.3)	332	(15.8)	122	(14.4)	28	(10.4)	2,115	(18.7)	–
Hemodialysis	3,515	(78.3)	2,934	(81.7)	1,770	(84.2)	727	(85.6)	240	(89.6)	9,186	(81.3)	–
Health security system													0.0499
National Health Insurance	4,026	(89.6)	3,228	(89.9)	1,872	(89.1)	744	(87.6)	228	(85.1)	10,098	(89.4)	–
Medical Aid	465	(10.4)	363	(10.1)	230	(10.9)	105	(12.4)	40	(14.9)	1,203	(10.6)	–
Comorbidities													
Diabetes mellitus	2,769	(61.7)	2,021	(56.3)	1,031	(49.0)	353	(41.6)	90	(33.6)	6,264	(55.4)	0.0000
Myocardial infarction	230	(5.1)	220	(6.1)	135	(6.4)	44	(5.2)	14	(5.2)	643	(5.7)	0.1587
Congestive heart failure	775	(17.3)	672	(18.7)	463	(22.0)	183	(21.6)	65	(24.3)	2,158	(19.1)	0.0000
Peripheral vascular disease	342	(7.6)	302	(8.4)	201	(9.6)	72	(8.5)	21	(7.8)	938)	(8.3	0.4549
Cerebrovascular disease	816	(18.2)	674	(18.8)	414	(19.7)	166	(19.6)	57	(21.3)	2,127	(18.8)	0.4549
Dementia	79	(1.8)	102	(2.8)	100	(4.8)	50	(5.9)	20	(7.5)	351	(3.1)	0.0000
Chronic pulmonary disease	877	(19.5)	810	(22.6)	545	(25.9)	209	(24.6)	70	(26.1)	2,511	(22.2)	0.0000
Connective tissue disease	141	(3.1)	105	(2.9)	73	(3.5)	29	(3.4)	9	(3.4)	357	(3.2)	0.8180
Peptic ulcer disease	726	(16.2)	637	(17.7)	383	(18.2)	141	(16.6)	41	(15.3)	1,928	(17.1)	0.1699
Hemiparesis	92	(2.0)	77	(2.1)	42	(2.0)	14	(1.6)	4	(1.5)	229	(2.0)	0.8673
Liver disease	424	(9.4)	312	(8.7)	171	(8.1)	65	(7.7)	17	(6.3)	989	(8.8)	0.1405
Any cancer	341	(7.6)	309	(8.6)	195	(9.3)	73	(8.6)	18	(6.7)	936	(8.3)	0.1351
Modified CCI													0.2483
0~1	1,463	(32.6)	1,142	(31.8)	675	(32.1)	290	(34.2)	90	(33.6)	3,660	(32.4)	–
2~3	1,589	(35.4)	1,246	(34.7)	722	(34.3)	310	(36.5)	104	(38.8)	3,971	(35.1)	–
≥4	1,439	(32.0)	1,203	(33.5)	705	(33.5)	249	(29.3)	74	(27.6)	3,670	(32.5)	–

*Statistical differences according to age group were calculated in χ^2 test.
ITT, intention-to-treat; CCI, Charlson comorbidity index.

mortality, such as dementia, disability, and various cardiovascular diseases [1,6,7].

Median survival after dialysis initiation was reported to be only 24.9 months among patients aged 80 or more in the United States [1]. In addition, a recent French study showed that median survival among patients aged 75 years or more had improved from 1.6 years in a 2002–2004 cohort to 2.6 years in a 2005–2007 cohort [8]. However, these studies derived from a Western population. A substantial number of evidences have suggested that there are significant differences in the overall and cardiovascular mortalities in dialysis patients across racial and ethnic groups [9,10]. To date, however, no studies have been reported on the survival rate and the factors affecting mortality in Asian elderly ESRD patients.

In this study, we evaluated survival rate and elucidated predictors associated with the mortality among elderly Korean patients initiating dialysis.

Methods

Ethics Statement

This investigation was conducted according to the principles expressed in the Declaration of Helsinki. The institutional review board at the Korean Health Insurance Review and Assessment Service (HIRA) approved the survey of the study population (No. 3159, 2012).

Data Source and Study Population

All data used in the study was obtained from the database of Korean Health Insurance Review and Assessment Service

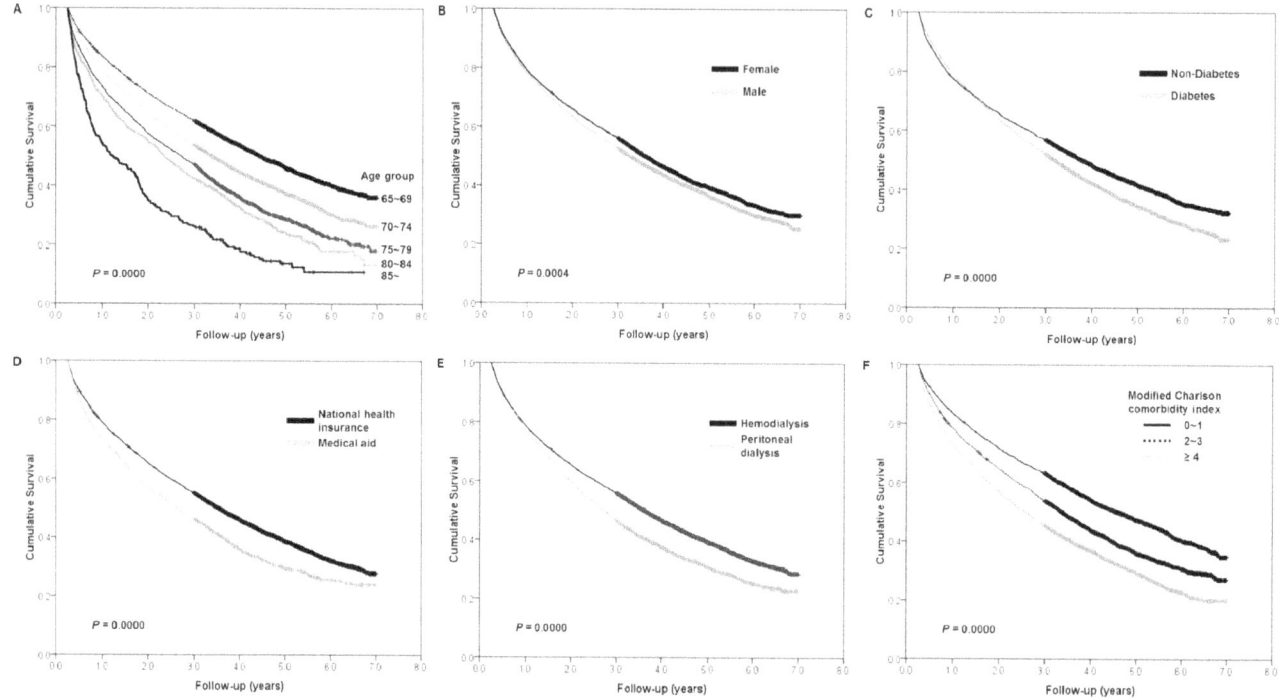

Figure 1. Kaplan-Meier survival curves and comparisons of survival rates by log-rank test. (A) Mortality rates gradually increased with the increment of age categories ($P = 0.0000$). (B) Females showed better survival rate compared to males ($P = 0.0004$). (C) Survival rate was better for patients without diabetes than that with diabetics ($P = 0.0000$). (D) Patients covered by National Health Insurance experienced higher better survival rate compared to Medical Aid beneficiaries ($P = 0.0000$). (E) Patients on hemodialysis experienced significant survival benefit over patients on peritoneal dialysis in the intention-to-treat analysis ($P = 0.0000$). (F) As the modified Charlson comorbidity index for end-stage renal disease patients increased, survival rates significantly decreased ($P = 0.0000$).

(HIRA). In South Korea, all citizens are obliged to join the National Health Security System, which is composed of National Health Insurance and Medical Aid, and is overseen by the Ministry of Health and Welfare.

All medical care expenses for dialysis are reimbursed by HIRA [11,12]. As such, we were able to identify every ESRD patient in the whole of South Korean population and analyzed the data for all ESRD patients who had started dialysis. We collected data such as unique de-identified number for each patient, age, sex, the type of insurance, list of diagnoses according to the International Classification of Diseases (ICD-10), and kidney transplantation. In addition, the end-point of time to death was confirmed by the Certificate Database (the recorded data of the reasons for changes in eligibility for National Health Insurance or Medical Aid, the death, or emigration) as well as through the National Health Insurance Claims Database.

The comorbidities of each subject were identified by screening the medical history data for the year leading up to the initiation of dialysis therapy. The list of analyzed comorbidities was determined based on suggestions from Charlson et al. [13], and patients were divided into 3 groups [grade $0{\sim}1$ (mild comorbidity), $2{\sim}3$ (moderate comorbidity), and ≥ 4 (severe comorbidity)] according to the modified Charlson Comorbidity Index for ESRD patients [14]. ICD-10 codes were used according to the proposed algorithms by Quan et al. [15].

We included data from patients aged 65 years or older who started hemodialysis (HD) or peritoneal dialysis (PD) between January 1, 2005 and December 31, 2008. Patients who survived

less than 90 days from the date of dialysis initiation were excluded, and the patients who underwent kidney transplantation or were not deceased until December 31, 2011 were censored.

For the comparison of survival rates between patients on HD and PD, we used both the intention-to-treat (ITT) and as-treated (AT) analyses. The patients were classified according to the treatment modality at the 90th day after commencement of dialysis in ITT analysis, or at the 60th day before death or censoring in the AT analysis.

Statistical Analysis

Statistical analysis was performed using SPSS software for Windows, version 15.0 (SPSS Inc., Chicago, IL, USA). All data were expressed as mean ± SD or number (%) unless otherwise specified. P-values <0.05 were considered statistically significant.

Baseline characteristics of ESRD patients according to age categories were compared using Pearson chi-square test for categorical variables. Kaplan-Meier survival curves were calculated, and the log-rank test was used for the comparison of unadjusted survival rates. In addition, we constructed life tables to estimate the cumulative proportion of survivors at the end of every 1-year-interval during the follow-up period. For delineating predictors for mortality, the Cox proportional hazard analysis was performed. Significant variables in univariate analyses were included for multivariate analysis, and a threshold was 0.10 for retention.

Table 2. Cumulative survival rate at each 1-year interval*.

Year	1	2	3	4	5	6	7
All	78.3	64.3	54.1	45.0	37.6	31.6	27.6
Sex							
Male	77.8	63.1	52.5	43.6	36.3	30.0	26.2
Female	78.9	65.8	56.0	46.5	39.2	33.5	29.3
Age groups							
65~69	83.5	71.2	61.8	53.4	45.9	40.0	35.7
70~74	78.6	64.3	53.5	44.5	37.5	30.9	26.4
75~79	73.1	57.3	47.1	35.9	28.4	22.3	18.4
80~84	70.1	54.7	42.2	33.1	24.1	18.4	15.1
85~	54.1	35.1	26.1	17.9	13.7	10.7	10.7
Dialysis modality (ITT)							
Hemodialysis	78.6	65.4	55.9	46.7	39.3	33.1	28.9
Peritoneal dialysis	76.9	59.7	46.5	37.5	30.5	25.2	22.1
Dialysis modality (AT)							
Hemodialysis	78.9	65.7	56.3	47.1	39.6	33.5	29.1
Peritoneal dialysis	75.1	57.5	43.6	34.4	28.3	22.8	20.3
Diabetes mellitus							
No	77.4	65.4	56.8	48.3	41.5	35.3	32.2
Yes	79.0	63.4	51.9	42.3	34.4	28.5	23.6
Modified CCI							
0~1	83.4	71.5	63.2	54.1	47.2	40.6	35.4
2~3	78.5	64.5	53.7	43.9	36.2	31.0	27.7
≥4	73.0	56.9	45.5	36.9	29.5	22.8	19.0

*All data are presented as percent (%).
ITT, intention-to-treat; AT, as-treated; CCI, Charlson comorbidity index.

Results

Baseline Characteristics

In total, 11,301 patients were included in this study. The number of elderly patients starting dialysis had increased from 2,517 in 2005 to 3,232 in 2008. The demographic characteristics are summarized in Table 1.

The mean age was 71.9±5.4 years (range, 65–96 years), and 6,138 (54.3%) were male. The median of follow-up duration was 37.8 months (range of 3–84 months). Patients were divided into 5 categories of age (65~69, 70~74, 75~79, 80~84, and 85 years or older), with 4,491 (39.7%), 3,591 (31.8%), 2,102 (18.6%), 849 (7.5%), and 268 (2.4%) patients in each group, respectively.

In the ITT analysis, 9,186 (81.3%) and 2,115 (18.7%) were managed with HD or PD at the 90th day after commencement of dialysis, respectively. The number of patients covered by National Health Insurance and Medical Aid was 10,098 (89.4%) and 1,203 (10.6%), respectively. During the follow-up period, 9 patients (0.1%) underwent kidney transplantation.

The number and proportion of patients with comorbid diseases diagnosed before or at the time of dialysis initiation are also described in Table 1.

The Survival Rates in Korean Elderly Patients Initiating Dialysis

Kaplan-Meier survival curves according to age categories, sex, diabetes mellitus, the type of insurance, dialysis modality, and the modified Charlson comorbidity index are shown in Figure 1, which were compared by the log-rank test. The unadjusted survival rates were described in Table 2.

The survival rates gradually decreased with increasing age; median survival was 53.1 months for the age group of 65~69 year, 40.6 months for 70~74 year, 32.6 months for 75~79 year, 28.0 months for 80~84 year, and 14.3 months for the age group over 85 years. The survival rate was decreased with increasing age groups (Figure 1A, $P=0.0000$). The unadjusted 5-year survival rate was 37.6% for all elderly dialysis patients, and the rate decreased with increasing age categories; 45.9% (65~69), 37.5% (70~74), 28.4% (75~79), 24.1% (80~84), and 13.7% (≥85 years) (Table 2).

The survival rate of female patients was significantly higher than that of male (Figure 1B, $P=0.0004$). Diabetes significantly affected on the survival outcomes (Figure 1C, $P=0.0000$). The type of insurance was also associated with the survival rate, which was higher for National Health Insurance subscribers than for Medical Aid beneficiaries (Figure 1D, $P=0.0000$). In the ITT analysis, survival was better for HD patients than for PD patients at all points along the follow-up period (5-year survival rates; 39.3% in the HD patients vs. 30.5% in the PD patients) (Figure 1E, $P=0.0000$), and the difference in survival rates remained in AT analysis (5-year survival rates; 39.6% in the HD patients vs. 28.3% in the PD patients). Furthermore, survival rates were gradually decreased with increasing the modified Charlson comorbidity index (Figure 1F, $P=0.0000$). The 5-year survival rate of patients with mild comorbidity (grade 0~1) was 47.2%, while it was significantly lower at 29.5% for patients with severe comorbidity (grade ≥4) (Table 2).

Predictors for All-cause Mortality

For the analysis of independent risk factors associated with all-cause mortality, the multivariate Cox proportional hazards analysis was performed with significant variables from univariate analyses (Table 3).

Age, female, Medical Aid, HD as an initial dialysis modality, comorbidities such as diabetes mellitus, myocardial infarction, congestive heart failure, peripheral vascular disease, cerebrovascular disease, dementia, chronic pulmonary disease, hemiparesis, liver disease, and any malignancy were significant independent predictors for mortality.

Furthermore, we compared hazard ratios of all independent predictors for mortality in the multivariate Cox analysis according to the age categories (Figure 2). For the simplicity in comparison, patients were divided into 3 categories of age (65~69, 70~79, and 80 years or older), with 4,491 (39.7%), 5,693 (50.4%), and 1,117 (9.9%) patients in each group, respectively. Age, peripheral vascular disease, and hemiparesis were the factors by which mortality risk gradually increased with increasing age groups. However, the influences of Medical Aid, peritoneal dialysis, diabetes mellitus, congestive heart failure, liver disease, and any malignancy on the mortality sequentially decreased with aging.

Discussion

In this study, we evaluated survival rates among elderly Korean ESRD patients initiating dialysis. More than 60% of elderly patients had survived for 2 years after initiation of dialysis. Even among the very elderly patients, the median survival was 28.0 months for patients 80~84 years of age; 14.3 months for patients 85~89 years of age; and 13.2 months for patients 90 years of age or older, respectively. The elderly dialysis patients in this study experienced a lower death rate when compared to that reported in

Table 3. Results of the Cox proportional hazards analysis for all-cause mortality.

	Univariate			Multivariate*		
	HR	95% CI	P-value	HR	95% CI	P-value
Age (per 1-yr increase)	1.05	1.04–1.05	0.0000	1.05	1.04–1.05	0.0000
Female (vs. Male)	0.92	0.87–0.96	0.0004	0.91	0.87–0.96	0.0002
Medical Aid (vs. National Health Insurance)	1.27	1.18–1.37	0.0000	1.25	1.16–1.34	0.0000
Hemodialysis (vs. Peritoneal dialysis)[†]	0.81	0.76–0.85	0.0000	0.75	0.71–0.80	0.0000
Diabetes mellitus	1.17	1.11–1.22	0.0000	1.24	1.18–1.30	0.0000
Myocardial Infarction	1.39	1.26–1.53	0.0000	1.23	1.12–1.36	0.0000
Congestive heart failure	1.30	1.23–1.37	0.0000	1.21	1.14–1.28	0.0000
Peripheral vascular disease	1.19	1.09–1.29	0.0000	1.11	1.02–1.21	0.0142
Cerebrovascular disease	1.42	1.34–1.51	0.0000	1.34	1.26–1.42	0.0000
Dementia	1.64	1.45–1.86	0.0000	1.30	1.15–1.48	0.0000
Chronic pulmonary disease	1.15	1.09–1.21	0.0000	1.09	1.03–1.16	0.0017
Connective tissue disease	1.08	0.95–1.23	0.2571	–	–	–
Peptic ulcer disease	0.97	0.91–1.04	0.4181	–	–	–
Hemiparesis	1.42	1.22–1.65	0.0000	1.20	1.03–1.41	0.0228
Liver disease	1.09	1.00–1.18	0.0401	1.09	1.00–1.18	0.0427
Any malignancy	1.47	1.35–1.59	0.0000	1.48	1.36–1.60	0.0000

*All-cause mortality was adjusted for all parameters with <0.10 of P-value in the univariate analysis.
[†]Mortality rates between patients on hemodialysis and those on peritoneal dialysis were compared in the intention-to-treat analysis.
HR, hazard ratio; CI, confidence interval.

a previous study of US octogenarians and nonagenarians starting dialysis, in which median survival rate was 15.6 months for patients aged 80~84 year; 11.6 months for patients aged 85~89 year; and 8.4 months for patients aged 90 year or older [1]. Several studies have also reported that median survival of the patients older than 75 years was around 2 years after the first dialysis [16,17,18]. In addition, a UK study of dialysis patients aged 70 or older found that overall 1-yr survival was 71% [19], which is slightly different from the results of this study (74.8% of oveall survival rate at 1 year among patients aged 70 or older).

There has been a controversy regarding initiation of dialysis in very elderly patients. Although a randomized controlled study is the most reliable and informative method of comparing outcomes between conservative care and dialysis initiation, such a trial is difficult to perform due to ethical concerns. When standardized mortality ratios were calculated in comparison with the general population, the ratio for the dialysis patients decreased from 26.7 in the 18- to 44-year-old group to 3.5 in the ≥85-year-old group, which implicated that older ESRD patients experienced less excess mortality, and age per se is more important factors for mortality in the elderly than in the younger age group [6]. Moreover, elderly patients have various chronic medical diseases concurrently, which have profound effects on their survival [20]. Therefore, very elderly patients may not always be considered as suitable candidates for dialysis. In this study, age and various comorbidities were the main determinants for mortality, which is consistent with previous reports. However, we suggest that the benefit and risk of dialysis initiation should be weighed in each patient because survival rate for elderly ESRD patients is not dismal in Korea and because the individualization strategy using predictors for mortality is feasible.

Although life expectancy is usually greater for females than for males in the general population, sex has not been considered as a risk factor for death in ESRD patients [4,6,19]. In this study,

however, the survival rate of female was higher than that of male in Kaplan-Meier analysis, and female still conferred a relative survival benefit over male after adjustment for baseline variables. Because there was no distinct reason for the difference across the sex, we suggest that racial/ethnic difference could be taken into account.

In a previous report, diabetes was not an independent predictor for mortality in an older patient group [19], while it was a significant risk factor for mortality in the present study. In addition, myocardial infarction, cerebrovascular disease, or chronic obstructive pulmonary disease were also independent risk factors for mortality in our study. Diabetes could take more time to influence mortality rates compared to concomitant comorbidities such as various vascular diseases. Thus, aging per se may offset the effect of diabetes on mortality in the very elderly patients. In this study, patients between 65 and 69 accounted for 39.7% of the total participants. Therefore, it was assumed that these comorbidities still had a significant effect on mortality because life expectancy was long enough to be affected.

The National Health Security System of South Korea consists of National Health Insurance and Medical Aid, which respectively provide healthcare coverage for 96.3% and 3.7% of the whole population in 2006 [21]. The Medical Aid Program was established for low-income households, thus it roughly represented lower socioeconomic status in this study. Several studies have proved that low socioeconomic status was related with poor outcomes in patients with chronic kidney disease as well as patients on HD [22,23]. In accordance with these reports, mortality rate was significantly worse for the Medical Aid beneficiaries than for patients covered by National Health Insurance. This difference between insurance remained as a strong predictor for mortality even after adjustment for baseline covariates.

Although the debates continue on the choice of dialysis modality in elderly patients, HD is preferred over PD in many countries. In

	Age		HR (95% CI)	P-value
Age (per 1-yr increase)	65~69		1.03 (1.00-1.06)	0.0700
	70~79		1.05 (1.03-1.06)	0.0000
	80~		1.05 (1.03-1.08)	0.0000
Female (vs. Male)	65~69		0.91 (0.83-0.98)	0.0202
	70~79		0.93 (0.87-1.00)	0.0419
	80~		0.84 (0.73-0.96)	0.0131
Medical aid (vs. National health insurance)	65~69		1.53 (1.35-1.73)	0.0000
	70~79		1.20 (1.08-1.33)	0.0005
	80~		0.89 (0.72-1.09)	0.2632
Hemodialysis (vs. Peritoneal dialysis)*	65~69		0.71 (0.65-0.78)	0.0000
	70~79		0.76 (0.70-0.83)	0.0000
	80~		0.85 (0.70-1.03)	0.0983
Diabetes mellitus	65~69		1.41 (1.29-1.54)	0.0000
	70~79		1.22 (1.14-1.30)	0.0000
	80~		0.95 (0.83-1.10)	0.4932
Myocardial Infarction	65~69		1.21 (1.02-1.44)	0.0263
	70~79		1.28 (1.13-1.45)	0.0001
	80~		1.08 (0.80-1.45)	0.6166
Congestive heart failure	65~69		1.25 (1.13-1.38)	0.0000
	70~79		1.19 (1.10-1.29)	0.0000
	80~		1.18 (1.00-1.38)	0.0492
Peripheral vascular disease	65~69		1.02 (0.88-1.19)	0.7794
	70~79		1.11 (0.99-1.24)	0.0792
	80~		1.40 (1.10-1.79)	0.0056
Cerebrovascular disease	65~69		1.55 (1.40-1.71)	0.0000
	70~79		1.22 (1.12-1.32)	0.0000
	80~		1.37 (1.16-1.62)	0.0002
Dementia	65~69		1.33 (1.01-1.74)	0.0402
	70~79		1.41 (1.19-1.66)	0.0000
	80~		1.18 (0.89-1.57)	0.2370
Chronic pulmonary disease	65~69		1.15 (1.04-1.27)	0.0055
	70~79		1.04 (0.96-1.12)	0.3729
	80~		1.26 (1.07-1.47)	0.0044
Hemiparesis	65~69		0.98 (0.75-1.29)	0.9077
	70~79		1.24 (1.00-1.54)	0.0492
	80~		2.17 (1.34-3.52)	0.0016
Liver disease	65~69		1.26 (1.11-1.44)	0.0006
	70~79		1.05 (0.94-1.18)	0.4046
	80~		0.92 (0.70-1.20)	0.5272
Any malignancy	65~69		1.71 (1.49-1.97)	0.0000
	70~79		1.42 (1.27-1.58)	0.0000
	80~		1.27 (1.00-1.62)	0.0495

0   0.5   1.0   1.5   2.0

Figure 2. Comparision of hazard ratios of all independent predictors for mortality in the multivariate Cox analysis according to the age categories. Age, peripheral vascular disease, and hemiparesis were the factors by which mortality risk gradually increased with increasing age groups. However, the influences of Medical Aid, peritoneal dialysis, diabetes mellitus, congestive heart failure, liver disease, and any malignancy on the mortality sequentially decreased with aging. * Mortality rates between patients on hemodialysis and those on peritoneal dialysis were compared in the intention-to-treat analysis. HR, hazard ratio; CI, confidence interval.

our study, the use of HD was about 5 times greater than PD. HD patients experienced higher survival rate than PD patients during the follow-up period, and multivariate analysis revealed that the initial choice of HD had 25% survival benefit over PD. Previous studies have revealed that HD provided better survival outcomes than PD in elderly patients, especially after 180 days of dialysis initiation [23,24,25,26]. In addition, the registry data from Australia and New Zealand suggested that PD may be advantageous initially in younger patients (<60 years) without comorbidity [22]. The Dutch registry data noted survival advantage for PD in young non-diabetic patients [27]. These findings require more judicious approach in considering PD as an initial dialysis modality in elderly patients.

In this study, we accepted the chronological age of 65 years as a definition of 'the elderly'. However, the patients aged 65 years or older were thought to be wide-ranged and were likely to have different characteristics. In accordance with this assumption, there were significant differences in the independent predictors according to the age categories. Age *per se* and the factors affecting the degree of disability such as peripheral vascular disease or hemiparesis were more significant with increasing age groups. However, the influences of traditional risk factors such as socioeconomic status, dialysis modality, and comorbidities such as diabetes mellitus, congestive heart failure, liver disease, or any malignancy on the mortality sequentially decreased with aging.

As with other registry-based studies, this study also has limitations inherent to such study design. First, potential confounding factors for mortality were unavailable, such as data regarding residual renal function, critical laboratory results, biomarkers of inflammation or nutrition, and dialysis doses.

Second, we could not gather the cause of death for each individual. Finally, quality of life is as an important outcome variable as mortality rates in elderly patients, but this could not be evaluated in this study.

In spite of these limitations, our study has provided several clinically relevant points. Although there have been many reports on outcome in elderly ESRD patients, the findings from these studies could not be generalized to the populations outside of Western countries. Due to the large sample size that includes the entire population of dialysis patients with relatively long follow-up (up to 84 months) periods of this study, the results may be extrapolated to the current status of dialysis outcome in elderly Asian populations, albeit differences in policies or clinical practices do exist across the countries. In addition, Korean elderly ESRD patients were found to have distinctive predictors for mortality, such as sex, diabetes mellitus, and various comorbidities, which should be considered during decision-making for dialysis initiation.

Taken together, the findings suggest that survival outcomes in elderly patients initiating dialysis are different from those of previous reports, probably due to racial and ethnic differences. The results can help to provide relevant guidance on the individualization strategy in Asian elderly ESRD patients.

Author Contributions

Conceived and designed the experiments: SL JHR HSA HH SJK DHK KBC DRR. Analyzed the data: HK KHK YC YMP. Contributed reagents/materials/analysis tools: KHK HSA HH. Wrote the paper: SL JHR DRR.

References

1. Kurella M, Covinsky KE, Collins AJ, Chertow GM (2007) Octogenarians and nonagenarians starting dialysis in the United States. Ann Intern Med 146: 177–183.
2. U.S. Renal Data System (2012) Annual Data Report: Atlas of Chronic Kidney Disease and End-Stage Renal Disease in the United States. Available: http://www.usrds.org/atlas.aspx. Accessed 2 August 2013.
3. Canaud B, Tong L, Tentori F, Akiba T, Karaboyas A, et al. (2011) Clinical practices and outcomes in elderly hemodialysis patients: results from the Dialysis Outcomes and Practice Patterns Study (DOPPS). Clin J Am Soc Nephrol 6: 1651–1662.
4. Jin DC, Ha IS, Kim NH, Lee SW, Lee JS, et al. (2012) Brief Report: Renal replacement therapy in Korea, 2010. Kidney Res Clin Pract 31: 62–71.
5. Jin DC (2011) Current status of dialysis therapy in Korea. Korean J Intern Med 26: 123–131.
6. Villar E, Remontet L, Labeeuw M, Ecochard R (2007) Effect of age, gender, and diabetes on excess death in end-stage renal failure. J Am Soc Nephrol 18: 2125–2134.
7. Murtagh FE, Marsh JE, Donohoe P, Ekbal NJ, Sheerin NS, et al. (2007) Dialysis or not? A comparative survival study of patients over 75 years with chronic kidney disease stage 5. Nephrol Dial Transplant 22: 1955–1962.
8. Glaudet F, Hottelart C, Allard J, Allot V, Bocquentin F, et al. (2013) The clinical status and survival in elderly dialysis: example of the oldest region of France. BMC Nephrol 14: 131.
9. Yoshino M, Kuhlmann MK, Kotanko P, Greenwood RN, Pisoni RL, et al. (2006) International differences in dialysis mortality reflect background general population atherosclerotic cardiovascular mortality. J Am Soc Nephrol 17: 3510–3519.
10. Held PJ, Brunner F, Odaka M, Garcia JR, Port FK, et al. (1990) Five-year survival for end-stage renal disease patients in the United States, Europe, and Japan, 1982 to 1987. Am J Kidney Dis 15: 451–457.
11. Jeong HS (2011) Korea's National Health Insurance–lessons from the past three decades. Health Aff (Millwood) 30: 136–144.
12. Kwon S (2009) Thirty years of national health insurance in South Korea: lessons for achieving universal health care coverage. Health Policy Plan 24: 63–71.
13. Charlson ME, Pompei P, Ales KL, MacKenzie CR (1987) A new method of classifying prognostic comorbidity in longitudinal studies: development and validation. J Chronic Dis 40: 373–383.
14. Hemmelgarn BR, Manns BJ, Quan H, Ghali WA (2003) Adapting the Charlson Comorbidity Index for use in patients with ESRD. Am J Kidney Dis 42: 125–132.
15. Quan H, Sundararajan V, Halfon P, Fong A, Burnand B, et al. (2005) Coding algorithms for defining comorbidities in ICD-9-CM and ICD-10 administrative data. Med Care 43: 1130–1139.
16. Jager KJ, van Dijk PC, Dekker FW, Stengel B, Simpson K, et al. (2003) The epidemic of aging in renal replacement therapy: an update on elderly patients and their outcomes. Clin Nephrol 60: 352–360.
17. Letourneau I, Ouimet D, Dumont M, Pichette V, Leblanc M (2003) Renal replacement in end-stage renal disease patients over 75 years old. Am J Nephrol 23: 71–77.
18. Munshi SK, Vijayakumar N, Taub NA, Bhullar H, Lo TC, et al. (2001) Outcome of renal replacement therapy in the very elderly. Nephrol Dial Transplant 16: 128–133.
19. Lamping DL, Constantinovici N, Roderick P, Normand C, Henderson L, et al. (2000) Clinical outcomes, quality of life, and costs in the North Thames Dialysis Study of elderly people on dialysis: a prospective cohort study. Lancet 356: 1543–1550.
20. Jassal SV, Trpeski L, Zhu N, Fenton S, Hemmelgarn B (2007) Changes in survival among elderly patients initiating dialysis from 1990 to 1999. CMAJ 177: 1033–1038.
21. Song YJ (2009) The South Korean health care system. JMAJ 52: 206–209.
22. McDonald SP, Marshall MR, Johnson DW, Polkinghorne KR (2009) Relationship between Dialysis Modality and Mortality. J Am Soc Nephrol 20: 155–163.

24

The Associations of Uric Acid, Cardiovascular and All-Cause Mortality in Peritoneal Dialysis Patients

Jie Dong[1]*, Qing-Feng Han[2], Tong-Ying Zhu[3], Ye-Ping Ren[4], Jiang-Hua Chen[5], Hui-Ping Zhao[6], Meng-Hua Chen[7], Rong Xu[1], Yue Wang[2], Chuan-Ming Hao[3], Rui Zhang[4], Xiao-Hui Zhang[5], Mei Wang[6], Na Tian[7], Hai-Yan Wang[1]

1 Renal Division, Department of Medicine, Peking University First Hospital; Institute of Nephrology, Peking University; Key Laboratory of Renal Disease, Ministry of Health; Key Laboratory of Renal Disease, Ministry of Education; Beijing, China, 2 Department of Nephrology, Peking University Third Hospital, Beijing, China, 3 Department of Nephrology, Huashan Hospital of Fudan University, Shanghai, China, 4 Department of Nephrology, Second Affiliated Hospital of Harbin Medical University, Heilongjiang, China, 5 Kidney Disease Center, The First Affiliated Hospital, College of Medicine, Zhejiang University, Hangzhou, China, 6 Department of Nephrology, Peking University People's Hospital, Beijing, China, 7 Department of Nephrology, General Hospital of Ningxia Medical University, Ningxia, China

Abstract

Aims: To investigate whether uric acid (UA) is an independent predictor of cardiovascular (CV) and all-cause mortality in peritoneal dialysis (PD) patients after controlling for recognized CV risk factors.

Methods: A total of 2264 patients on chronic PD were collected from seven centers affiliated with the Socioeconomic Status on the Outcome of Peritoneal Dialysis (SSOP) Study. All demographic and laboratory data were recorded at baseline. Multivariate Cox regression was used to calculate the hazard ratio (HR) of CV and all-cause mortality with adjustments for recognized traditional and uremia-related CV factors.

Results: There were no significant differences in baseline characteristics between patients with (n = 2193) and without (n = 71) UA measured. Each 1 mg/dL of increase in UA was associated with higher all-cause mortality with 1.05(1.00~1.10) of HR and higher CV mortality with 1.12 (1.05~1.20) of HR after adjusting for age, gender and center size. The highest gender-specific tertile of UA predicted higher all-cause mortality with 1.23(1.00~1.52) of HR and higher CV mortality with 1.69 (1.21~2.38) of HR after adjusting for age, gender and center size. The predictive value of UA was stronger in patients younger than 65 years without CV disease or diabetes at baseline. The prognostic value of UA as both continuous and categorical variable weakened or disappeared after further adjusted for uremia-related and traditional CV risk factors.

Conclusions: The prognostic value of UA in CV and all-cause mortality was weak in PD patients generally, which was confounded by uremia-related and traditional CV risk factors.

Editor: Yan Li, Shanghai Institute of Hypertension, China

Funding: This study is supported in part by New Century Excellent Talents from The Education Department, China, Baxer Clinical Research Award from Baxter Corp, China, and an ISN Research Award from the ISN GO R&P Committee. The funders had no role in study design, data collection and analysis, decision to publish, or preparation of the manuscript.

Competing Interests: This study was partly funded by Baxter Corp and there are no patents, products in development or marketed products to declare. This does not alter adherence to all the PLOS ONE policies on sharing data and materials, as detailed online in the guide for authors.

* E-mail: dongjie@medmail.com.cn

Introduction

Increased cardiovascular (CV) events have been extensively documented in patients with end-stage renal disease (ESRD) including peritoneal dialysis (PD) and hemodialysis(HD) population [1,2]. CV events still accounts for approximately 40% of the annual mortality in dialysis patients [3]. Although numerous risk factors, categorized into traditional, uremic-related and non-traditional factors, have been recognized in recent years [4,5], series of meta-analysis have not been able to demonstrate significant effect of targeting some of factors such as hyperlipidemia [6], hyperhomocystinemia [7], oxidative stress [8] and hyperphosphatemia [9] on outcomes in this high-risk patient group. Exploring novel and potentially modifiable risk factors for CV and all-cause mortality is therefore urgent.

Uric acid (UA), as one of novel risk factors, has been paid more attention in recent years. In general population, previous studies have shown that UA is closely associated with hypertension, coronary heart disease and chronic kidney disease (CKD) [10–12]. High UA also could independently predict CV events and mortality for ones with chronic diseases including CKD [13–15]. For dialysis population, a few studies from HD population indicated inconsistent relationship between UA and outcomes, that is, UA is negatively or 'J-shaped' related to all-cause or CV mortality [16–19]. There is no specific data on UA and outcomes for PD population yet.

In the present study, we aimed to explore associations of UA, all-cause and CV mortality in a large-scale multi-center PD cohort. The prognostic value of UA would be compared between patients≥65 years and <65years, with or without CV disease

(CVD), diabetes and non-diabetes at baseline respectively. In addition, we determined whether associations of UA and outcomes would be changed after controlling for uremic-related factors(albumin, hemoglobin, residual renal function, phosphate etc) and traditional CV risk factors (hypertension, hyperlipidemia, obesity, diabetes, etc).

Methods

This is an affiliated study with the Socioeconomic Status on the Outcome of Peritoneal Dialysis (SSOP) Study, which is a retrospective multi-center cohort study as described in detail in our previous paper [20]. The ethics committee of Peking University First Hospital approved this study.

Centers enrollment

Centers which have professional PD doctors and PD nurses, and have well-developed databases of at least 3-years duration, recording baseline characteristics and follow-up data every 1~3 months for each patient in our country participated this study voluntarily. Totally 9 centers were qualified, and 7 of them agreed to participate providing about 70 percent of all incident patients from 9 centers. Enrolled centers were from 5 provinces and located at 4 geographical regions (north, northeast, northwest, or east) in China. Data from each center have been collected within the strict quality control framework and further inspected and optimized to keep integrity and accuracy of the database. All study investigators and staff members completed a training program that taught them the methods and processes of the study. A manual of detailed instructions for data collection was distributed.

Subjects selection

All the incident patients on chronic PD between the date of intact database creation and August 2011 were enrolled into this study. Each patient signed informed consent to agree their demographic and lab data to be used in future studies since they started PD therapy. All subjects began the PD program within one month after catheter implantation and were given lactate-buffered glucose dialysate with a twin-bag connection system (Baxter Healthcare, Guangzhou, China).

Data collection

Demographic and clinical data including age, gender, body mass index (BMI), socioeconomic status (income and education level, living condition, etc), primary renal disease, the presence of cardiovascular disease (CVD) and diabetes mellitus (DM) were collected at baseline. Center size was also recorded according to number of enrolled patients of each center. CVD was recorded if one of the following conditions was present: angina, class III–IV congestive heart failure (NYHA), trandient ischemic attack, history of myocardial infarction or cerebrovascular accident and peripheral arterial disease [21].

Blood pressures were measured according to the guidelines presented in the Seventh Report of the Joint National Committee on Prevention, Detection, Evaluation and Treatment of High Blood pressure [22]. Patients took antihypertensive medications and performed the bag exchange as usual at their home on the morning of each clinic visit. A skilled nurse using a mercury sphygmomanometer measured brachial blood pressure in sitting position after they had rested for at least 10 minutes in a quiet and peaceful room. Systolic and diastolic blood pressure, and calculated mean arterial pressure during the first 3 months were averaged for at least three times of readings.

Biochemistry data including hemoglobin, serum albumin, UA, lipids spectrum, glucose, calcium, phosphate and intact parathyroid hormone (iPTH) were examined using an automatic Hitachi chemistry analyzer. The first testing was completed within one month of PD at the first visit, and then repeatedly once a month. The mean values in the first 3 months were calculated. The coefficient of variation of UA from multiple measurements was 5.3% for subjects from Peking University First Hospital but not recorded for those from other hospitals. Serum UA was measured by the uricase method using the same autoanalyzer. Serum high sensitive C-reactive protein (CRP) was measured by immune rate nephelometric analysis. Dialysis adequacy and residual renal function (RRF) were measured after one month of dialysis therapy. RRF was defined as the mean of residual creatinine clearance and residual urea clearance. Dialysis adequacy was defined as total Kt/V and total creatinine clearance. Corrected calcium was calculated by standard equation: Corrected calcium = serum total calcium+0.02*(40-serum albumin in g/L).

Definition of outcome event

The outcomes were defined as cardiovascular and all-cause death. The cardiovascular death was defined as death due to myocardial infarction, congestive heart failure, cerebral bleeding, cerebral infarction, arrhythmia, peripheral arterial disease, and sudden death. In all analysis, we censored follow-up at trandferring to HD, loss to follow-up, renal trandplantation, or the end of the study (November 1, 2011).

Statistical analysis

Continuous data were presented as mean with SDs except for CRP and RRF, which were presented as median (interquartile range) because of a high skew. Categorical variables were presented as proportions. Patients' data were compared by using the t-test or ANOVA F-test for normally distributed continuous variables, chi-square test for categorical variables, and Mann-Whitney U test for skewed continuous variables. UA was trandformed into categorical variable by gender-specific tertiles or quartiles.

For determining associations of UA, CV and all-cause mortality, UA as continuous variable was first examined in Cox regression models after adjusting for age, gender and center size (model 1) for all participants, and then in subgroups such as patients≥65 years or <65 years, with or without CVD, with or without DM respectively. Next, we explored whether associations of UA and CV/all-cause mortality in all participants were confounded by traditional and uremia-related CVD factors. Uremia-related factors such as serum albumin, hemoglobin, phosphate, RRF and CRP (model 2), and additional traditional CV factors such as BMI, the history of diabetes or CVD, mean arterial pressure and LDL cholesterol(model 3) were constructed respectively. For these examinations, UA was also considered as categorical variable by gender-specific tertiles or quartiles respectively but only gender-specific tertiles of UA was shown in the context since similar linear trends were indicated. Gender was not included as the adjusted variable if UA is examined as the gender-specific variable.

We reported the multivariable adjusted hazards ratios (HRs) with 95% CIs. All probabilities were two-tailed, and the level of significance was set at 0.05. Statistical analysis was performed by SPSS for Windows software version 13.0 (SPSS Inc., Chicago, IL).

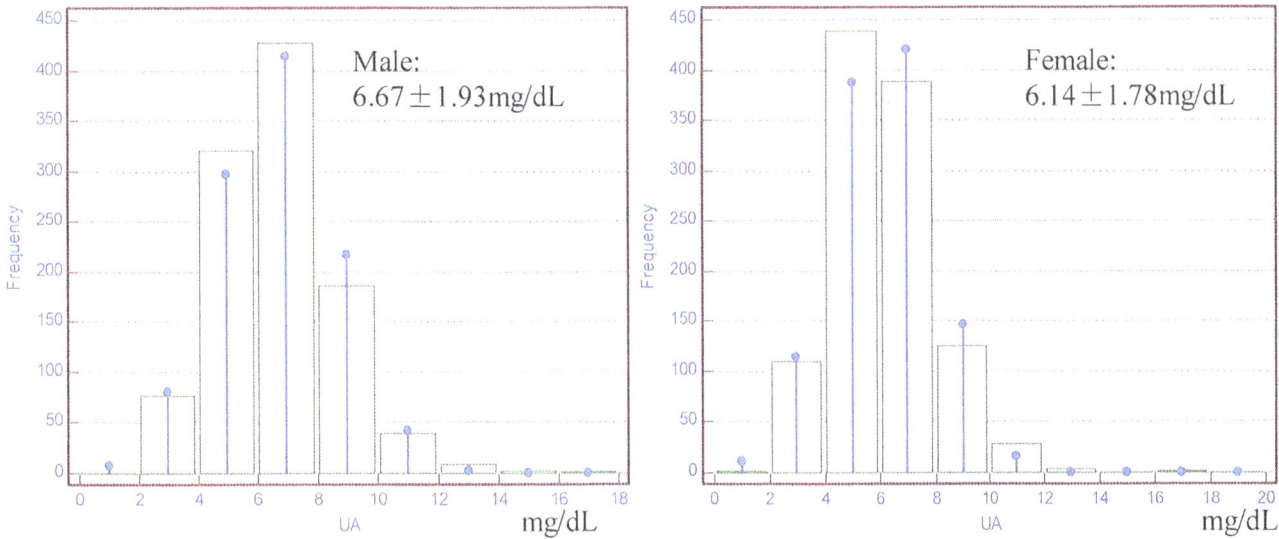

n=1078 for male, 1115 for female

Figure 1. The distribution chart of serum uric acid.

Results

Baseline characteristics and follow-up

A total of 2264 PD patients were collected, with a mean age of 58.1±15.5 years, BMI of 22.9±3.6 kg/m², 37.7% were diabetic and CVD was present in 41.5% of subjects at baseline. Chronic glomerulonephritis was the most common cause of ESRD (34.4%), followed by diabetic nephropathy (29.3%) and hypertensive nephropathy (15.5%). There were 71 of 2264 patients without UA values at baseline. The mean age, BMI, MBP, serum lipids, distribution of primary renal disease, CVD history, prevalence of DM were not significantly different between those who had measured UA and those who did not (2193 patients) (P>0.05). A total of 80 patients with inactive solid organ tumors at baseline were not excluded since their UA values were comparable to the remainders, and linear trends of UA and outcomes were not changed when they were excluded. Thereafter, 2193 patients were included in the final analysis.

The median follow-up time was 26.5(13.6~43.6) months. At the end of study, of 586 (26.7% of 2193) patients who died, 231 cases (39.4%) were due to CVD, 140 cases (23.8%) were due to infection, and other causes of death included malignancy (11.9%), gastrointestinal bleeding (4.3%), severe malnutrition (4.8%), miscellaneous (5.1%), and undefined (10.6%). Of 231 patients who died from CVD, the leading cause was myocardial infarction (52 cases, 22.5%), followed by congestive heart failure (19.0%), cerebral bleeding (14.3%), cerebral infarction (12.9%), sudden death (9.5%), arrhythmia (4.8%), peripheral arterial disease (1.3%), and undefined causes (15.1%).

UA and clinic characteristics

The mean values of UA were 6.41±1.87 mg/dL for the whole cohort. The normal distribution of UA in male and female was shown respectively in **Fig. 1**. The clinical characteristics and biochemistry data of patients by gender-specific tertiles of UA were represented in **Table 1**. Patients with higher UA were more likely to be younger and obese. The prevalence of CVD was highest but diabetes was lowest in high tertile group. Systolic and diastolic blood pressure, serum albumin, urea nitrogen, creatinine, phosphate, and parathyroid hormone levels increased, but corrected calcium, hemoglobin and total Kt/V decreased in the middle/high tertiles. Serum CRP, triglycerides, total cholesterol, HDL and LDL cholesterol, total Ccr and RRF levels were not significantly different between groups (P>0.05).

The association between UA and outcome

The associations between UA and outcomes were analyzed. First, UA was examined as a continuous variable. Each 1 mg/dL of increase in UA was associated with higher all-cause mortality with 1.05(1.00~1.10) of HR(P=0.05) and higher CV mortality with 1.12 (1.05~1.20) of HR(P=0.001) after adjusting for age, gender and center size (**Tables 2 and 3**). We further divided patients into subgroups, i.e.age≥65 years and <65years, with and without CVD, DM and non-DM respectively. For CV mortality rather than all-cause mortality, the prognostic value of UA was significant in low-risk groups such as patients with age<65 years, without CVD or DM at baseline rather than in their counterpars respectively (**Figs. 2 and 3**). Next, UA was examined as categorical variable by gender-specific tertiles and quartiles (data not shown for the latter). The highest gender-specific tertile of UA predicted higher all-cause mortality with 1.23(1.00~1.52) of HR(P=0.04) and higher CV mortality with 1.69 (1.21~2.38) of HR(P=0.002) after adjusting for age, gender and center size compared to low tertile of UA. However, the associations of UA and CVD/all-cause mortality weakened after further adjusted for uremia-related factors including serum albumin, hemoglobin, phosphate, and CRP, and disappeared with additional adjustement for traditional CV factors such as CVD history, DM, body mass index, and LDL cholestrol (**Table 2 and 3**).

Table 1. Clinical characteristics and biochemistry data of patients by gender-specific tertiles of UA.

Variables	Tertile 1 M: 2.09~5.79 mg/dL FM: 1.74~5.37 mg/dL	Tertile 2 M: 5.80~7.38 mg/dL FM: 5.38~6.65 mg/dL	Tertile 3 M: 7.39~16.7 mg/dL FM: 6.66~8.08 mg/dL	P values$^{\&}$
N	731	731	731	—
Age, yrs	61.9±15.1***	57.7±15.4$^{\Delta\Delta\Delta}$	54.7±15.3$^{\#\#\#}$	<0.001
Male (%)	49.2	49	49.2	0.99
BMI, Kg/m^2	22.4±3.5***	23.3±3.6	23.1±3.7$^{\#\#\#}$	<0.001
Diabetes (%)	40.2	40.6$^{\Delta\Delta}$	32.8$^{\#\#}$	0.003
CVD history (%)	34.8**	42.7	46.6$^{\#\#\#}$	<0.001
Systolic blood pressure, mmHg	133.5±22.5**	137.8±18.9	138.7±16.5$^{\#\#\#}$	<0.001
Diastolic blood pressure, mmHg	78.4±12.9**	80.5±12.9	82.1±11.2$^{\#\#}$	<0.001
Triglycerides, mmol/L	1.84±1.28	1.94±1.29	1.87±1.08	0.23
Total cholesterol, mmol/L	4.92±1.27	4.97±1.28	4.82±1.23	0.08
HDL cholesterol, mmol/L	1.16±0.38	1.13±0.35	1.14±0.37	0.2
LDL cholesterol, mmol/L	2.71±0.89	2.71±0.96	2.69±0.93	0.97
Albumin, g/L	33.9±5.4***	35.6±5.1$^{\Delta\Delta}$	36.5±5.2$^{\#\#\#}$	<0.001
Hemoglogin, g/dL	103.6±19.5	104.2±18.6	101.7±19.8	0.04
UA, mg/dL	4.5±0.8***	6.3±0.5$^{\Delta\Delta\Delta}$	8.4±1.4$^{\#\#\#}$	<0.001
Urea nitrogen, mmol/L	17.7±6.3***	21.0±6.3$^{\Delta\Delta\Delta}$	23.1±7.1$^{\#\#\#}$	<0.001
Creatinine, umol/L	621.8±242.8***	695.0±246.9$^{\Delta\Delta\Delta}$	728.9±274.5$^{\#\#\#}$	<0.001
Corrected calcium, mmol/L	2.29±0.25	2.29±0.25$^{\Delta\Delta\Delta}$	2.25±0.24$^{\#\#\#}$	<0.001
Parathyroid hormone, pg/ml	157.8 (74.5, 318.9)	163.5(75.9, 314.8)$^{\Delta}$	196.8(91.8, 345.7)$^{\#}$	0.02
Phosphate, mmol/L	1.4±0.4***	1.6±0.4$^{\Delta\Delta\Delta}$	1.7±0.5$^{\#\#\#}$	<0.001
CRP, mg/L	3.1(1.2, 6.9)	2.6(1.0, 7.8)	2.8(1.0, 7.5)	0.32
Total Kt/V	2.19±0.65***	2.01±0.60	1.95±0.63$^{\#\#\#}$	<0.001
Total Ccr, L/w/1.73m2	76.2±30.9	73.5±33.6	73.3±30.3	0.23
RRF, ml/min	3.1(1.4, 5.2)	3.2(1.6, 5.2)	3.7(1.8, 5.8)	0.16

Abbreviations: M, male; FM, female; UA, uric acid; BMI, body mass index; CVD, cardiovascular disease; CRP, C-reactive protein; Ccr, creatinie clearance; RRF, residual renal function.
$^{\&}$P for comparisons among tertiles.
*P<0.05, **P<0.01, ***P<0.001 for Tertile 1 vs Tertile 2.
$^{\Delta}$P<0.05, $^{\Delta\Delta}$P<0.01, $^{\Delta\Delta\Delta}$P<0.001 for Tertile 2 vs Tertile 3.
$^{\#}$P<0.05, $^{\#\#}$P<0.01, $^{\#\#\#}$P<0.01 for Tertile 1 vs Tertile 3.

Discussion

In contrast to previous studies on HD patients showing a negative or 'J-shaped' relationship between UA and mortality [16–19], the present PD study did ont indicate similar trends between UA and CV or all-cause mortality. One may suspect that it is due to that the mean UA values in this cohort is quite different. This hypothesis is easily denied since the mean UA values(6.4 mg/dL) for our participants were very close to those reported in HD patients [16–19,23]. It was also hypothesized that the inverse association of UA and outcome previously reported is confounded by nutrition status as indicated from DOPPS data [19]. From our data, although serum UA was also closely associated with higher body mass index, serum albumin, creatinine, phosphorous and better residual renal function, we could not observe a similar trend to HD patients.

The inconsistent trend of UA and outcomes was more likely to be explained by its dual effects on CV outcomes. Excess UA is closely related to components of metabolic syndrome, endothelial dysfunction, inflammation, oxidative stress and activated renin-angiotensin-aldosterone system in general population and patients with CKD [16,24–29]. On the other hand, both in vitro and in vivo studies have shown UA to be a powerful free radical scavenger in humand and could be expected to offer a number of benefits within the cardiovascular system [30,31].Therefore, the final trend for the association of UA and outcomes for a specific population might depend on the balance between the protective and toxic effects of UA. In addition, hyperuricaemia is significantly associated with the rate of decline of RRF [32], and RRF play a critical role in predicting CV events and all-cause death in PD population [33], which might partly contribute to the weakly negative associations of hyperuricaemia and outcomes for our PD patients.

Another interesting finding from our data is that the prognostic value of UA in CV mortality only existed in relatively low-risk patients including ones younger than 65 years, without CVD or DM at the start of PD therapy. This phenomenon has been indicated in previous data. For example, UA levels at either

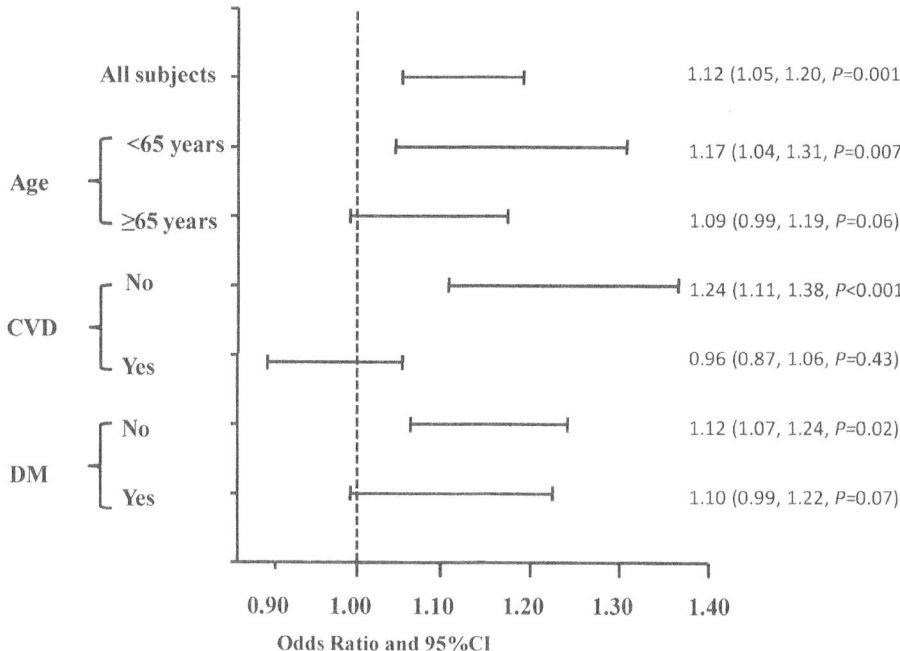

Figure 2. Risk of CVD mortality in all subjects and subgroups. Subgroups were divided by age ≥65 years or <65 years, with or without CVD or DM at baseline. All models are adjusted for age, gender and center size. Abbreviations: UA, uric acid; CDV, cardiovascular disease; DM, diabetes.

extremes predicted higher risk for cardiovascular mortality in general population, which was stronger in subgroups without DM, hypertension, coronary heart disease, stroke, heart failure and CKD [34]. The association between UA and renal function decline was more obvious in subgroups without hypertension and DM from a Chinese population [35]. Inverse associations of serum UA and morbidity of acute ischemic stroke were observed only in non-DM hemodialysis patients [36]. The potential cause for this

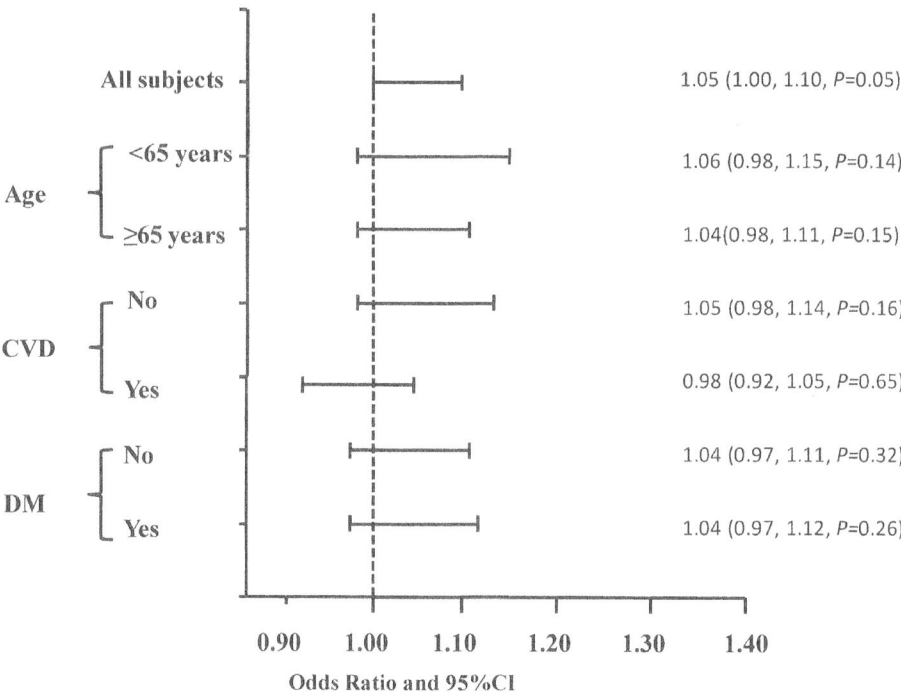

Figure 3. Risk of all-cause mortality in all subjects and subgroups. Subgroups were divided by age ≥65 years or <65 years, with or without CVD or DM at baseline. All models are adjusted for age, gender and center size. Abbreviations: UA, uric acid; CDV, cardiovascular disease; DM, diabetes.

Table 2. The prognostic values of UA as continuous or categorical variable for all-cause mortality.

Subjects	Age, gender-adjusted in Model 1		Multivariate-adjusted in Model 2		Multivariate-adjusted in Model 3	
	Hazard ratio (95% CI)	P	Hazard ratio (95% CI)	P	Hazard ratio (95% CI)	P
UA (per 1 mg/dL increase)	1.05(1.00~1.10)	0.05	1.05(0.98~1.12)	0.15	1.05(0.96~1.14)	0.34
Gender-specific tertiles of UA						
Tertile 1	Reference		Reference		Reference	
Tertile 2	1.09(0.89~1.33)	0.41	1.26 (0.97~1.65)	0.09	1.23 (0.90~1.70)	0.19
Tertile 3	1.23 (1.00~1.52)	0.04	1.30 (0.98~1.75)	0.07	1.21 (0.85~1.73)	0.3

Abbreviation: UA, uric acid; CI, confidence interval.
Model 1: age,center size-adjusted, gender-adjusted only UA as continuous variable.
Model 2: age,residual renal function, serum albumin, hemoglobin,phosphate, C-reactive protein and center size-adjusted, gender-adjusted only UA as continuous variable.
Model 3: age, residual renal function, serum albumin, hemoglobin,phosphate, C-reactive protein, the histroy of cardiovascular disease,diabetes, body mass index, mean arterial pressure, LDL cholestrol and center size-adjusted, gender-adjusted only UA as continuous variable.

phenomena is not clear but it might be relevant to concomitant confounders for CV mortality muting the association of UA and outcome in high-risk subjects. This finding also call us to pay more attention to low-risk subjects with elevated UA value.

Our data further indicated that the association of UA and CV/all-cause mortality was not independent, but rather related to concomitant uremia-related and traditional CV risk factors for PD population. This finding is in accordance with previous data from general population [37–40] and patients with CKD [41,42], showing that independent role of UA weakened or abolished after controlling for some traditional or non-traditional factors. Recently, Chen et al also showed that the association between UA and acute ischemic stroke was confounded by demographic characteristics and malnutrition-microinflammation syndrome in Chinese HD patients [36]. Therefore, whether hyperuricemia represents a marker or a cause for CV events and mortality is still not clear for CKD population [43,44]. Interventional studies should focus on this area to demonstrate if CKD patients would benefit from interventions lowering the elevated UA value.

Our large-scale multi-center cohort study gave us a valuable chance to observe the weak association of UA and CV/all-cause mortality in PD population for the first time. All participants were enrolled from 'core' PD centers of medical school affiliated hospital, which ensure the integrity and accuracy of clinical data for statistical adjustments. Second, multiple measurements of baseline laboratory were averaged, leading to more reliable data. Only 3.1% of participants missing UA values is also a merit. By contrast, most studies only have one single-point measurement [13,15–17,19,36] or relatively higher percentage of missing values [19].

This study also has several of limitations. First of all, for observational studies where associations do not prove causality, residual confounding cannot entirely be excluded. As a retrospective study, the quality of data collection must have been affected by many uncontrolled factors. There was even no information about the diuretics and/or allopurinol treatment. Smoking habits, alcohol consumption and other non-traditional CV factors were not entirely examined. Howerver, if confounding occurred, it would result in underestimation of the association but not change our main findings at all. In addition, we should be aware of the possibilities of ascertainment bias (totally 3.1% eligible patients were not included).

In conclusion, we suggested that high UA is weakly associated with CV and all-cause mortality for PD population. More large-scale PD cohort studies are needed to verify our findings. Whether high UA levels should be modified for PD patients as done for CKD patients is to be determined.

Table 3. The prognostic values of UA as continuous or categorical variable for cardiovascular mortality.

Subjects	Age, gender-adjusted in Model 1		Multivariate-adjusted in Model 2		Multivariate-adjusted in Model 3	
	Hazard ratio (95% CI)	P	Hazard ratio (95% CI)	P	Hazard ratio (95% CI)	P
UA (per 1 mg/dL increase)	1.12(1.05, 1.20)	0.001	1.05(0.95, 1.17)	0.35	1.04(0.89, 1.20)	0.65
Gender-specific tertiles of UA						
Tertile 1	Reference		Reference		Reference	
Tertile 2	1.56(1.13, 2.15)	0.007	1.48(0.96, 2.29)	0.08	1.29(0.75, 2.23)	0.35
Tertile 3	1.69(1.21, 2.38)	0.002	1.50(0.93, 2.41)	0.09	1.35(0.74, 2.46)	0.33

Abbreviation: UA, uric acid; CI, confidence interval.
Model 1: Age, center size-adjusted, gender-adjusted only UA as continuous variable.
Model 2: Age, residual renal function, serum albumin, hemoglobin,phosphate, C-reactive protein and center size-adjusted, gender-adjusted only UA as continuous variable.
Model 3: Age, residual renal function, serum albumin, hemoglobin,phosphate, C-reactive protein, the history of cardiovascular disease, diabetes, body mass index, mean arterial pressure, LDL cholestrol and center size-adjusted, gender-adjusted only UA as continuous variable.

Acknowledgments

The authors express their appreciation to the patients, doctors, and nursing staff of the peritoneal dialysis center of Peking University First Hospital, Division of Nephrology of Peking University Third Hospital, Division of Nephrology of Huashan Hospital, Fudan University, Division of Nephrology of the second affiliated hospital of Harbin Medical University, Division of Nephrology of Peking University People's Hospital, Division of Nephrology of the first affiliated hospital of Zhejiang University School of Medicine, Division of Nephrology of General Hospital of NingXia Medical University, for their participation in this study.

Author Contributions

Conceived and designed the experiments: JD HYW. Performed the experiments: JD QFH TYZ YPR JHC HPZ MHC RX YW CMH RZ XHZ MW NT. Analyzed the data: JD RX. Contributed reagents/materials/analysis tools: JD RX. Wrote the paper: JD.

References

1. Sarnak MJ, Levey AS, Schoolwerth AC, Coresh J, Culleton B, et al. (2003) Kidney disease as a risk factor for development of cardiovascular disease: a statement from the American Heart Association Councils on Kidney in Cardiovascular Disease, High Blood Pressure Research, Clinical Cardiology, and Epidemiology and Prevention. Hypertension 42: 1050–1065.
2. Elsayed EF, Tighiouart H, Griffith J, Kurth T, Levey AS, et al. (2007) Cardiovascular disease and subsequent kidney disease. Arch Intern Med 167: 1130–1136.
3. USRDS Annual Data Report. Available: http://www.usrds.org/2011/view/v2_04.asp. Accessed 2013 Jun 3.
4. Muntner P, He J, Astor BC, Folsom AR, Coresh J (2005) Traditional and nontraditional risk factors predict coronary heart disease in chronic kidney disease: results from the atherosclerosis risk in communities study. J Am Soc Nephrol 16: 529–538.
5. Stenvinkel P, Carrero JJ, Axelsson J, Lindholm B, Heimburger O, et al. (2008) Emerging biomarkers for evaluating cardiovascular risk in the chronic kidney disease patient: how do new pieces fit into the uremic puzzle? Clin J Am Soc Nephrol 3: 505–521.
6. Navaneethan SD, Nigwekar SU, Perkovic V, Johnson DW, Craig JC, et al. (2009) HMG CoA reductase inhibitors (statins) for dialysis patients. Cochrane Database Syst Rev: CD004289.
7. Pan Y, Guo LL, Cai LL, Zhu XJ, Shu JL, et al. (2012) Homocysteine-lowering therapy does not lead to reduction in cardiovascular outcomes in chronic kidney disease patients: a meta-analysis of randomised, controlled trials. Br J Nutr 108: 400–407.
8. Jun M, Venkataraman V, Razavian M, Cooper B, Zoungas S, et al. (2012) Antioxidants for chronic kidney disease. Cochrane Database Syst Rev 10: CD008176.
9. Palmer SC, Nistor I, Craig JC, Pellegrini F, Messa P, et al. (2013) Cinacalcet in patients with chronic kidney disease: a cumulative meta-analysis of randomized controlled trials. PLoS Med 10: e1001436.
10. Johnson RJ, Kang DH, Feig D, Kivlighn S, Kanellis J, et al. (2003) Is there a pathogenetic role for uric acid in hypertension and cardiovascular and renal disease? Hypertension 41: 1183–1190.
11. Jonasson T, Ohlin AK, Gottsater A, Hultberg B, Ohlin H (2005) Plasma homocysteine and markers for oxidative stress and inflammation in patients with coronary artery disease-a prospective randomized study of vitamin supplementation. Clin Chem Lab Med 43: 628–634.
12. Niskanen LK, Laaksonen DE, Nyyssonen K, Alfthan G, Lakka HM, et al. (2004) Uric acid level as a risk factor for cardiovascular and all-cause mortality in middle-aged men: a prospective cohort study. Arch Intern Med 164: 1546–1551.
13. Madero M, Sarnak MJ, Wang X, Greene T, Beck GJ, et al. (2009) Uric acid and long-term outcomes in CKD. Am J Kidney Dis 53: 796–803.
14. Chen J, Mohler ER 3rd, Xie D, Shlipak MG, Townsend RR, et al. (2012) Risk factors for peripheral arterial disease among patients with chronic kidney disease. Am J Cardiol 110: 136–141.
15. Kanbay M, Yilmaz MI, Sonmez A, Solak Y, Saglam M, et al. (2012) Serum uric acid independently predicts cardiovascular events in advanced nephropathy. Am J Nephrol 36: 324–331.
16. Suliman ME, Johnson RJ, Garcia-Lopez E, Qureshi AR, Molinaei H, et al. (2006) J-shaped mortality relationship for uric acid in CKD. Am J Kidney Dis 48: 761–771.
17. Lee SM, Lee AL, Winters TJ, Tam E, Jaleel M, et al. (2009) Low serum uric acid level is a risk factor for death in incident hemodialysis patients. Am J Nephrol 29: 79–85.
18. Hsu SP, Pai MF, Peng YS, Chiang CK, Ho TI, et al. (2004) Serum uric acid levels show a 'J-shaped' association with all-cause mortality in haemodialysis patients. Nephrol Dial Trandplant 19: 457–462.
19. Latif W, Karaboyas A, Tong L, Winchester JF, Arrington CJ, et al. (2011) Uric acid levels and all-cause and cardiovascular mortality in the hemodialysis population. Clin J Am Soc Nephrol 6: 2470–2477.
20. Xu R, Han QF, Zhu TY, Ren YP, Chen JH, et al. (2012) Impact of individual and environmental socioeconomic status on peritoneal dialysis outcomes: a retrospective multicenter cohort study. PLoS One 7: e50766.
21. Smith SC Jr, Jackson R, Pearson TA, Fuster V, Yusuf S, et al. (2004) Principles for national and regional guidelines on cardiovascular disease prevention: a scientific statement from the World Heart and Stroke Forum. Circulation 109: 3112–3121.
22. Chobanian AV, Bakris GL, Black HR, Cushman WC, Green LA, et al. (2003) The Seventh Report of the Joint National Committee on Prevention, Detection, Evaluation, and Treatment of High Blood Pressure: the JNC 7 report. JAMA 289: 2560–2572.
23. Garg JP, Chasan-Taber S, Blair A, Plone M, Bommer J, et al. (2005) Effects of sevelamer and calcium-based phosphate binders on uric acid concentrations in patients undergoing hemodialysis: a randomized clinical trial. Arthritis Rheum 52: 290–295.
24. Alexander RW (1994) Inflammation and coronary artery disease. N Engl J Med 331: 468–469.
25. Iuliano L (2001) The oxidant stress hypothesis of atherogenesis. Lipids 36 Suppl: S41–44.
26. Caravaca F, Martin MV, Barroso S, Cancho B, Arrobas M, et al. (2005) [Serum uric acid and C-reactive protein levels in patients with chronic kidney disease]. Nefrologia 25: 645–654.
27. Khosla UM, Zharikov S, Finch JL, Nakagawa T, Roncal C, et al. (2005) Hyperuricemia induces endothelial dysfunction. Kidney Int 67: 1739–1742.
28. Kanbay M, Yilmaz MI, Sonmez A, Turgut F, Saglam M, et al. (2011) Serum uric acid level and endothelial dysfunction in patients with nondiabetic chronic kidney disease. Am J Nephrol 33: 298–304.
29. Melendez-Ramirez G, Perez-Mendez O, Lopez-Osorio C, Kuri-Alfaro J, Espinola-Zavaleta N (2012) Effect of the treatment with allopurinol on the endothelial function in patients with hyperuricemia. Endocr Res 37: 1–6.
30. Nieto FJ, Iribarren C, Gross MD, Comstock GW, Cutler RG (2000) Uric acid and serum antioxidant capacity: a reaction to atherosclerosis? Atherosclerosis 148: 131–139.
31. Suzuki T (2007) Nitrosation of uric acid induced by nitric oxide under aerobic conditions. Nitric Oxide 16: 266–273.
32. Park JT, Kim DK, Chang TI, Kim HW, Chang JH, et al. (2009) Uric acid is associated with the rate of residual renal function decline in peritoneal dialysis patients. Nephrol Dial Trandplant 24: 3520–3525.
33. Wang AY (2007) The "heart" of peritoneal dialysis. Perit Dial Int 27 Suppl 2: S228–232.
34. Kuo CF, See LC, Yu KH, Chou IJ, Chiou MJ, et al. (2013) Significance of serum uric acid levels on the risk of all-cause and cardiovascular mortality. Rheumatology (Oxford) 52: 127–134.
35. Zhang L, Wang F, Wang X, Liu L, Wang H (2012) The association between plasma uric acid and renal function decline in a Chinese population-based cohort. Nephrol Dial Trandplant 27: 1836–1839.
36. Chen Y, Ding X, Teng J, Zou J, Zhong Y, et al. (2011) Serum uric acid is inversely related to acute ischemic stroke morbidity in hemodialysis patients. Am J Nephrol 33: 97–104.
37. Culleton BF, Larson MG, Kannel WB, Levy D (1999) Serum uric acid and risk for cardiovascular disease and death: the Framingham Heart Study. Ann Intern Med 131: 7–13.
38. Moriarity JT, Folsom AR, Iribarren C, Nieto FJ, Rosamond WD (2000) Serum uric acid and risk of coronary heart disease: Atherosclerosis Risk in Communities (ARIC) Study. Ann Epidemiol 10: 136–143.
39. Wen CP, David Cheng TY, Chan HT, Tsai MK, Chung WS, et al. (2010) Is high serum uric acid a risk marker or a target for treatment? Examination of its independent effect in a large cohort with low cardiovascular risk. Am J Kidney Dis 56: 273–288.
40. Wannamethee SG, Shaper AG, Whincup PH (1997) Serum urate and the risk of major coronary heart disease events. Heart 78: 147–153.
41. Navaneethan SD, Beddhu S (2009) Associations of serum uric acid with cardiovascular events and mortality in moderate chronic kidney disease. Nephrol Dial Trandplant 24: 1260–1266.
42. Liu WC, Hung CC, Chen SC, Yeh SM, Lin MY, et al. (2012) Association of hyperuricemia with renal outcomes, cardiovascular disease, and mortality. Clin J Am Soc Nephrol 7: 541–548.
43. Tangri N, Weiner DE (2010) Uric acid, CKD, and cardiovascular disease: confounders, culprits, and circles. Am J Kidney Dis 56: 247–250.
44. Badve SV, Brown F, Hawley CM, Johnson DW, Kanellis J, et al. (2011) Challenges of conducting a trial of uric-acid-lowering therapy in CKD. Nat Rev Nephrol 7: 295–300.

25

The Relationship of Initial Transferrin Saturation to Cardiovascular Parameters and Outcomes in Patients Initiating Dialysis

Hyang Mo Koo[1], **Chan Ho Kim**[1], **Fa Mee Doh**[1], **Mi Jung Lee**[1], **Eun Jin Kim**[1], **Jae Hyun Han**[1], **Ji Suk Han**[1], **Hyung Jung Oh**[1], **Jung Tak Park**[1], **Seung Hyeok Han**[1], **Tae-Hyun Yoo**[1], **Shin-Wook Kang**[1,2]*

1 Department of Internal Medicine, Yonsei University College of Medicine, Seoul, Korea, **2** Brain Korea 21 PLUS Project for Medical Science, Yonsei University, Seoul, Korea

Abstract

Background: The prognostic importance of anemia for cardiovascular (CV) events and mortality has been extensively investigated. However, little is known about the impact of transferrin saturation (TSAT), a marker reflecting the availability of iron for erythropoiesis, on clinical outcome in dialysis patients.

Methods: A total of 879 anemic incident dialysis patients were recruited from the Clinical Research Center for End-Stage Renal Disease in Korea and were divided into 3 groups according to baseline TSAT of ≤20%, 20–40%, and >40%.

Results: There were no differences in hemoglobin levels and the proportion of patients on erythropoiesis-stimulating agents or iron supplements among the 3 groups. During a mean follow-up duration of 19.3 months, 51 (5.8%) patients died. CV composite (11.71 vs. 5.55 events/100 patient-years, P = 0.001) and all-cause mortality rates (5.38 vs. 2.31 events/100 patient-years, P = 0.016) were significantly higher in patients with TSAT ≤20% compared to those with TSAT 20–40% (reference group). Cox regression analysis revealed that patients with TSAT ≤20% had 1.62- and 2.19-fold higher risks for CV composite outcome (P = 0.046) and all-cause mortality (P = 0.030). Moreover, TSAT ≤20% was significantly associated with left ventricular hypertrophy [odds ratio (OR) = 1.46], high-sensitivity C-reactive protein ≥3 mg/dL (OR = 2.09), N-terminal pro B-type natriuretic peptide ≥10000 pg/mL (OR = 2.04), and troponin-T≥0.1 ng/mL (OR = 2.02), on logistic regression analysis.

Conclusions: Low TSAT was a significant independent risk factor for adverse clinical outcome in incident dialysis patients with anemia, which may be partly attributed to cardiac dysfunction and inflammation.

Editor: James Connor, The Pennsylvania State University Hershey Medical Center, United States of America

Funding: None of the authors received any significant primary financial arrangements with commercial companies that produce or sell products or with competitors of such companies. This study was supported by a grant of the Korea Healthcare Technology R&D Project, Ministry for Health, Welfare & Family Affairs, Republic of Korea (HI10C2020). The funders had no role in study design, data collection and analysis, decision to publish, or preparation of the manuscript.

Competing Interests: The authors have declared that no competing interests exist.

* E-mail: kswkidney@yuhs.ac

Introduction

Anemia is prevalent in patients with chronic kidney disease (CKD), and develops during the early stages of the disease and worsens as renal function declines [1,2]. It is well known that anemia is closely linked with fatigue, exercise intolerance, and poor quality of life. In addition, anemia has been demonstrated to be an independent risk factor for left ventricular hypertrophy (LVH), congestive heart failure (CHF), and cardiovascular (CV) mortality [3–5]. In CKD patients, anemia is also associated with the progression of renal dysfunction [6,7].

Anemia in CKD patients is attributed to inadequate production of erythropoietin, iron and/or folate deficiency, secondary hyperparathyroidism, chronic inflammation, and bone marrow suppression due to uremic toxins [8]. Among these factors except for erythropoietin deficiency, iron deficiency is the leading cause of anemia in patients with CKD. Therefore clinicians must determine patients' iron levels not only at the start of erythropoi-

esis-stimulating agent (ESA) therapy but also monitor iron levels during ESA treatment in this population [9,10]. To evaluate iron status, serum iron concentrations, transferrin saturation (TSAT); the ratio of serum iron to total iron-binding capacity (TIBC), multiplied by 100, and serum ferritin levels are commonly used. While serum iron concentrations and TSAT reflect the amount of iron available for erythropoiesis, serum ferritin levels are the only marker of total body iron stores. Ferritin levels also are greatly influenced by nutritional and/or inflammatory status and do not correlate well with bone marrow findings in patients with various chronic diseases [11]. Considering these findings, TSAT <20% and serum ferritin concentrations <100 ng/mL are regarded as absolute iron deficiency, and TSAT <20% and serum ferritin levels >100 ng/mL as relative iron deficiency [9,11].

Iron is an essential nutrient. It plays critical roles in binding and transporting oxygen, oxidative metabolism by serving as a component of the mitochondrial respiratory chain proteins, and the synthesis of DNA and protein [12]. Therefore, iron deficiency may result in numerous pathologies, especially in cells with high energy demands, such as cardiomyocytes [13,14]. In addition to its association with poor cognitive function, reduced exercise performance, and decreased quality of life, previous studies have found that absolute or relative iron deficiency, regardless of the presence of anemia, is an independent predictor of adverse clinical outcomes, including a progression of CHF and mortality, in patients with CHF [15–18]. These findings suggest that lack of circulating available iron has a direct deleterious effect on the heart.

Since CV disease is the most common cause of morbidity and mortality in patients with end-stage renal disease (ESRD), it follows that iron deficiency may have a negative impact on the clinical outcome of ESRD patients. However, to date, this effect has never been evaluated in this population. In the present study, therefore, we investigated whether low TSAT was a significant predictor of CV mortality/composite outcome and all-cause mortality in Korean incident dialysis patients from the Clinical Research Center (CRC) for ESRD. The relationships of TSAT with echocardiographic parameters and cardiac biomarkers were also defined in these patients.

Patients and Methods

Ethics statement

This study was carried out in accordance with the Declaration of Helsinki and study protocol was approved by the Institutional Review Board of each participating hospital's Clinical Trial Center (CTC); Kyungpook National University Hospital CTC, Youngnam University Medical Center CTC, Dong-A University Medical Center CTC, Busan National University Hospital CTC, Inje University Pusan Paik Hospital CTC, Ulsan University Hospital CTC, Seoul National University Hospital CTC, Seoul National University Bundang Hospital CTC, Seoul National University Boramae Hospital CTC, Gachon University Gil Medical Center CTC, Yonsei University Health System CTC, National Health Insurance Corporation Ilsan Hospital CTC, Ehwa Womens University Mokdong Hospital CTC, Kwandong University College of Medicine Myongi Hospital CTC, Kangnam Severance Hospital CTC, The Catholic University of Korea Seoul St. Mary's Hospital CTC, The Catholic University of Korea Yeouido St. Mary's Hospital CTC, The Catholic University of Korea Bucheon St. Mary's Hospital CTC, The Catholic University of Korea St. Vincent's Hospital CTC, The Catholic University of Korea Uijeongbu St. Mary's Hospital CTC, Chung-Ang University Health System CTC, Chonnam National University Hospital CTC, Chungnam National University Hospital CTC, Chungbuk National University Hospital CTC, Chonbuk National University Hospital CTC, and Cheju Halla General Hospital CTC. All patients provided their written informed consent before entering the study.

Patients

Initial recruitment for this prospective observational multicenter study included all ESRD patients who started dialysis between August 1, 2008 and December 31, 2012 at 27 centers of the CRC for ESRD in Korea. Among these patients, we excluded those who were younger than 18 years old, had a history of kidney transplantation prior to dialysis therapy, had an underlying active malignancy or acute infection, or died within 3 months of the initiation of dialysis. Patients who were not anemic; anemia was defined as Hb <13 g/dL in men and <12 g/dL in women according to World Health Organization (WHO) criteria [19],

had a recent bleeding episode, or had insufficient baseline data were also excluded from the study. Ultimately, a total of 879 incident dialysis patients were included in the final analysis.

Data Collection

Demographic and clinical data were recorded at the time of study entry, including age, gender, body mass index (BMI) calculated as weight/height^2, primary renal disease, comorbidities, and medications. Coronary arterial disease (CAD) was defined as a history of angioplasty, coronary artery bypass grafts, myocardial infarction, or angina, while peripheral arterial disease (PAD) was defined as a history of claudication, ischemic limb loss and/or ulceration, or peripheral revascularization procedure. At the time of study entry and every 3 months thereafter, laboratory data were measured from fasting blood samples, which were drawn prior to the start of hemodialysis (HD) on the day of a midweek session in HD patients and at 2-hours after the first peritoneal dialysis (PD) exchange with 1.5% dextrose dialysate in PD patients. The estimated glomerular filtration rate (eGFR) was calculated using the four-variable Modification of Diet in Renal Disease study (MDRD) and Chronic Kidney Disease Epidemiology Collaboration study (CKD-EPI) equations [20]. In addition, a 24-hour urine collection was performed to determine residual urine volume, and 24-hour urinary protein, urea, and creatinine excretion. Nutritional status was also evaluated by the subjective global assessment (SGA) score [21]. The quality of life was assessed using a Korean version of Kidney Disease Quality of Life Short Form (KDQOL-SF, version 1.3) [22].

Echocardiography was performed on a non-dialysis day in HD patients and in the morning with an empty abdomen in PD patients, close to the time of discharge, based on the imaging protocol recommended by the American Society of Echocardiography. Left atrial dimension (LAD) was assessed at the end of the ventricular systole at the level of the aortic valve, according to the leading-edge-to-leading-edge convention. Left ventricular (LV) mass was determined using the method described by Devereux et al. [23], and the LV mass index (LVMI) was calculated by dividing LV mass by body surface area. LV hypertrophy (LVH) was defined as a LVMI >131 g/m^2 for men and >100 g/m^2 for women [24]. LV systolic function was estimated by the LV ejection fraction (LVEF) using a modified biplane Simpson's method from the apical two-chamber and four-chamber views. Inter-ventricular septal thickness (IST), left ventricular posterior wall thickness (LVPWT), and left ventricular dimensions (LVEDD, LVESD) were also measured at the end of both the diastolic and systolic phases. Multiple reproducibility, inter-reader reliability, intra-reader reliability, and reader drift analyses were performed at a core echocardiography laboratory (Kyungpook National University, Daegu, Korea) on a random sample of 3% of the entire cohort each year. The intra-class correlation coefficients for the echocardiographic measures were 0.773 for LAD, 0.745 for LVMI, and 0.842 for LVEF.

Outcome measures

For the current study, all mortality and hospitalization event records were retrieved from the CRC for ESRD database and carefully reviewed. The primary endpoints were CV mortality and CV composite outcome (death and hospitalization), and the secondary endpoint was all-cause mortality. CV event was considered death or hospitalization from myocardial infarction/ischemia, congestive heart failure, pulmonary edema, or cerebrovascular disorder.

Statistical analysis

Statistical analysis was performed using SPSS for Windows, version 18.0 (SPSS Inc., Chicago, IL, USA). Data are expressed as mean ± standard deviation or median (interquartile range) for continuous variables, and as a number (percentage) for categorical variables. Normality of distribution was assessed by the Shapiro-Wilk test. Patients were categorized into 3 groups according to TSAT concentrations; ≤20%, 20–40%, and >40%. Patient demographics, clinical characteristics, and laboratory findings were compared among the three groups using ANOVA or Kruskal-Wallis test for continuous variables and the chi-square test for categorical variables. Cumulative survival curves for CV mortality, CV composite outcome, and all-cause mortality were created by the Kaplan-Meier method, and between-group survival was compared by a log-rank test. The independent prognostic power of TSAT for clinical outcomes was ascertained by multivariate Cox proportional hazards regression analysis, which included only the variables of a P-value <0.10 on the univariate analysis. Binary logistic regression analysis was conducted to determine the independent predictive value of TSAT for echocardiographic parameters (LVEF <60%, LVH, LVEDD ≥ 55 mm, LVESD ≥35 mm, and LAD ≥40 mm) and inflammatory and cardiac biomarkers [high-sensitivity C-reactive protein (hs-CRP) ≥3 mg/dL, N-terminal pro B-type natriuretic peptide (NT-proBNP) ≥10000 pg/mL, and cardiac troponin-T (cTnT) ≥ 0.1 ng/mL]. A P-value of less than 0.05 was considered statistically significant.

Results

Baseline characteristics

The baseline demographics and clinical characteristics are shown in Table 1. The mean age was 56.4±14.5 years, and 59.6% of patients were male. The most common cause of ESRD was diabetes (DM, 52.7%), followed by hypertension (16.5%). A total of 645 patients (73.4%) were treated with HD and 234 patients (26.6%) with PD. The mean values of hemoglobin (Hb) and TSAT were 8.6±1.4 g/dL and 28.4±16.0%, respectively, and the median levels of ferritin were 201.3 (103.5–363.4) ng/mL.

When patients were divided into three groups according to baseline TSAT concentrations, age, sex, the proportion of patients on HD, the presence of DM and CV diseases, and KDQOL-SF scores were comparable among the three groups. There were also no differences in the proportions of patients on renin-angiotensin system (RAS) blockers, ESA, and supplementary iron. However, beta-blockers were more frequently prescribed in the lowest TSAT group compared to the other groups (P = 0.019) (Table 1). Even though only one third of patients (n = 319, 36.3%) were on iron therapy at the time of dialysis commencement, 166 patients with TSAT ≤20% (58.9%) were newly treated with iron agents after the initiation of dialysis. Therefore, 261 patients (92.6%) with initial TSAT ≤20% were on iron therapy at 3-month.

Within the laboratory and echocardiographic findings, blood urea nitrogen and creatinine levels were significantly lower in the lowest TSAT group compared to the highest TSAT group (P< 0.001), whereas serum calcium, bicarbonate, and triglyceride concentrations were significantly higher (P<0.05). There were also significant gradual increases in serum iron and ferritin concentrations and a significant gradual decrease in TIBC levels across the TSAT groups (P<0.001). However, eGFR and Hb concentrations were not significantly different among the three groups. Meanwhile, hs-CRP and NT-proBNP levels were significantly higher in the lowest TSAT group compared to the other two groups (P<

0.001 and P = 0.011, respectively). Echocardiographic parameters were comparable among the three groups (Table 2).

CV mortality, CV composite outcome, and all-cause mortality according to TSAT concentrations

During a mean follow-up duration of 19.3±11.8 months, 51 patients (5.8%) died. Among them, 29 patients (3.3%) died from CV causes and 12 (1.4%) from infection.

Compared to the reference group (TSAT 20–40%), CV composite and all-cause mortality rates were significantly higher in patients with TSAT ≤20% (CV composite: 11.71 vs. 5.55 events per 100 patient-yr, P = 0.001; all-cause mortality: 5.38 vs. 2.31 events per 100 patient-yr, P = 0.016). In contrast, there was no significant difference in CV mortality rates among the three groups (Table 3). Kaplan-Meier analysis also showed that the CV composite and all-cause mortality rates were significantly higher in patients with TSAT ≤20% compared to the other two groups (P = 0.009 and P = 0.046, respectively) (Figure 1). However, there was no significant difference in the CV composite and all-cause mortality rates between the reference and TSAT >40% groups.

Multivariate Cox-proportional hazard regression analysis revealed that patients in the lowest TSAT group had 1.62- and 2.19-fold higher risks for CV composite outcome and all-cause mortality, respectively, even after adjusting for demographic characteristics, laboratory findings, and echocardiographic parameters (P = 0.046 and P = 0.030, respectively) (Table 4).

In another analysis, we simply dichotomized patients into 'low' and 'normal to high' TSAT groups based on TSAT concentrations of 20%, and compared the clinical outcomes between the two groups. The 'low' TSAT group had significantly higher rates of CV composite (11.71 vs. 6.15 events per 100 patient-yr, P<0.001) and all-cause mortality (5.38 vs. 2.74 events per 100 patient-yr, P = 0.008) than patients with TSAT >20%, and the hazard ratios (HRs) were 1.53 and 2.04, respectively, on the multivariate Cox regression analysis (Table S1 and S2, and Figure S1).

Relationships between TSAT and echocardiographic parameters

In binary logistic regression analysis for echocardiographic parameters, TSAT ≤20% was demonstrated to be significantly associated with LVH [odds ratio (OR) = 1.46, P = 0.048]. The ORs of TSAT ≤20% for LVEF <60%, LVEDD ≥55 mm, LVESD ≥35 mm, and LAD ≥40 mm were also increased, but did not reach statistical significances (Table 5).

Based on these results, we performed an additional multivariate linear regression analysis for LVMI. Along with diastolic blood pressure, underlying CV disease, SGA score, smoking status, serum Hb and albumin concentrations, and usage of RAS blockers, calcium-based phosphate binders, and iron agents, TSAT ≤20% was a significant independent determinant of LVMI (R = 7.151, P = 0.044) (Table S3).

Relationships between TSAT and serum inflammatory and cardiac biomarkers

Binary logistic regression analysis revealed that there were significant independent associations of TSAT ≤20% with hs-CRP ≥3 mg/dL (OR = 2.09, P = 0.003), NT-proBNP ≥10,000 pg/mL (OR = 2.04, P = 0.011), and cTnT ≥0.1 ng/mL (OR = 2.02, P = 0.023) (Table 6).

In an additional multivariate linear regression analysis, TSAT ≤20% was found to be a significant determinant of natural log values (Ln) of hs-CRP levels (R = 0.304, P<0.001), but not of Ln

Table 1. Baseline demographic and clinical characteristics of the patients.

Variables	Total	TSAT ≤20%	TSAT 20–40%	TSAT >40%	P
N	879	282	431	166	
Age (years)	56.4±14.5	57.1±14.0	56.4±14.2	55.3±16.2	0.414
Sex (Male)	524 (59.6)	162 (57.4)	258(59.9)	104 (62.7)	0.550
BMI (kg/m^2)	23.2±3.7	23.3±3.7	23.4±3.8	22.6±3.3	0.097
Systolic BP (mmHg)	142.4±24.7	142.2±24.7	142.7±25.4	141.7±22.9	0.898
Diastolic BP (mmHg)	77.6±15.2	76.9±15.0	77.8±15.3	78.1±15.1	0.666
Heart rate (beat per minute)	76.7±13.6	76.9±13.0	76.8±13.1	76.2±15.7	0.845
Dialysis modality (HD)	645 (73.4)	212 (75.2)	310 (71.9)	123 (74.1)	0.614
Follow-up duration (months)	19.3±11.8	19.8±11.6	19.3±11.7	18.6±12.3	0.562
Smoking status					0.878
Current smoker	103 (11.7)	31 (11.0)	51 (11.8)	21 (12.7)	
Ex-smoker	291 (33.1)	92 (32.6)	143 (33.2)	56 (33.7)	
Non-smoker	467 (53.1)	155 (55.0)	225 (52.2)	87 (52.4)	
Unknown	18 (2.0)	4 (1.4)	12 (2.8)	2 (1.2)	
Primary cause of end-stage renal disease					0.151
Diabetes	463 (52.7)	162 (57.4)	228 (52.9)	73 (44.0)	
HTN/Large vessel disease	145 (16.5)	43 (15.2)	75 (17.4)	27 (16.3)	
Glomerulonephritis	147 (16.7)	38 (13.5)	67 (15.5)	42 (25.3)	
Interstitial nephritis	9 (1.0)	3 (1.1)	5 (1.2)	1 (0.6)	
Hereditary/Congenital disease	15 (1.7)	7 (2.5)	6 (1.4)	2 (1.2)	
Others	43 (4.9)	11 (3.9)	24 (5.6)	8 (4.8)	
Unknown	57 (6.5)	18 (6.4)	26 (6.0)	13 (7.8)	
Comorbid disease					
Chronic lung disease	72 (8.2)	20 (7.1)	32 (7.4)	20 (12.0)	0.130
CAD	127 (14.4)	48 (17.0)	57 (13.2)	22 (13.3)	0.329
PAD	65 (7.4)	22 (7.8)	36 (8.4)	7 (4.2)	0.213
CVA	92 (10.5)	29 (10.3)	47 (10.9)	16 (9.6)	0.896
CHF	127 (14.4)	42 (14.9)	65 (15.1)	20 (12.0)	0.619
Arrhythmia	25 (2.8)	6 (2.1)	17 (3.9)	2 (1.2)	0.153
Diabetes	486 (55.3)	167 (59.2)	239 (55.5)	80 (48.2)	0.076
Connective tissue disease	85 (9.7)	25 (8.9)	43 (10.0)	17 (10.2)	0.853
Liver disease	81 (9.2)	17 (6.0)	39 (9.0)	25 (15.1)	0.006
CVD*	298 (33.9)	102 (36.2)	141 (32.7)	55 (33.1)	0.618
Cardiac disease†	224 (25.5)	78 (27.7)	107 (24.8)	39 (23.5)	0.563
Modified CCI	5.1±2.6	5.1±2.5	5.1±2.6	4.9±2.6	0.665
SGA >1	278 (31.6)	84 (29.8)	144 (33.4)	50 (30.1)	0.535
KDQOL-SF score	60.1±14.9	60.1±14.8	60.5±15.2	59.0±14.3	0.696
Medications					
RAS blockers	528 (60.1)	167 (59.2)	259 (60.1)	102 (61.4)	0.898
Diuretics	461 (52.4)	150 (53.2)	225 (52.2)	86 (51.8)	0.951
Beta blocker	477 (54.3)	170 (60.3)	229 (53.1)	78 (47.0)	0.019
CCB	549 (62.5)	183 (64.9)	263 (61.0)	103 (62.0)	0.576
Nitrate	34 (3.9)	10 (3.5)	13 (3.0)	11 (6.6)	0.116
Aspirin	214 (24.3)	81 (28.7)	98 (22.7)	35 (21.1)	0.106
Clopidogrel	73 (8.3)	31 (11.0)	30 (7.0)	12 (7.2)	0.139
Vitamin D	124 (14.1)	39 (13.8)	70 (16.2)	25 (15.1)	0.680
Ca based P-binders	472 (53.7)	164 (58.2)	224 (52.0)	84 (50.6)	0.182
ESA	282 (32.1)	83 (29.4)	148 (34.3)	51 (30.7)	0.358
Iron agent	319 (36.3)	95 (33.7)	160 (37.1)	64 (38.6)	0.516

Table 2. Laboratory and echocardiographic findings of the patients.

Variables	Total	TSAT ≤20%	TSAT 20–40%	TSAT >40%	P
Baseline laboratory data					
WBC (/µL)	7239.1±2936.6	7637.2±3080.2	7055.1±2793.8	7039.6±2997.5	0.022
Hemoglobin (g/dL)	8.55±1.43	8.54±1.34	8.47±1.41	8.44±1.61	0.604
ALP (IU/L)	78.0 (59.0–109.0)	80.0 (60.0–109.0)	75.0 (57.0–105.0)	80.5 (59.0–115.3)	0.065
Ca (mg/dL)	8.22±1.08	8.32±0.96	8.22±1.05	8.06±1.30	0.048
P (mg/dL)	5.61±1.38	5.59±1.08	5.60±1.36	5.81±1.81	0.106
Ca x P product	45.4±15.1	45.4±13.7	45.3±14.9	46.1±17.7	0.239
Uric acid (mg/dL)	8.36±2.13	8.25±2.06	8.40±2.07	8.50±2.35	0.260
Glucose (mg/dL)	140.9±37.4	141.6±40.7	141.9±39.5	137.0±25.1	0.747
HbA1c (%)	6.12±0.81	6.12±0.90	6.16±0.75	6.02±0.81	0.570
Protein (g/dL)	6.05±0.80	6.08±0.76	6.03±0.82	6.06±0.82	0.702
Albumin (g/dL)	3.32±0.59	3.29±0.59	3.33±0.57	3.35±0.61	0.522
BUN (mg/dL)	82.7±26.8	76.6±22.7	82.3±25.7	94.4±33.4	<0.001
Creatinine (mg/dL)	8.52±3.52	7.97±2.58	8.42±3.32	9.73±4.98	<0.001
GFR-MDRD (mL/min/1.73m2)	7.12±3.13	7.40±3.42	7.18±3.14	6.51±2.54	0.080
GFR-EPI (mL/min/1.73m2)	7.29±2.94	7.47±2.76	7.39±3.16	6.72±2.60	0.111
Sodium (mEq/L)	137.2±4.9	137.0±4.6	137.3±5.0	137.4±5.0	0.763
Potassium(mEq/L)	4.67±0.95	4.61±0.95	4.66±0.93	4.79±1.01	0.115
Bicarbonate (mmol/L)	19.0±5.6	19.3±5.3	19.1±5.5	17.9±6.5	0.037
Intact-PTH (pg/mL)	203.9 (119.0–341.4)	198.7 (119.4–326.7)	210.0 (112.6–329.3)	209.9 (129.1–379.9)	0.413
Serum iron (µg/dL)	60.5±32.0	29.8±8.9	61.2±14.6	110.6±33.9	<0.001
TIBC (µg/dL)	217.7±44.0	227.7±51.9	216.5±39.5	204.2±37.2	<0.001
TSAT (%)	28.4±16.0	13.2±4.2	28.4±5.6	54.3±13.0	<0.001
Ferritin (ng/mL)	201.3 (103.5–363.4)	122.6 (64.3–274.1)	216.2 (121.6–369.8)	294.4 (190.3–479.9)	<0.001
Total cholesterol (mg/dL)	155.2±46.3	153.9±44.8	156.7±46.9	151.5±47.3	0.219
Triglyceride (mg/dL)	127.1±54.8	127.3±64.9	129.2±51.0	116.7±43.6	0.035
LDL-cholesterol (mg/dL)	89.3±32.0	87.8±29.3	92.6±34.7	83.6±28.6	0.044
HDL-cholesterol (mg/dL)	38.6±12.5	38.4±11.9	38.3±12.2	39.9±14.2	0.380
hs-CRP (mg/dL)	0.32 (0.08–1.46)	0.71 (0.15–2.09)	0.24 (0.06–0.99)	0.25 (0.07–1.20)	<0.001
Troponin-T (ng/mL)	0.056 (0.025–0.110)	0.057 (0.027–0.125)	0.059 (0.025–0.106)	0.046 (0.021–0.096)	0.409
NT-proBNP (pg/mL)	6505.4 (1576.7–25840.0)	11012.0 (1998.0–30000.0)	5969.5 (1364.0–21882.8)	4903.0 (1269.0–25151.5)	0.011
24-hr urine study					
Urea (mg/dL)	220.0 (142.0–327.4)	190.1 (136.8–293.5)	238.8 (152.5–347.3)	206.7 (127.8–325.1)	0.018
Creatinine (mg/dL)	54.1 (38.0–86.6)	51.5 (36.4–76.0)	55.9 (38.4–91.3)	56.2 (36.6–84.1)	0.119
Protein (mg/day)	1180.5 (418.1–2794.5)	1153.0 (426.2–3150.5)	1305.6 (393.0–2951.7)	1053.0 (383.0–2604.0)	0.723
Volume (mL/day)	970.0 (600.0–1400.0)	990.0 (525.0–1445.0)	985.0 (600.0–1450.0)	880.0 (600.0–1300.0)	0.367
Echocardiographic parameters					
LVPWT (cm)	1.20±0.29	1.21±0.29	1.19±0.29	1.20±0.27	0.737
IST (cm)	1.15±0.22	1.17±0.24	1.14±0.22	1.13±0.20	0.095
LVESD (cm)	3.51±0.72	3.58±0.75	3.48±0.71	3.43±0.69	0.062
LVEDD (cm)	5.16±0.61	5.20±0.61	5.15±0.60	5.12±0.63	0.329
LAD (cm)	4.22±0.71	4.27±0.71	4.22±0.71	4.13±0.69	0.131
LVMI (g/m2)	146.7±43.4	151.7±46.1	144.2±42.1	144.5±41.6	0.117
LVEF (%)	58.2±11.3	57.3±12.3	58.3±11.1	59.3±10.3	0.206

Abbreviations: WBC, white blood cell; ALP, alkaline phosphatase; Ca, calcium; P, phosphorus; HbA1C, hemoglobin A1C; BUN, blood urea nitrogen; GFR, glomerular filtration rate; MDRD, Modification of Diet in Renal Disease; EPI, Chronic Kidney Disease Epidemiology Collaboration Equation; PTH, parathyroid hormone;TIBC, total iron binding capacity; TSAT, transferrin saturation; LDL, low density lipoprotein; HDL, high density lipoprotein; hs-CRP, high-sensitivity C-reactive protein; NT-proBNP, N-terminal pro B-type natriuretic peptide; LVPWT, left ventricular posterior wall thickness; IST, inter-ventricularseptalthickness; LVESD, left ventricular end-systolic dimension; LVEDD, left ventricular end-diastolic dimension; LAD, left atrial dimension; LVMI, left ventricular mass index; LVEF, left ventricular ejection fraction.

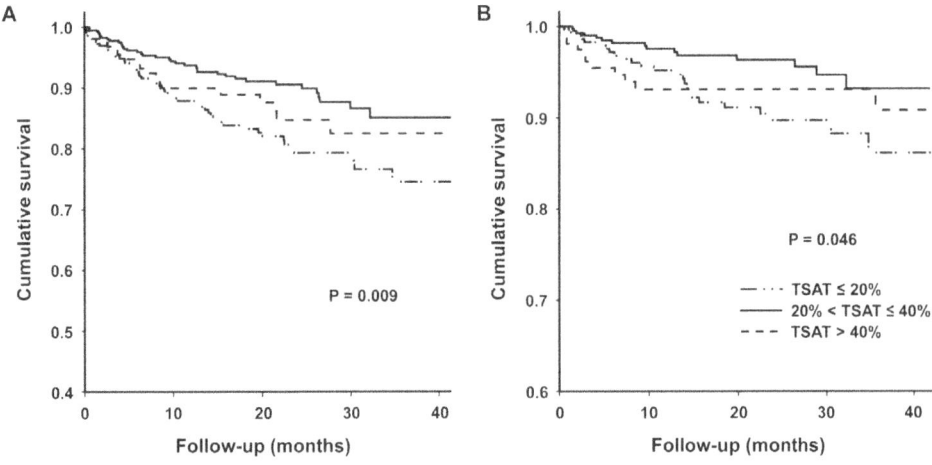

Figure 1. Kaplan-Meier curves for CV composite outcome (A) and all-cause mortality (B) according to baseline TSAT concentrations. The CV composites and all-cause mortality rates were significantly higher in patients with TSAT ≤20% compared to the other two groups. *Abbreviation:* CV, cardiovascular; TSAT, transferrin saturation.

NT-proBNP (R = 0.229, P = 0.134) and Ln cTnT concentrations (R = 0.092, P = 0.406) (Table S4).

Discussion

TSAT is one of the available markers reflecting the adequacy of iron for erythropoiesis and is closely correlated with Hb levels [9,11]. Even though a number of studies have shown that anemia is an independent risk factor for CV events and mortality in ESRD patients, as well as in the general population [3,4,7,25], the impact of TSAT on clinical outcome has never been explored in dialysis patients. In the current study on incident dialysis patients with anemia, we demonstrate for the first time that the lowest TSAT group has significantly higher risk for CV composite outcome and all-cause mortality, irrespective of Hb concentrations. In addition, TSAT ≤20% was significantly associated with LVMI and hs-CRP levels. These findings suggest that the adverse clinical outcomes in patients with 'low' TSAT are partly attributed to LVH and inflammation.

Iron deficiency is the most frequent cause of anemia in the general population. In ESRD patients, a decrease in the production of erythropoietin is the main factor contributing to anemia, but iron deficiency anemia (IDA) is also prevalent [8]. Even though anemia has been demonstrated to be an independent risk factor for renal function deterioration and CV morbidity/mortality in patients with CKD [4,7,25], the results of some previous studies on the impact of anemia correction on the clinical

outcome of CKD/ESRD patients have not been promising, except for some improvement in quality of life [26–28]. Similarly, anemia is common in patients with CHF, most of which are attributed to 'anemia of chronic disease' or iron deficiency [5,29,30]. Numerous previous studies demonstrated that anemia was associated with impaired functional capacity and poor quality of life in CHF patients, which were ameliorated by elimination of the anemia [31,32]. However, a body of evidence indicating that anemia correction has a beneficial effect on CV mortality in these patients is lacking. Based on these findings, it is still debatable whether adverse clinical outcomes in anemic patients are attributed to anemia per se or other factors contributing to anemia.

Iron is essential for normal cell physiology. In addition to its critical role in erythropoiesis, iron is involved in the process of oxygen transport and storage, oxidative metabolism including ATP (adenosine triphosphate) production at the mitochondrial electron transport chain in the form of cytochrome (a, b, c) and iron-sulfur-containing dehydrogenases, and the synthesis and/or degradation of RNA and DNA. Therefore, iron deficiency can lead to not only anemia but also various cellular dysfunctions, especially in high energy-requiring cells such as cardiomyocytes and renal cells. In the clinical field, reduced oxidative capacity caused by cytochrome dysfunction can manifest as fatigue, impaired prolonged exercise, malnutrition, and cardiac dysfunction [12,33,34]. A previous study by Dong et al. [13] showed that heart weight and size were significantly increased, and the left

Table 3. Comparisons of clinical outcomes according to the TSAT concentrations.

| | TSAT ≤20% | | 20% < TSAT ≤40% | | TSAT >40% | | |
	N (%)	Rates (per 100 patient-yr)	N (%)	Rates (per 100 patient-yr)	N (%)	Rates (per 100 patient-yr)	P
CV mortality	12 (4.3%)	2.58	10 (2.3%)	1.44	7 (4.2%)	2.73	0.281
CV composite	51 (18.1%)	11.71	37 (8.6%)	5.55	19 (11.4%)	7.78	0.001
All-cause mortality	25 (8.9%)	5.38	16 (3.7%)	2.31	10 (6.0%)	3.90	0.016

*Composite: composite of death and hospitalization.
Abbreviations: TSAT, transferrin saturation; CV, cardiovascular.

Table 4. Hazard ratios and 95% confidence intervals for primary and secondary endpoints according to baseline TSAT concentrations (Cox-proportional hazard regression analysis).

	CV mortality			CV composite			All-cause mortality		
	HR	95% CI	P	HR	95% CI	P	HR	95% CI	P
Unadjusted									
TSAT ≤20%	1.798	0.777–4.161	0.171	1.918	1.256–2.929	0.003	2.117	1.130–3.965	0.019
20% < TSAT ≤40%	1	-	-	1	-	-	1	-	-
TSAT >40%	1.881	0.716–4.941	0.200	1.420	0.817–2.469	0.214	1.714	0.778–3.777	0.182
Adjusted for demographics									
TSAT ≤20%	1.651	0.710–3.841	0.245	1.729	1.123–2.661	0.013	2.278	1.190–4.363	0.013
20% < TSAT ≤40%	1	-	-	1	-	-	1	-	-
TSAT >40%	1.785	0.675–4.724	0.243	1.499	0.859–2.616	0.154	1.749	0.760–4.026	0.189
Adjusted for demographics and medications									
TSAT ≤20%	1.635	0.701–3.813	0.255	1.645	1.066–2.539	0.025	2.002	1.041–3.852	0.038
20% < TSAT ≤40%	1	-	-	1	-	-	1	-	-
TSAT >40%	1.797	0.679–4.755	0.238	1.488	0.851–2.603	0.163	1.814	0.790–4.165	0.160
Adjusted for demographics, medications, and laboratory parameters									
TSAT ≤20%	1.448	0.608–3.445	0.403	1.668	1.049–2.652	0.030	2.128	1.057–4.283	0.034
20% < TSAT ≤40%	1	-	-	1	-	-	1	-	-
TSAT >40%	1.587	0.583–4.315	0.366	1.323	0.751–2.331	0.332	1.432	0.613–3.343	0.407
Adjusted for demographics, medications, laboratory parameters, and echocardiographic findings									
TSAT ≤20%	1.383	0.555–3.448	0.486	1.616	1.008–2.607	0.046	2.193	1.081–4.450	0.030
20% < TSAT ≤40%	1	-	-	1	-	-	1	-	-
TSAT >40%	1.687	0.580–4.908	0.337	1.212	0.673–2.185	0.522	1.292	0.533–3.129	0.571

*Composite: composite of death and hospitalization.
*CV mortality was sequentially adjusted for demographics (age, diabetes, underlying cardiovascular disease, and subjective global assessment score), medications (aspirin), laboratory parameters (albumin, glucose, alkaline phosphatase, and log transformed high-sensitivity C-reactive protein), and echocardiographic findings (left ventricular mass index and left ventricular ejection fraction).
*CV composite was sequentially adjusted for demographics (age, systolic blood pressure, diabetes, and underlying cardiovascular disease), medications (aspirin, clopidogrel, vitamin D, and erythropoiesis-stimulating agents), laboratory parameters (calcium, glucose, potassium, log transformed ferritin, and log transformed high-sensitivity C-reactive protein), and echocardiographic findings (left ventricular mass index and left ventricular ejection fraction).
*All-cause mortality was sequentially adjusted for demographics (body mass index, Charlson Comorbidity Index, and subjective global assessment score), medications (aspirin, clopidogrel, and vitamin D), laboratory parameters (alkaline phosphatase, calcium, glucose, log transformed ferritin, and log transformed high-sensitivity C-reactive protein), and echocardiographic findings (left ventricular mass index and left ventricular ejection fraction).
Abbreviations: TSAT, transferrin saturation; CV, cardiovascular; HR, hazard ratio; CI, confidence interval.

ventricular dimension and chamber volume were significantly enhanced, in rats fed an iron-deficient diet for 12 weeks. Mitochondrial swelling and abnormal sarcomere structure were also observed in ventricular tissues of the iron-deficient rats. These findings inferred that iron deficiency per se might induce cardiac dysfunction and morphological aberration. Moreover, another recent study demonstrated that patients with advanced CHF displayed significantly lower serum iron concentrations and TSAT compared to healthy controls. This study also showed that myocardial iron content and myocardial mRNA expression of the type 1 transferrin receptor, a key molecule in cellular iron transport, were significantly reduced in CHF versus non-CHF samples, suggesting a linkage among the presence of iron depletion in the failing heart, anemia, and adverse prognosis in CHF [35]. However, since hematocrit or Hb levels were significantly lower in the iron-deficiency groups in those two studies, it was difficult to conclude whether iron deficiency had a direct unfavorable impact on the heart.

Recently, Jankowska et al. [15] found that iron deficiency, defined as ferritin <100 μg/L or ferritin 100-300 μg/L with TSAT <20%, rather than anemia, was an independent risk factor for poor clinical outcome in 546 patients with stable

systolic CHF. Patients with iron deficiency had significantly lower survival rates, either when death and heart transplantation or death alone were considered events in both univariate and multivariate Cox regression models, whereas anemia was a significant predictor of adverse clinical outcome only in univariate analysis. Based on these findings, they suggested that iron deficiency had a direct deleterious effect on cardiomyocytes. The results of the present study also showed that clinical outcome was significantly worse in the lowest TSAT group, despite comparable Hb concentrations, and that TSAT ≤20% was a significant independent risk factor for CV composite outcome and all-cause mortality. Taken together, we surmise that the association between 'low' TSAT and adverse clinical outcome in incident dialysis patients is a consequence of iron deficiency rather than anemia in the heart, which may be partly attributed to mitochondrial cytochrome dysfunction.

In a similar context, several clinical trials have shown the beneficial effect of iron replacement therapy in CHF patients with anemia. The first randomized trial was performed by Toblli et al. [31] to evaluate the effect of intravenous iron therapy in anemic patients with CHF and CKD, and demonstrated that iron supplements substantially reduced NT-proBNP and inflammatory

Table 5. Odds ratios and 95% confidence intervals for echocardiographic parameters according to baseline TSAT concentrations (Logistic regression analysis).

	Unadjusted			Adjusted		
	OR	95% CI	P	OR	95% CI	P
Left ventricular ejection fraction <60%						
TSAT ≤20%	1.435	1.068–1.926	0.016	1.313	0.910–1.895	0.146
20% < TSAT ≤40%	1	-	-	1	-	-
TSAT >40%	0.969	0.689–1.363	0.857	0.715	0.466–1.096	0.124
Left ventricular hypertrophy						
TSAT ≤20%	1.482	1.065–2.062	0.020	1.455	1.003–2.110	0.048
20% < TSAT ≤40%	1	-	-	1	-	-
TSAT >40%	0.838	0.574–1.224	0.361	0.931	0.604–1.435	0.747
Left ventricular end-diastolic dimension ≥55 mm						
TSAT ≤20%	1.363	0.981–1.892	0.065	1.258	0.849–1.862	0.252
20% < TSAT ≤40%	1	-	-	1	-	-
TSAT >40%	0.941	0.624–1.418	0.770	0.765	0.474–1.235	0.274
Left ventricular end-systolic dimension ≥35 mm						
TSAT ≤20%	1.346	0.995–1.821	0.054	1.341	0.935–1.924	0.111
20% < TSAT ≤40%	1	-	-	1	-	-
TSAT >40%	0.888	0.617–1.277	0.522	0.687	0.449–1.052	0.084
Left atrial dimension ≥40 mm						
TSAT ≤20%	1.456	1.051–2.015	0.024	1.145	0.777–1.689	0.494
20% < TSAT ≤40%	1	-	-	1	-	-
TSAT >40%	0.835	0.578–1.205	0.335	0.725	0.468–1.124	0.150

*Left ventricular ejection fraction was adjusted for sex, body mass index, heart rates, underlying diabetes and cardiovascular disease, hemoglobin, serum glucose, albumin, and creatinine levels, log transformed high-sensitivity C-reactive protein, and usage of diuretics, beta blockers, and vitamin D.
*Left ventricular hypertrophy was adjusted for sex, diastolic blood pressure, underlying cardiac disease, subjective global assessment score, hemoglobin, serum calcium, and albumin concentrations, and usage of renin-angiotensin system blockers and beta blockers.
*Left ventricular end-diastolic dimension was adjusted for sex, body mass index, underlying diabetes and cardiac disease, smoking status, hemoglobin, serum phosphorus and albumin levels, log transformed high-sensitivity C-reactive protein, and usage of renin-angiotensin system blockers and beta blockers.
*Left ventricular end-systolic dimension was adjusted for sex, diastolic blood pressure, underlying cardiovascular disease, smoking status, hemoglobin, serum phosphorus, albumin, and creatinine concentrations, log transformed high-sensitivity C-reactive protein, and usage of renin-angiotensin system blockers and beta blockers.
*Left atrial dimension was adjusted for age, sex, pulse pressure, underlying diabetes and cardiac disease, smoking status, hemoglobin, serum albumin levels, log transformed high-sensitivity C-reactive protein, and usage of diuretics, beta blockers, calcium channel blockers, and aspirin.
Abbreviations: TSAT, transferrin saturation; OR, odds ratio; CI, confidence interval.

status in these patients, along with an improvement in LVEF, New York Heart Association (NYHA) functional class, exercise capacity, and quality of life. However, they found that Hb levels were also significantly increased in the treatment group compared to the placebo group. Recently, two prospective randomized controlled trials showed that the correction of iron deficiency with intravenous iron conferred symptomatic benefits in patients with CHF [36,37]. Compared to the control group, patient global assessment, exercise capacity, and NYHA functional class were significantly improved in the iron-treated group regardless of the presence of anemia, suggesting that iron deficiency per se was detrimental to the heart. Considering the results of our study, further studies on the use of intravenous iron in incident ESRD patients with 'low' TSAT will be necessary to clarify whether iron therapy can improve the clinical outcome of these patients, as in CHF patients.

Meanwhile, an excess of iron can be toxic because it has the ability to accept and donate electrons by exchanging between ferrous and ferric forms. During this exchange, active free iron undergoes "Fenton and Haber-Weiss reaction", causing oxidative stress and organic biomolecule oxidation by releasing hydroxyl radicals and other reactive oxygen species (ROS) [38,39]. Furthermore, in the vasculature, ROS produced at the endothelium by excessive iron is known to promote the thrombotic complications [33]. Even though ferritin concentration is usually considered a marker of iron store and has been demonstrated to be an independent predictor of clinical outcomes in not only the general population but also specific patients groups, several previous studies have found that TSAT, an indicator of a predisposition for iron overload, is also a significant prognostic factor in the general population. A cohort study using data from the First Health and Nutrition Examination Survey I (NHANES I) merged with the NHANES I Epidemiologic Follow Up Study showed that all-cause mortality was significantly increased in patients with a serum TSAT of more than 55% compared with those with saturations below this cutoff [HR = 1.60, 95% confidence interval (CI) = 1.17–2.21], on a Cox proportional hazard regression analysis [40]. In addition, Ellervik et al. [41] examined mortality according to baseline TSAT in two Danish population-based follow-up studies and demonstrated that the cumulative survival was significantly reduced in individuals with TSAT ≥50% vs. <50% (P<0.0001). In that study, there was a

Table 6. Odds ratios and 95% confidence intervals for serum inflammatory and cardiac biomarkers according to baseline TSAT concentrations (Logistic regression analysis).

	Unadjusted			Adjusted		
	OR	95% CI	P	OR	95% CI	P
hs-CRP ≥3 mg/dL						
TSAT ≤20%	1.772	1.162–2.702	0.008	2.087	1.292–3.372	0.003
20% < TSAT ≤40%	1	-	-	1	-	-
TSAT >40%	0.980	0.558–1.722	0.945	0.817	0.443–1.506	0.517
NT-proBNP ≥10000 pg/mL						
TSAT ≤20%	1.630	1.124–2.363	0.010	2.039	1.181–3.521	0.011
20% < TSAT ≤40%	1	-	-	1	-	-
TSAT >40%	0.640	0.400–1.023	0.062	0.328	0.171–0.629	0.001
Troponin-T ≥0.1 ng/mL						
TSAT ≤20%	1.498	1.004–2.235	0.048	2.019	1.104–3.691	0.023
20% < TSAT ≤40%	1	-	-	1	-	-
TSAT >40%	0.876	0.518–1.484	0.623	0.989	0.484–2.024	0.976

*hs-CRP was adjusted for Charlson Comorbidity Index, subjective global assessment score, smoking status, hemoglobin, serum calcium, glucose, albumin, and sodium concentrations, and log transformed ferritin.
*NT-proBNP was adjusted for diastolic blood pressure, underlying diabetes and cardiac disease, hemoglobin, serum glucose, albumin, creatinine, and sodium levels, log transformed high-sensitivity C-reactive protein, log transformed ferritin, log transformed troponin-T, and usage of renin-angiotensin system blockers, diuretics, and beta blockers.
*Troponin-T was adjusted for sex, systolic blood pressure, underlying diabetes and cardiac disease, subjective global assessment score, hemoglobin, serum calcium, glucose, and albumin concentrations, log transformed high-sensitivity C-reactive protein, log transformed ferritin, log transformed 24-hr urine volume, left atrial dimension, left ventricular mass index, left ventricular ejection fraction, and usage of diuretics and nitrate.
Abbreviations: hs-CRP, high-sensitivity C-reactive protein; NT-proBNP, N-terminal pro B-type natriuretic peptide; TSAT, transferrin saturation; OR, odds ratio; CI, confidence interval.

stepwise increase in all-cause mortality, with the first significant increased risk conferred by TSAT ≥40%. Based on these findings, we tried to elucidate the impact of iron deficiency as well as a proxy of iron overload, and thus categorized patients into 3 groups based on TSAT; ≤20% (low), 20–40% (normal), and >40% (high). Even though HRs for clinical outcomes; CV mortality, CV composite, and all-cause mortality; were slightly increased in patients with TSAT >40%, there were no statistical significances. In another analysis conducted after dichotomizing the study subjects into just 'low' and 'normal to high' TSAT groups, patients with TSAT ≤20% showed significantly higher rates of CV composite outcome and all-cause mortality, and the HRs for each outcome were 1.53 and 2.04, respectively, which were comparable with those of the original analysis. These data indirectly implicate the lack of statistical difference between the reference group and subjects with TSAT >40%, and further

clarify our finding of low TSAT (≤20%) as a risk factor for adverse clinical outcomes.

LVH is a well-known powerful independent predictor of CV morbidity and mortality in patients with ESRD. Furthermore, a change in LVH has been identified as a strong prognostic factor in these patients. A previous prospective study on prevalent HD patients revealed that the rates of LVMI increase were significantly higher in patients with incident CV events than in those without such events and that cardiovascular event-free survival in patients with changes in LVMI below the 25th percentile was significantly higher than in those with changes above the 75th percentile [42]. Similarly, in a cohort study of 153 incident ESRD patients receiving HD, a reduction in LV mass during a mean follow-up duration of 54 months resulted in significant decreases in all-cause and CV mortality. In that study, LV mass reduction was also independently associated with improved patient survival, even after adjustment for confounding variables [43]. On the other hand, uremia-related nontraditional risk factors, including inflammation and oxidative stress, were implicated in the pathogenesis of CV disease in dialysis patients [44]. Since accumulating evidence indicates that inflammation is an integral part of the development and progression of atherosclerosis, it has been proposed that hs-CRP concentrations are closely linked to the presence of CV disease. In addition, numerous previous studies have found that serum hs-CRP levels are predictive of CV mortality, as well as future CV events, in not only the general population but also ESRD patients [45,46]. In this study, LVMI and serum hs-CRP concentrations were higher in the lowest TSAT group compared to the other two groups. Moreover, TSAT ≤20% was found to be a significant determinant of LVMI and Ln hs-CRP concentrations in multivariate linear regression analysis. Taken together, the impact of 'low' TSAT on clinical outcome in our patients seems to be partly mediated by LVH and inflammation.

Several shortcomings of the current study should be discussed. First, since the study subjects were all Korean incident ESRD patients, the association of TSAT with mortality and composite outcome may not be generalizable to other populations. Second, because only the baseline laboratory and echocardiographic measurements were used for the analysis, it was difficult to demonstrate the impact of the changes of TSAT on patients' clinical outcomes. Third, even though CV disease was the leading cause of death in our subjects, CV mortality was comparable among the three groups in spite of a significant difference in all-cause mortality, which may be attributed to 'low' CV mortality rates in the current study compared to those in previous studies on Western ESRD patients. We propose that the difference is mainly attributed to disparate ethnicities as the mortality rates of our patients were not significantly different from those of Japanese dialysis patients [47]. Fourth, we stratified the patients based on TSAT only, without considering ferritin levels, indicating that patients with TSAT ≤20% may not be purely iron deficient. Since ferritin is an acute-phase reactant, high ferritin concentrations with low TSAT may imply a condition of iron sequestration, which is a characteristic of 'anemia of chronic disease'. In the present study, in fact, there was a significant correlation between serum ferritin levels and Ln hs-CRP concentrations (r = 0.368, P<0.001), whereas Hb levels did not correlate with serum ferritin concentrations (r = 0.002, P = 0.954). Fifth, TSAT is also known to be influenced by nutritional status. TIBC may be decreased due to reduced transferrin synthesis in the setting of malnutrition and chronic disease, resulting in high TSAT, disproportionate to the iron content [11]. However, serum albumin levels were not significantly different among the three groups, suggesting that TSAT was not largely affected by nutritional status in our patients. Sixth, data for transfusion were not available. So, we excluded patients who had a history of acute/recent bleeding in the analysis. Lastly, about one-third of patients were already taking iron or ESA agents at the time of inclusion. Nevertheless, the proportions of patients taking those medications were not significantly different among the three groups, and multivariate analysis was conducted after adjusting for these factors. Despite these limitations, to our knowledge, the current study is the first study to investigate the impact of TSAT at the time of dialysis initiation on clinical outcome in a large and single-ethnicity incident dialysis patient cohort. Further studies will be needed to elucidate whether serial monitoring, rather than a single measurement of TSAT, is helpful in identifying ESRD patients at a high risk of all-cause and CV morbidity and mortality and whether iron supplements are beneficial to clinical outcome in 'low' TSAT patients.

In conclusion, 'low' TSAT was a significant independent risk factor for CV composite outcome and all-cause mortality in incident dialysis patients with anemia. Furthermore, TSAT $\leq 20\%$ was significantly associated with LVMI and hs-CRP concentrations. These findings suggest that the adverse clinical outcomes in patients with 'low' TSAT are partly attributed to LVH and inflammation.

Supporting Information

Figure S1 Kaplan-Meier curves for CV composite outcome (A) and all-cause mortality (B) according to

References

1. Robinson BE (2006) Epidemiology of chronic kidney disease and anemia. J Am Med Dir Assoc 7: S3-6; quiz S17–21.
2. McClellan W, Aronoff SL, Bolton WK, Hood S, Lorber DL, et al. (2004) The prevalence of anemia in patients with chronic kidney disease. Curr Med Res Opin 20: 1501–1510.
3. Vlagopoulos PT, Tighiouart H, Weiner DE, Griffith J, Pettit D, et al. (2005) Anemia as a risk factor for cardiovascular disease and all-cause mortality in diabetes: the impact of chronic kidney disease. J Am Soc Nephrol 16: 3403–3410.
4. Portoles J, Lopez-Gomez JM, Aljama P (2007) A prospective multicentre study of the role of anaemia as a risk factor in haemodialysis patients: the MAR Study. Nephrol Dial Transplant 22: 500–507.
5. Tang YD, Katz SD (2006) Anemia in chronic heart failure: prevalence, etiology, clinical correlates, and treatment options. Circulation 113: 2454–2461.
6. Keane WF, Brenner BM, de Zeeuw D, Grunfeld JP, McGill J, et al. (2003) The risk of developing end-stage renal disease in patients with type 2 diabetes and nephropathy: the RENAAL study. Kidney Int 63: 1499–1507.
7. Kovesdy CP, Trivedi BK, Kalantar-Zadeh K, Anderson JE (2006) Association of anemia with outcomes in men with moderate and severe chronic kidney disease. Kidney Int 69: 560–564.
8. Weiss G, Goodnough LT (2005) Anemia of chronic disease. N Engl J Med 352: 1011–1023.
9. (2006) KDOQI Clinical Practice Guidelines and Clinical Practice Recommendations for Anemia in Chronic Kidney Disease. Am J Kidney Dis 47: S11–145.
10. (2012) KDIGO Clinical Practice Guideline for Anemia in Chronic Kidney Disease. Kidney international supplements 2: 282–335.
11. Wish JB (2006) Assessing iron status: beyond serum ferritin and transferrin saturation. Clin J Am Soc Nephrol 1 Suppl 1: S4–8.
12. Wang J, Pantopoulos K (2011) Regulation of cellular iron metabolism. Biochem J 434: 365–381.
13. Dong F, Zhang X, Culver B, Chew HG Jr., Kelley RO, et al. (2005) Dietary iron deficiency induces ventricular dilation, mitochondrial ultrastructural aberrations and cytochrome c release: involvement of nitric oxide synthase and protein tyrosine nitration. Clin Sci (Lond) 109: 277–286.
14. Naito Y, Tsujino T, Matsumoto M, Sakoda T, Ohyanagi M, et al. (2009) Adaptive response of the heart to long-term anemia induced by iron deficiency. Am J Physiol Heart Circ Physiol 296: H585–593.
15. Jankowska EA, Rozentryt P, Witkowska A, Nowak J, Hartmann O, et al. (2010) Iron deficiency: an ominous sign in patients with systolic chronic heart failure. Eur Heart J 31: 1872–1880.
16. van Veldhuisen DJ, Anker SD, Ponikowski P, Macdougall IC (2011) Anemia and iron deficiency in heart failure: mechanisms and therapeutic approaches. Nat Rev Cardiol 8: 485–493.
17. Okonko DO, Mandal AK, Missouris CG, Poole-Wilson PA (2011) Disordered iron homeostasis in chronic heart failure: prevalence, predictors, and relation to anemia, exercise capacity, and survival. J Am Coll Cardiol 58: 1241–1251.
18. Jankowska EA, von Haehling S, Anker SD, Macdougall IC, Ponikowski P (2013) Iron deficiency and heart failure: diagnostic dilemmas and therapeutic perspectives. Eur Heart J 34: 816–829.
19. Beutler E, Waalen J (2006) The definition of anemia: what is the lower limit of normal of the blood hemoglobin concentration? Blood 107: 1747–1750.
20. Michels WM, Grootendorst DC, Verduijn M, Elliott EG, Dekker FW, et al. (2010) Performance of the Cockcroft-Gault, MDRD, and new CKD-EPI formulas in relation to GFR, age, and body size. Clin J Am Soc Nephrol 5: 1003–1009.
21. Steiber AL, Kalantar-Zadeh K, Secker D, McCarthy M, Sehgal A, et al. (2004) Subjective Global Assessment in chronic kidney disease: a review. J Ren Nutr 14: 191–200.
22. Park HJ, Kim S, Yong JS, Han SS, Yang DH, et al. (2007) Reliability and validity of the Korean version of Kidney Disease Quality of Life instrument (KDQOL-SF). Tohoku J Exp Med 211: 321–329.
23. Devereux RB, Alonso DR, Lutas EM, Gottlieb GJ, Campo E, et al. (1986) Echocardiographic assessment of left ventricular hypertrophy: comparison to necropsy findings. Am J Cardiol 57: 450–458.
24. Liao Y, Cooper RS, Durazo-Arvizu R, Mensah GA, Ghali JK (1997) Prediction of mortality risk by different methods of indexation for left ventricular mass. J Am Coll Cardiol 29: 641–647.
25. Li S, Collins AJ (2004) Association of hematocrit value with cardiovascular morbidity and mortality in incident hemodialysis patients. Kidney Int 65: 626–633.
26. Drueke TB, Locatelli F, Clyne N, Eckardt KU, Macdougall IC, et al. (2006) Normalization of hemoglobin level in patients with chronic kidney disease and anemia. N Engl J Med 355: 2071–2084.
27. Singh AK, Szczech L, Tang KL, Barnhart H, Sapp S, et al. (2006) Correction of anemia with epoetin alfa in chronic kidney disease. N Engl J Med 355: 2085–2098.
28. Pfeffer MA, Burdmann EA, Chen CY, Cooper ME, de Zeeuw D, et al. (2009) A trial of darbepoetin alfa in type 2 diabetes and chronic kidney disease. N Engl J Med 361: 2019–2032.
29. Anand IS (2008) Anemia and chronic heart failure implications and treatment options. J Am Coll Cardiol 52: 501–511.

baseline TSAT concentrations. The CV composites and all-cause mortality rates were significantly higher in patients with TSAT $\leq 20\%$ compared to patients with TSAT $>20\%$. *Abbreviation:* CV, cardiovascular; TSAT, transferrin saturation.

Table S1 Comparisons of clinical outcomes between patients with TSAT $\leq 20\%$ and TSAT $>20\%$.

Table S2 Hazard ratios and 95% confidence intervals for primary and secondary endpoints according to baseline TSAT concentrations (Cox-proportional hazard regression analysis).

Table S3 Multivariate linear regression analysis for left ventricular mass index.

Table S4 Multivariate linear regression analyses for inflammatory and cardiac biomarkers.

Author Contributions

Conceived and designed the experiments: HMK SWK. Performed the experiments: HMK EJK JHH JSH. Analyzed the data: HMK CHK FMD MJL. Contributed reagents/materials/analysis tools: HMK HJO JTP SHH THY. Wrote the paper: HMK SWK.

30. Nanas JN, Matsouka C, Karageorgopoulos D, Leonti A, Tsolakis E, et al. (2006) Etiology of anemia in patients with advanced heart failure. J Am Coll Cardiol 48: 2485–2489.

31. Toblli JE, Lombrana A, Duarte P, Di Gennaro F (2007) Intravenous iron reduces NT-pro-brain natriuretic peptide in anemic patients with chronic heart failure and renal insufficiency. J Am Coll Cardiol 50: 1657–1665.

32. Silverberg DS, Wexler D, Iaina A, Schwartz D (2008) The role of correction of anaemia in patients with congestive heart failure: a short review. Eur J Heart Fail 10: 819–823.

33. Franchini M, Targher G, Montagnana M, Lippi G (2008) Iron and thrombosis. Ann Hematol 87: 167–173.

34. Dallman PR (1986) Biochemical basis for the manifestations of iron deficiency. Annu Rev Nutr 6: 13–40.

35. Maeder MT, Khammy O, dos Remedios C, Kaye DM (2011) Myocardial and systemic iron depletion in heart failure implications for anemia accompanying heart failure. J Am Coll Cardiol 58: 474–480.

36. Anker SD, Comin Colet J, Filippatos G, Willenheimer R, Dickstein K, et al. (2009) Ferric carboxymaltose in patients with heart failure and iron deficiency. N Engl J Med 361: 2436–2448.

37. Comin-Colet J, Lainscak M, Dickstein K, Filippatos GS, Johnson P, et al. (2013) The effect of intravenous ferric carboxymaltose on health-related quality of life in patients with chronic heart failure and iron deficiency: a subanalysis of the FAIR-HF study. Eur Heart J 34: 30–38.

38. Murphy CJ, Oudit GY (2010) Iron-overload cardiomyopathy: pathophysiology, diagnosis, and treatment. J Card Fail 16: 888–900.

39. Kremastinos DT, Farmakis D (2011) Iron overload cardiomyopathy in clinical practice. Circulation 124: 2253–2263.

40. Mainous AG 3rd, Gill JM, Carek PJ (2004) Elevated serum transferrin saturation and mortality. Ann Fam Med 2: 133–138.

41. Ellervik C, Tybjaerg-Hansen A, Nordestgaard BG (2011) Total mortality by transferrin saturation levels: two general population studies and a metaanalysis. Clin Chem 57: 459–466.

42. Zoccali C, Benedetto FA, Mallamaci F, Tripepi G, Giacone G, et al. (2004) Left ventricular mass monitoring in the follow-up of dialysis patients: prognostic value of left ventricular hypertrophy progression. Kidney Int 65: 1492–1498.

43. London GM, Pannier B, Guerin AP, Blacher J, Marchais SJ, et al. (2001) Alterations of left ventricular hypertrophy in and survival of patients receiving hemodialysis: follow-up of an interventional study. J Am Soc Nephrol 12: 2759–2767.

44. Cachofeiro V, Goicochea M, de Vinuesa SG, Oubina P, Lahera V, et al. (2008) Oxidative stress and inflammation, a link between chronic kidney disease and cardiovascular disease. Kidney Int Suppl: S4–9.

45. Danesh J, Wheeler JG, Hirschfield GM, Eda S, Eiriksdottir G, et al. (2004) C-reactive protein and other circulating markers of inflammation in the prediction of coronary heart disease. N Engl J Med 350: 1387–1397.

46. Han SS, Ahn JM, Chin HJ, Chae DW, Oh KH, et al. (2010) Impact of C-reactive protein and pulse pressure evaluated at the start of peritoneal dialysis on cardiovascular events in the course of treatment with peritoneal dialysis. Perit Dial Int 30: 300–310.

47. Robinson BM, Port FK (2009) International hemodialysis patient outcomes comparisons revisited: the role of practice patterns and other factors. Clin J Am Soc Nephrol 4 Suppl 1: S12–17.

26

Are Non-cardiac Surgeries Safe for Dialysis Patients? – A Population-Based Retrospective Cohort Study

Yih-Giun Cherng[1,2], Chien-Chang Liao[2,3,4], Tso-Hsiao Chen[5], Duan Xiao[6], Chih-Hsiung Wu[7❥], Ta-Liang Chen[2,3,4]❥

1 Department of Anesthesiology, Shuang Ho Hospital, affiliated with Taipei Medical University, New Taipei City, Taiwan, **2** Department of Anesthesiology, School of Medicine, College of Medicine, Taipei Medical University, Taipei, Taiwan, **3** Department of Anesthesiology, Taipei Medical University Hospital, Taipei, Taiwan, **4** Health Policy Research Center, Taipei Medical University Hospital, Taipei, Taiwan, **5** Department of Nephrology, Wan Fang Medical Center, affiliated with Department of Internal Medicine, College of Medicine, Taipei Medical University, Taipei, Taiwan, **6** Department of Coloproctology, the Second People's Hospital of Shi-Fang City, Shi-Fang City, Sichuan Province, People Republic of China, **7** Department of Surgery, Shuang Ho Hospital, affiliated with Taipei Medical University, New Taipei City, Taiwan

Abstract

Background: End-stage renal disease represents a risk complex that complicates surgical results. The surgical outcomes of dialysis patients have been studied in specific fields, but the global features of postoperative adverse outcomes in dialysis patients receiving non-cardiac surgeries have not been examined.

Methods: Taiwan's National Health Insurance Research Database was used to study 8,937 patients under regular dialysis with 8,937 propensity-score matched-pair controls receiving non-cardiac surgery between 2004 and 2007. We investigated the influence of hemodialysis and peritoneal dialysis, effects of hypertension and diabetes, and impact of additional comorbidities on postoperative adverse outcomes.

Results: Postoperative mortality in dialysis patients was higher than in controls (odds ratio [OR] 3.33, 95% confidence interval [CI] 2.56 to 4.33) when receiving non-cardiac surgeries. Complications such as acute myocardial infarction, pneumonia, bleeding, and septicemia were significantly increased. Postoperative mortality was significantly increased among peritoneal dialysis patients (OR 2.71, 95% CI 1.70 to 4.31) and hemodialysis patients (OR 3.42, 95% CI 2.62 to 4.47) than in controls. Dialysis patients with both hypertension and diabetes had the highest risk of postoperative complications; these risks increased with number of preoperative medical conditions. Patients under dialysis also showed significantly increased length of hospitalization, more ICU stays and higher medical expenditures.

Conclusion: Surgical patients under dialysis encountered significantly higher postoperative complications and mortality than controls when receiving non-cardiac surgeries. Different dialysis techniques, pre-existing hypertension/diabetes, and various comorbidities had complication-specific impacts on surgical adverse outcomes. These findings can help surgical teams provide better risk assessment and postoperative care for dialysis patients.

Editor: Jane-Lise Samuel, Inserm, France

Funding: This research was supported by a Foundation for Anesthesia Education and Research fellowship grant through Taipei Medical University Hospital without conflict of interest. The funders had no role in study design, data collection and analysis, decision to publish, or preparation of the manuscript.

Competing Interests: The authors have declared that no competing interests exist.

* E-mail: tlc@tmu.edu.tw

❥ These authors contributed equally to this work.

Introduction

Renal function impairment is a chronic and progressive process that is usually a complication of hypertension, diabetes mellitus, glomerulonephritis, drug abuse or other etiologies such as heavy metal intoxication [1–4]. Advanced renal dysfunction results in end-stage renal disease (ESRD), which may render patients dialysis-dependent. Chronic kidney disease can be considered a pre-ESRD stage whose prevalence during this period in Taiwan was usually underestimated due to lack of public awareness [5,6]. Health care for patients with chronic kidney disease or ESRD is usually a complicated task due to their diverse etiologies, coexisting diseases, complications and types of dialysis [5,7]. The issues of patient awareness, socio-economic status, compliance with ther-

apy, vascular accessibility and nutritional and hormonal balance might also further increase the complexity of dialysis patient care [8,9].

As expected, overall mortality of dialysis-dependent patients is much higher than of non-dialysis populations, especially due to cardiovascular diseases and their complications [1,10,11]. Recent improvement in dialysis techniques, such as more frequent dialysis and more effective retained solutes removal, have provided uremic patients with longer survival times and better life quality [12–15]. With the prolongation of lifespan, dialysis-dependent patients are more likely to undergo surgical procedures. As for postoperative complications and mortality, most studies were confined to cardiovascular surgeries and procedures [16–18]; investigations on other surgeries were few with limited sample sizes [19,20]. Accordingly, global postoperative outcomes for dialysis patients exposed to non-cardiac surgery on a population-based scale were not well defined.

Taiwan has noted the world's highest prevalence rate of ESRD during 2001–2007, with a total of 53,242 ESRD subjects undergoing dialysis treatment by 2008 [1] and the estimated prevalence rate of chronic kidney disease for adults aged 20 years and older over the period from 1994 to 2006 was 11.93% [5]. We conducted a retrospective nationwide population-based study among dialysis-dependent surgical patients receiving non-cardiac surgery to illustrate the global features of postoperative complications and mortality, the impact of peritoneal dialysis (PD) or hemodialysis (HD), coexisting with hypertension or diabetes mellitus, and additional medical conditions on postoperative adverse outcomes.

Methods

Data Sources and Study Population

This study used reimbursement claims data from Taiwan's National Health Insurance, a universal insurance program started in March 1995. More than 99% of 22.6 million Taiwan residents are enrolled in this system. Taiwan's National Health Research Institutes established a National Health Insurance Research Database (NHIRD) to record all beneficiaries' inpatient and outpatient medical services. Information in the database includes patients' demographics, primary and secondary disease diagnoses, procedures, prescriptions and medical expenditures. The NHIRD's validity has been documented [21] and research from this database has been published in our previous work and by many others [22,23]. For confidentiality, the electronic database was decoded with patient identifications scrambled to protect privacy for further public access. The study was evaluated and approved by the NHIRD research committee.

We examined medical claims and identified 8,937 surgical patients with preoperative regular HD or PD from 2,010,412 persons who underwent major inpatient surgeries between 2004 and 2007. Receiving HD or PD at least three times per week for more than three months before the index surgery was defined as preoperative regular dialysis in this study [24,25]. We used propensity-score to select matched-controls randomly by age, sex, teaching hospital, coexisting disease, type of surgery and anesthesia from surgical patient populations without a history of preoperative renal dialysis. Major inpatient surgeries are defined as surgeries requiring general, epidural or spinal anesthesia and hospitalization for more than one day.

We used propensity-score matched-pairs analyses to determine the adjusted association of preoperative renal dialysis with the primary outcome (30-day mortality). We developed a non-parsimonious multivariable logistic regression model to estimate a propensity score for preoperative renal dialysis, irrespective of outcome. Clinical significance guided the initial choice of covariates in this model: age, sex, coexisting medical conditions (included hypertension, stroke, chronic obstructive pulmonary diseases, myocardial infarction, diabetes, congestive heart failure, peripheral vascular disease, and emergency operation), teaching hospital, types of surgery, and types of anesthesia. According to a statistical research on the development of propensity score [26], we used a structured iterative approach to refine this model, with the goal of achieving covariate balance within the matched-pairs. The chi-square tests were used to measure covariate balance and a p-value <0.05 was suggested to represent meaningful covariate imbalance. We matched renal-dialysis patients to non-dialysis patients using a greedy-matching algorithm with a calliper width of 0.2 SD of the log odds of the estimated propensity score. This method could remove 98% of the bias from measured covariates [27,28].

Outcome Measures

We evaluated coexisting medical illnesses of study subjects including acute myocardial infarction, acute renal failure, chronic obstructive pulmonary disease, congestive heart failure, hypertension, diabetes mellitus, peripheral vascular disease and stroke within the preoperative 24-month period using medical claims data. Parameters of medical services used, such as surgeries performed in teaching hospitals or not and emergency operations, were also considered as surgical functional status. Six major postoperative complications (acute myocardial infarction, deep wound infection, pneumonia, postoperative bleeding, septicemia and stroke) and subsequent overall in-hospital mortality within 30 days after index surgery were the study's primary outcomes [29]. Information collected on surgical admission included length of hospital and intensive care unit stays. We considered the patients in specific groups who's length of hospitalization were above the lower limit of the highest quintile of length of stay (≥18 days in this study) among the overall patients and divided by number of patients in each group as the percent of increased length of stay. The same definition was applied to percentage of increased medical expenditures. The ICU stay and increased length of stay were also identified as adverse outcomes. According to the *International Classification of Diseases, 9th Revision, Clinical Modification* (ICD-9-CM) we defined comorbidities and postoperative complications including hypertension (ICD-9-CM 401–405), chronic obstructive pulmonary disease (ICD-9-CM 490–496), diabetes mellitus (ICD-9-CM 250), stroke (ICD-9-CM 430–438), acute myocardial infarction (ICD-9-CM 410), congestive heart failure (ICD-9-CM 428), peripheral vascular disease (ICD-9-CM 443), postoperative bleeding (ICD-9-CM 998.0, 998.1 and 998.2), pneumonia (ICD-9-CM 480–486), septicemia (ICD-9-CM 038, 998.5) and deep wound infection (ICD-9-CM 958).

To assess dialysis type-specific effects on postoperative complications and mortality, we categorized preoperative dialysis into HD and PD. The differential effects of preoperative hypertension and diabetes mellitus and of numbers of coexisting medical conditions on postoperative complications and mortality were also evaluated among surgical patients receiving dialysis.

Data Analysis

We compared postoperative complication and mortality rates between surgical patients with and without preoperative dialysis using Chi-square tests and descriptive parameters concerning demographic status, coexisting medical conditions, operation in teaching hospital or not, and types of surgery and anesthesia. Odds ratios (ORs) and 95% confidence intervals (CIs) for increased length of stay, ICU stay, 30-day postoperative complications and mortality associated with preoperative dialysis (HD or PD) were estimated in multivariate logistic regressions by adjusting operation in teaching hospital or not, preoperative coexisting medical conditions, and types of surgery and anesthesia. We also calculated the adjusted ORs and 95% CIs for surgical adverse outcomes associated with number of coexisting diseases and the effects of hypertension and diabetes. All analyses were performed using SAS statistical software (version 9.1 for Windows; SAS Institute). The results were considered statistically significant when 2-tailed p<0.05.

Results

Under propensity-score matched method, there was no significant difference in sociodemographic factors, co-existing medical conditions, types of surgery and types of anesthesia between patients with and without dialysis (Table 1). Compared with controls, patients with preoperative regular dialysis showed higher rates of postoperative acute myocardial infarction (1.23% vs. 0.69%, p<0.0001), pneumonia (7.23% vs. 4.73%, p<0.0001), bleeding (4.92% vs. 3.55%, p<0.0001), septicemia (10.98% vs. 4.46%, p<0.0001), overall postoperative complication rate (25.95% vs. 18.44%, p<0.0001) and significantly higher 30-day postoperative mortality rate (2.64% vs. 0.85%, p<0.0001) (Table 2). Incidence of increased length of hospitalization, ICU stay, and increased medical expenditure was higher in dialysis patients than in non-dialysis patients. After adjustment for age, sex, teaching hospital, coexisting disease and type of surgery and anesthesia, surgical patients with preoperative regular dialysis exhibited significantly higher risk of postoperative complications including acute myocardial infarction (OR 1.85; 95% CI 1.35 to 2.54), pneumonia (OR 1.70, 95% CI 1.49 to 1.94), postoperative bleeding (OR 1.40, 95% CI 1.21 to 1.63), septicemia (OR 2.83, 95% CI 2.50 to 3.20) and overall complications (OR 1.70, 95% CI 1.58 to 1.84). The corresponding OR for 30-day postoperative mortality was 3.33 (95% CI 2.56 to 4.33). The ORs of preoperative dialysis associated with increased length of stay, ICU stay and increased medical expenditure were 2.20 (95% CI 2.03 to 2.38), 2.37 (95% CI 2.20 to 2.55), and 2.91 (95% CI 2.68 to 3.16), respectively.

Considering 30-day postoperative mortality among patients receiving different types of renal dialysis, surgical patients had higher risk when receiving regular preoperative PD (OR 2.71, 95% CI 1.70 to 4.31) or HD (OR 3.42, 95% CI 2.62 to 4.47) when compared with surgical patients without dialysis. As for postoperative complications, preoperative HD or PD significantly increased risk of postoperative pneumonia, postoperative bleeding, septicemia and overall complications without significant differences between PD and HD (Table 3). HD patients had no significant higher mortality after surgery compared with PD patients (OR = 1.26, 95% CI 0.82–1.94) (not showed in the tables).

Among patients with regular dialysis, those who had both hypertension and diabetes were at the highest risk of 30-day postoperative pneumonia (OR 1.68, 95% CI 1.19 to 2.38), septicemia (OR 1.45, 95% CI 1.09 to 1.93), stroke (OR 1.89, 95% CI 1.27 to 2.81) and overall major complications (OR 1.74, 95% CI 1.43 to 2.13) compared with patients without diabetes or hypertension (Table 4). The highest risks of increased length of stay (OR 1.78, 95% CI 1.46 to 2.17), ICU stay (OR 1.22, 95% CI 1.02 to 1.44) and increased medical expenditure (OR 1.44, 95% CI 1.21 to 1.73) were also found in patients with hypertension and diabetes compared with patients without diabetes or hypertension.

Among surgical patients with preoperative renal dialysis, the number of preoperative co-existing medical illnesses was associated with postoperative adverse outcomes including postoperative bleeding, septicemia, stroke and overall complications. The risks of increased length of hospitalization, ICU stay and increased medical expenditure were positively correlated with the number of preoperative co-existing diseases among surgical patients with preoperative renal dialysis (Table 5).

Discussion

After adjusting the covariates under propensity-score matched method in this large-scale population-based study, ESRD patients with preoperative dialysis therapy, either PD or HD, encountered

Table 1. Characteristics of surgical patients with renal dialysis and controls.*

	Controls, N = 8937		Dialysis, N = 8937		p
Sex	n	(%)	n	(%)	1.00
Female	4892	(54.7)	4892	(54.7)	
Male	4045	(45.3)	4045	(45.3)	
Age, years					0.34
20–29	136	(1.5)	161	(1.8)	
30–39	425	(4.8)	450	(5.0)	
40–49	1157	(13.0)	1193	(13.4)	
50–59	2044	(22.9)	2080	(23.3)	
60–69	2296	(25.7)	2286	(25.6)	
70–79	2148	(24.0)	2093	(23.4)	
≥80	731	(8.2)	674	(7.5)	
Operation in teaching hospital					0.34
No	329	(3.7)	353	(4.0)	
Yes	8608	(96.3)	8584	(96.0)	
Coexisting medical conditions					
Hypertension	7558	(84.6)	7518	(84.1)	0.41
Stroke	1654	(18.5)	1637	(18.3)	0.74
COPD	3276	(36.7)	3268	(36.6)	0.90
Myocardial infarction	3965	(44.4)	3930	(44.0)	0.59
Diabetes	4628	(51.8)	4589	(51.4)	0.55
Congestive heart failure	3387	(37.9)	3399	(38.0)	0.85
Peripheral vascular disease	692	(7.7)	730	(8.2)	0.29
Emergency operation	455	(5.1)	507	(5.7)	0.08
Types of surgery					0.91
Skin	580	(6.5)	604	(6.8)	
Breast	75	(0.8)	82	(0.9)	
Musculoskeletal	2768	(31.0)	2750	(30.8)	
Respiratory	388	(4.3)	382	(4.3)	
Digestive	1871	(20.9)	1888	(21.1)	
Kidney, ureter, bladder	1269	(14.2)	1283	(14.4)	
Delivery, CS, abortion	28	(0.3)	28	(0.3)	
Neurosurgery	764	(8.6)	709	(7.9)	
Eye	155	(1.7)	171	(1.9)	
Others	1039	(11.6)	1040	(11.6)	
Types of anesthesia					0.43
General	6872	(76.9)	6828	(76.4)	
Epidural or spinal	2065	(23.1)	2109	(23.6)	

*Renal dialysis: at least three times per week lasting more than three months for dialysis therapy within the 24-month preoperative period.
COPD, chronic obstructive pulmonary disease; CS, caesarean section.

significantly higher postoperative complication and mortality rates compared with controls when receiving non-cardiac surgery, and facing significantly high risks of acute myocardial infarction, pneumonia, bleeding and septicemia. Compared with dialysis patients with neither hypertension nor diabetes mellitus, dialysis patients with hypertension and diabetes mellitus were found to

Table 2. Risk of 30-day postoperative mortality and complications among controls and patients with preoperative regular dialysis receiving non-cardiac surgery.

Adverse outcomes	Control, %	Dialysis, %	Multivariate* OR	(95% CI)
30-day postoperative mortality	0.85	2.64	3.33	(2.56–4.33)
Postoperative complications				
Acute myocardial infarction	0.69	1.23	1.85	(1.35–2.54)
Deep wound infection	0.85	0.54	0.62	(0.43–0.89)
Pneumonia	4.73	7.23	1.70	(1.49–1.94)
Postoperative bleeding	3.55	4.92	1.40	(1.21–1.63)
Septicemia	4.46	10.98	2.83	(2.50–3.20)
Stroke	8.11	7.43	0.94	(0.83–1.06)
Any of above	18.44	25.95	1.70	(1.58–1.84)
Increased length of stay†	13.92	24.57	2.20	(2.03–2.38)
ICU stay	20.06	33.47	2.37	(2.20–2.55)
Elevated medical expenditure	12.58	27.41	2.91	(2.68–3.16)

*Adjusted for age, sex, teaching hospital, coexisting disease and type of surgery and anesthesia.
†Increased length of stay: patients in specific groups who's length of hospitalization were above the lower limit of the highest quintile of length of stay (≥18 days in this study) among the overall patients and divided by number of patients in each group as the percent of increased length of stay.
OR, odds ratio; CI, confidence interval; ICU, intensive care unit.

have the highest relative risks for postoperative complications among groups. Increasing numbers of medical conditions were linked with incremental increases in rates for overall postoperative

complications, and medical utility when compared with dialysis patients without additional comorbidities.

Discrepancies were noted between the risks for systemic infection (pneumonia and septicemia) and deep wound infection among patients under dialysis management in our data and previous studies [19,20]. This might be explained by recent improvements in restrictive fluid management for surgical patients under dialysis therapy. During the last decade, worldwide acceptance of restrictive fluid regimens applied to surgical patients receiving major operations such as thoracic surgery resulted in significant decreases in pulmonary morbidity [30,31]. The restrictive fluid strategy for surgical patients further provided better outcomes than liberal fluid regimen in overall postoperative morbidity [32]. Cardiopulmonary and tissue-healing complications were also significantly reduced under a limited fluid administration regimen for patients receiving elective colorectal surgeries [33]. Most patients would receive dialysis treatment followed by restriction of perioperative fluid before elective surgery, and surgeons keep patients in a relatively dehydrated status to limit the potential risk of local/deep wound infection [34]. However, further prospective study is needed for an evidence-based explanation.

When kidney dysfunction progresses to ESRD, patients must choose a type of renal dialysis, PD or HD, for replacement therapy depending on patients' preference, economic status, geographic location and severity of comorbid illnesses [35]. Although the patients maintained on HD seem to have a higher comorbid burden than those on PD, outcome benefits were still equivocal [35–38]. The impact of different types of renal dialysis on surgical adverse outcomes in large scale has not been documented previously. After adjustment of patients' demographics and comorbidities with propensity-score matched-pair controls, we demonstrated that surgical patients under HD had relatively higher risk of in-hospital mortality than the PD group when compared with non-dialysis controls. As for postoperative complications, patients with HD showed similar risks in overall

Table 3. Risk of postoperative 30-day mortality and complications among surgical patients with peritoneal or hemodialysis versus controls.*

Adverse outcomes	Controls OR	(95% CI)	Peritoneal dialysis OR	(95% CI)	Hemodialysis OR	(95% CI)
30-day postoperative mortality	1.00	(reference)	2.71	(1.70–4.31)	3.42	(2.62–4.47)
Postoperative complications						
Acute myocardial infarction	1.00	(reference)	1.63	(0.87–3.06)	1.88	(1.37–2.59)
Deep wound infection	1.00	(reference)	0.28	(0.09–0.90)	0.67	(0.46–0.97)
Pneumonia	1.00	(reference)	1.73	(1.34–2.23)	1.70	(1.48–1.94)
Postoperative bleeding	1.00	(reference)	2.29	(1.82–2.87)	1.24	(1.06–1.45)
Septicemia	1.00	(reference)	2.73	(2.20–3.40)	2.85	(2.51–3.23)
Stroke	1.00	(reference)	0.96	(0.74–1.24)	0.93	(0.82–1.06)
Any of above	1.00	(reference)	1.86	(1.61–2.15)	1.68	(1.55–1.82)
Increased length of stay	1.00	(reference)	2.31	(1.99–2.68)	2.18	(2.01–2.37)
ICU stay	1.00	(reference)	2.27	(1.98–2.61)	2.38	(2.20–2.57)
Elevated medical expenditure	1.00	(reference)	2.78	(2.41–3.22)	2.94	(2.70–3.19)

*Adjusted for age, sex, teaching hospital, coexisting disease and type of surgery and anesthesia.
†The highest quintile of length of stay during the surgical admission (the patient percentage for each group belonging to the highest quintile of length of stay [≥18 days] of the total patients as percentage of increased length of stay).
OR, odds ratio; CI, confidence interval; ICU, intensive care unit.

Table 4. Postoperative mortality and complications associated with hypertension or diabetes mellitus in surgical patients with preoperative regular dialysis.*

	Hypertension		No		Yes		No		Yes	
	Diabetes		No		No		Yes		Yes	
	OR	(95% CI)	OR	(95% CI)	OR	(95% CI)	OR	(95% CI)	OR	(95% CI)
Postoperative 30-day mortality	1.00	(reference)	0.93	(0.56–1.55)	1.48	(0.68–3.25)	1.09	(0.65–1.81)		
Postoperative 30-day complications										
Acute myocardial infarction	1.00	(reference)	1.11	(0.45–2.75)	1.40	(0.34–5.70)	1.82	(0.76–4.39)		
Deep wound infection	1.00	(reference)	1.57	(0.35–7.15)	2.57	(0.35–18.9)	2.53	(0.57–11.3)		
Pneumonia	1.00	(reference)	1.17	(0.83–1.66)	1.48	(0.84–2.59)	1.68	(1.19–2.38)		
Postoperative bleeding	1.00	(reference)	1.51	(1.03–2.20)	1.45	(0.76–2.76)	1.50	(1.01–2.22)		
Septicemia	1.00	(reference)	1.06	(0.79–1.41)	1.53	(0.98–2.39)	1.45	(1.09–1.93)		
Stroke	1.00	(reference)	1.89	(1.27–2.79)	1.54	(0.80–2.95)	1.89	(1.27–2.81)		
Any of above	1.00	(reference)	1.32	(1.08–1.61)	1.58	(1.14–2.20)	1.74	(1.43–2.13)		
Increased length of stay[†]	1.00	(reference)	1.04	(0.85–1.27)	1.62	(1.18–2.24)	1.78	(1.46–2.17)		
ICU stay	1.00	(reference)	0.94	(0.80–1.11)	1.24	(0.92–1.67)	1.22	(1.02–1.44)		
Elevated medical expenditure	1.00	(reference)	1.03	(0.87–1.23)	1.47	(1.08–2.01)	1.44	(1.21–1.73)		

*Adjusted for age, sex, teaching hospital, coexisting disease and type of surgery and anesthesia.
[†]The highest quintile of length of stay during the surgical admission (the patient percentage for each group belonged to the highest quintile of length of stay [≥18 days] of the total patients as percentage of increased length of stay).
OR, odds ratio; CI, confidence interval; ICU, intensive care unit.

complications when compared with patients with PD except for acute myocardial infarction.

Comorbidities may predispose uremic patients to higher mortality and morbidity [39]. However, the impact of complex pre-existing comorbidities, as shown by numbers or types, on surgical outcomes in ESRD patients had not been well demon-strated. In our data, surgical dialysis patients with hypertension and diabetes mellitus exhibited the highest complication rates than patients with either hypertension or diabetes or neither. According to the 2005 annual data report by Taiwan's renal registry, causes other than chronic glomerulonephritis, chronic interstitial nephri-tis, hypertension or diabetes mellitus constituted a high proportion,

Table 5. Postoperative mortality and complications associated with additional coexisting diseases in surgical patients with preoperative regular dialysis.

	Number of co-existing diseases*									
	0		1		2		3		4	
	OR	(95% CI)	OR	(95% CI)	OR	(95% CI)	OR	(95% CI)	OR	(95% CI)
Postoperative 30-day mortality	1.00	(reference)	0.82	(0.38–1.76)	1.24	(0.62–2.48)	0.94	(0.46–1.91)	1.47	(0.75–2.89)
Postoperative 30-day complications										
Acute myocardial infarction	1.00	(reference)	NA[‡]		NA[‡]		NA[‡]		NA[‡]	
Deep wound infection	1.00	(reference)	NA[‡]		NA[‡]		NA[‡]		NA[‡]	
Pneumonia	1.00	(reference)	0.73	(0.46–1.15)	0.70	(0.45–1.08)	1.04	(0.69–1.58)	1.35	(0.91–2.02)
Postoperative bleeding	1.00	(reference)	1.66	(0.96–2.86)	2.04	(1.20–3.46)	1.61	(0.94–2.77)	2.12	(1.25–3.58)
Septicemia	1.00	(reference)	1.40	(0.89–2.20)	1.56	(1.01–2.40)	1.90	(1.24–2.91)	2.63	(1.73–3.99)
Stroke	1.00	(reference)	1.26	(0.74–2.15)	1.45	(0.87–2.40)	2.27	(1.38–3.74)	2.83	(1.74–4.60)
Any of above	1.00	(reference)	1.30	(0.98–1.72)	1.42	(1.08–1.86)	1.87	(1.43–2.44)	2.61	(2.01–3.39)
Increased length of stay[†]	1.00	(reference)	1.12	(0.84–1.48)	1.26	(0.96–1.65)	1.66	(1.27–2.17)	2.59	(2.00–3.36)
ICU stay	1.00	(reference)	0.90	(0.72–1.13)	0.99	(0.80–1.23)	1.21	(0.97–1.50)	1.54	(1.25–1.91)
Elevated medical expenditure	1.00	(reference)	1.12	(0.89–1.41)	1.08	(0.86–1.36)	1.32	(1.05–1.65)	1.83	(1.47–2.28)

*Adjusted for age, sex, teaching hospital, coexisting disease and types of surgery and anesthesia.
[†]The highest quintile of length of stay during the surgical admission (patient percentage for each group belonging to the highest quintile of length of stay [≥18 days] of the total patients as percentage of increased length of stay).
[‡]NA, Not available due to small sample size.
OR, odds ratio; CI, confidence interval; ICU, intensive care unit; NA, not available.

24.6% of ESRD, in prevalent dialysis patients [10]. The disparity in etiology other than common medical conditions might partially explain the relatively lower mortality of ESRD patients in Taiwan (118.2 per thousand dialysis patients) in comparison with that in the United States (236 per thousand dialysis patients) [1,10]. Similar conditions also exist in the Western world with environmental pollutants and drug abuse [2–4]. A possible explanation for this phenomenon might be attributed to etiologies other than hypertension and diabetes for this specific population. First, Orientals such as Taiwanese people were frequent users of traditional alternative medicine, and habitually received herbal remedies [3,40]. Another reason might be chronic use of self-prescribed over-the-counter analgesics such as aspirin, acetaminophen or conventional non-steroidal anti-inflammatory drugs which were universal [2]. Long-term exposure to these medications might result in chronic kidney disease and subsequent ESRD [2,3]. Renal impairment due to heavy metal intoxication should also be taken into consideration because environmental pollutants are ingested with water, food or herbal drugs; this is a critical health issue in Taiwan and over the world [4]. Lin et al. showed that low-level environmental lead exposure can accelerate progression of renal dysfunction in patients without diabetes mellitus or hypertension [4].

Patients with both hypertension and diabetes mellitus had higher risks over the non-hypertensive, non-diabetic group in postoperative pneumonia and septicemia, but these risks were not significantly different in patients with hypertension or diabetes alone. Patients with both hypertension and diabetes mellitus also had the significant risk in postoperative adverse outcomes. These results indicate the combination of hypertension and diabetes might have an additive influence surpassing each disease's individual effect on postoperative outcomes, especially systemic infection (pneumonia and septicemia) and cerebrovascular events. In contrast, dialysis patients without hypertension or diabetes exhibited lower morbidity rate, and it can be explained by difference in etiological severity between diabetes/hypertension, herbal drugs, analgesics, heavy metal intoxication and etc. In our data, the combined effect of hypertension and diabetes increased the risk of deep wound infection without statistical significance and the independent association between diabetes and deep wound infection in dialysis surgical patients is still controversial.

Several limitations of this study must be addressed. First, the study is retrospective, and the database did not disclose detailed information regarding characteristics or severity of dialysis, such as specific etiology and definite duration of dialysis. The administrative database also lacked detailed profiles of dialysis management including dialysis time, type of dialysate, use of specific drugs and body weight changes. All of these factors might relate to surgical risks in patients under regular maintenance dialysis. In addition, detailed variables concerning the perioperative risks of surgery and anesthesia are not available in this database, such as preoperative laboratory data, blood pressure, oxygenation status, total blood loss, transfusions, and the use of prophylaxis antibiotics or inotropes. With such a large sample size in this study, we assumed that the influence of all of these covariates was evenly distributed between groups and bias would be diminished. Third, the study's design and grouping of hemodialysis versus peritoneal dialysis, hypertension versus diabetes mellitus, and categorization by the numbers of comorbidities, are all procedure- or diagnosis-oriented. Thus the study can validate only the association of factors and outcomes, not causation. Finally, our retrospective study did not achieve randomized distribution between groups. In spite of meticulous adjustment of major covariates, this non-randomization might still influence risk estimations and need further investigation.

In this nationwide population-based study using Taiwan's National Health Insurance Research Database with propensity-score matched method, we found significant increases in postoperative mortality and complication rates among surgical patients with preoperative regular dialysis underwent non-cardiac surgeries, either HD or PD. Increasing numbers of comorbidities, including hypertension or diabetes, may predispose these patients to higher rates of postoperative complications. Our findings suggested that meticulous preoperative assessment, optimal control for diabetes and hypertension, early recognition of morbidities and appropriate interventions might reduce adverse outcomes in dialysis patients receiving non-cardiac surgery.

Author Contributions

Conceived and designed the experiments: YGC CCL TLC. Performed the experiments: CCL CHW TLC. Analyzed the data: YGC CCL THC DX CHW TLC. Contributed reagents/materials/analysis tools: CCL DX CHW TLC. Wrote the paper: YGC TLC.

References

1. National Institute of Diabetes and Digestive and Kidney Diseases (2010) U.S. Renal Data System. USRDS 2010 annual data report. Atlas of chronic kidney disease and end-stage renal disease in the United States. Bethesda, MD: National Institutes of Health, National Institute of Diabetes and Digestive and Kidney Diseases.

2. Kuo HW, Tsai SS, Tiao MM, Liu YC, Lee IM, et al. (2010) Analgesic use and the risk for progression of chronic kidney disease. Pharmacoepidemiol Drug Saf 19: 745–751.

3. Guh JY, Chen HC, Tsai JF, Chuang LY (2007) Herbal therapy is associated with the risk of CKD in adults not using analgesics in Taiwan. Am J Kidney Dis 49: 626–633.

4. Lin JL, Lin-Tan DT, Hsu KH, Yu CC (2003) Environmental lead exposure and progression of chronic renal diseases in patients without diabetes. N Engl J Med 348: 277–286.

5. Wen CP, Cheng TYD, Tsai MK, Chang YC, Chan HT, et al. (2008) All-cause mortality attributable to chronic kidney disease: a prospective cohort study based on 462293 adults in Taiwan. Lancet 371: 2173–2182.

6. Kuo HW, Tsai SS, Tiao MM, Yang CY (2007) Epidemiological features of CKD in Taiwan. Am J Kidney Dis 49: 46–55.

7. Ifudu O (1998) Care of patients undergoing hemodialysis. N Engl J Med 339: 1054–1062.

8. Himmelfarb J, Ikizler TA (2010) Hemodialysis. N Engl J Med 363: 1833–1845.

9. Yang WC, Hwang SJ, Chiang SS, Chen HF, Tsai ST (2001) The impact of diabetes on economic costs in dialysis patients: experiences in Taiwan. Diabetes Res Clin Pract 54 Suppl 1: S47–S54.

10. Huang CC (2008) Taiwan renal registry- 2005 annual data report. Acta Nephrologica 22: 215–228.

11. de Jager DJ, Grootendorst DC, Jager KJ, van Dijk PC, Tomas LM, et al. (2009) Cardiovascular and noncardiovascular mortality among patients starting dialysis. JAMA 302: 1782–1789.

12. Meyer TW, Hostetter TH (2007) Uremia. N Engl J Med 357: 1316–1325.

13. Pastan S, Bailey J (1998) Dialysis therapy. N Engl J Med 338: 1428–1437.

14. Schiffl H, Lang SM, Fischer R (2002) Daily hemodialysis and the outcome of acute renal failure. N Engl J Med 346: 305–310.

15. The FHN trial group (2010) In-center hemodialysis six times per week versus three times per week. N Engl J Med 363: 2287–2300.

16. Bechtel JF, Detter C, Fischlein T, Krabatsch T, Osswald BR, et al. (2008) Cardiac surgery in patients on dialysis: decreased 30-day mortality, unchanged overall survival. Ann Thorac Surg 85: 147–153.

17. Penta de Peppo A, Nardi P, De Paulis R, Pellegrino A, Forlani S, et al. (2002) Cardiac surgery in moderate to end-stage renal failure: analysis of risk factors. Ann Thorac Surg 74: 378–383.

18. Herzog CA, Ma JZ, Collins AJ (2002) Comparative survival of dialysis patients in the United States after coronary angioplasty, coronary artery stenting, and coronary artery bypass surgery and impact on diabetes. Circulation 106: 2207–2211.

19. Yu YH, Chen WJ, Chen LH, Niu CC, Fu TS, et al. (2011) Posterior instrumented lumbar spinal surgery in uremic patients under maintenance hemodialysis. Spine 36: 660–666.

20. Drolet S, Maclean AR, Myers RP, Shaheen AA, Elijah Dixon E, et al. (2010) Morbidity and mortality following colorectal surgery in patients with end-stage renal failure: a population-based study. Dis Colon Rectum 53: 1508–1516.

21. Cheng CL, Kao YHY, Lin SJ, Lee CH, Lai ML (2011) Validation of the National Health Insurance Research Database with ischemic stroke cases in Taiwan. Pharmacoepidemiol Drug Saf 20: 236–242.

22. Lin JA, Liao CC, Chang CC, Chang H, Chen TL (2011) Postoperative adverse outcomes in intellectually disabled surgical patients: a nationwide population-based study. PLoS One 6: e26977.

23. Liao CC, Shen WW, Chang CC, Chang H, Chen TL (2013) Surgical adverse outcomes in patients with schizophrenia: a population-based study. Ann Surg 257: 433–438.

24. Perrinet M, Décaudin B, Champs BB, Heran I, Urbina MA, et al. (2010) Chronic dialysis-associated anaemia in end-stage renal disease: analysis of management in two French centres. J Clin Pharm Ther 35: 395–400.

25. Lin HF, Li YH, Wang CH, Chou CL, Kuo DJ, et al. (2011) Increased risk of cancer in chronic dialysis patients: a population-based cohort study in Taiwan. Nephrol Dial Transplant 27: 1585–1590.

26. Austin PC (2007) Propensity-score matching in the cardiovascular surgery literature from 2004 to 2006: a systematic review and suggestions for improvement. J Thorac Cardiovasc Surg 134: 1128–1135.

27. Rosenbaum PR, Rubin DB (1985) Constructing a control group using multivariate matched sampling methods that incorporate the propensity score. Am Stat 39: 33–38.

28. Wijeysundera DN, Beattie WS, Austin PC, Hux JE, Laupacis A (2008) Epidural anaesthesia and survival after intermediate-to-high risk non-cardiac surgery: a population-based cohort study. Lancet 372: 562–569.

29. Khuri SF, Henderson WG, DePalma RG, Mosca C, Healey NA, et al. (2005) Determinants of long-term survival after major surgery and the adverse effect of postoperative complications. Ann Surg 242: 326–341.

30. Parquin F, Marchal M, Mehiri S, Hervé P, Lescot B (1996) Post-pneumonectomy pulmonary edema: analysis and risk factors. Eur J Cardiothorac Surg 10: 929–933.

31. Slinger PD (1995) Perioperative fluid management for thoracic surgery: the puzzle of postpneumonectomy pulmonary edema. J Cardiothorac Vasc Anesth 9: 442–451.

32. Nisanevich V, Felsenstein I, Almogy G, Weissman C, Einav S, et al. (2005) Effect of intraoperative fluid management on outcome after intraabdominal surgery. Anesthesiology 103: 25–32.

33. Brandstrup B, Tonnesen H, Beier-Holgersen R, Hjortso E, Ording H, et al. (2003) Effects of intravenous fluid restriction on postoperative complications: comparison of two perioperative fluid regimens. Ann Surg 238: 641–648.

34. Miller RD, Eriksson LI, Fleisher LA, Wiener-Kronish JP, Young WL (2009) Miller's Anesthesia. In: Roizen MF, Fleisher LA, editors. Anesthetic implications of concurrent Diseases. Philadelphia, PA: Churchill Livingstone. 1067–1149.

35. Murphy SW, Foley RN, Barrett BJ, Kent GM, Morgan J, et al. (2000) Comparative mortality of hemodialysis and peritoneal dialysis in Canada. Kidney Int 57: 1720–1726.

36. Noordzij M, Korevaar JC, Bos WJ, Boeschoten EW, Dekker FW, et al. (2006) Mineral metabolism and cardiovascular morbidity and mortality risk: peritoneal dialysis patients compared with haemodialysis patients. Nephrol Dial Transplant 21: 2513–2520.

37. Winkelmayer WC, Glynn RJ, Mittleman MA, Levin R, Pliskin JS, et al. (2002) Comparing mortality of elderly patients on hemodialysis versus peritoneal dialysis: a propensity score approach. J Am Soc Nephrol 13: 2353–2362.

38. Jaar BG, Coresh J, Plantinga LC, Fink NE, Klag MJ, et al. (2005) Comparing the risk for death with peritoneal dialysis and hemodialysis in a national cohort of patients with chronic kidney disease. Ann Intern Med 143: 174–183.

39. Prichard SS (2000) Comorbidities and their impact on outcome in patients with end-stage renal disease. Kidney Int 57: S100–S104.

40. Tsai SY, Tseng HF, Tan HF, Chien YS, Chang CC (2009) End-stage renal disease in Taiwan: a case-control study. J Epidemiol 19: 169–176.

27

Progression of Aortic Arch Calcification over 1 Year is an Independent Predictor of Mortality in Incident Peritoneal Dialysis Patients

Mi Jung Lee[1], Dong Ho Shin[1], Seung Jun Kim[1], Hyung Jung Oh[1], Dong Eun Yoo[1], Kwang Il Ko[1], Hyang Mo Koo[1], Chan Ho Kim[1], Fa Mee Doh[1], Jung Tak Park[1], Seung Hyeok Han[1], Tae-Hyun Yoo[1,2], Kyu Hun Choi[1], Shin-Wook Kang[1,2]*

1 Department of Internal Medicine, College of Medicine, Yonsei University, Seoul, Korea, **2** Severance Biomedical Science Institute, Brain Korea 21, Yonsei University, Seoul, Korea

Abstract

Backgrounds and Aims: The presence and progression of vascular calcification have been demonstrated as important risk factors for mortality in dialysis patients. However, since the majority of subjects included in most previous studies were hemodialysis patients, limited information was available in peritoneal dialysis (PD) patients. Therefore, the aim of this study was to investigate the prevalence of aortic arch calcification (AoAC) and prognostic value of AoAC progression in PD patients.

Methods: We prospectively determined AoAC by chest X-ray at PD start and after 12 months, and evaluated the impact of AoAC progression on mortality in 415 incident PD patients.

Results: Of 415 patients, 169 patients (40.7%) had AoAC at baseline with a mean of $18.1 \pm 11.2\%$. The presence of baseline AoAC was an independent predictor of all-cause [Hazard ratio (HR): 2.181, 95% confidence interval (CI): 1.336–3.561, $P = 0.002$] and cardiovascular mortality (HR: 3.582, 95% CI: 1.577–8.132, $P = 0.002$). Among 363 patients with follow-up chest X-rays at 12 months after PD start, the proportion of patients with AoAC progression was significantly higher in patients with baseline AoAC (64.2 vs. 5.3%, $P < 0.001$). Moreover, all-cause and cardiovascular death rates were significantly higher in the progression groups than in the non-progression group ($P < 0.001$). Multivariate Cox analysis revealed that AoAC progression was an independent predictor for all-cause (HR: 2.625, 95% CI: 1.150–5.991, $P = 0.022$) and cardiovascular mortality (HR: 4.008, 95% CI: 1.079–14.890, $P = 0.038$) in patients with AoAC at baseline.

Conclusions: The presence and progression of AoAC assessed by chest X-ray were independently associated with unfavorable outcomes in incident PD patients. Regular follow-up by chest X-ray could be a simple and useful method to stratify mortality risk in these patients.

Editor: Hugo ten Cate, Maastricht University Medical Center, The Netherlands

Funding: This work was supported by the Brain Korea 21 Project for Medical Science, Yonsei University, by the National Research Foundation of Korea grant funded by the Korea government (MEST) (No. 2011-0030711), and by a grant of the Korea Healthcare Technology Research & Development project, Ministry ofHealth and Welfare, Republic of Korea (A102065). The funders had no role in study design, data collection and analysis, decision to publish, or preparation of the manuscript.

Competing Interests: The authors have declared that no competing interests exist.

* E-mail: kswkidney@yumc.yonsei.ac.kr

Introduction

Cardiovascular disease is the most common cause of morbidity and mortality in patients with end-stage renal disease (ESRD) [1]. Since traditional risk factors, such as advanced age, hypertension, diabetes, smoking, and dyslipidemia, cannot fully account for the high prevalence of cardiovascular disease, uremia-related factors, including inflammation and oxidative stress, have been implicated in the pathogenesis of cardiovascular disease in ESRD patients [2]. Recently, accumulating evidence has shown that disturbances in calcium-phosphorus metabolism also play a pivotal role in cardiovascular disease, partly via the development of vascular calcification [2,3,4].

Vascular calcification is not uncommon in general elderly population; 20–30% of people older than 65 years have calcification in the aorta [5]. In patients with chronic kidney disease (CKD), this proportion is reported to be substantially higher; more than one half of CKD patients even before the start of dialysis and up to 80–90% of ESRD patients have some form of vascular calcification [6,7]. Previous studies have revealed vascular calcification is independently associated with all-cause and cardiovascular mortality in both general population and ESRD [3,8,9,10,11]. Moreover, since vascular calcification progresses rapidly in dialysis patients, ESRD patients with the progression of vascular calcification are demonstrated to have an unfavorable outcome [12]. Therefore, not only the identification of vascular calcification but also risk stratification of patients by the changes in vascular calcification may be important for clinicians to manage dialysis patients.

To date, a number of techniques are available to detect vascular calcification. Electron beam computed tomography (EBCT), multi-slice CT (MSCT), planar X-ray (such as plain X-ray of lateral abdomen, pelvis, and hands), 2D ultrasonography, and echocardiography have been used to assess vascular calcification [6,9,10,13,14,15,16,17]. Among these, EBCT and MSCT are well-validated noninvasive imaging methods that are considered the golden standard for quantifying vascular calcification. However, EBCT and MSCT cannot be routinely performed due to the relatively high cost of testing and exposure to a high radiation dose [16]. Recently, aortic arch calcification (AoAC) in plain chest X-rays was found to reflect the magnitude of whole aortic calcification in general population and dialysis patients [15,16]. In addition, several previous studies showed that AoAC was an independent predictor of cardiovascular events and that AoAC progression was significantly associated with increased cardiovascular mortality in patients with ESRD [3,11,18,19]. However, since the majority of subjects included in most previous studies were ESRD patients on hemodialysis (HD), little is known about the prevalence, natural history, and prognostic value of vascular calcification in peritoneal dialysis (PD) patients. In the present study, we investigated the prevalence of AoAC at PD initiation and the frequencies of AoAC progression or regression during the first year after PD. The impact of AoAC progression on all-cause and cardiovascular mortality was also determined.

Methods

Ethics Statement

The study was carried out in accordance with the Declaration of Helsinki and approved by the Institutional Review Board of Yonsei University Health System Clinical Trial Center. We obtained informed written consent from all participants involved in our study.

Patients

All consecutive ESRD patients over 18 years of age who started PD at Yonsei University Health System between January 2005 and June 2010 were initially included in this prospective observational study. Among a total of 530 incident PD patients, patients with PD duration of less than 3 months, active infection, malignancy, and decompensated liver cirrhosis were excluded. Thus, the remaining 415 patients were included in the final analysis.

Demographic and Clinical Data Collection

A well-trained examiner used a questionnaire at the time of PD start to collect demographic data. Traditional cardiovascular risk factors such as age, hypertension, diabetes mellitus, smoking history, and previous history of cardiovascular disease were recorded. In smokers, the amount of smoking was expressed as pack-years; the product of the number of cigarette packs consumed per day by the duration of smoking (years). Cardiovascular disease was defined as a history of coronary, cerebrovascular, or peripheral vascular disease: coronary disease was defined as a history of angioplasty, coronary artery bypass grafts, myocardial infarction, or angina and cerebrovascular disease as a history of transient ischemic attack, stroke, or carotid endarterectomy, while peripheral vascular disease was defined as a history of claudication, ischemic limb loss and/or ulceration, or peripheral revasculariza-

tion procedure. Patients were weighed in light clothing and height was measured with no shoes. Body mass index (BMI) was calculated as weight/height^2 (kg/m^2). Blood was drawn after a 12-hour overnight fasting, and the following laboratory data were measured from blood samples: hemoglobin, blood urea nitrogen, creatinine, calcium, phosphorus, albumin, total cholesterol, triglyceride, low density lipoprotein (LDL)-cholesterol, high density lipoprotein (HDL)-cholesterol, and intact parathyroid hormone (iPTH) concentrations. In addition, high sensitivity C-reactive protein (hs-CRP) levels were determined by a latex-enhanced immunoephelometric method using a BN II analyzer (Dade Behring, Newark, DE, USA). To reflect the actual situation, usual overnight dialysate volume and glucose concentrations were not changed for this study. Kt/V urea was determined from the total loss of urea nitrogen in spent dialysate using PD Adequest 2.0 for Windows software (Baxter Healthcare, Deerfield, Illinois, USA). The modified peritoneal equilibration test was performed with 4.25% glucose dialysis solution as described previously [20] and the dialysate-to-plasma creatinine (D/P Cr) and glucose (D/D0 glucose) concentration ratios at 4 hours of dwell were used to describe the peritoneal transport characteristics; high, high average, low average, and low.

Assessment of AoAC by Chest X-ray

To determine AoAC extent, two trained medical doctors blinded to the patients' clinical data reviewed posterior-anterior plain chest X-rays taken at the start of PD using a specific scale developed by Ogawa et al [16]. This scale, which divides the aortic arch into 16 sections by circumference, was attached to the aortic arch on chest X-rays and the number of sectors was divided by 16. AoAC scores (AoACS) were calculated after multiplication by 100 to express results as a percentage. To confirm the intra-reader variability, randomly selected 100 chest X-rays were reexamined by the same reader. The median intra-class correlation coefficient for AoACS was 0.91 [95% confidence interval (CI): 0.71 to 0.99] and 0.90 (95% CI: 0.69 to 0.98) in two readers. In addition, any discrepancies between the two observers were resolved by an independent third reader. Progression of AoAC was defined as an increase in AoACS on the follow-up chest X-ray taken 1 year after PD initiation.

Follow-up and Endpoints

All patients included in this study were regularly followed-up at the PD clinic, and all deaths and hospitalization were recorded in the serious adverse events database. Mortality events were retrieved from the database and carefully reviewed to determine all-cause and cardiovascular mortality. Cardiovascular mortality was considered death from myocardial infarction or ischemia, congestive heart failure, pulmonary edema, and cerebral hemorrhage or vascular disorder.

Among 415 patients, follow-up chest X-rays at 12 months were not available in 52 patients; 30 died within 12 months of PD start, 11 changed dialysis modality to HD, 9 underwent kidney transplantation, and 2 were transferred to other PD units. Therefore, the association between the progression of AoAC and survival was analyzed in 363 patients.

Statistical Analysis

Statistical analysis was performed using SPSS for Windows version 18.0 (SPSS Inc., Chicago, IL, USA). Continuous variables were expressed as mean ± SD, and categorical variables were expressed as a number (percentage). Since hs-CRP did not yield a Gaussian distribution, log values were used. In the first analysis, 415 patients were divided into two groups according to the presence of AoAC at baseline. To determine differences between the two groups, a Student's t-test and the chi-square test were performed for continuous variables and categorical variables, respectively. Multivariate binary logistic regression models were used to identify significant determinants of AoAC presence at PD initiation. Cumulative survival curves were generated by the Kaplan-Meier method, and between-group survival was compared by a log-rank test. Independent prognostic values of AoAC at baseline for all-cause and cardiovascular mortality were ascertained by Cox proportional hazards models, which included only the significant variables in univariate analysis. Meanwhile, the progression of AoAC was focused in the second analysis. In the second analysis, mean values of the biochemical parameters during the first year of PD were used. Pearson's correlation analysis was performed to estimate association between the changes in AoACS and other continuous variables. Multivariate binary logistic regression models, which included significant variables in univariate analysis, were constructed to determine significant independent predictors of AoAC progression. Subgroup analysis was also performed according to the presence of baseline AoAC. The impact of AoAC progression on patient outcome was examined by the Kaplan-Meier method and Cox proportional hazards regression analysis. Significant variables in univariate analysis, traditional risk factors (age, sex, and diabetes mellitus), and factors associated with inflammation and nutrition (serum hs-CRP and albumin concentrations) were included in multivariate Cox proportional hazard models. A P value less than 0.05 was considered statistically significant.

Results

Clinical Characteristics According to the Presence of AoAC at Baseline

Baseline patient characteristics according to the presence of AoAC at baseline are shown in Table 1. The mean age was 55.8 ± 13.8 years (21–80 years), and 234 patients (56.3%) were male. Of 415 patients, 169 patients (40.7%) had AoAC at baseline with a mean AoACS of $18.1 \pm 11.2\%$. Diabetic nephropathy was the most common cause of ESRD, followed by chronic glomerulonephritis in both groups. The mean age, the proportion of patients with diabetes and previous history of cardiovascular disease, and the proportion of patients taking lipid-lowering agents and β-blockers were significantly higher in patients with AoAC at baseline. In addition, compared to patients without baseline AoAC, total cholesterol, iPTH, and albumin concentrations were significantly lower, while hs-CRP levels were significantly higher in the baseline AoAC present group. Moreover, even though the proportion of smoker was significantly lower, the mean amount of smoking was significantly greater in patients with baseline AoAC. Among 224 patients (53.9%), who performed echocardiography at baseline, the ejection fraction was significantly lower in patients with baseline AoAC compared to the baseline AoAC absent group. On the other hand, there were no significant differences in peritoneal membrane transport characteristics, weekly Kt/V urea, systolic blood pressure, BMI, calcium-phosphate (Ca x P) product values, and the use of phosphate binders between the two groups.

Association of Various Parameters with the Presence of AoAC at Baseline

In univariate analysis, age, diabetes mellitus, previous history of cardiovascular disease, smoking, lipid-lowering therapy, serum

Table 1. Baseline characteristics of the patients with and without aortic arch calcification (AoAC).

Characteristics	With AoAC	Without AoAC	P
Number (%)	169 (40.7%)	246 (59.3%)	
Age (years)	66.7±9.3	52.1±13.1	<0.001
Male, n (%)	88 (52.0%)	146 (59.3%)	NS
Diabetes mellitus, n (%)	104 (61.5%)	92 (37.3%)	<0.001
Primary renal disease, n (%)			NS
Glomerulonephritis	38 (22.4%)	73 (29.6%)	
Diabetes mellitus	86 (50.9%)	84 (34.1%)	
Hypertensive nephrosclerosis	12 (7.1%)	21 (8.5%)	
Polycystic kidney disease	1 (0.6%)	4 (1.6%)	
Others/Unknown	32 (18.9%)	64 (26.0%)	
Peritoneal equilibration test, n (%)			NS
High	7 (4.1%)	24 (9.8%)	
High average	123 (72.7%)	126 (51.2%)	
Low average	34 (20.1%)	90 (36.5%)	
Low	5 (2.9%)	6 (2.4%)	
Kt/V urea (per week)	2.3±0.5	2.5±0.7	NS
Cardiovascular disease, n (%)	94 (55.6%)	51 (20.7%)	<0.001
Ejection fraction (%)	52.8±17.5	61.4±9.8	0.03
History of smoking, n (%)	41 (24.2%)	87 (35.3%)	0.02
Amount of smoking (pack-years)	35.1±24.0	24.1±18.2	0.03
Systolic blood pressure (mmHg)	139.3±21.8	139.8±19.8	NS
BMI (kg/m^2)	22.6±3.0	22.6±3.1	NS
Hemoglobin (g/dL)	9.2±1.4	9.2±1.6	NS
Total cholesterol (mg/dL)	147.7±43.5	158.8±43.4	0.02
Ca × P product (mg^2/dL^2)	41.6±12.7	43.9±12.6	NS
iPTH (pg/mL)	138.4±123.8	213.5±176.0	<0.001
Albumin (g/dL)	3.4±0.5	3.5±0.6	0.008
Log hs-CRP (mg/L)	0.1±0.6	−0.2±0.9	<0.001
Lipid-lowering therapy, n (%)	80 (47.3%)	65 (26.4%)	<0.001
Antihypertensive drugs, n (%)			
RAS blockers	128 (75.7%)	189 (76.8%)	NS
Beta-blockers	105 (62.1%)	111 (45.1%)	0.03
Calcium channel blockers	107 (63.3%)	150 (60.9%)	NS
Phosphate binders, n (%)			NS
Calcium-based	88 (52.0%)	126 (51.2%)	
Non calcium-based	13 (7.6%)	19 (7.7%)	

Data are expressed as mean ± standard deviation or number of patients (percent).
Kt/V, fractional urea clearance; BMI, body mass index; Ca, calcium; P, phosphate; iPTH, intact parathyroid hormone; hs-CRP, high sensitivity C-reative protein; RAS, Renin-angiotensin system; NS, not significant.

albumin, iPTH, and hs-CRP concentrations were significantly associated with the presence of AoAC at baseline. Multivariate binary logistic regression analysis revealed that age [odds ratio (OR): 1.101, 95% CI: 1.066–1.138, $P<0.001$] and previous history of cardiovascular disease (OR: 2.084, 95% CI: 1.006–4.314, $P=0.048$) were significant independent factors associated with the presence of AoAC at baseline.

Presence of AoAC at Baseline as an Independent Risk Factor for All-cause and Cardiovascular Mortality

During a mean follow-up duration of 34.2±20.4 months, 90 patients (21.7%) died. Among them, 39 patients (43.3%) died from cardiovascular causes. Both the all-cause and cardiovascular mortality-free survival rates were significantly lower in patients with baseline AoAC (log-rank test, $P<0.001$) (Figure 1). Univariate Cox proportional hazard analysis showed older age, presence of diabetes and previous cardiovascular disease, usage of lipid-lowering medication, increased Ca × P products and hs-CRP levels, decreased albumin concetrations, and presence of AoAC at baseline were significant risk factors for all-cause and cardiovascular mortality. In multivariate Cox analysis, the presence of baseline AoAC was revealed as a significant independent predictor of all-cause [Hazard ratio (HR): 2.181, 95% CI: 1.336–3.561, $P=0.002$] and cardiovascular mortality (HR: 3.582, 95% CI: 1.577–8.132, $P=0.002$). Previous history of cardiovascular disease and higher hs-CRP levels were also found to be independent risk factors for all-cause and cardiovascular mortality. In contrast, older age was independently associated only with all-cause mortality (Table 2).

Progression of AoAC: Subgroup Analysis According to the Presence of Baseline AoAC

Follow-up chest X-rays at 12 months after PD start were available in 363 patients. Among them, 140 patients (38.5%) had AoAC at baseline and 223 patients (61.5%) did not. The progression of AoAC was significantly more observed in patients with AoAC at baseline ($P<0.001$). Among 140 patients with AoAC at baseline, 90 patients (64.2%) experienced AoAC progression, whereas AoAC progressed in only 12 (5.3%) out of 223 patients without baseline AoAC. Two hundred eleven patients with AoACS of zero at baseline remained free of AoAC during the 12-month follow-up.

Pearson's correlation analysis revealed that changes in AoACS were significantly associated with baseline AoACS ($r=0.389$, $P<0.001$), age ($r=0.301$, $P<0.001$), and time-averaged hs-CRP ($r=0.167$, $P=0.001$) and calcium concentrations ($r=0.124$, $P=0.02$). In multivariate binary logistic regression analysis,

Table 2. Multivariate Cox's proportional hazard models of baseline aortic arch calcification (AoAC) all-cause and cardiovascular mortality.

	All- cause mortality			Cardiovascular mortality		
	HR	95% CI	P	HR	95% CI	P
Age (years)	1.048	1.022–1.074	<0.001	1.028	0.988–1.069	NS
Male gender	1.136	0.660–1.954	NS	0.554	0.254–1.206	NS
Diabetes mellitus	1.071	0.679–1.690	NS	0.772	0.389–1.532	NS
Cardiovascular disease	2.000	1.143–3.500	0.015	3.807	1.441–10.054	0.007
History of smoking	0.928	0.520–1.657	NS	0.522	0.226–1.209	NS
Lipid-lowering therapy	1.027	0.629–1.676	NS	1.453	0.688–3.071	NS
Ca×P (mg^2/dL^2)	0.989	0.970–1.007	NS	1.002	0.972–1.032	NS
Albumin (g/dL)	0.763	0.520–1.118	NS	0.707	0.389–1.285	NS
Log hs-CRP (mg/L)	1.725	1.257–2.367	<0.001	1.769	1.044–2.996	0.034
Baseline AoAC	2.181	1.336–3.561	0.002	3.582	1.577–8.132	0.002

Ca, calcium; P, phosphate; hs-CRP, high sensitivity C-reative protein; HR, hazard ratio; CI, confidence interval; NS, not significant.

baseline AoACS (OR: 1.803, 95% CI: 1.383–2.349, $P<0.001$), age (OR: 1.058, 95% CI: 1.016–1.101, $P=0.006$), and hs-CRP levels (OR: 1.904, 95% CI: 1.180–3.070, $P=0.008$) were found to be independent risk factors associated with AoAC progression. Since the baseline AoACS was significantly correlated with AoAC progression, subgroup analysis was performed to clarify the independent predictor for AoAC progression in patients with and without baseline AoAC. In patients with AoAC at baseline, there was a significant correlation between hs-CRP concentrations and the changes in AoACS ($r=0.248$, $P=0.02$), while changes in AoACS were significantly associated with age ($r=0.124$, $P=0.04$) and hs-CRP levels ($r=0.126$, $P=0.036$) in patents without baseline AoAC. However, the changes in Ca × P products and

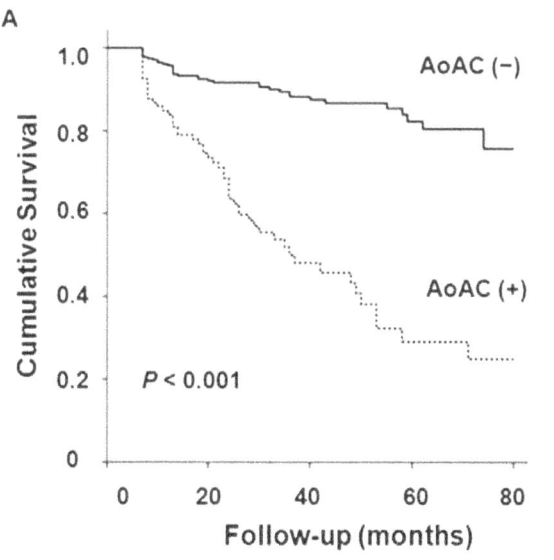
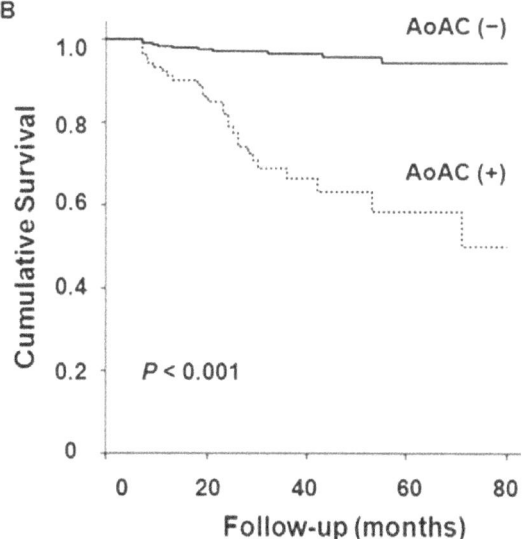

Figure 1. Kaplan-Meier analysis of (A) all-cause and (B) cardiovascular mortality in 415 patients. Patients with baseline aortic arch calcification (AoAC) showed significantly higher all-cause and cardiovascular mortality than those without (both log-rank test, $P<0.001$).

iPTH concentrations did not correlate with changes in AoACS in both subgroups.

Similar findings were observed in binary logistic regression analysis. In patients with AoAC at baseline, univariate analysis reavealed that diabetes mellitus, previous cardiovascular disease, lipid-lowering therapy, hs-CRP levels, and baseline AoACS were significantly associated with AoAC progression. In multivariate binary logistic regression models, baseline AoACS (OR: 1.234, 95% CI: 1.104–5.197, $P = 0.027$) and hs-CRP levels (OR: 2.238, 95% CI: 1.051–4.767, $P = 0.037$) were independent predictors of AoAC progression after adjustment for confounders. On the other hand, in patients without baseline AoAC, age, previous cardiovascular disease, the use of lipid-lowering drugs, and hs-CRP levels were significant predictors of AoAC progression in univariate analysis. Multivariate binary logistic regression models demonstrated that age (OR: 1.063, 95% CI: 1.014–1.113, $P = 0.002$) and hs-CRP concentrations (OR: 1.294, 95% CI: 1.019–4.581, $P = 0.035$) were significant risk factors for AoAC progression. However, peritoneal membrane transport characteristics, weekly Kt/V urea, Ca x P products, iPTH concentrations, and the use of phosphate binders were not significantly associated with AoAC progression in both subgroups.

Progression of AoAC as an Independent Risk Factor for Mortality

In patients with AoAC at baseline, all-cause and cardiovascular death rates were significantly higher in the AoAC progression group (19.8 vs. 8.6 and 11.0 vs. 3.8 per 100 Person-Years, respectively, $P < 0.001$). Results were similar even when the analysis was performed using only patients without baseline AoAC. In the progression groups, all-cause and cardiovascular death rates were 11.1 and 4.4 per 100 Person-Years, respectively. These rates were significantly higher than those of the non-progression group (2.2 and 0.6 per 100 Person-Years, respectively, $P < 0.001$) (Table 3).

Kaplan-Meier analysis and Cox proportional hazard models (Figure 2 and Table 4) were used to determine the prognostic

value of AoAC progression on mortality. In patients with baseline AoAC, patients with AoAC progression had significantly lower all-cause and cardiovascular mortality-free survival rates compared to patients without progression (log-rank test, $P = 0.002$ and 0.016, respectively). In addition, AoAC progression along with previous history of cardiovascular disease and hs-CRP levels was found to be significantly associated with all-cause and cardiovascular mortality in univariate Cox analysis. However, multivariate Cox proportional hazard analysis revealed that AoAC progression was an independent predictor of all-cause (HR: 2.625, 95% CI: 1.15–5.991, $P = 0.022$) and cardiovascular mortality (HR: 4.008, 95% CI: 1.079–14.890, $P = 0.038$). Similarly, in the subgroup of patients without baseline AoAC, Kaplan-Meier analysis showed that patients with AoAC progression had significantly higher risks for all-cause ($P < 0.001$) and cardiovascular mortality ($P = 0.003$). Moreover, in univariate analysis, age, previous history of cardiovascular disease, the use of lipid-lowering drugs, and hs-CRP concentrations as well as AoAC progression were demonstrated to be significant risk factors for all-cause and cardiovascular mortality. However, subsequent multivariate Cox proportional hazard models found that AoAC progression was a significant independent predictor of all-cause mortality (HR: 3.408, 95% CI: 1.028–11.300, $P = 0.045$), but not of cardiovascular mortality (HR: 5.935, 95% CI: 0.912–36.995, $P = 0.057$).

Discussion

Vascular calcification is common in ESRD patients and closely linked with cardiovascular disease, the leading cause of death in this population [1,5,8,9,10,11]. In this study, we demonstrate that AoAC presence at the initiation of dialysis is a significant predictor for all-cause and cardiovascular mortality in a relatively large number of incident PD patients. In addition, AoAC progression was found to be associated with patient outcome, irrespective of the presence of AoAC at baseline.

Accumulating evidence has shown that vascular calcification is highly prevalent in ESRD patients [6,7] and that it is associated with increased vascular stiffness and decreased vascular compli-

Table 3. All-cause and cardiovascular death rates according to the presence of aortic arch calcification (AoAC) at baseline and progression of AoAC.

	No. of events /No. of patients	Follow-up, No. of Person-Years	Event rate per 100 Person-Years
All-cause death			
Baseline AoAC present group ($n = 140$)			
Progression (+)	27/90	136.3	19.8
Progression (−)	9/50	104.6	8.6
Baseline AoAC absent group ($n = 223$)			
Progression (+)	5/12	45.0	11.1
Progression (−)	19/211	863.3	2.2
Cardiovascular death			
Baseline AoAC present group ($n = 140$)			
Progression (+)	15/90	136.3	11.0
Progression (−)	4/50	105.2	3.8
Baseline AoAC absent group ($n = 223$)			
Progression (+)	2/12	45.4	4.4
Progression (−)	6/211	998.3	0.6

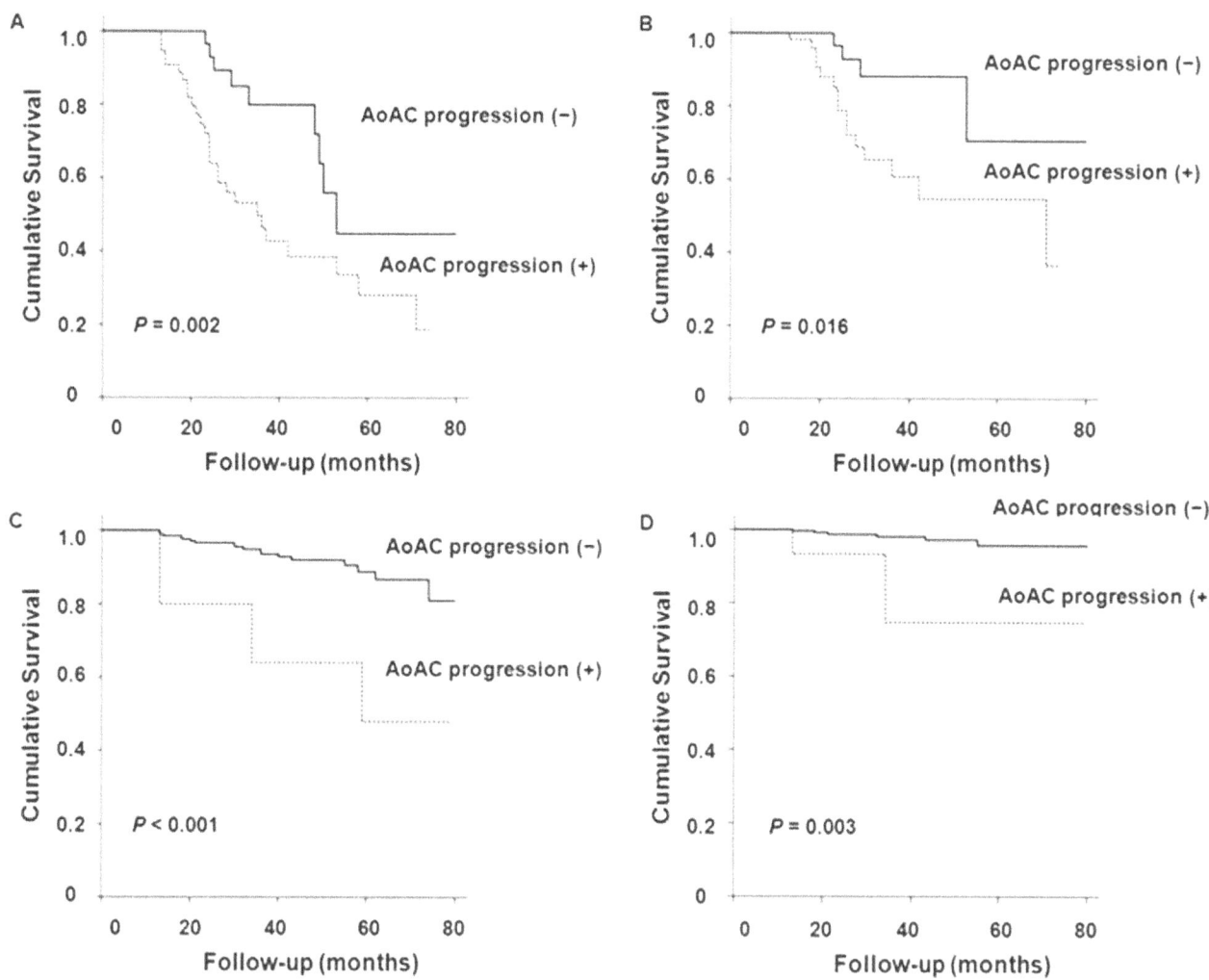

Figure 2. Kaplan-Meier analysis of aortic arch calcification (AoAC) progression for all-cause and cardiovascular mortality according to baseline AoAC subgroups. In baseline AoAC present group, patients with AoAC progression showed significantly higher all-cause (A) and cardiovascular (B) mortality (log-rank test, $P = 0.002$ and $P = 0.016$, respectively). Patients with AoAC progression in baseline AoAC absent group also showed significantly higher all-cause (C) and cardiovascular (D) mortality ($P < 0.001$ and $P = 0.003$, respectively).

ance, resulting in left ventricular (LV) hypertrophy and LV diastolic dysfunction [21,22]. Furthermore, arterial stiffness leads to a decrease in diastolic blood pressure, which can compromise coronary perfusion to increase LV mass, irrespective of preexisting coronary artery disease [23,24]. Based on these findings, some investigators have suggested that vascular calcification may contribute in part to significantly high cardiovascular mortality in ESRD. In accordance with most previous studies, this study showed AoAC presence at the start of PD was a significant independent predictor of all-cause and cardiovascular mortality in incident PD patients [3,11,18].

The prevalence of AoAC at baseline was 40.7% in this study, which was much lower than that of most previous studies from Western countries [2,3,13,14,25]. In the study by Ogawa et al [11], however, only 50.6% of 401 prevalent HD patients with dialysis duration of more than 8 years had AoAC. A study on 184 Korean incident dialysis patients also showed that AoAC was present in 41.3% before initial dialysis, which is comparable with the results of our study [26]. Taken together, the prevalence of vascular calcification in ESRD patients seems to be highly variable depending on not only the screening technique but also the studied

population, such as ethnicity and BMI. Meanwhile, the proportion of smokers was significantly lower in patients with AoAC at baseline in this study. Most previous studies demonstrated that smoking was a significant risk factor for AoAC and that a dose-response relationship was observed between the amount of smoking and AoAC [27,28]. Moreover, several studies revealed that smoking cessation decreased the risk of AoAC in some light ex-smokers [28,29]. Considering these findings, we surmised that that the amount of smoking might be a possible explanation for the discrepancy in the association between smoking status and the risk of AoAC, and therefore re-evaluated the data of cigarette consumption and calculated pack-years of smoking in smokers. In result, compared to the baseline AoAC absent group, the mean amount of smoking was significantly higher in patients with baseline AoAC despite lower proportion of smokers. Furthermore, when smokers were dichotomized by the median value of the amount of smoking, the proportion of patients with AoAC at baseline was significantly higher in heavy smokers compared to light smoker group (26.2% vs. 13.4%, $P = 0.04$). Based on these findings, it was presumed that not only the smoking status but also the amount of smoking could affect the risk of AoAC. However,

Table 4. Cox's proportional hazard models of aortic arch calcification (AoAC) progression for all-cause and cardiovascular mortality.

	Unadjusted		Adjusted	
	HR (95% CI)	P	HR (95% CI)	P
Baseline AoAC present group (*n*=140)				
All-cause mortality				
AoAC progression	2.679 (1.255–5.717)	0.011	[a]2.625 (1.15–5.991)	0.022
Cardiovascular mortality				
AoAC progression	3.506 (1.16–10.598)	0.026	[a]4.008 (1.079–14.890)	0.038
Baseline AoAC absent group (*n*=223)				
All-cause mortality				
AoAC progression	5.017 (1.853–13.587)	0.002	[b]3.408 (1.028–11.300)	0.045
Cardiovascular mortality				
AoAC progression	7.026 (1.408–35.053)	0.017	[b]5.935 (0.912–36.995)	NS

[a]Adjusted: adjusted for age, sex, presence of diabetes mellitus, previous cardiovascular disease, log high sensitivity C-reative protein, and albumin levels.
[b]Adjusted: adjusted for age, sex, presence of diabetes mellitus, previous cardiovascular disease, lipid-lowering therapy, log high sensitivity C-reactive protein, and albumin levels.
HR, hazard ratio; CI, confidence interval; NS, not significant.

due to limited information about detailed smoking status (ex- or current smoker), the relationship of the smoking status and the amount of smoking with AoAC could not be thoroughly clarified in this study.

Compared to previous studies on the association of various parameters with vascular calcification and the clinical consequences of vascular calcification, the risk factors for the progression of vascular calcification are largely unexplored in dialysis patients. In addition, impacts of the vascular calcification progression on these patients' outcome have not been elucidated. A previous study by Sigrist et al [14] investigated the independent factors associated with the progression of vascular calcification and the influence of it on mortality over 24 months in 134 patients with stage 4 and 5 CKD. It found that progressive calcification was associated with age, male gender, and serum alkaline phosphatase levels. Similarly, the NECOSAD study showed that age, hypercalcemia, hyperparathyroidism, and the interval between the first and last assessed AoACS were significantly linked with an increase in calcification score over time [3]. Kim et al [26] also found that age, dialysis duration, and the presence of AoAC were related to AoAC progression. However, in those studies, about two-thirds of patients were HD patients. In addition, changes in calcification score were significantly higher in HD patients than in PD patients. Moreover, the interval between the first and last measurement of AoACS was inconsistent in the NECOSAD study [3]. In this study, only incident PD patients were included and the interval between the first and follow-up AoACS assessment was 12 months in all patients. Therefore, the results of the aforementioned studies may not be applicable to ours. Even though age was significantly associated with AoAC progression in our subjects, when analysis was preformed separately according to the baseline AoAC presence, the association of age and AoACS with progression remained meaningful only in patients without baseline AoAC. Considering that age was significantly higher in patients with baseline AoAC than in patients without, we surmised that the effect of age on AoAC progression might be lessened in elderly incident PD patients who already had AoAC.

In the present study, AoAC progression was an independent predictor of unfavorable outcome in incident PD patients, which is

in agreement with the results of most previous studies [3,11,18]. However, the mechanism by which AoAC progression influences mortality in ESRD patients has not been fully understood. We suppose that a different type of vascular calcification can be one of the possible mechanisms. London et al [9] examined the impact of intimal and medial calcification on the prognosis in prevalent HD patients and found that arterial medial calcification (AMC) was a much stronger predictor of mortality than arterial intimal calcification in these patients. On the other hand, it is well known that chronic inflammation, malnutrition, and atherosclerosis are closely linked with each other in ESRD patients [30]. Furthermore, the current study demonstrated that AoAC progression was observed even in patients without baseline AoAC and that AoAC progression was significantly associated with elevated hs-CRP levels in both baseline AoAC present and absent groups. Based on these findings, we surmised that AoAC progression was associated with AMC progression specific to dialysis therapy. A previous study also revealed that the reason of higher mortality in patients with AMC was attributed to increased arterial stiffness [31]. Increased arterial stiffness may cause vessel wall damage, atherosclerosis, and high pulse pressure, which were independent prognostic factors in ESRD [9,31].

Mounting evidence has shown a close interrelationship among malnutrition, inflammation, and atherosclerosis [30]. In addition, atherosclerosis is closely associated with vascular and cardiac valvular calcification [32,33]. Based on these findings, chronic inflammation has also been suggested to be implicated in the pathogenesis and progression of vascular calcification in dialysis patients and we also found that hs-CRP concentrations were significantly associated with the changes in AoACS in incident PD patients, irrespective of the presence of baseline AoAC. However, the association of hs-CRP levels with the progression of vascular calcification was not consistent. Previous studies demonstrated that CRP was independently associated with the progression of coronary artery calcification over a 24-month period in 40 prevalent HD patients and was identified as an independent risk factor for the progression of abdominal aortic calcification over 3 years in 71 prevalent HD patients [34,35]. In contrast, other studies failed to identify association between CRP levels and the progression of vascular calcification in HD and/or PD patients [3,36]. We surmised that failure to find this association was due to a small number of patients, combined analysis of patients with diverse dialysis modalities, and missing values. Since other circulating markers of inflammation and various calcification activators and inhibitors (such as bone morphogenetic proteins, matrix GIa-protein, fetuin-A, and osteoprotegerin) were not measured in this study [32,37,38,39], our results that hs-CRP is the only non-traditional predictor of AoAC progression should be interpreted with caution.

Conclusions

The present study shows that the presence of AoAC assessed by chest X-ray at the start of dialysis and the progression of AoAC

during the first 12 months of dialysis were significant independent risk factors for mortality in incident PD patients. Taken together, regular follow-up by chest X-ray could be a simple and useful tool to stratify mortality risk in these patients. In addition, efforts to prevent development of vascular calcification and to attenuate progression of vascular calcification are needed to improve these patients' outcomes.

Author Contributions

Conceived and designed the experiments: MJL SWK. Analyzed the data: DHS SJK HJO DEY. Wrote the paper: MJL SWK. Carried out data collection: KIK HMK CHK FMD JTP. Participated in the interpretation of data: SHH THY KHC.

References

1. Foley RN, Parfrey PS, Sarnak MJ (1998) Clinical epidemiology of cardiovascular disease in chronic renal disease. Am J Kidney Dis 32: S112–119.
2. Block GA, Klassen PS, Lazarus JM, Ofsthun N, Lowrie EG, et al. (2004) Mineral metabolism, mortality, and morbidity in maintenance hemodialysis. J Am Soc Nephrol 15: 2208–2218.
3. Noordzij M, Cranenburg EM, Engelsman LF, Hermans MM, Boeschoten EW, et al. (2011) Progression of aortic calcification is associated with disorders of mineral metabolism and mortality in chronic dialysis patients. Nephrol Dial Transplant 26: 1662–1669.
4. Shanahan CM, Crouthamel MH, Kapustin A, Giachelli CM (2011) Arterial calcification in chronic kidney disease: key roles for calcium and phosphate. Circ Res 109: 697–711.
5. Iribarren C, Sidney S, Sternfeld B, Browner WS (2000) Calcification of the aortic arch: risk factors and association with coronary heart disease, stroke, and peripheral vascular disease. JAMA 283: 2810–2815.
6. Blacher J, Guerin AP, Pannier B, Marchais SJ, London GM (2001) Arterial calcifications, arterial stiffness, and cardiovascular risk in end-stage renal disease. Hypertension 38: 938–942.
7. Garland JS, Holden RM, Groome PA, Lam M, Nolan RL, et al. (2008) Prevalence and associations of coronary artery calcification in patients with stages 3 to 5 CKD without cardiovascular disease. Am J Kidney Dis 52: 849–858.
8. Witteman JC, Kok FJ, van Saase JL, Valkenburg HA (1986) Aortic calcification as a predictor of cardiovascular mortality. Lancet 2: 1120–1122.
9. London GM, Guerin AP, Marchais SJ, Metivier F, Pannier B, et al. (2003) Arterial media calcification in end-stage renal disease: impact on all-cause and cardiovascular mortality. Nephrol Dial Transplant 18: 1731–1740.
10. Okuno S, Ishimura E, Kitatani K, Fujino Y, Kohno K, et al. (2007) Presence of abdominal aortic calcification is significantly associated with all-cause and cardiovascular mortality in maintenance hemodialysis patients. Am J Kidney Dis 49: 417–425.
11. Ogawa T, Ishida H, Akamatsu M, Matsuda N, Fujiu A, et al. (2010) Progression of aortic arch calcification and all-cause and cardiovascular mortality in chronic hemodialysis patients. Int Urol Nephrol 42: 187–194.
12. Braun J, Oldendorf M, Moshage W, Heidler R, Zeitler E, et al. (1996) Electron beam computed tomography in the evaluation of cardiac calcification in chronic dialysis patients. Am J Kidney Dis 27: 394–401.
13. Chertow GM, Burke SK, Raggi P (2002) Sevelamer attenuates the progression of coronary and aortic calcification in hemodialysis patients. Kidney Int 62: 245–252.
14. Sigrist MK, Taal MW, Bungay P, McIntyre CW (2007) Progressive vascular calcification over 2 years is associated with arterial stiffening and increased mortality in patients with stages 4 and 5 chronic kidney disease. Clin J Am Soc Nephrol 2: 1241–1248.
15. Hashimoto H, Iijima K, Hashimoto M, Son BK, Ota H, et al. (2009) Validity and usefulness of aortic arch calcification in chest X-ray. J Atheroscler Thromb 16: 256–264.
16. Ogawa T, Ishida H, Matsuda N, Fujiu A, Matsuda A, et al. (2009) Simple evaluation of aortic arch calcification by chest radiography in hemodialysis patients. Hemodial Int 13: 301–306.
17. Karohl C, Gascon LD, Raggi P (2011) Noninvasive imaging for assessment of calcification in chronic kidney disease. Nat Rev Nephrol 7: 567–577.
18. Inoue T, Ogawa T, Ishida H, Ando Y, Nitta K (2011) Aortic arch calcification evaluated on chest X-ray is a strong independent predictor of cardiovascular events in chronic hemodialysis patients. Heart Vessels.
19. Kurita N, Hosokawa N, Nomura S, Maeda Y, Uchihara H, et al. (2011) A simple four-grade score for aortic arch calcification by posteroanterior chest X-ray is associated with cardiovascular disease in haemodialysis patients. Nephrol Dial Transplant 26: 1747–1748.
20. Twardowski ZJ (1989) Clinical value of standardized equilibration tests in CAPD patients. Blood Purif 7: 95–108.

21. Nitta K, Akiba T, Uchida K, Otsubo S, Otsubo Y, et al. (2004) Left ventricular hypertrophy is associated with arterial stiffness and vascular calcification in hemodialysis patients. Hypertens Res 27: 47–52.
22. Temmar M, Liabeuf S, Renard C, Czernichow S, Esper NE, et al. (2010) Pulse wave velocity and vascular calcification at different stages of chronic kidney disease. J Hypertens 28: 163–169.
23. Foley RN, Parfrey PS, Harnett JD, Kent GM, Martin CJ, et al. (1995) Clinical and echocardiographic disease in patients starting end-stage renal disease therapy. Kidney Int 47: 186–192.
24. Drueke TB, Massy ZA (2010) Atherosclerosis in CKD: differences from the general population. Nat Rev Nephrol 6: 723–735.
25. Sigrist M, Bungay P, Taal MW, McIntyre CW (2006) Vascular calcification and cardiovascular function in chronic kidney disease. Nephrol Dial Transplant 21: 707–714.
26. Kim HG, Song SW, Kim TY, Kim YO (2011) Risk factors for progression of aortic arch calcification in patients on maintenance hemodialysis and peritoneal dialysis. Hemodial Int 15: 460–467.
27. Taniwaki H, Ishimura E, Tabata T, Tsujimoto Y, Shioi A, et al. (2005) Aortic calcification in haemodialysis patients with diabetes mellitus. Nephrol Dial Transplant 20: 2472–2478.
28. Jiang CQ, Lao XQ, Yin P, Thomas GN, Zhang WS, et al. (2009) Smoking, smoking cessation and aortic arch calcification in older Chinese: the Guangzhou Biobank Cohort Study. Atherosclerosis 202: 529–534.
29. Woodward M, Lam TH, Barzi F, Patel A, Gu D, et al. (2005) Smoking, quitting, and the risk of cardiovascular disease among women and men in the Asia-Pacific region. Int J Epidemiol 34: 1036–1045.
30. Turkmen K, Kayikcioglu H, Ozbek O, Solak Y, Kayrak M, et al. (2011) The relationship between epicardial adipose tissue and malnutrition, inflammation, atherosclerosis/calcification syndrome in ESRD patients. Clin J Am Soc Nephrol 6: 1920–1925.
31. Klassen PS, Lowrie EG, Reddan DN, DeLong ER, Coladonato JA, et al. (2002) Association between pulse pressure and mortality in patients undergoing maintenance hemodialysis. JAMA 287: 1548–1555.
32. Wang AY, Woo J, Lam CW, Wang M, Chan IH, et al. (2005) Associations of serum fetuin-A with malnutrition, inflammation, atherosclerosis and valvular calcification syndrome and outcome in peritoneal dialysis patients. Nephrol Dial Transplant 20: 1676–1685.
33. Leskinen Y, Paana T, Saha H, Groundstroem K, Lehtimaki T, et al. (2009) Valvular calcification and its relationship to atherosclerosis in chronic kidney disease. J Heart Valve Dis 18: 429–438.
34. Jung HH, Kim SW, Han H (2006) Inflammation, mineral metabolism and progressive coronary artery calcification in patients on haemodialysis. Nephrol Dial Transplant 21: 1915–1920.
35. Yamada K, Fujimoto S, Nishiura R, Komatsu H, Tatsumoto M, et al. (2007) Risk factors of the progression of abdominal aortic calcification in patients on chronic haemodialysis. Nephrol Dial Transplant 22: 2032–2037.
36. Ammirati AL, Dalboni MA, Cendoroglo M, Draibe SA, Santos RD, et al. (2007) The progression and impact of vascular calcification in peritoneal dialysis patients. Perit Dial Int 27: 340–346.
37. Momiyama Y, Ohmori R, Fayad ZA, Kihara T, Tanaka N, et al. (2010) Associations between plasma osteopontin levels and the severities of coronary and aortic atherosclerosis. Atherosclerosis 210: 668–670.
38. Koo HM, Do HM, Kim EJ, Lee MJ, Shin DH, et al. (2011) Elevated osteoprotegerin is associated with inflammation, malnutrition and new onset cardiovascular events in peritoneal dialysis patients. Atherosclerosis 219: 925–930.
39. Rana JS, Gransar H, Wong ND, Shaw L, Pencina M, et al. (2012) Comparative Value of Coronary Artery Calcium and Multiple Blood Biomarkers for Prognostication of Cardiovascular Events. Am J Cardiol.

Permissions

The contributors of this book come from diverse backgrounds, making this book a truly international effort. This book will bring forth new frontiers with its revolutionizing research information and detailed analysis of the nascent developments around the world.

We would like to thank all the contributing authors for lending their expertise to make the book truly unique. They have played a crucial role in the development of this book. Without their invaluable contributions this book wouldn't have been possible. They have made vital efforts to compile up to date information on the varied aspects of this subject to make this book a valuable addition to the collection of many professionals and students.

This book was conceptualized with the vision of imparting up-to-date information and advanced data in this field. To ensure the same, a matchless editorial board was set up. Every individual on the board went through rigorous rounds of assessment to prove their worth. After which they invested a large part of their time researching and compiling the most relevant data for our readers.

The editorial board has been involved in producing this book since its inception. They have spent rigorous hours researching and exploring the diverse topics which have resulted in the successful publishing of this book. They have passed on their knowledge of decades through this book. To expedite this challenging task, the publisher supported the team at every step. A small team of assistant editors was also appointed to further simplify the editing procedure and attain best results for the readers.

Apart from the editorial board, the designing team has also invested a significant amount of their time in understanding the subject and creating the most relevant covers. They scrutinized every image to scout for the most suitable representation of the subject and create an appropriate cover for the book.

The publishing team has been an ardent support to the editorial, designing and production team. Their endless efforts to recruit the best for this project, has resulted in the accomplishment of this book. They are a veteran in the field of academics and their pool of knowledge is as vast as their experience in printing. Their expertise and guidance has proved useful at every step. Their uncompromising quality standards have made this book an exceptional effort. Their encouragement from time to time has been an inspiration for everyone.

The publisher and the editorial board hope that this book will prove to be a valuable piece of knowledge for researchers, students, practitioners and scholars across the globe.

List of Contributors

Ghazaleh Gouya, Michael Wolzt
Department of Clinical Pharmacology, Medical University Vienna, Vienna, Austria

Gisela Sturm, Claudia Lamina, Florian Kronenberg
Division of Genetic Epidemiology, Department of Medical Genetics, Molecular and Clinical Pharmacology, Innsbruck Medical University, Innsbruck, Austria

Emanuel Zitt, Florian Knoll
Department of Nephrology and Dialysis, Academic Teaching Hospital Feldkirch, Feldkirch, Austria

Karl Lhotta, Ulrich Neyer
Department of Nephrology and Dialysis, Academic Teaching Hospital Feldkirch, Feldkirch, Austria
Vorarlberg Institute for Vascular Investigation and Treatment (VIVIT), Feldkirch, Austria

Friederike Lins, Otto Freistätter
Vorarlberg Institute for Vascular Investigation and Treatment (VIVIT), Feldkirch, Austria

Joachim Struck
Research Department, B.R.A.H.M.S GmbH (Part of ThermoFisher Scientific), Hennigsdorf/Berlin, Germany

Jin-Bor Chen, Wen-Chin Lee
Division of Nephrology, Department of Internal Medicine, Mitochondrial Research Unit, Kaohsiung Chang Gung Memorial Hospital, Chang Gung University College of Medicine, Kaohsiung, Taiwan

Yi-Hsin Yang
School of Pharmacy, Kaohsiung Medical University, Kaohsiung, Taiwan

Chia-Wei Liou, Tsu-Kung Lin
Department of Neurology and Mitochondrial Research Unit, Kaohsiung Chang Gung Memorial Hospital and Chang Gung University College of Medicine, Kaohsiung, Taiwan

Yueh-Hua Chung
Institute of Biomedical Sciences, National Sun Yat-Sen University, Kaohsiung, Taiwan

Yeh Chuang
Department of Chemical Engineering & Institute of Biotechnology and Chemical Engineering, I-Shou University, Kaohsiung, Taiwan

Li- Cheng-Hong Yang
Department of Electronic Engineering, National Kaohsiung University of Applied Sciences, Kaohsiung, Taiwan

Hsueh-Wei Chang
Department of Biomedical Science and Environmental Biology, Kaohsiung Medical University, Taiwan
Center of Excellence for Environmental Medicine, Cancer Center, Kaohsiung Medical University Hospital, Kaohsiung Medical University, Kaohsiung, Taiwan

Chun-Fu Lai, Pei-Chen Wu, Chia-Ter Chao, Tze-Wah Kao, Tun-Jun Tsai, Kwan-Dun Wu
Division of Nephrology, Department of Internal Medicine, National Taiwan University Hospital, Taipei, Taiwan

Vin-Cent Wu
Division of Nephrology, Department of Internal Medicine, National Taiwan University Hospital, Taipei, Taiwan
NSARF: National Taiwan University Hospital Study Group on Acute Renal Failure, Taipei, Taiwan

Chih-Chung Shiao
Division of Nephrology, Department of Internal Medicine, Saint Mary's Hospital and Saint Mary's Medicine, Nursing and Management College, Yilan, Taiwan

Yu-Feng Lin, Guang-Huar Young, Yin-Yi Han
Department of Traumatology, National Taiwan University Hospital, Taipei, Taiwan

Wen-Je Ko
Department of Traumatology, National Taiwan University Hospital, Taipei, Taiwan
Department of Surgery, National Taiwan University Hospital, Taipei, Taiwan

Fu- Chang Hu
International Harvard Statistical Consulting Company, Taipei, Taiwan

Tao-Min Huang
Division of Nephrology, Department of Internal Medicine, Yun-Lin Branch, Douliou City, Yun-Lin County, Taiwan

Yu-Chang Yeh
Department of Anesthesiology, National Taiwan University Hospital, Taipei, Taiwan

I-Jung Tsai
Department of Pediatrics, National Taiwan University Hospital, Taipei, Taiwan

Wen-Chung Wu
Section of Internal Medicine, Miao-Li Hospital, Department of Health, Miao-Li, Taiwan

Chun-Cheng Hou
Department of Internal medicine, Min-Sheng Hospital, Tao-Yuan, Taiwan

Valéria C. Ferreira, Carlos F. M. A. Rodrigues
Nefroclínica de Uberlândia, Minas Gerais, Brazil,

Sebastião R. Ferreira-Filho, Gilberto R. Machado
Nefroclínica de Uberlândia, Minas Gerais, Brazil
Federal University of Uberlândia, Minas Gerais, Brazil

Thyago Proença de Moraes, Roberto Pecoits-Filho, Marcia Olandoski
Center for Health and Biological Sciences, Pontifícia Universidade Católica do Paraná, Curitiba, Brazil,

José C. Divino-Filho
Baxter Healthcare, Division of Baxter Novum and Renal Medicine, CLINTEC, Karolinska Institute, Stockholm, Sweden,

Christopher McIntyre
Faculty of Medicine & Health Sciences, University of Nottingham, Nottingham, United Kingdom,

Laura E. A. Harrison, James O. Burton
Department of Renal Medicine, Royal Derby Hospital, Derby, United Kingdom

Christopher W. McIntyre
Department of Renal Medicine, Royal Derby Hospital, Derby, United Kingdom
School of Graduate Entry Medicine and Health, University of Nottingham, Derby, United Kingdom

Cheuk-Chun Szeto, Philip K. T. Li
Department of Medicine and Therapeutics, Chinese University of Hong Kong, Hong Kong, China

Greg Knoll
Division of Nephrology, Kidney Research Center, Ottawa Hospital Research Institute, Ottawa, Ontario, Canada,
Clinical Epidemiology Program, Ottawa Hospital Research Institute, Ottawa, Ontario, Canada

Swapnil Hiremath
Division of Nephrology, Kidney Research Center, Ottawa Hospital Research Institute, Ottawa, Ontario, Canada

Clinical Epidemiology Program, Ottawa Hospital Research Institute, Ottawa, Ontario, Canada
Department of Health Policy and Management, Harvard School of Public Health, Boston, Massachusetts, United States of America

Milton C. Weinstein
Department of Health Policy and Management, Harvard School of Public Health, Boston, Massachusetts, United States of America

Linda Dunford, Michael J. Carr, Jonathan Dean, Allison Waters, Jeff Connell, Suzie Coughlan, William W. Hall
Ireland Vietnam Blood-Borne Virus Initiative (IVVI), Dublin, Ireland and Ha Noi Vietnam
National Virus Reference Laboratory, University College Dublin, Dublin, Ireland

Linh Thuy Nguyen, Thu Hong Ta Thi, Lan Anh Bui Thi, Huy Duong Do, Thu Thuy Duong Thi, Ha Thu Nguyen, Trinh Thi Diem Do, Quynh Phuong Luu, Lan Anh Nguyen Thi, Hien Tran Nguyen
Ireland Vietnam Blood-Borne Virus Initiative (IVVI), Dublin, Ireland and Ha Noi Vietnam
Laboratory for Molecular Diagnostics, National Institute of Hygiene and Epidemiology, Ha Noi, Vietnam

Carlo A. Gaillard
Department of Nephrology, VU Medical Center, Amsterdam, The Netherlands

Neelke C. van der Weerd
Department of Nephrology, VU Medical Center, Amsterdam, The Netherlands
Department of Nephrology, Academic Medical Center, University of Amsterdam, Amsterdam, The Netherlands

Piet M. ter Wee, Menso J. Nube´, Muriel P. C. Grooteman
Department of Nephrology, VU Medical Center, Amsterdam, The Netherlands
Institute for Cardiovascular Research VU Medical Center (ICaR-VU), VU Medical Center, Amsterdam, The Netherlands

E. Lars Penne
Department of Nephrology, VU Medical Center, Amsterdam, The Netherlands
Department of Nephrology, University Medical Center Utrecht, Utrecht, The Netherlands

Michiel L. Bots
Julius Center for Health Sciences and Primary Care, University Medical Center Utrecht, Utrecht, The Netherlands

Marinus A. van den Dorpel
Department of Internal Medicine, Maasstad Hospital, Rotterdam, The Netherlands

Claire H. den Hoedt
Department of Internal Medicine, Maasstad Hospital, Rotterdam, The Netherlands
Department of Nephrology, University Medical Center Utrecht, Utrecht, The Netherlands

Albert H. A. Mazairac, Peter J. Blankestijn
Department of Nephrology, University Medical Center Utrecht, Utrecht, The Netherlands

Jack F. M. Wetzels
Department of Nephrology, Radboud University Nijmegen Medical Center, Nijmegen, The Netherlands

Erwin T. Wiegerinck, Dorine W. Swinkels
Department of Laboratory Medicine, Laboratory of Genetic, Endocrine and Metabolic Diseases, Radboud University Nijmegen Medical Center, Nijmegen, The Netherlands
Hepcidinanalysis.com, Radboud University Nijmegen Medical Center, Nijmegen, The Netherlands

Yoke Mun Chan
Institute of Gerontology, University Putra Malaysia, Serdang, Malaysia
Department of Nutrition and Dietetics, Faculty of Medicine and Health Sciences, University Putra Malaysia, Serdang, Malaysia

Mohd Shariff Zalilah
Department of Nutrition and Dietetics, Faculty of Medicine and Health Sciences, University Putra Malaysia, Serdang, Malaysia

Sing Ziunn Hii
Viva Life Science Private Limited, Petaling Jaya, Malaysia

Kalliopi Zafeiropoulou, Apostolos Polykratis, Stella Karabina, Panagiotis Katsoris
Department of Biology, University of Patras, Patras, Achaia, Greece

Theodora Bita, John Vlachojannis
Department of Internal Medicine-Nephrology, University Hospital of Patras, Patras, Achaia, Greece

Vin-Cent Wu, Chia-Ter Chao, Shao-Yu Yang, Chun-Fu Lai, Yung-Ming Chen, Kwan-Dun Wu
Division of Nephrology, Department of Internal Medicine, National Taiwan University Hospital, Taipei, Taiwan

Tao-Min Huang
Division of Nephrology, Department of Internal Medicine, Yun-Lin Branch, National Taiwan University Hospital, Douliou, Taiwan

Pei-Chen Wu
Division of Nephrology, Department of Internal Medicine, Da Chien General Hospital, Miaoli, Taiwan

Wei-Jie Wang
Department of Internal Medicine, Taoyuan General Hospital, Department of Health, Executive Yuan, Taoyuan, Taiwan

Yih-Sharng Chen, Ron-Bin Hsu, Guang-Huar Young, Shoei-Shen Wang, Pi-Ru Tsai
Department of Surgery, National Taiwan University Hospital, Taipei, Taiwan

Wen-Je Ko
Department of Surgery, National Taiwan University Hospital, Taipei, Taiwan
Department of Raumatology, National Taiwan University Hospital, Taipei, Taiwan

Chih-Chung Shiao
Division of Nephrology, Department of Internal Medicine, Saint Mary's Hospital and Saint Mary's Medicine, Nursing and Management College, Luodong, Yilan

Fu-Chang Hu
International Harvard Statistical Consulting Company, Taipei, Taiwan

Yu-Feng Lin, Yin-Yi Han
Department of Raumatology, National Taiwan University Hospital, Taipei, Taiwan

Ting-Ting Chao
Medical Research Center, Cardinal Tien Hospital, Fu Jen Catholic University College of Medicine, Taipei, Taiwan

Zaida Noemy Cabrera Jimenez, Benedito Jorge Pereira, João Egidio Romão Jr, Sonia Cristina da Silva Makida, Hugo Abensur, Rosa Maria Affonso Moyses, Rosilene Motta Elias
Renal Division, Internal Medicine, Hospital das Clínicas, University of São Paulo School of Medicine, São Paulo, Brazil

Seung Jun Kim, Hyung Jung Oh, Dong Eun Yoo, Dong Ho Shin, Mi Jung Lee, Hyoung Rae Kim, Jung Tak Park, Seung Hyeok Han, Tae-Hyun Yoo, Kyu Hun Choi
Department of Internal Medicine, College of Medicine, Yonsei University, Seoul, Korea

Shin-Wook Kang
Department of Internal Medicine, College of Medicine, Yonsei University, Seoul, Korea
Severance Biomedical Science Institute, Brain Korea 21, Yonsei University, Seoul, Korea

Allison Tong
Centre for Kidney Research, Children's Hospital at Westmead, Westmead, Australia

Jonathan C. Craig
Centre for Kidney Research, Children's Hospital at Westmead, Westmead, Australia
School of Public Health, University of Sydney, Sydney, Australia

Germaine Wong, Angela C. Webster
Centre for Kidney Research, Children's Hospital at Westmead, Westmead, Australia
School of Public Health, University of Sydney, Sydney, Australia
Centre for Transplant and Renal Research, Westmead Hospital, Sydney, Australia

Kirsten Howard
School of Public Health, University of Sydney, Sydney, Australia

Jeremy R. Chapman
Centre for Transplant and Renal Research, Westmead Hospital, Sydney, Australia

Steven Chadban
Central Clinical School, University of Sydney, Sydney, Australia

Nicholas Cross
Department of Nephrology,Christchurch Hospital, Christchurch, New Zealand

Berthold Hocher, Christoph Reichetzeder
Institute of Nutritional Science, University of Potsdam, Potsdam-Rehbrücke, Germany

Franz Paul Armbruster, Stanka Stoeva, Hans Jürgen Grön
Immundiagnostik AG, Bensheim, Germany

Ina Lieker, Dmytro Khadzhynov, Torsten Slowinski
Department of Nephrology, Charité-Mitte, Berlin, Germany

Heinz Jürgen Roth
Department of Endocrinology/Oncology, Limbach Laboratory, Heidelberg, Germany

Dong Eun Yoo, Jung Tak Park, Hyung Jung Oh, Seung Jun Kim, Mi Jung Lee, Dong Ho Shin, Seung Hyeok Han, Tae-Hyun Yoo, Kyu Hun Choi, Shin-Wook Kang
Department of Internal Medicine, College of Medicine, Brain Korea 21 for Medical Science, Severance Biomedical Science Institute, Yonsei University, Seoul, Korea

Ferruh Artunc andreas Peter, Claus Thamer, Peter Weyrich, Hans-Ulrich Haering
Department of Internal Medicine, Division of Endocrinology, Diabetology, Vascular Disease, Nephrology and Clinical Chemistry, University of Tuebingen, Germany

Christian Mueller, Tobias Breidthardt, Raphael Twerenbold
Department of Internal Medicine, Division of Cardiology, University of Basel, Basel, Switzerland

Bjoern Friedrich
Department of Internal Medicine, Division of Endocrinology, Diabetology, Vascular Disease, Nephrology and Clinical Chemistry, University of Tuebingen, Germany
Dialysis Center, Leonberg, Germany

Viknesh Selvarajah
Clinical Pharmacology Unit, Department of Medicine, University of Cambridge, Cambridge, United Kingdom
Department of Nephrology, Cambridge University Hospitals NHS Foundation Trust, Cambridge, United Kingdom

Sanjay Ojha
Department of Nephrology, Cambridge University Hospitals NHS Foundation Trust, Cambridge, United Kingdom

Laura Pasea
Centre for Applied Medical Statistics, Department of Public Health and Primary Care, Institute of Public Health, University of Cambridge, Cambridge, United Kingdom

Ian B. Wilkinson, Laurie A. Tomlinson
Cambridge Clinical Trials Unit, University of Cambridge, Cambridge, United Kingdom

Szu-Chun Hung
Division of Nephrology, Buddhist Tzu Chi General Hospital, Taipei Branch, Taipei, Taiwan

Yao-Ping Lin
Division of Nephrology, Department of Medicine and Immunology Research Center, Taipei Veterans General Hospital, Taipei, Taiwan

Der-Cherng Tarng
Division of Nephrology, Department of Medicine and Immunology Research Center, Taipei Veterans General Hospital, Taipei, Taiwan
Department and Institute of Physiology, School of Medicine, National Yang-Ming University, Taipei, Taiwan

Hsin-Lei Huang, Hsiao-Fung Pu
Department and Institute of Physiology, School of Medicine, National Yang-Ming University, Taipei, Taiwan

Ming-Yen Lin
Division of Nephrology, Department of Internal Medicine, Kaohsiung Medical University Hospital, Kaohsiung, Taiwan

Ping-Hsun Wu
Division of Nephrology, Department of Internal Medicine, Kaohsiung Medical University Hospital, Kaohsiung, Taiwan
Department of Internal Medicine, College of Medicine, Kaohsiung Medical University, Kaohsiung, Taiwan

Mei-Chuan Kuo, Yi-Wen Chiu, Shang- Jyh Hwang, Hung-Chun Chen
Division of Nephrology, Department of Internal Medicine, Kaohsiung Medical University Hospital, Kaohsiung, Taiwan
Faculty of Renal Care, College of Medicine, Kaohsiung Medical University, Kaohsiung, Taiwan

Tzu-Chi Lee
Department of Family Medicine, Kaohsiung Medical University Hospital, Kaohsiung, Taiwan

Yi-Ting Lin
Department of Family Medicine, Kaohsiung Medical University Hospital, Kaohsiung, Taiwan
Department of Public Health, College of Medicine, Kaohsiung Medical University, Kaohsiung, Taiwan

Ira M. Mostovaya, Albert H. A. Mazairac, Peter J. Blankestijn
Department of Nephrology, University Medical Center Utrecht, Utrecht, the Netherlands

Claire H. den Hoedt
Department of Nephrology, University Medical Center Utrecht, Utrecht, the Netherlands
Department of Internal Medicine, Maasstad Hospital, Rotterdam, the Netherlands

E. Lars Penne, Neelke C. van der Weerd
Department of Nephrology, University Medical Center Utrecht, Utrecht, the Netherlands
Department of Nephrology, Vrije Universiteit Medical Center, Amsterdam, the Netherlands

Michiel L. Bots
Julius Center for Health Sciences and Primary Care, University Medical Center Utrecht, Utrecht, the Netherlands

Marinus A. van den Dorpel
Department of Internal Medicine, Maasstad Hospital, Rotterdam, the Netherlands

Roel Goldschmeding
Department of Pathology, University Medical Center Utrecht, Utrecht, the Netherlands

Otto Kamp
Department of Cardiology, Vrije Universiteit Medical Center, Amsterdam, the Netherlands

Rene´e Levesque
Department of Nephrology, Centre Hospitalier de l'Universite´de Montre´al St. Luc Hospital, Montre´al, Canada

Muriel P. C. Grooteman, Piet M. ter Wee, Menso J. Nube´
Department of Nephrology, Vrije Universiteit Medical Center, Amsterdam, the Netherlands
Institute for Cardiovascular Research Vrije Universiteit Medical Center, Vrije Universiteit Medical Center, Amsterdam, the Netherlands

Dorine W. Swinkels
Department of Laboratory Medicine, Laboratory of Genetic, Endocrine and Metabolic diseases, Radboud University Medical Centre Nijmegen, the Netherlands

Rukshana C. Shroff, Karen L. Price, Maria Kolatsi-Joannou, Alexandra F. Todd, Lesley Rees, David A. Long
Nephro-Urology Unit, UCL Institute of Child Health and Great Ormond Street Hospital for Children NHS Trust, London, United Kingdom

David Wells
Department of Chemical Pathology, Great Ormond Street Hospital for Children NHS Trust, London, United Kingdom

John Deanfield
National Centre for Cardiovascular Disease Prevention and Outcomes, University College London, London, United Kingdom

Richard J. Johnson
Division of Renal Diseases and Hypertension, University of Colorado, Denver, Colorado, United States of America

Adrian S. Woolf
Institute of Human Development, University of Manchester and the Royal Manchester Children's Hospital, Manchester, United Kingdom

Shina Lee, Jung-Hwa Ryu, Seung-Jung Kim, Duk-Hee Kang, Kyu Bok Choi, Dong-Ryeol Ryu
Department of Internal Medicine, School of Medicine, Ewha Womans University, Seoul, Korea,

Hyunwook Kim
Department of Internal Medicine, Wonkwang University College of Medicine Sanbon Hospital, Gunpo, Korea

Kyoung Hoon Kim
Department of Public Health, Graduate School, Korea University, Seoul, Korea

Hyeong Sik Ahn
Department of Preventive Medicine, College of Medicine, Korea University, Seoul, Korea

Hoo Jae Hann, Yongjae Cho, Young Mi Park
Ewha Medical Research Institute, School of Medicine, Ewha Womans University, Seoul, Korea

Jie Dong, Rong Xu, Hai-Yan Wang
Renal Division, Department of Medicine, Peking University First Hospital; Institute of Nephrology, Peking University; Key Laboratory of Renal Disease, Ministry of Health; Key Laboratory of Renal Disease, Ministry of Education; Beijing, China

Qing-Feng Han, Yue Wang
Department of Nephrology, Peking University Third Hospital, Beijing, China

Tong-Ying Zhu, Chuan-Ming Hao
Department of Nephrology, Huashan Hospital of Fudan University, Shanghai, China

Ye-Ping Ren, Rui Zhang
Department of Nephrology, Second Affiliated Hospital of Harbin Medical University, Heilongjiang, China

Jiang-Hua Chen, Xiao-Hui Zhang
Kidney Disease Center, The First Affiliated Hospital, College of Medicine, Zhejiang University, Hangzhou, China

Hui-Ping Zhao, Mei Wang
Department of Nephrology, Peking University People's Hospital, Beijing, China

Meng-Hua Chen, Na Tian
Department of Nephrology, General Hospital of Ningxia Medical University, Ningxia, China

Hyang Mo Koo, Chan Ho Kim, Fa Mee Doh, Mi Jung Lee, Eun Jin Kim, Jae Hyun Han, Ji Suk Han, Hyung Jung Oh, Jung Tak Park, Seung Hyeok Han, Tae-Hyun Yoo
Department of Internal Medicine, Yonsei University College of Medicine, Seoul, Korea

Shin-Wook Kang
Department of Internal Medicine, Yonsei University College of Medicine, Seoul, Korea
Brain Korea 21 PLUS Project for Medical Science, Yonsei University, Seoul, Korea

Yih-Giun Cherng
Department of Anesthesiology, Shuang Ho Hospital, affiliated with Taipei Medical University, New Taipei City, Taiwan
Department of Anesthesiology, School of Medicine, College of Medicine, Taipei Medical University, Taipei, Taiwan

Chien-Chang Liao, Ta-Liang Chen
Department of Anesthesiology, School of Medicine, College of Medicine, Taipei Medical University, Taipei, Taiwan
Department of Anesthesiology, Taipei Medical University Hospital, Taipei, Taiwan
Health Policy Research Center, Taipei Medical University Hospital, Taipei, Taiwan

Tso-Hsiao Chen
Department of Nephrology, Wan Fang Medical Center, affiliated with Department of Internal Medicine, College of Medicine, Taipei Medical University, Taipei, Taiwan

Duan Xiao
Department of Coloproctology, the Second People's Hospital of Shi-Fang City, Shi-Fang City, Sichuan Province, People Republic of China

Chih-Hsiung Wu
Department of Surgery, Shuang Ho Hospital, affiliated with Taipei Medical University, New Taipei City, Taiwan

Mi Jung Lee, Dong Ho Shin, Seung Jun Kim, Hyung Jung Oh, Dong Eun Yoo, Kwang Il Ko, Hyang Mo Koo, Chan Ho Kim, Fa Mee Doh, Jung Tak Park, Seung Hyeok Han, Kyu Hun Choi
Department of Internal Medicine, College of Medicine, Yonsei University, Seoul, Korea

Tae-Hyun Yoo, Shin-Wook Kang
Department of Internal Medicine, College of Medicine, Yonsei University, Seoul, Korea
Severance Biomedical Science Institute, Brain Korea 21, Yonsei University, Seoul, Korea

Index

www.ingramcontent.com/pod-product-compliance
Lightning Source LLC
Chambersburg PA
CBHW080412190526
45161CB00003B/213